BARTS AND THE LONDON

SCHOOL OF MEDICINE AND DENTISTRY

WHITECHAPEL LIBRARY,TURNER STREET, LONDON E1 2AD
020 7882 7110

ONE WEEK LOAN

Book are to be returned on or before the last date below,
otherwise fines may be charged.

Progress in Pain Research and Management
Volume 27

Psychosocial Aspects of Pain:
A Handbook for Health Care Providers

Mission Statement of IASP Press®

The International Association for the Study of Pain (IASP) is a nonprofit, interdisciplinary organization devoted to understanding the mechanisms of pain and improving the care of patients with pain through research, education, and communication. The organization includes scientists and health care professionals dedicated to these goals. The IASP sponsors scientific meetings and publishes newsletters, technical bulletins, the journal *Pain,* and books.

The goal of IASP Press is to provide the IASP membership with timely, high-quality, attractive, low-cost publications relevant to the problem of pain. These publications are also intended to appeal to a wider audience of scientists and clinicians interested in the problem of pain.

Progress in Pain Research and Management
Volume 27

Psychosocial Aspects of Pain: A Handbook for Health Care Providers

Editors

Robert H. Dworkin, PhD

Department of Anesthesiology,
University of Rochester School of Medicine and Dentistry,
Rochester, New York, USA

William S. Breitbart, MD

Department of Psychiatry and Behavioral Sciences,
Memorial Sloan-Kettering Cancer Center,
and Weill Medical College, Cornell University,
New York, New York, USA

IASP PRESS® • SEATTLE

Timely topics in pain research and treatment have been selected for publication, but the information provided and opinions expressed have not involved any verification of the findings, conclusions, and opinions by IASP®. Thus, opinions expressed in *Psychosocial Aspects of Pain: A Handbook for Health Care Providers* do not necessarily reflect those of IASP or of the Officers and Councillors.

No responsibility is assumed by IASP for any injury and/or damage to persons or property as a matter of product liability, negligence, or from any use of any methods, products, instruction, or ideas contained in the material herein. Because of the rapid advances in the medical sciences, the publisher recommends that there should be independent verification of diagnoses and drug dosages.

Library of Congress Cataloging-in-Publication Data

Psychosocial aspects of pain : a handbook for health care providers / editors, Robert H. Dworkin, William S. Breitbart.
    p. cm. -- (Progress in pain research and management ; v. 27)
  ISBN 0-931092-48-5 (alk. paper)
   1. Pain--Handbooks, manuals, etc. 2. Pain--Psychological aspects---Handbooks, manuals, etc. 3. Pain--Patients--Psychology--Handbooks, manuals, etc. I. Dworkin, Robert H. II. Breitbart, William, 1951- III. Series.

RB127.P875 2003
616'.0472--dc22

2003060582

Published by:

IASP Press
International Association for the Study of Pain
909 NE 43rd Street, Suite 306
Seattle, WA 98105-6020 USA
Fax: 206-547-1703
www.iasp-pain.org
www.painbooks.org

Printed in the United States of America

Contents

Part IV: Complex Disorders

Part V: Specific Populations

Part VI: Special Issues

Contributing Authors

Frank Andrasik, PhD *Institute for Human and Machine Cognition, University of West Florida, Pensacola, Florida, USA*

J. Hampton Atkinson, Jr., MD *Psychiatry Services, VA San Diego Healthcare System, San Diego, California; and Department of Psychiatry, School of Medicine, University of California, San Diego, La Jolla, California, USA*

William S. Breitbart, MD *Department of Psychiatry and Behavioral Sciences, Memorial Sloan-Kettering Cancer Center, and Weill Medical College, Cornell University School of Medicine, New York, New York, USA*

Stephen Bruehl, PhD *Department of Anesthesiology, Vanderbilt University School of Medicine, Nashville, Tennessee, USA*

Lisa C. Campbell, PhD *Department of Psychiatry, Duke University Medical Center, Durham, North Carolina, USA*

Lucille A. Cardella, PhD *The Abacus Group, Cranston, Rhode Island, USA*

James W. Carson, PhD *Department of Psychiatry, Duke University Medical Center, Durham, North Carolina, USA*

C. Richard Chapman, PhD *Pain Research Center, Department of Anesthesiology, School of Medicine, University of Utah, Salt Lake City, Utah, USA*

Ok Yung Chung, MD, MBA *Department of Anesthesiology, Vanderbilt University School of Medicine, Nashville, Tennessee, USA*

Robert H. Dworkin, PhD *Department of Anesthesiology, University of Rochester School of Medicine and Dentistry, Rochester, New York, USA*

Robert R. Edwards, PhD *Department of Psychiatry and Behavioral Sciences, Johns Hopkins University School of Medicine, Baltimore, Maryland, USA*

Michael J. Farrell, PhD *National Ageing Research Institute, Parkville, Victoria, Australia; currently Howard Florey Institute, National Neuroscience Facility, University of Melbourne, Parkville, Victoria, Australia*

Howard L. Fields, MD, PhD *Department of Neurology, University of California, San Francisco, San Francisco, California, USA*

Herta Flor, PhD *Department of Clinical and Cognitive Neuroscience at the University of Heidelberg, Central Institute of Mental Health, Mannheim, Germany*

Rollin M. Gallagher, MD, MCP *Pain Center, Departments of Psychiatry and Anesthesiology, College of Medicine, and School of Public Health, Drexel University, Philadelphia, Pennsylvania, USA; currently Department of Pain Medicine, Veterans Hospital of Philadelphia, and Departments of Psychiatry and Anesthesiology, University of Pennsylvania, Philadelphia, Pennsylvania, USA*

Robert J. Gatchel, PhD *Department of Psychiatry, The University of Texas Southwestern Medical Center at Dallas, Dallas, Texas, USA*

Michael E. Geisser, PhD *The Spine Program, Department of Physical Medicine and Rehabilitation, University of Michigan Medical Center, Ann Arbor, Michigan, USA*

Stephen J. Gibson, PhD *National Ageing Research Institute, Parkville, Victoria, Australia*

Jennifer Haythornthwaite, PhD *Department of Psychiatry and Behavioral Sciences, Johns Hopkins University School of Medicine, Baltimore, Maryland, USA*

Leslie J. Heinberg, PhD *Department of Psychiatry, Case Western Reserve University School of Medicine, Cleveland, Ohio, USA*

Christiane Hermann, PhD *Department of Clinical and Cognitive Neuroscience at the University of Heidelberg, Central Institute of Mental Health, Mannheim, Germany*

Vicenzio Holder-Perkins, MD *Inpatient Psychiatric Services and Department of Psychiatry and Behavioral Sciences, The George Washington University, Washington, DC, USA*

Kenneth A. Holroyd, PhD *Psychology Department, Ohio University, Athens, Ohio, USA*

Robert N. Jamison, PhD *Pain Management Center, Brigham and Women's Hospital, and Departments of Anesthesia and Psychiatry, Harvard Medical School, Boston, Massachusetts, USA*

Francis J. Keefe, PhD *Department of Psychiatry, Duke University Medical Center, Durham, North Carolina, USA*

Robert D. Kerns, PhD *VA Connecticut Healthcare System, West Haven, Connecticut; and Yale University School of Medicine, New Haven, Connecticut, USA*

Kenneth L. Kirsh, PhD *Symptom Management and Palliative Care Program, Markey Cancer Center, University of Kentucky, Lexington, Kentucky, USA*

Jon D. Levine, MD, PhD *Department of Oral and Maxillofacial Surgery, University of California, San Francisco, San Francisco, California, USA*

Ann Matt Maddrey, PhD *Department of Psychiatry, The University of Texas Southwestern Medical Center at Dallas, Dallas, Texas, USA*

Patrick J. McGrath, OC, PhD, FRCS *Departments of Psychology, Pediatrics, and Psychiatry, Dalhousie University; and Pediatric Pain Service, IWK Health Centre, Halifax, Nova Scotia, Canada*

Jonathan M. Meyer, MD *Psychiatry Services, VA San Diego Healthcare System, San Diego, California; and Department of Psychiatry, School of Medicine, University of California, San Diego, La Jolla, California, USA*

Christine Miaskowski, RN, PhD, FAAN *Department of Physiological Nursing, University of California, San Francisco, San Francisco, California, USA*

Stephen Morley, PhD *Academic Unit of Psychiatry and Behavioural Sciences, School of Medicine, University of Leeds, Leeds, United Kingdom*

Richard Ohrbach, DDS, PhD *Department of Oral Diagnostic Sciences, University at Buffalo, Buffalo, New York, USA*

Akiko Okifuji, PhD *Department of Anesthesiology, School of Medicine, University of Utah, Salt Lake City, Utah, USA*

John D. Otis, PhD *VA Boston Healthcare System and Boston University School of Medicine, Boston, Massachusetts, USA*

Steven D. Passik, PhD *Symptom Management and Palliative Care Program, Markey Cancer Center, University of Kentucky, Lexington, Kentucky, USA*

David Payne, PhD *Department of Psychiatry and Behavioral Sciences, Memorial Sloan-Kettering Cancer Center, and Weill Medical College, Cornell University School of Medicine, New York, New York, USA*

Ellen L. Poleshuck, PhD *Department of Psychiatry, University of Rochester School of Medicine and Dentistry, Rochester, New York, USA*

Richard C. Robinson, PhD *Department of Psychiatry, The University of Texas Southwestern Medical Center at Dallas, Dallas, Texas, USA*

Jeffrey Sherman, PhD *Department of Oral Medicine, School of Dentistry, University of Washington, Seattle, Washington, USA*

Mark A. Slater, PhD *Psychiatry Services, VA San Diego Healthcare System, San Diego, California; and Department of Psychiatry, School of Medicine, University of California, San Diego, La Jolla, California, USA*

Mark Sullivan, MD, PhD *Department of Psychiatry and Behavioral Sciences, School of Medicine, University of Washington, Seattle, Washington, USA*

Raymond C. Tait, PhD *Department of Psychiatry, Saint Louis University School of Medicine, St. Louis, Missouri, USA*

Dennis C. Turk, PhD *Department of Anesthesiology, University of Washington School of Medicine, Seattle, Washington, USA*

Sunil Verma, MBBS *Pain Center and Department of Psychiatry, College of Medicine, Drexel University, Philadelphia, Pennsylvania, USA*

Sandra J. Waters, PhD *Department of Psychiatry, Duke University Medical Center, Durham, North Carolina, USA*

Amanda C. de C. Williams, PhD *INPUT Pain Management Unit, Guy's and St. Thomas' Hospital, London, United Kingdom*

David A. Williams, PhD *Division of Rheumatology, Department of Medicine, University of Michigan, Ann Arbor, Michigan, USA*

Thomas Wise, MD *Department of Psychiatry and Behavioral Sciences, Johns Hopkins University School of Medicine, Baltimore, Maryland; and Department of Psychiatry, Inova Fairfax Hospital, Falls Church, Virginia, USA*

Preface

Psychosocial Aspects of Pain: A Handbook for Health Care Providers is intended to serve as a comprehensive resource for health care providers who would like to become knowledgeable about the psychological, psychiatric, and social aspects of pain. Other books on these topics have targeted psychologists, psychiatrists, and other mental health specialists. This volume, however, has been prepared for all the other clinicians in the health care professions—including physicians, nurses, and physical therapists—who would like to learn more about psychosocial issues in the evaluation and treatment of patients with painful conditions. Interest in these aspects of pain and in the particular challenges that often arise in treating pain patients is widespread in health care, and this handbook provides a collection of focused reviews of the psychosocial aspects of pain.

The chapters in Part I provide the foundation for the rest of the volume. These chapters review biological, psychological, and social influences on pain and discuss biopsychosocial models of their interaction. Such models not only have demonstrated validity in research but can also be very valuable in understanding the complexity of pain experienced in the clinical setting. Methods for evaluating the numerous factors that influence patients' experience of both acute and chronic pain are discussed in Part II. The chapters in this section review the issues that must be considered in evaluating patients with pain and describe specific measures that can be used to accomplish a comprehensive and accurate assessment.

Beginning with a chapter that discusses the multiple perspectives that must be considered in determining the goals of pain treatment, Part III also includes three chapters on psychological and psychiatric treatments for pain. These chapters were written with two objectives—to provide overviews of the psychological and psychiatric treatments that are available for pain patients and, perhaps more importantly, to present various components of psychiatric and psychological treatment approaches that can be used by all clinicians, regardless of their specialty.

All chronic pain syndromes share the potential to cause suffering and major disruptions in patients' lives, but they are also all unique in the specific issues that must be considered in their evaluation and treatment. The chapters in Part IV review several types of chronic pain that often present particularly complex challenges for clinicians. Pain in children, older individuals, and those with drug abuse problems is addressed in Part V. These groups of patients can be especially prevalent in primary care and pain treatment settings, and there is ample reason to believe that pain in the young, the old, and those with drug abuse histories is very often misunderstood and undertreated.

There are numerous specific psychosocial issues that are often of great interest to clinicians who evaluate and treat painful conditions, and we have selected six of these for the final section of this volume. The chapters in Part VI address a set of questions that are asked frequently in discussions of the psychology of pain and present the results of recent research that has begun to provide some answers. Knowledge of the causes, treatment, and prevention of both acute and chronic pain will grow rapidly in the future and will build on the advances discussed in this volume. There can be little doubt that such progress will continue to improve the care of patients with pain.

We are indebted to a number of individuals in helping us complete this volume. In his former capacity as Editor-in-Chief of IASP Press, Howard Fields, MD, PhD, provided the encouragement to begin this project and enthusiastically supported it. The current IASP Press Editor-in-Chief, M. Catherine Bushnell, PhD, kept us on track and greatly helped in bringing the volume to completion. Elizabeth Endres and Roberta Scholz provided valuable assistance at different stages of the project, and made editing this book a smooth and easy process. Finally, it is a pleasure to acknowledge our deep gratitude for our wives and children, Sharon Gordon and Lili and Jordan Dworkin, as well as Rachel Epstein Breitbart and Samuel Breitbart, who understand that although we love our work and it sometimes keeps us away from them, it is their love for us and our love for them that really brings us happiness.

ROBERT H. DWORKIN, PHD

WILLIAM S. BREITBART, MD

Part I

Conceptualizing Pain

Psychosocial Aspects of Pain: A Handbook for Health Care Providers, Progress in Pain Research and Management, Vol. 27, edited by Robert H. Dworkin and William S. Breitbart, IASP Press, Seattle, © 2004.

1

Pain: Basic Mechanisms and Conscious Experience

C. Richard Chapman[a] and Akiko Okifuji[b]

[a]*Pain Research Center and* [b]*Department of Anesthesiology, School of Medicine, University of Utah, Salt Lake City, Utah, USA*

Pain is among the most complex of human experiences, and yet most didactic descriptions of pain mechanisms are simplistic. Many writers and lecturers commonly speak of pain receptors, refer to the transmission of signals of tissue injury as pain messages or even pain sensations, and trace the pathways of transmission along labeled lines to the cortex, where the messages are "realized" as pain. Although this simple model has generated some valuable basic science over the years, it cannot account satisfactorily for clinical pain states. Young health care professionals armed with knowledge at this level are often bewildered when confronted with the challenge of assessing and managing clinical pain problems, which are usually rich in neurological and psychological complexity.

Fortunately, research on the neurophysiology of pain, functional brain imaging studies of persons in pain, and consciousness studies are yielding converging evidence that narrows the gap between measurable neurological and psychological function. This convergence shows that simplistic models of pain as a specific sensory message, subject to modulation along the way but destined for arrival at the somatosensory cortex, are no longer viable. Pain is not a primitive sensory message somehow recognized by the cortex but rather the end product of massive distributed and parallel processing within the brain. It has emotional and cognitive features because it is the end product of central processing in brain areas that produce the interdependent processes of emotion and cognition. Moreover, pain occurs in the context of other experience that the brain is generating moment by moment, and involves motor function such as facial expression and the tendency to fight or escape. In humans the brain integrates pain into an immediate social context.

The specification of pathways for nociceptive transmission has an enduring place in the study of pain, but its role is limited. It is necessary but not sufficient. Signals contribute to the experience of pain, but they are not sensory experiences waiting for realization at the cortex. They do not arrive at final destinations and enter consciousness. Current evidence suggests instead that signals trigger several higher-order processes that operate in parallel. The brain integrates these processes with other ongoing functions to form a coherent immediate awareness, sets up appropriate adaptive or protective behaviors, and feeds all of this forward into a broader, purposive psychological context that involves personal agency and sense of self.

This chapter offers a view of pain mechanisms that emphasizes higher-order mechanisms of emotion and cognition. It begins with a brief overview of the peripheral mechanisms that detect and signal tissue damage. It then describes multiple pathways of first-order central transmission, which implicate emotion-generating structures in the perception of pain. A brief review of evidence from functional brain imaging studies confirms this mechanism. A review of brain mechanisms related to emotion and stress suggests that pain involves complex psychological processes. The chapter concludes with a brief overview of the cognitive-emotional aspects of pain that emerge from central processing.

DETECTION OF TISSUE INJURY

Sensory end organs that detect and signal tissue trauma, termed nociceptors, are the free nerve endings of either myelinated, small-diameter (Aδ) or unmyelinated (C) fiber axons (Besson and Chaouch 1987; Heppelmann et al. 1991; Willis and Westlund 1997; Riedel and Neeck 2001). Aδ fibers conduct more rapidly (4–44 m/s vs. roughly 0.5–1 m/s) and generate a different quality of sensation than do C fibers. Aδ fibers produce brief, sharp, pricking pain sensations while C fibers typically generate burning or aching sensations. Pin-prick at the foot will produce first a fast pain with a bright, sharp quality that lasts no more than 50 ms followed by a painless interval of approximately 1 second, and then a slow pain with a burning quality that lasts roughly 1 second. Aδ fibers mediate the fast pain and C fibers the slow pain.

Nerve fibers, including nociceptors, signal stimulus intensity according to how many fibers a stimulus excites and the frequency of their action potentials. For a given nerve fiber, the stronger the stimulus, the higher the firing frequency. A peripheral nerve may include fibers of various diameters from different types of receptors and so exhibit a compound action potential of overlapping frequencies.

Nociceptors innervate skin, muscle, fascia, joints, tendons, periosteum, teeth, meninges, blood vessels, and visceral organs. As sensory mechanisms, these tissues group into cutaneous, deep, and visceral types. The quality of the pain that ensues from nociceptive activation varies across these types. Most cutaneous pain is well localized, sharp, and pricking or burning. Deep tissue pain usually seems diffuse and dull or aching, although deep tissues can produce bright, sharp pains under certain conditions (e.g., muscle rupture). Visceral pain is very diffuse, often referred to the body surface in confusing ways, long-lasting, and frequently associated with a queasy quality that most people describe as "sickening." Severe visceral pain typically produces an accompaniment of profuse sweating, nausea, and vomiting.

Most nociceptors are polymodal, responding to mechanical stimuli such as crush, extreme thermal changes, and chemical irritation. They encode localization and stimulus intensity. However, visceral nociceptors do not respond to cutting, pinching, or burning. Instead, they respond to abnormal distension or contraction of the muscle walls of hollow viscera, the rapid stretching of capsules of solid organs, anoxemia of smooth muscles, traction or compression of vessels or ligaments, and chemical irritation (Gebhart and Ness 1991). Pain originating in visceral nociception commonly manifests as a pain on the surface of the body (termed *referred pain*), and sometimes the location of the pain is distant from the site of pathology. Ischemia in heart muscle, for example, causes pain that patients often experience in the pectoral muscles of the chest or as radiating down the left arm into the little finger and ring finger.

With repeated noxious stimulation, nociceptors may sensitize, lowering their threshold for firing, decreasing their response latency, and persisting in their firing after a stimulus event terminates (McMahon and Koltzenburg 1990; Willis 1993). The site of injury itself become extraordinarily sensitive, or hyperalgesic, and surrounding, uninjured tissue becomes increasingly sensitive as a result of central nervous system (CNS) changes in a process called peripheral sensitization.

In most cases of natural injury, inflammation develops at the site of the injury as a protective response. The process of inflammation sensitizes nociceptors and thereby increases their signal-generating capability (Woolf 1989). Increased blood flow produce redness and heat, and increased vascular permeability causes local swelling. The production of various mediating substances including bradykinin and certain types of prostaglandins can alter the chemical environment of nociceptors, lowering their thresholds for firing and in some cases recruiting other fibers to function as nociceptors. Thus, injured peripheral tissues can become extraordinarily sensitive because of local chemical changes.

Sensitization of nociceptors is a major factor in many clinical pain states (Alexander and Black 1992). It amplifies the intensity of noxious signals arising in damaged tissue, falsely representing the threat of a minor or harmless stimulus delivered to the tissue. A key feature of sensitization is that it can awaken nociceptors that are otherwise silent—so-called *sleeping nociceptors* (McMahon and Koltzenburg 1990). Furthermore, it can recruit sensory endings that are normally not nociceptive (Aβ fibers) to function as nociceptors. Ordinarily, these end organs will not respond to harmless sensory stimuli, but noxious events or chemical changes can sensitize them so that they function thereafter as nociceptors.

Not all pain is a consequence of nociception. Some painful conditions, collectively termed *neuropathic pain,* arise from injury or dysfunction of the peripheral or central nervous systems (Woolf and Mannion 1999). When pain originates in disturbed neural function, such as neurogenic inflammation, it is *neurogenic* in origin. Patients with neurogenic pain may experience ongoing or episodic electrical sensations or paresthesias, painful paroxysms, or a general hypersensitivity that makes harmless stimuli exquisitely painful (Davar and Maciewicz 1989; Bowsher 1991; Elliott 1994; Galer 1995). Neuropathic pain arises from damage to or pathological changes in the peripheral or central nervous system. Injury to a peripheral nerve can produce pathophysiological changes in electrical excitability that generate abnormal ongoing and evoked discharge (Devor 1991). Changes in the afferent impulse barrage can induce long-term shifts of central synaptic excitability as well as changes in spinal cord cell excitability (Wall 1991).

Neuropathic pain takes many forms. Chronic nerve root compression, such as a herniated disk, can generate pain by causing severe demyelination and fibrosis (Boulu and Benoist 1996). Certain mono- and polyneuropathies associated with diabetes (Boulton 1992) or alcoholism (Koike et al. 2001) sometimes produce persisting pain. In addition, pain can arise from iatrogenic or adventitious injury to peripheral nerves or neural plexuses (Vecht et al. 1989) or to central structures such as the spinal cord (Siddall et al. 1995). Severed nerves occasionally form neuromas that generate abnormal impulse discharge (Fried et al. 1991). Not all neuropathy is painful; why some lesions produce pain and others do not is still an enigma. The quality of pain may require the generation of certain abnormal discharge patterns.

TRANSMISSION OF INJURY SIGNALS

The centripetal transmission of noxious signals takes place in the spinal cord. Nociceptive afferents enter the spinal cord primarily through the dorsal route, terminating principally in lamina I (the marginal zone) but also in laminae II (the substantia gelatinosa) and V of the dorsal horn (Craig 1991). The spinal and medullary dorsal horns are much more than simple relay stations; these complex structures participate directly in sensory processing, performing local abstraction, integration, selection, and appropriate dispersion of afferent impulses (Perl 1984; Jänig 1987; Willis 1988; Bonica 1990). Upon entry, nociceptive afferents synapse with projection neurons that convey information to higher centers, with facilitatory interneurons that relay input to projection neurons, and with inhibitory interneurons that modulate the flow of nociceptive signals to higher centers (Jessell and Kelly 1991). Similar neural processing occurs in the spinal cord and the medullary dorsal horn.

The spinal cord contains a complex network of interneurons. These interneurons not only relay signals to higher levels of the CNS but also modulate signal transmission and initiate motor reflexes. Peripheral trauma can sensitize dorsal horn nociceptive neurons, making them excessively responsive to normal inputs (Woolf and Wall 1986; Woolf and King 1990; Willis and Westlund 1997). The exaggerated response of transmission cells in the spinal cord is central sensitization. Enduring central sensitization could cause persisting pain.

There are two principal types of projection neurons in the spinal cord: nociceptive-specific (NS) and multireceptive or wide-dynamic-range (WDR) neurons (Jänig 1987). NS neurons respond only to tissue trauma signals, while WDR neurons respond to stimuli of increasing intensity. Ascending tracts include spinothalamic, spinoreticular, spinomesencephalic, spinocervical, and postsynaptic dorsal cord tracts. Willis and Westlund (1997) and Besson and Chaouch (1987) provide useful reviews of nociceptive transmission mechanisms.

THE SPINOTHALAMIC AND SPINOCERVICAL TRACTS

The thalamus receives and integrates nociceptive and other signals, encoding information about type, temporal pattern, intensity, and localization of tissue trauma. It comprises several functionally distinct nuclei that are reciprocally connected to many parts of the limbic system and the cortex (Willis and Westlund 1997). Medial and ventrobasal thalamic nuclei relay

noxious signals to the primary (S1) and secondary (S2) somatosensory cortices, where refined localization and discrimination occur. In classical teaching about pain, the "appreciation of pain" occurs in these cortical areas. The
thalamus interacts bidirectionally with both limbic and cortical structures
such as the somatosensory cortices. The spinothalamic pathway with its
cortical connections makes possible the sensory features of pain. The spinocervical tract, like the spinothalamic tract, conveys signals to the thalamus.

SPINOLIMBIC TRACTS: SPINOHYPOTHALAMIC
AND SPINOAMYGDALAR

The spinohypothalamic tract conveys nociceptive messaging to both the
lateral and medial hypothalamus, which is effectively the control center of
the limbic brain (Burstein et al. 1988, 1991). The spinoamygdalar tract
extends to the central nucleus of the amygdala (Bernard and Besson 1990).

THE SPINOMESENCEPHALIC TRACT

The spinomesencephalic tract comprises several projections that terminate in multiple midbrain nuclei, including the periaqueductal gray, the red
nucleus, the nucleus cuniformis, and the Edinger-Westphal nucleus (Willis
and Westlund 1997). Some of these structures contribute to descending modulation of nociceptive signaling, particularly the nucleus raphe magnus, the
periaqueductal gray, and the solitary nucleus. Activation of the pathways
descending from these and related structures can result in the attenuation of
nociceptive traffic at the dorsal horn of the spinal cord. Direct electrical
stimulation of these areas, administration of opioid drugs, and the release of
endogenous opioid-like compounds (endorphins) can create analgesia via
this pathway. Moreover, increases in blood pressure provoke the carotid
baroreceptors, which in turn activate the solitary nucleus, which triggers the
descending nociception-inhibiting pathway. This process attenuates nociceptive traffic from the dorsal horn to the brain.

THE SPINORETICULAR TRACT

The spinoreticular tract contains somatosensory and viscerosensory afferent pathways that arrive at different levels of the brain stem. Spinoreticular
axons possess receptive fields that resemble those of spinothalamic tract
neurons projecting to the medial thalamus; like their spinothalamic counterparts, they transmit tissue injury information (Villanueva et al. 1990; Craig
1992). Most spinoreticular neurons carry nociceptive signals, and many of

them respond preferentially to noxious activity (Bowsher 1976; Bing et al. 1990).

The spinoreticular pathway plays a role in the emotional dimension of pain. Nociceptive signals reach multiple structures including the locus ceruleus, which sends extensive noradrenergic projections to diffuse areas of the limbic brain, the hypothalamus, and the cerebellum. One of the projections originating in the locus ceruleus, the dorsal noradrenergic bundle, extends to many limbic and cortical areas. Activation of this pathway tends to produce hypervigilance, negative emotional arousal, and behavior consistent with anxiety and threat.

BRAIN IMAGING AND PAIN

Until the early 1990s, when brain imaging in humans became possible, pain research relied upon "bottom-up" research strategies that identified and line-labeled pathways of transmission occasioned by noxious stimulation. Positron emission tomography (PET) and functional magnetic imaging (fMRI) have provided a "top-down" view of pain perception. More than 130 studies involving brain imaging support the hypothesis that painful stimulation activates central structures associated with emotion—namely, the limbic brain. Most are PET studies of regional cerebral blood flow (rCBF). Changes in rCBF index synaptic activity in specific brain regions.

Reviews by Casey (2000), Ingvar (1999), Davis (2000), Hudson (2000), Bromm (2001), and Treede et al. (2000) indicate that persons experiencing clinical and laboratory pain show activity in the lenticular nucleus, the thalamus, the somatosensory cortices, the insular cortex, various frontal cortical areas, the cerebellum, the cingulate cortex, and the anterior cingulate cortex (as well as other limbic structures). Many of these same structures are active during self-generated emotions.

Some brain imagers interpret limbic activation as a reaction to pain, which reduces to activation in the somatosensory cortex. Others prefer to think of it in terms of thalamocortical and thalamolimbic loops occasioned by thalamic activation. The "bottom-up" evidence, however, strongly indicates that nociceptive signals have multiple destinations; that they trigger multiple neural networks that perform preconscious processing; and that pain emerges from massive, distributed parallel processing in areas that concomitantly generate sensation, emotion, and cognition. If this is the case, then pain is inherently a complex perception, psychological in nature, as opposed to a primitive sensation that triggers complex psychological reactions.

NOCICEPTION AND THE LIMBIC BRAIN

The limbic brain is the central mechanism of emotion. MacLean (1952) introduced the somewhat controversial term "limbic system" and characterized its functions. He later identified three main subdivisions of the limbic brain—amygdala, septum, and thalamocingulate (MacLean 1990)—that represent sources of afferents to parts of limbic cortex. MacLean postulated that the limbic brain responds to two basic types of input: interoceptive and exteroceptive. These descriptors refer to sensory information from internal and external environments, respectively. Because nociception by definition involves signals of tissue trauma, it excites the limbic brain via interoceptive signaling.

Central sensory and affective pain processes share common sensory mechanisms in the periphery. Aδ and C fibers serve as tissue trauma transducers (nociceptors) for both processes, the chemical products of inflammation sensitize these nociceptors, and peripheral neuropathic mechanisms such as ectopic firing excite both processes. In some cases neuropathic mechanisms may substitute for nociception as we classically define it, producing afferent signal volleys that appear, to the CNS, like signals originating in nociceptors. Differentiation of sensory and affective processing begins at the dorsal horn of the spinal cord. Sensory transmission follows spinothalamic and spinocervical pathways, while transmission destined for affective processing takes place in spinoreticular and hypothalamic pathways. Complex interconnections between the thalamus and limbic brain probably play a part as well.

Although other processes governed predominantly by other neurotransmitters almost certainly play important roles in the complex experience of emotion during pain, we emphasize the role of central noradrenergic processing and the medial forebrain bundle here. This limited perspective offers the advantage of simplicity, and the literature on the role of central noradrenergic pathways in anxiety, panic, stress, and post-traumatic stress disorder provides a strong basis (Bremner et al. 1996; Charney and Deutch 1996). Noradrenergic processing involves primarily the medial forebrain bundle that subdivides into two central noradrenergic pathways: the dorsal and ventral noradrenergic bundles.

THE LOCUS CERULEUS AND THE DORSAL NORADRENERGIC BUNDLE

Substantial evidence supports the hypothesis that noradrenergic brain pathways are major mechanisms of anxiety and stress (Bremner et al. 1996).

Most noradrenergic neurons originate in the locus ceruleus (LC). This pontine nucleus resides bilaterally near the wall of the fourth ventricle. The LC has three major projections: ascending, descending, and cerebellar. The ascending projection, the dorsal noradrenergic bundle (DNB), is the most extensive and important pathway for our purposes (Fillenz 1990). Projecting from the LC throughout limbic brain and to all of the neocortex, the DNB accounts for about 70% of all brain norepinephrine (Svensson 1987). The LC gives rise to most central noradrenergic fibers in the spinal cord, hypothalamus, thalamus, and hippocampus (Aston-Jones et al. 1985, 1991), and in addition, it projects to the limbic cortex and neocortex. Consequently, the LC exerts a powerful influence on higher-level brain activity.

The *noradrenergic stress response hypothesis* holds that any stimulus that threatens the biological, psychological, or psychosocial integrity of the individual increases the firing rate of the LC, in which in turn results in increased release and turnover of norepinephrine in the brain areas involved in noradrenergic innervation. Studies show that the LC reacts to signaling from sensory stimuli that potentially threaten the biological integrity of the individual or signal damage to that integrity (Svensson 1987). Spinal cord lamina one cells terminate in the LC (Craig 1992). The major sources of LC afferent input are the paragigantocellularis and prepositus hypoglossi nuclei in the medulla, but destruction of these nuclei does not block LC response to somatosensory stimuli (Rasmussen and Aghajanian 1989). Other sources of afferent input to the LC include the lateral hypothalamus, the amygdala, and the solitary nucleus. Whether nociception stimulates the LC directly or indirectly is still uncertain.

Nociception inevitably and reliably increases activity in neurons of the LC (Korf et al. 1974; Stone 1975; Morilak et al. 1987; Svensson 1987). Notably, this response does not require cognitively mediated attentional control because it occurs in anesthetized animals. Foote et al. (1983) reported that slow, tonic spontaneous activity at the LC in rats changed under anesthesia in response to noxious stimulation. Experimentally induced phasic LC activation produces alarm and apparent fear in primates (Redmond and Huang 1979), and lesions of the LC eliminate normal heart rate increases to threatening stimuli (Redmond 1977). In a resting animal, LC neurons discharge in a slow, phasic manner (Rasmussen et al. 1986).

The LC reacts consistently, but does not respond exclusively, to nociception. LC firing rates increase following nonpainful but threatening events such as strong cardiovascular stimulation (Elam et al. 1985; Morilak et al. 1987) and certain visceral events such as distension of the bladder, stomach, colon, or rectum (Aston-Jones et al. 1985; Svensson 1987). Highly novel and sudden stimuli that could represent potential threat, such as loud clicks or flashes of light, can also excite the LC in experimental animals (Rasmussen et al. 1986). Thus, the LC responds to biologically threatening or potentially threatening events, of which tissue injury is a significant subset. Amaral and Sinnamon (1977) described the LC as a central analogue of the sympathetic ganglia. Viewed in this way, it is an extension of the autonomic protective mechanism described above.

Invasive studies confirm the linkage between LC activity and threat. Direct activation of the DNB and associated limbic structures in laboratory animals produces sympathetic nervous system response and elicits emotional behaviors such as defensive threat, fright, enhanced startle, freezing, and vocalization (McNaughton and Mason 1980). This response indicates that enhanced activity in these pathways corresponds to negative emotional arousal and behaviors appropriate to perceived threat. LC firing rates increase two- to three-fold during the defense response elicited in a cat that has perceived a dog (Barrett et al. 1987). Moreover, infusion of norepinephrine into the hypothalamus of an awake cat elicits a defensive rage reaction that includes activation of the LC noradrenergic system. In general, the mammalian defense response involves increased regional turnover and release of norepinephrine in the brain regions innervated by the LC. The LC response to threat, therefore, may be a component of the partly "prewired" patterns associated with the defense response.

Increased alertness is a key element in early stages of the defense response. Normally, activity in the LC increases alertness. Tonically enhanced LC and DNB discharge corresponds to hypervigilance and emotionality (Foote et al. 1983; Butler et al. 1990; Bremner et al. 1996). The DNB is the mechanism for vigilance and defensive orientation to affectively relevant and novel stimuli. It also regulates attentional processes and facilitates motor responses (Elam et al. 1986; Foote and Morrison 1987; Gray 1987; Svensson 1987). In this sense, the LC influences the stream of consciousness on an ongoing basis and readies the individual to respond quickly and effectively to a threat when it occurs.

The LC and DNB support biological survival by making possible global vigilance for threatening and harmful stimuli. Siegel and Rogawski (1988) hypothesized a link between the LC noradrenergic system and vigilance, focusing on rapid eye movement (REM) sleep. They noted that LC noradrenergic neurons maintain continuous activity in both the normal waking state and non-REM sleep, but during REM sleep these neurons virtually cease discharge activity. Moreover, an increase in REM sleep ensues both after lesion of the DNB or following administration of clonidine, an α_2-adrenoceptor agonist. Because LC inactivation during REM sleep permits rebuilding of noradrenergic stores, this phase of sleep may be necessary preparation for sustained periods of high alertness during subsequent waking. Siegel and Rogawski contended that "a principal function of NE [norepinephrine] in the CNS is to facilitate the excitability of target neurons to specific high priority signals." Conversely, reduced LC activity periods during REM sleep allow time for a suppression of sympathetic tone.

Both adaptation and sensitization can alter the LC response to threat. Abercrombie and Jacobs (1987a,b) demonstrated a noradrenergically mediated increase in heart rate in cats exposed to white noise. Elevated heart rate decreased with repeated exposure, as did LC activation and circulating levels of norepinephrine. Libet and Gleason (1994) found that stimulation via permanently implanted LC electrodes did not elicit indefinite anxiety. This finding indicates that the brain either adapts to LC excitation or engages a compensatory response to excessive LC activation under some circumstances. In addition, central noradrenergic responsiveness changes as a function of learning. In the cat, pairing a stimulus with a noxious air puff results in increased LC firing with subsequent presentations of the stimulus, but previous pairing of that stimulus with a food reward produces no alteration in LC firing rates with repeated presentation (Rasmussen et al. 1986). These studies show that, despite its apparently "prewired" behavioral subroutines, the noradrenergic brain shows substantial neuroplasticity. The emotional response of animals and humans to a painful stimulus is adaptive and can change as a function of experience.

From a different perspective, Bremner et al. (1996) postulated that chronic stress can affect regional norepinephrine turnover and thus contribute to the *response sensitization* evident in panic disorder and post-traumatic stress disorder. Chronic exposure to a stressor (including ongoing nociception) could create a situation in which noradrenergic synthesis cannot keep up with demand, thus depleting brain norepinephrine levels. Animals exposed to inescapable shock demonstrate greater LC responsiveness to an excitatory stimulus than do animals that have experienced escapable shock (Weiss and Simson 1986). In addition, such animals display "learned helplessness" behaviors—they cease trying to adapt to, or cope with, the source of shock (Seligman et al. 1980). From an evolutionary perspective, this behavior is a failure of the defense response as adaptation; it represents surrender to suffering. Extrapolating this and related observations to patients, Bremner and colleagues (1996) suggested that persons who have once encountered overwhelming stress and suffered exhaustion of central noradrenergic resources may respond excessively to similar stressors that they encounter later.

THE AUTONOMIC NERVOUS SYSTEM AND EMOTION

The autonomic nervous system (ANS) plays an important role in regulating the constancy of the internal environment, and it does so in a feedback-regulated manner under the direction of the hypothalamus, the solitary nucleus, the amygdala, and other CNS structures (LeDoux 1986, 1996). In general, it regulates activities that are not normally under voluntary control. The hypothalamus is the principal integrator of autonomic activity. Stimulation of the hypothalamus elicits highly integrated patterns of response that involve the limbic system and other structures (Morgane 1981). Autonomic activity contributes to the pathophysiology of chronic pain (Benarroch 2001). It is also an important feature of the emotional aspect of pain (Chapman et al. 2002).

Many researchers hold that the ANS comprises three divisions—the sympathetic, the parasympathetic, and the enteric (Dodd and Role 1991; Burnstock and Hoyle 1992). Others subsume the enteric under the other two divisions. Broadly, the sympathetic nervous system (SNS) makes possible the arousal needed for fight and flight reactions, while the parasympathetic system governs basal heart rate, metabolism, and respiration. The enteric nervous system innervates the viscera via a complex network of interconnected plexuses.

The sympathetic and parasympathetic systems are largely mutual physiological antagonists—if one system inhibits a function, the other typically augments it. There are, however, important exceptions to this rule that demonstrate complementary or integratory relationships. The mechanism most heavily involved in the affective response to tissue trauma is the SNS.

During emergency or injury to the body, the hypothalamus uses the SNS to increase cardiac output, respiration rate, and blood glucose. It also regulates body temperature, causes piloerection, alters muscle tone, provides compensatory responses to hemorrhage, and dilates pupils. These responses are part of a coordinated, well-orchestrated pattern called the defense response (Cannon 1929; Sokolov 1963, 1990; Donaldson et al. 2003). It resembles the better-known orienting response in some respects, but it can only occur following a strong stimulus that is noxious or frankly painful. It sets the stage for escape or confrontation, thus serving to protect the organism from danger. In a conscious cat, both electrical stimulation of the hypothalamus and infusion of norepinephrine into the hypothalamus elicit a rage reaction with hissing, snarling, and attack posture with claw exposure, accompanied by a pattern of SNS arousal (Hess 1936; Hilton 1966; Barrett et al. 1987). Circulating epinephrine produced by the adrenal medulla during activation of the hypothalamic-pituitary-adrenocortical (HPA) axis accentuates the defense response, fear responses, and aversive emotional arousal in general.

Because the defense response and related changes are involuntary, we generally perceive them as something that the environment does to us. We generally describe such physiological changes, not as the bodily responses that they are, but rather as feelings. We might describe a threatening and physiologically arousing event by saying: "It scared me" or "It made me really mad."

Phenomenologically, feelings seem to happen to us; we do not "do" them in the sense that we think thoughts or choose actions. They are not volitional. Emotions are who we are in a given circumstance rather than choices we make, and we commonly interpret events and circumstances in terms of the emotions that they elicit. ANS arousal, therefore, plays a major role in the complex psychological experience of injury and is a part of that experience.

Early views of the ANS followed the lead of Cannon (1929) and held that emergency responses and all forms of intense aversive arousal are un-differentiated, diffuse patterns of sympathetic activation. While this belief is broadly true, research has shown that definable patterns characterize emotional arousal, and that these patterns are related to the emotion involved, the motor activity required, and perhaps the context (LeDoux 1986, 1996). An investigator attempting to understand how humans experience emotions must remember that the brain not only recognizes patterns of arousal; it also creates them.

One of the primary mechanisms in the creation of emotion is feedback-dependent sympathetic efferent activation. The ANS has both afferent and efferent functions. The afferent mechanisms signal changes in the viscera and other organs, while efferent activity conveys commands to those organs. Consequently, the ANS can maintain feedback loops related to viscera, muscle, blood flow, and other responses. The visceral feedback system ex-emplifies this process. In addition, feedback can occur via the endocrine system, which under the control of the ANS releases neurohormones into the systemic circulation. Because feedback involves both autonomic afferents and endocrine responses, and because some feedback occurs at the level of unconscious homeostatic balance and other feedback involves awareness, the issue of how visceral change contributes to the creation of an emotional state is complex. The mechanisms are almost certainly pattern-dependent, dynamical, and at least partly specific to the emotion involved. Moreover, they occur in parallel with sensory information processing.

The feedback concept is central to emotion research: awareness of physiological changes elicited by a stimulus is a primary mechanism of emotion. The psychiatric patient presenting with panic attack, phobia, or anxiety is reporting a subjective state based on patterns of physiological signals and not an existential crisis that takes place somewhere in the domain of the mind, somehow apart from the body. Similarly, the medical patient expressing emotional distress during a painful procedure, or during uncontrolled postoperative pain, is experiencing the sensory features of that pain against the background of strong sympathetic arousal signals.

The concept of feedback underscores an essential point: nociception stimulus does not have purely sensory effects. It undergoes parallel processing at the affective level. When a neural signal involves threat to biological integrity, it elicits strong patterns of sympathetic and neuroendocrine response. These, in turn, contribute to the awareness of the perceiver. Sensory processing provides information about the environment, but this information exists in awareness against a background of emotional arousal, either positive or negative, and that arousal may vary from mild to extreme.

THE VENTRAL NORADRENERGIC BUNDLE AND THE HYPOTHALAMIC-PITUITARY-ADRENOCORTICAL AXIS

The ventral noradrenergic bundle (VNB) originates in the LC and enters the medial forebrain bundle. Neurons in the medullary reticular formation project to the hypothalamus via the VNB (Sumal et al. 1983). Sawchenko and Swanson (1982) identified two VNB-linked noradrenergic and adrenergic pathways to the paraventricular hypothalamus in the rat: the A1 region of the ventral medulla (lateral reticular nucleus, LRN), and the A2 region of the dorsal vagal complex (the nucleus tractus solitarius, or solitary nucleus), which receives visceral afferents. These medullary neuronal complexes supply 90% of catecholaminergic innervation to the paraventricular hypothalamus via the VNB (Assenmacher et al. 1987).

The noradrenergic axons in the VNB respond to noxious stimulation (Svensson 1987), as does the hypothalamus itself (Kanosue et al. 1984). Moreover, nociception-transmitting neurons at all segmental levels of the spinal cord project to medial and lateral hypothalamus and several telencephalic regions (Burstein et al. 1988, 1991; Willis and Westlund 1997). These projections link tissue injury and the hypothalamic response, as do hormonal messengers in some circumstances.

The hypothalamic paraventricular nucleus (PVN) coordinates the HPA axis. Neurons of the PVN receive afferent information from several reticular areas including the ventrolateral medulla, dorsal raphe nucleus, nucleus raphe magnus, LC, dorsomedial nucleus, and nucleus tractus solitarius (Sawchenko and Swanson 1982; Peschanski and Weil-Fugacza 1987; Lopez et al. 1991). Still other afferents project to the PVN from the hippocampus, septum, and amygdala (Feldman et al. 1995). Nearly all hypothalamic and preoptic nuclei send projections to the PVN. This pattern suggests that limbic connections mediate endocrine responses during stress. Feldman et al. noted that limbic stimulation always increases adrenocortical activity in rats.

In responding to potentially or frankly injurious stimuli, the PVN initiates a complex series of events regulated by feedback mechanisms. These processes ready the organism for extraordinary behaviors that will maximize its chances to cope with the threat at hand (Selye 1978). While laboratory studies often involve highly controlled and specific noxious stimulation, real-life tissue trauma usually involves a spectrum of afferent activity, and the pattern of activity may be a greater determinant of the stress response than the specific receptor system involved (Lilly and Gann 1992). Traumatic injury, for example, might involve complex signaling from the site of injury including inflammatory mediators, baroreceptor signals from blood volume changes, and hypercapnia. Tissue trauma normally initiates many physiological changes in addition to nociception.

Diminished nociceptive transmission during stress or injury helps people and animals to cope with threat without the distraction of pain. Laboratory studies with rodents indicate that animals placed in restraint or subjected to cold water develop analgesia (Amir and Amit 1979; Bodnar et al. 1979; Kelly et al. 1993). Lesioning the PVN attenuates such stress-induced analgesia (Truesdell and Bodnar 1987).

The medullary mechanisms involved in this phenomenon are complex and include the response of the solitary nucleus to baroreceptor stimulation (Ghione 1996). Stressor-induced increases in blood pressure stimulate carotid baroreceptors, and these in turn activate the solitary nucleus, which then initiates activity in descending pathways that gate incoming nociceptive traffic at the dorsal horn of the spinal cord. This mechanism links psychophysiological response to a stressor with endogenous pain modulation.

Some investigators emphasize that neuroendocrine arousal mechanisms are not limited to emergency situations, even though most research emphasizes that such situations elicit them (Henry 1986; Grant et al. 1988). In complex social contexts, submission, dominance, and other transactions can elicit neuroendocrine and autonomic responses, modified perhaps by learning and memory. Neuroendocrine processes thus may accompany all sorts of emotion-eliciting situations.

The hypothalamic PVN supports stress-related autonomic arousal through neural as well as hormonal pathways. It sends direct projections to the sympathetic intermediolateral cell column in the thoracolumbar spinal cord and the parasympathetic vagal complex, both sources of preganglionic autonomic outflow (Krukoff 1990). In addition, it signals release of epinephrine and norepinephrine from the adrenal medulla. Release of adrenocorticotrophic hormone, while not instantaneous, is quite rapid: it occurs within about 15 seconds (Sapolsky 1992). These considerations implicate the HPA axis in the neuroendocrinological and autonomic manifestations of emotion associated with tissue trauma.

In addition to controlling neuroendocrine and ANS reactivity, the HPA axis coordinates emotional arousal with behavior (Panksepp 1986). As noted above, stimulation of the hypothalamus can elicit well-organized action patterns, including defensive threat behaviors and autonomic arousal (Jänig 1985). The existence of demonstrable behavioral subroutines in animals suggests that the hypothalamus plays a key role in matching behavioral reactions and bodily adjustments to challenging circumstances or biologically relevant stimuli. Moreover, stress hormones at high levels, especially glucocorticoids, may affect central emotional arousal, lowering startle thresholds and influencing cognition (Sapolsky 1992). Saphier (1987) observed that cortisol altered the firing rate of neurons in the limbic forebrain. Clearly, stress regulation is a complex, feedback-dependent, and coordinated process. The hypothalamus appears to take executive responsibility for coordinating behavioral readiness with physiological capability, awareness, and cognitive function.

Chapman and Gavrin (1999) suggested that prolonged nociception may cause a sustained, maladaptive stress response in patients. Signs and symptoms of this response include fatigue, dysphoria, myalgia, nonrestorative sleep, somatic hypervigilance, reduced appetite and libido, impaired physical functioning, and poor concentration. In this way, the emotional dimension of persisting pain may, through its physiological manifestation, contribute heavily to the disability associated with chronic or unrelieved cancer pain.

COGNITIVE FACTORS

So far, we have established that pain is not just an end-point of noxious sensory signaling but an integrated perceptual experience. Pain is highly individual because countless unique personal factors influence the formation of perception. Reviewing the diverse range of psychological influences that can affect pain is beyond the scope of this chapter. However, in this section we review specific neurocognitive factors that create a phenomenology of pain unique to each person.

ATTENTION

Attention directs limited perceptual resources to selected aspect internal and external environment, in the service of goal-directed activity or protection. Focused attention to one thing usually results in distraction from another. Intuitively, we all know that we experience less pain if we are actively engaged in a distraction task while an injury is occurring. We repeatedly hear stories such as athletes continuing to play despite serious injury, feeling significant pain only after the game. Modification of attention is one of the most commonly used nonpharmacological methods for pain control for children undergoing invasive medical procedures (Kuttner 1989).

Neuroimaging research investigating attention and pain suggests that attentional processes modulate pain perception at multiple brain areas. For example, distracted subjects show attenuated activity in the somatosensory region, periaqueductal gray, and anterior cingulate cortex while engaging in a cognitively distracting task (Longe et al. 2001; Bantick et al. 2002). Alternatively, when patients with chronic phantom pain following unilateral arm amputation underwent hypnotic suggestions to have their "phantom" arm in a painful position, they reported greater pain than with suggestions for comfortable positioning. In addition, suggestions for painful positioning seemed to activate the somatomotor cortex and the posterior aspect of the anterior cingulate cortex (Willoch et al. 2002). These results may pertain to the reliably observed phenomenon that chronic pain patients exhibit persistent hypervigilance for interoceptive sensory events, particularly noxious events.

EXPECTATION/ANTICIPATION

Human laboratory pain research has repeatedly demonstrated alteration of experimentally induced pain with manipulation of subjects' expectations. Beliefs about pain interact with attention to, and appraisal of, sensory events. Thus, subjects who expect a noxious experience may allocate greater attention to, and interpret sensory experience as more aversive, than those who do not.

At the neural level, research suggests that top-down mechanisms related to expectation may contribute to the modulation of pain. A study using functional magnetic resonance imaging (fMRI) demonstrated that learned anticipation of pain evokes increased activity in the primary somatosensory cortex, even in the absence of a noxious event (Porro et al. 2002).

To some extent, patients respond to medical conditions according to their subjective ideas about illness and their symptoms. Health care providers

ow that patients having similar pain
fer greatly in their beliefs about their
d not merely the objective characteristics
ice behavior and emotions.

rate views of their physical states, and these
ovide the basis for action plans and coping. Be-
of a pain and one's ability to function despite dis-
. aspects of expectations about pain. For example, a
cog. tion that one has a very serious, debilitating condition,
that dis. a necessary aspect of pain, that activity is dangerous, and
that pain is . acceptable excuse for neglecting responsibilities will most likely result in significant deactivation and deconditioning. Deconditioned individuals with such belief systems may experience greater pain with exercise, further reinforcing the belief that activity is dangerous and harmful.

From the psychobehavioral perspective, certain beliefs lead to maladaptive coping, increased suffering, and greater disability. Patients who believe that their pain is likely to persist may be passive in their coping efforts and fail to make use of strategies that can help them cope with pain. Patients who consider their pain to be an unexplainable mystery may negatively evaluate their own abilities to control or decrease the pain, and they are less likely to rate their coping strategies as effective (Williams and Keefe 1991).

APPRAISALS

When a new pain occurs, a person will actively attempt to "make sense" of the newly recognized sensory experience. Consider the case of a woman who wakes up one morning with pain in the upper back. In one scenario, she attributes the backache to muscular strain from gardening the previous day. In comparison, interpretation of the back pain as signaling a herniated disk, possibly requiring surgery, could lead to a very different response. Thus, although the amount of nociceptive input may be equivalent, cognitive appraisals contribute significantly to the modulatory process leading into the phenomenology of pain. Different interpretations, like different qualities of pain, lead to different behavioral consequences. If the interpretation is that back pain comes from excessive exercise, then there might be little emotional arousal. The response might be to take some over-the-counter analgesics, take a hot shower, and rest. However, fears of a herniated disk will most likely generate significant worry and a doctor visit.

Maladaptive cognition, or cognitive error, contributes to the distress and disability associated with pain. One extreme type of cognitive error, catastrophizing, is associated with severe disability and poor outcome of chronic pain treatment (Sullivan et al. 1998; Severeijns et al. 2001). Catastrophizing refers to the generation of negative thoughts about one's plight and interpreting even minor problems as major catastrophes. This type of negative appraisal appears to be a particularly potent way of thinking that influences pain and disability. Several acute and chronic pain studies indicate that patients who spontaneously use catastrophizing thoughts report greater pain than those who do not catastrophize (Buckelew et al. 1992; Hadjistavropoulos and Craig 1994). Turk et al. (1983) state that "what appears to distinguish low from high pain tolerant individuals is their cognitive processing, catastrophizing thoughts and feelings that precede, accompany, and follow aversive stimulation."

How individuals appraise their bodily conditions affects their physiology (Flor and Turk 1989). For example, headache patients exhibit elevated skin conductance in response to seeing words describing migraine headaches displayed on a screen (Jamner and Tursky 1987). Similarly, elevated muscle tension is commonly observed in patients who are asked to think about pain in the pain-afflicted regions (Flor et al. 1985). Such tension occurs only under stressful or pain-related conditions in the symptom-specific regions. If, for example, back patients are not discussing their pain, their electromyographic values in the paraspinal areas are comparable to those of healthy controls.

Manipulation of cognitive appraisal may engage central modulatory processes. Therapeutic manipulation using cognitive coping via modification of pain appraisals reduces pain complaints. Bandura and colleagues (1987) demonstrated that naloxone blocks the therapeutic benefits of cognitive coping. This finding suggests that higher level brain activity, including cortical activity, can activate neuromodulatory processes at deeper brain levels. Bandura and colleagues concluded that the physical mechanism by which cognitive coping influences pain perception may at least be partially mediated by endogenous opioids.

SUMMARY

Our brief review of how attentional, anticipatory, and appraisal processes influence pain clearly indicates that these cognitive factors are an integrated aspect of human pain experience. Recent advances in imaging technologies lend supportive knowledge and suggest that cognitive activities are a part of the central processes that modulate pain. Fig. 1 illustrates this concept.

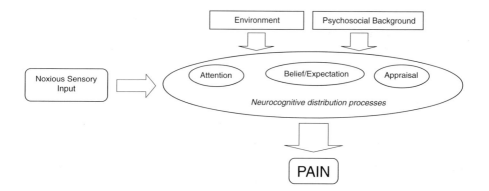

Fig. 1. The cognitive repertoire involved in the processing of pain.

Over time, every person develops cognitive repertoires for attending to, anticipating, and appraising injurious events and noxious sensory signals. These repertoires, uniquely defined by the cultural and environmental factors specific to the individual, are dynamic, constantly evolving with new and repeated occasions of pain and guiding their interpretation at any given moment. Pain is, in part, the end product of cognitive processing involving multiple repertoires.

REFERENCES

Abercrombie ED, Jacobs BL. Single-unit response of noradrenergic neurons in the locus coeruleus of freely moving cats. I. Acutely presented stressful and nonstressful stimuli. *J Neurosci* 1987a; *7*(9):2837–2843.

Abercrombie ED, Jacobs BL. Single-unit response of noradrenergic neurons in the locus coeruleus of freely moving cats. II. Adaptation to chronically presented stressful stimuli. *J Neurosci* 1987b; *7*(9):2844–2848.

Amaral DB, Sinnamon HM. The locus coeruleus: neurobiology of a central noradrenergic nucleus. *Prog Neurobiol* 1977; 9:147–196.

Amir S, Amit Z. The pituitary gland mediates acute and chronic pain responsiveness in stressed and non-stressed rats. *Life Sci* 1979; 24:439–448.

Assenmacher I, Szafarczyk A, Alonso G, Ixart G, Barbanel G. Physiology of neuropathways affecting CRH secretion. In: Ganong WF, Dallman MF, Roberts JL (Eds). *The Hypothalamic-Pituitary-Adrenal Axis Revisited*, Annals of the New York Academy of Sciences, Vol. 512. New York: New York Academy of Sciences, 1987, pp 149–161.

Aston-Jones G, Foote SL, Segal M. Impulse conduction properties of noradrenergic locus coeruleus axons projecting to monkey cerebrocortex. *Neuroscience* 1985; 15:765–777.

Aston-Jones G, Shipley MT, Chouvet G, et al. Afferent regulation of locus coeruleus neurons: anatomy, physiology and pharmacology. *Prog Brain Res* 1991; 88:47–75.

Bandura A, O'Leary A, Taylor CB, Gauthier J, Gossard D. Perceived self-efficacy and pain control: opioid and nonopioid mechanisms. *J Pers Soc Psychol* 1987; 53:563–571.

Bantick SJ, Wise RG, Ploghaus A, et al. Imaging how attention modulates pain in humans using functional MRI. *Brain* 2002; 125:310–319.

Barrett JA, Shaikh MB, Edinger H, Siegel A. The effects of intrahypothalamic injections of norepinephrine upon affective defense behavior in the cat. *Brain Res* 1987; 426(2):381–384.

Benarroch EE. Pain-autonomic interactions: a selective review. *Clin Auton Res* 2001; 11(6):343–349.

Bernard JF, Besson JM. The spino(trigemino)pontoamygdaloid pathway: electrophysiological evidence for an involvement in pain processes. *J Neurophysiol* 1990; 63(3):473–490.

Besson JM, Chaouch A. Peripheral and spinal mechanisms of nociception. *Psychol Rev* 1987; 67:67–185.

Bing Z, Villanueva L, Le Bars D. Ascending pathways in the spinal cord involved in the activation of subnucleus reticularis dorsalis neurons in the medulla of the rat. *J Neurophysiol* 1990; 63:424–438.

Bodnar RJ, Glusman M, Brutus M, Spiaggia A, Kelly D. Analgesia induced by cold-water stress: attenuation following hypophysectomy. *Physiol Behav* 1979; 23:53–62.

Bonica JJ (Ed). *The Management of Pain,* 2nd ed. Philadelphia: Lea & Febiger, 1990.

Boulton A. What causes neuropathic pain? *J Diabetes Complications* 1992; 6(1):58–63.

Boulu P, Benoist M. Recent data on the pathophysiology of nerve root compression and pain. *Rev Rhum Engl Ed* 1996; 63(5):358–363.

Bowsher D. Role of the reticular formation in responses to noxious stimulation. *Pain* 1976; 2:361–378.

Bowsher D. Neurogenic pain syndromes and their management. *Br Med Bull* 1991; 47(3):644–666.

Bremner JD, Krystal JH, Southwick SM, Charney DS. Noradrenergic mechanisms in stress and anxiety: I. Preclinical studies. *Synapse* 1996; 23(1):28–38.

Bromm B. Brain images of pain. *News Physiol Sci* 2001; 16:244–249.

Buckelew SP, Conway RC, Shutty MS, et al. Spontaneous coping strategies to manage acute pain and anxiety during electrodiagnostic studies. *Arch Phys Med Rehabil* 1992; 73:594–598.

Burnstock G, Hoyle CHV (Eds). *Autonomic Neuroeffector Mechanisms.* Philadelphia: Harwood Academic, 1992.

Burstein R, Cliffer KD, Giesler GJ (Eds). *The Spinohypothalamic and Spinotelecephalic Tracts: Direct Nociceptive Projections from the Spinal Cord to the Hypothalamus and Telencephalon.* New York: Elsevier, 1988.

Burstein R, Dado RJ, Cliffer KD, Giesler GJJ. Physiological characterization of spino-hypothalamic tract neurons in the lumbar enlargement of rats. *J Neurophysiol* 1991; 66(1):261–284.

Butler PD, Weiss JM, Stout JC, Nemeroff CB. Corticotropin-releasing factor produces fear-enhancing and behavioral activating effects following infusion into the locus coeruleus. *J Neurosci* 1990;10:176–183.

Cannon WB. *Bodily Changes in Pain, Hunger, Fear and Rage.* New York: Appleton, 1929.

Casey KL. Concepts of pain mechanisms: the contribution of functional imaging of the human brain. *Prog Brain Res* 2000; 129:277–287.

Chapman CR, Gavrin J. Suffering the contributions of persisting pain. *Lancet* 1999; 353:2233–2237.

Chapman CR, Donaldson GW, Nakamura Y, et al. Psychophysiological causal model of pain report validity. *J Pain* 2002; 3(2):143–155.

Charney DS, Deutch A. A functional neuroanatomy of anxiety and fear: implications for the pathophysiology and treatment of anxiety disorders. *Crit Rev Neurobiol* 1996; 10(3-4):419–446.

Craig AD. Supraspinal pathways and mechanisms relevant to central pain. In: Casey KL (Ed). *Pain and Central Nervous System Disease: The Central Pain Syndromes.* New York: Raven Press, 1991, pp 157–170.

Craig AD. Spinal and trigeminal lamina I input to the locus coeruleus anterogradely labeled with *Phaseolus vulgaris* leucoagglutinin (PHA-L) in the cat and the monkey. *Brain Res* 1992; 584(1–2):325–328.

Davar G, Maciewicz RJ. Deafferentation pain syndromes. *Neurol Clin* 1989; 7(2):289–304.

Davis KDE. The neural circuitry of pain as explored with functional MRI. *Neurol Res* 2000; 22(3):313–317.

Devor M. Neuropathic pain and injured nerve: peripheral mechanisms. *Br Med Bull* 1991; 47(3):619–630.

Dodd J, Role LW. The anatomic nervous system. In: Kandel ER, Schwartz JH, Jessell TM (Eds). *Principles of Neural Science*, 3rd ed. New York: Elsevier, 1991, pp 761–775.

Donaldson GW, Chapman CR, Nakamura Y, et al. Pain and the defense response structural equation modeling reveals a coordinated psychophysiological response to increasing painful stimulation. *Pain* 2003; 102: 97–108.

Elam M, Svensson TH, Thoren P. Differentiated cardiovascular afferent regulation of locus coeruleus neurons and sympathetic nerves. *Brain Res* 1985; 358:77–84.

Elam M, Svensson TH, Thoren P. Locus coeruleus neurons and sympathetic nerves: activation by cutaneous sensory afferents. *Brain Res* 1986; 366:254–261.

Elliott KJ. Taxonomy and mechanisms of neuropathic pain. *Semin Neurol* 1994; 14(3):195–205.

Feldman S, Conforti N, Weidenfeld J. Limbic pathways and hypothalamic neurotransmitters mediating adrenocortical responses to neural stimuli. *Neurosci Biobehav Rev* 1995; 19(2):235–240.

Fillenz M. *Noradrenergic Neurons*. Cambridge: Cambridge University Press, 1990.

Flor H, Turk DC. Psychophysiology of chronic pain: do chronic pain patients exhibit symptom-specific psychophysiological responses? *Psychol Bull* 1989; 105:215–259.

Flor H, Turk DC, Birbaumer N. Assessment of stress-related psychophysiological reactions in chronic back pain patients. *J Consult Clin Psychol* 1985; 53:354–364.

Foote SL, Morrison JH. Extrathalamic modulation of corticofunction. *Annu Rev Neurosci* 1987; 10:67–95.

Foote SL, Bloom FE, Aston-Jones G. Nucleus locus ceruleus: new evidence of anatomical and physiological specificity. *Physiol Rev* 1983; 63:844–914.

Fried K, Govrin LR, Rosenthal F, Ellisman MH, Devor M. Ultrastructure of afferent axon endings in a neuroma. *J Neurocytol* 1991; 20(8):682–701.

Galer BS. Neuropathic pain of peripheral origin: advances in pharmacologic treatment. *Neurology* 1995; 45(12 Suppl 9):S17–25.

Gebhart GF, Ness TJ. Central mechanisms of visceral pain. *Can J Physiol Pharmacol* 1991; 69(5):627–634.

Ghione S. Hypertension-associated hypalgesia: evidence in experimental animals and humans, pathophysiological mechanisms, and potential clinical consequences. *Hypertension* 1996; 28(3):494–504.

Grant SJ, Aston-Jones G, Redmond DE Jr. Responses of primate locus coeruleus neurons to simple and complex sensory stimuli. *Brain Res Bull* 1988; 21(3):401–410.

Gray JA. *The Psychology of Fear and Stress,* 2nd ed. Cambridge: Cambridge University Press, 1987.

Hadjistavropoulos HD, Craig KD. Acute and chronic low back pain: cognitive, affective, and behavioral dimensions. *J Consult Clin Psychol* 1994; 62:341–349.

Henry JP. Neuroendocrine patterns of emotional response. In: Plutchik R, Kellerman H (Eds). *Emotion: Theory, Research and Practice,* Vol. 3. Orlando: Academic Press, 1986, pp 37–60.

Heppelmann B, Messlinger K, Schaible HG, Schmidt RF. Nociception and pain. *Curr Opin Neurobiol* 1991; 1(2):192–197.

Hess WR. Hypothalamus und die Zantren des autonomen Nervensystems: Physiologie. *Archiv Psychiatrie Nervenkrankheiten* 1936; 104:548–557.

Hilton SM. Hypothalamic regulation of the cardiovascular system. *Br Med Bull* 1966; 22:243–248.

Hudson AJ. Pain perception and response: central nervous system mechanisms. *Can J Neurol Sci* 2000; 27(1):2–16.

Ingvar M. Pain and functional imaging. *Philos Trans R Soc Lond B Biol Sci* 1999; 354(1387):1347–1358.

Jamner L, Tursky B. Discrimination between intensity and affective pain descriptors: a psycho-physiological evaluation. *Pain* 1987; 30:271–283.

Jänig W. Systemic and specific autonomic reactions in pain: efferent, afferent and endocrine components. *Eur J Anaesth* 1985; 2:319–346.

Jänig W. Neuronal mechanisms of pain with special emphasis on visceral and deep somatic pain. *Acta Neurochir Suppl (Wien)* 1987; 38:16–32.

Jessell TM, Kelly DD. Pain and analgesia. In: Kandel ER, Schwarta JH, Jessell TM (Eds). *Principles of Neural Science,* 3rd ed. New York: Elsevier, 1991, pp 385–398.

Kanosue K, Nakayama T, Ishikawa Y, Imai-Matsumura K. Responses of hypothalamic and thalamic neurons to noxious and scrotal thermal stimulation in rats. *J Thermobiol* 1984; 9:11–13.

Kelly DD, Silverman AJ, Glusman M, Bodner RJ. Characterization of pituitary mediation of stress-induced antinociception in rats. *Physiol Behav* 1993; 53:769–775.

Koike H, Mori K, Misu K, et al. Painful alcoholic polyneuropathy with predominant small fiber loss and normal thiamine status. *Neurology* 2001; 56:1727–1732.

Korf J, Bunney BS, Aghajanian GK. Noradrenergic neurons: morphine inhibition of spontaneous activity. *Eur J Pharmacol* 1974; 25:165–169.

Krukoff TL. Neuropeptide regulation of autonomic outflow at the sympathetic preganglionic neuron: anatomical and neurochemical specificity. *Ann N Y Acad Sci* 1990; 579:162–167.

Kuttner L. Management of young children's acute pain and anxiety during invasive medical procedures. *Pediatrician* 1989; 16:39–44.

LeDoux JE. The neurobiology of emotion. In: LeDoux JE, Hirst W (Eds). *Mind and Brain: Dialogs in Cognitive Neuroscience.* Cambridge: Cambridge University Press, 1986, pp 301–354.

LeDoux JE. *The Emotional Brain: The Mysterious Underpinnings of Emotional Life.* New York: Simon & Schuster, 1996, p 384.

Libet B, Gleason CA. The human locus coeruleus and anxiogenesis. *Brain Res* 1994; 634(1):178–180.

Lilly MP, Gann DS. The hypothalamic-pituitary-adrenal-immune axis: a critical assessment. *Arch Surg* 1992; 127(12):1463–1474.

Longe SE, Wise R, Bantick S, et al. Counter-stimulatory effects on pain perception and processing are significantly altered by attention: an fMRI study. *Neuroreport* 2001; 12:2021–2025.

Lopez JF, Young EA, Herman JP, Akil H, Watson SJ. Regulatory biology of the HPA axis: an integrative approach. In: Risch SC (Ed). *Central Nervous System Peptide Mechanisms in Stress and Depression.* Washington, DC: American Psychiatric Press, 1991, pp 1–52.

MacLean PD. Some psychiatric implications of physiological studies on frontotemporal portion of limbic system (visceral brain). *Electroencehalogr Clin Neurophysiol* 1952; 4:407–418.

MacLean PD. *The Triune Brain in Evolution: Role in Paleocerebral Functions.* New York: Plenum Press, 1990.

McMahon S, Koltzenburg M. The changing role of primary afferent neurons in pain. *Pain* 1990; 43:269–272.

McNaughton N, Mason ST. The neuropsychology and neuropharmacology of the dorsal ascending noradrenergic bundle—a review. *Prog Neurobiol* 1980; 14:157–219.

Morgane PJ. Historical and modern concepts of hypothalamic organization and function. In: Morgane PJ, Panksepp J (Eds). *Handbook of the Hypothalamus,* Vol. 1. New York: Marcel Dekker, 1981, pp 1–64.

Morilak DA, Fornal CA, Jacobs BL. Effects of physiological manipulations on locus coeruleus neuronal activity in freely moving cats. II. Cardiovascular challenge. *Brain Res* 1987; 422:24–31.

Panksepp J. The anatomy of emotions. In: Plutchik R, Kellerman H (Eds). *Emotion: Theory, Research and Experience,* Vol. 3. Orlando: Academic Press, 1986, pp 91–124.

Perl ER. Characterization of nociception and their activation of neurons in the superficial dorsal horn: first steps for the sensation of pain. In: Kruger L, Liebeskind JC (Eds). *Neural Mechanisms of Pain,* Advances in Pain Research and Therapy, Vol. 6. New York: Raven Press, 1984, pp 23–52.

Peschanski M, Weil-Fugacza J. Aminergic and cholinergic afferents to the thalamus: experimental data with reference to pain pathways. In: Besson JM, Guilbaud G, Paschanski M (Eds). *Thalamus and Pain.* Amsterdam: Excerpta Medica, 1987, pp 127–154.

Porro CA, Baraldi P, Pagnoni G, et al. Does anticipation of pain affect cortical nociceptive systems? *J Neurosci* 2002; 22:3206–3214.

Rasmussen K, Aghajanian GK. Withdrawal-induced activation of locus coeruleus neurons in opiate-dependent rats: attenuation by lesions of the nucleus paragigantocellularis. *Brain Res* 1989; 505(2):346–350.

Rasmussen K, Morilak DA, Jacobs BL. Single unit activity of locus coeruleus neurons in the freely moving cat. I. During naturalistic behaviors and in response to simple and complex stimuli. *Brain Res* 1986; 371(2):324–334.

Redmond DEJ. Alteration in the functions of the nucleus locus coeruleus: a possible model for studies of anxiety. In: Hannin I, Usdin E (Eds). *Animal Models in Psychiatry and Neurology.* New York: Pergamon Press, 1977, pp 293–306.

Redmond DEJ, Huang YG. Current concepts. II. New evidence for a locus coeruleus-norepinephrine connection with anxiety. *Life Sci* 1979; 25:2149–2162.

Riedel W, Neeck G. Nociception, pain, and antinociception: current concepts. *Z Rheumatol* 2001; 60(6):404–415.

Saphier D. Cortisol alters firing rate and synaptic responses of limbic forebrain units. *Brain Res Bull* 1987; 19:519–524.

Sapolsky RM. *Stress, the Aging Brain, and the Mechanisms of Neuron Death.* Cambridge: MIT Press, 1992.

Sawchenko PE, Swanson LW. The organization of noradrenergic pathways from the brain stem to the paraventricular and supraoptic nuclei in the rat. *Brain Res* 1982; 273(3):275–325.

Seligman ME, Weiss J, Weinraub M, Schulman A. Coping behavior: learned helplessness, physiological change and learned inactivity. *Behav Res Ther* 1980; 18:459–512.

Selye H. *The Stress of Life.* New York: McGraw-Hill, 1978.

Severeijns R, Vlaeyen JW, van den Hout MA, Weber WE. Pain catastrophizing predicts pain intensity, disability and psychological distress independent of the level of physical impairment. *Clin J Pain* 2001; 17:165–172.

Siddall PJ, Taylor D, Cousins MJ. Pain associated with spinal cord injury. *Curr Opin Neurol* 1995; 8(6):447–450.

Siegel JM, Rogawski MA. A function for REM sleep: regulation of noradrenergic receptor sensitivity. *Brain Res Rev* 1988; 13:213–233.

Sokolov EN. *Perception and the Conditioned Reflex.* Oxford: Pergamon Press, 1963.

Sokolov EN. The orienting response, and future directions of its development. *Pavlov J Biol Sci* 1990; 25(3):142–150.

Stone EA. Stress and catecholamines. In: Friedhoff AJ (Ed). *Catecholamines and Behavior,* Vol. 2. New York: Plenum Press, 1975, pp 31–72.

Sullivan MJ, Stanish W, Waite H, Sullivan M, Trip DA. Catastrophizing, pain, and disability in patients with soft-tissue injuries. *Pain* 1998; 77:253–260.

Sumal KK, Blessing WW, Joh TH, Reis DJ, Pickel VM. Synaptic interaction of vagal afference and catecholaminergic neurons in the rat nucleus tractus solitarius. *J Brain Res* 1983; 277:31–40.

Svensson TH. Peripheral, autonomic regulation of locus coeruleus noradrenergic neurons in brain: putative implications for psychiatry and psychopharmacology. *Psychopharmacology* 1987; 92:1–7.

Treede RD, Apkarian AV, Bromm B, Greenspan JD, Lenz FA. Cortical representation of pain: functional characterization of nociceptive areas near the lateral sulcus. *Pain* 2000; 87(2):113–119.

Truesdell LS, Bodner RJ. Reduction in cold-water swim analgesia following hypothalamic paraventricular nucleus lesions. *Physiol Behav* 1987; 39:727–731.

Turk D, Meichenbaum M, Genest M. *Pain and Behavioral Medicine: A Cognitive-Behavioral Perspective.* New York: Guilford, 1983.

Vecht CJ, Van de Brand HJ, Wajer OJ. Post-axillary dissection pain in breast cancer due to lesion of the intercostobrachial nerve. *Pain* 1989; 38(2):171–176.

Villanueva L, Cliffer KD, Sorkin LS, Le Bars D, Willis WDJ. Convergence of heterotopic nociceptive information onto neurons of caudal medullary reticular formation in monkey (*Macaca fascicularis*). *J Neurophysiol* 1990; 63:1118–1127.

Wall PD. Neuropathic pain and injured nerve: central mechanisms. *Br Med Bull* 1991; 47(3):631–643.

Weiss JM, Simson PG. Depression in an animal model: focus on the locus ceruleus. *Ciba Found Symp* 1986; 123:191–215.

Williams DA, Keefe FJ. Pain beliefs and the use of cognitive-behavioral coping strategies. *Pain* 1991; 46:185–190.

Willis WD. Dorsal horn neurophysiology of pain. *Ann New York Acad Sci* 1988; 531:76–89.

Willis WD. Mechanisms of somatic pain. In: Chapman, CR, Foley KM (Eds). *Current and Emerging Issues in Cancer Pain.* New York: Raven Press, 1993, pp 67–81.

Willis WD, Westlund KN. Neuroanatomy of the pain system and of the pathways that modulate pain. *J Clin Neurophysiol* 1997; 14:2–31.

Willoch F, Rosen G, Tolle TR, et al. Phantom limb pain in the human brain: unraveling neural circuitries of phantom limb sensations using positron emission tomography. *Ann Neurol* 2002; 48:842–849.

Woolf CJ. Recent advances in the pathophysiology of acute pain. *Br J Anaesth* 1989; 63(2):139–146.

Woolf CJ, King AE. Dynamic alterations in the cutaneous mechanoreceptive fields of dorsal horn neurons in the rat spinal cord. *J Neurosci* 1990; 10(8):2717–2726.

Woolf CJ, Mannion RJ. Neuropathic pain: aetiology, symptoms, mechanisms, and management. *Lancet* 1999; 353(9168):1959–1964.

Woolf CJ, Wall PD. Relative effectiveness of C primary afferent fibers of different origins in evoking a prolonged facilitation of the flexor reflex in the rat. *J Neurosci* 1986; 6(5):1433–1442.

Correspondence to: C. Richard Chapman, PhD, Pain Research Center, Department of Anesthesiology, University of Utah School of Medicine, 615 Arapeen Drive, Suite 200, Salt Lake City, UT 84108, USA. Tel: 801-585-0458; Fax: 801-585-7694; email: crc20@utah.edu.

Psychosocial Aspects of Pain: A Handbook for Health Care Providers, Progress in Pain Research and Management, Vol. 27, edited by Robert H. Dworkin and William S. Breitbart, IASP Press, Seattle, © 2004.

2

The Influence of Family and Culture on Pain

John D. Otis,[a] Lucille A. Cardella,[b] and Robert D. Kerns[c]

[a]VA Boston Healthcare System and Boston University School of Medicine, Boston, Massachusetts, USA; [b]The Abacus Group, Cranston, Rhode Island, USA; [c]VA Connecticut Healthcare System, West Haven, Connecticut, and Yale University School of Medicine, New Haven, Connecticut, USA

Research consistently indicates that the family can be an influential source of learning and support across the entire lifespan (Turk and Kerns 1985; Ramsey 1989). For example, family factors play a significant role in shaping the development and course of a variety of disorders seen in childhood (Johnson 1998). In addition, family interactions are influential in shaping the course and adjustment of adults with psychological issues and medical diagnoses, and of those undergoing medical procedures (Fox 1989; Rodrigue et al. 1999; Marriott et al. 2000). Within the chronic pain literature, substantial empirical evidence supports the role of psychosocial factors in the experience of pain (Robinson and Riley 1998). Most recently, interest has developed among many chronic pain researchers in exploring the ways in which family interactions can influence the experience and course of chronic pain conditions.

Of particular importance in understanding the influence of the family on the experience of chronic pain is the cultural background and context of the family. Culture, defined as the behavioral and attitudinal norms of a group of people and the systems of meaning in which they take place, shapes a person's (or family's) beliefs and behaviors related to illness, health care practices, help-seeking behaviors, and receptiveness to medical interventions. Culture also shapes efforts to make sense of symptoms and suffering (Kirmayer et al. 1994). Cultural factors related to the experience of pain can influence pain expression, the language used to describe pain, coping responses, beliefs about pain and suffering, and perceptions of the health care system (Lasch 2000). Culture can also influence the types of medical treatments that are considered acceptable. Within each cultural group, variations in symptom attribution may affect the clinical presentation, course, and outcome of many disorders, including pain disorders (Kirmayer et al. 1994).

This chapter provides a critical review and synthesis of the literature on the relationship between the family and its cultural context and pain. We first provide an overview of some of the most influential, integrative theoretical conceptualizations of the influences of family interactions and social context on pain. We then discuss how existing research on family interaction, culture, and ethnicity may influence a person's ways of coping with pain, and in turn, how this information might affect the provision of appropriate, culturally sensitive treatment for pain that may also incorporate family members. Finally, we summarize the existing research on culture and pain and delineate central questions and issues that should guide future research efforts. Thus, this chapter aims to provide a consolidation and close scrutiny of this burgeoning area of theory and research, beginning to outline what it is that we know and highlighting the many questions still left unanswered.

THE FAMILY AND PAIN: THEORETICAL CONCEPTUALIZATIONS

The experience of chronic pain does not occur in isolation from other parts of a person's life. It often has a significant impact on the things people with chronic pain complaints are able to do (e.g., their ability to work or engage in recreational activities), on how they think and feel about themselves (e.g., "I'm not the person I was before this happened"), and on the ways in which they interact with significant others, including family members. In turn, an individual's environment and the family's actions in response to a family member's pain can have a significant influence on how, and to what extent, pain effects the patient's life. While family systems models of health and illness were initially helpful in guiding thought about the role of the family in chronic pain (Patterson and Garwick 1994), none of these models has had widespread influence on the field due to their complexity, difficulties in operationalizing key constructs, and the absence of empirical data supporting the effectiveness of interventions based on the models (Kerns and Weiss 1994; Kerns and Otis, in press). However, two models of behavior have been investigated that can help to explain some of the patterns of family interactions that are characteristically seen in patients receiving clinical treatment for a chronic pain condition.

THE OPERANT-BEHAVIORAL MODEL

The learning model of operant conditioning states that all overt behaviors are significantly influenced by their consequences and by the context in which they occur (Goldfried and Davidson 1994). This model has underpinned research focusing on the role of the social and family environment in the development and maintenance of chronic pain (Fordyce 1976). Central to the model is the idea that observable "pain behaviors" (e.g., complaining, grimacing, and bracing oneself) may be maintained via contingent social reinforcement, perhaps in the form of a sympathetic response from a significant other, even in the absence of continued nociception (see Table I for a list of common pain behaviors). Significant others, including family members and health care providers, play potentially crucial roles as primary sources of social reinforcement for pain behaviors, to the detriment of alternative, health-promoting "well behaviors" such as working and exercising. It is important to note that the overt expression of pain behaviors is only one part of the overall pain presentation, which also includes cognitive and subjective responses to pain (Sanders 1985). Inpatient treatment programs designed to reduce pain behaviors have met with success; however, their cost and the questionable maintenance of improved outcomes over time have decreased their appeal to insurance companies. At the present time, we lack more detailed descriptions of the hypothesized role of the family, empirical examinations of the importance of pain-related family interactions, and family-based outpatient interventions consistent with the operant model.

Table I
Common types of pain behaviors

Verbal Pain Responses
Expressions of hurting
Complaining
Moaning, sighing
Expressions of pain through subjective intensity ratings
Nonverbal Pain Responses
Grimacing
Bracing and guarding
Limping
Rubbing
Use of a cane
Activity Level
Sitting or lying down
Pain Management
Consumption of medications and use of therapeutic devices to control pain

THE COGNITIVE-BEHAVIORAL TRANSACTIONAL MODEL

In response to the limitations of the operant-behavioral model, a cognitive-behavioral transactional model of the role of the family in the course of chronic illness has been described in which the social (family) context is considered the key environment in which adaptation or maladaptation occurs in response to a chronic pain condition (Kerns and Weiss 1994; Kerns 1995; Kerns et al. 2002). According to this model, the experience of chronic pain is a function of the interaction between an individual's prior vulnerabilities in biological, behavioral, cognitive, and affective domains and the specific challenges or stresses of the painful condition. This interaction takes place in a social (family) environment that selectively reinforces positive or negative outcomes. Consistent with a cognitive-behavioral perspective on chronic pain (Turk et al. 1983), the model hypothesizes that the family actively seeks out and evaluates information about the painful condition and makes judgments about its ability to meet the associated challenges. The family also develops a relatively fixed set of beliefs about concepts such as illness, pain, disability, and ability to cope. These beliefs affect the family's appraisal of ongoing experiences in living with the individual with chronic pain, and influence both the individual's and the family's responses to the perceived challenges. This process ultimately determines their level of adaptation. The family's level of flexibility in adopting new strategies for coping with the challenges of chronic pain, together with its more characteristic patterns of responding to stress, further mediates the response. Finally, the family's appraisals of its success in mastering the challenges and in promoting optimal outcomes contribute to future responding. This later step in the appraisal-coping process will determine whether or not the response is repeated. Perceptions of failed efforts to manage the painful condition will most likely enhance the intensity of the perceived threat of the condition, perhaps contributing to a heightened level of perceived pain, increased disability, and greater affective distress. Conversely, perceptions of success in coping will most likely moderate the experience of pain, increase confidence in the family's ability to respond effectively in the future, and reinforce the repeated use of similar strategies.

RESEARCH ON THE ROLE OF FAMILY AND PAIN

The operant model has contributed to the development of psychometrically sound instruments for the assessment of pain-relevant interactions with significant others (Kerns et al. 1985; Kerns and Rosenberg 1995). The model also has facilitated the development of direct observational methods for pain (Romano et al. 1992). Research supports the hypothesis that positive attention from a spouse (e.g., making the patient comfortable in a chair or taking away duties) that is contingent on a patient's expressions of pain is associated with higher reported levels of pain and pain behaviors (Block et al. 1980; Kerns et al. 1990, 1991; Lousberg et al. 1992), higher frequency of observed pain behaviors (Lousberg et al. 1992; Romano et al. 1992; Paulsen and Altmaier 1995), and reports of greater disability and interference with daily life (Flor et al. 1989; Turk et al. 1992). In addition, a high frequency of negative responding to pain from a spouse (e.g., yelling, complaining, or name calling) is reliably associated with depressive symptom severity and other demonstrations of affective distress (Kerns et al. 1990, 1991). Evidence is also emerging that gender and level of global marital satisfaction (Flor et al. 1989; Turk et al. 1992) as well as depressive symptom severity and level of pain (Romano et al. 1995) may serve to moderate these relationships. Future research in this area could examine more complex patterns of pain-relevant interactions and the role of cognitive appraisal in these interactions in an effort to improve the prediction of pain and disability (Weiss and Kerns 1995).

Although the cognitive-behavioral transactional model is important in elucidating interactions between the chronic pain patient and his or her family, there have been no reports to date of controlled empirical evaluations of family therapy for chronic pain, and only a few that have examined the efficacy of couples treatment (Kerns and Otis, in press). While there is support for the conclusion that chronic pain commonly has a negative impact on the family and its members, the data are not unequivocal (Roy 2001). For example, while there is some evidence of marital and sexual dysfunction, increased prevalence of psychophysiological disorders, and elevated affective distress (particularly depression) among the partners of individuals with chronic pain (Maruta et al. 1981; Ahern et al. 1985; Feuerstein et al. 1985; Flor et al. 1987), it is not clear that families of chronic pain patients experience a higher level of distress or other problems relative to families of other chronically ill individuals.

While global differences in coping and functioning in some families relative to others have not been identified, more sophisticated examinations of family beliefs and appraisals may yield potential mediators or moderators of these processes and outcomes. Of particular interest in this regard will be investigations of factors and processes that are reliably associated with the attitudes, beliefs, and appraisals that may ultimately influence the family's response to the patient's experience of pain, and in a reciprocal and dynamic process, modify the patient's adaptation to pain. Explicit attention to the cultural context of the family, in particular, may serve to significantly advance our ability to understand, and ultimately to influence, the course of adjustment and adaptation to pain.

CLINICAL IMPLICATIONS AND RECOMMENDATIONS

The models presented identify several potential target areas for assessment, including the domains of the chronic pain experience (e.g., pain, disability, and affective distress), pain-associated challenges or stressors for the family and its members, and historical information about personal and family resources and supports available for coping with the challenges. The assessment of the family's cognitions (e.g., attitudes, beliefs, and attributions) concerning the pain experience and of family members' behavioral and affective responses to the patient's pain is an important part of a comprehensive pain assessment. Clinicians can then develop a "timeline" of chronic pain development that examines the interactions between the pain with its associated challenges and the individual's and family's efforts to cope with them. On the basis of a comprehensive assessment, the clinician should be able to generate specific hypotheses about the nature of the problems being experienced and the factors that may be contributing to their maintenance over time. It is on the basis of this conceptualization that a multidimensional plan for treatment can be developed.

Ultimately, the health care provider, in collaboration with the family, can develop a pain management plan that targets identified problems and hypothesized factors contributing to the patient's experience of pain. For example, the treatment of one family may focus primarily on patterns of solicitous pain-relevant communication between the patient and the spouse, whereas treatment of a second family may specifically target the family's negative responses to the patient's expressions of pain. Given the complexity of the experience of chronic pain, a successful intervention plan will commonly incorporate multiple treatment targets and strategies. Optimally, the treatment plan and its implementation should remain consistent with the family's treatment goals. It is important to remember that pain patients are sometimes seen only after they have had years of pain that has dramatically affected their lives. Over time, family dynamics and roles, even those of the "disabled spouse," can become entrenched and highly resistant to change.

As with all cognitive-behavioral approaches to pain management, treatment should be time-limited and problem-focused. Interventions should encourage the development of an adaptive problem-solving approach to pain management, increase the effective use of available family resources, teach family members new adaptive coping skills, and help them to draw upon available external resources. Efforts to help family members reduce the stress and challenges of the painful condition and to reconceptualize the situation as less threatening constitute a second general goal. Reduction of the negative impact of the pain problem on the family and its members (including the individual with the chronic pain condition), and the promotion of adaptive family functioning and well-being, are the overarching or higher-order goals of this therapeutic approach.

The structure and functioning of a family system is likely to vary across individuals and over the course of time. Just as siblings, parents, and teachers can reinforce pain behaviors and disability in children, so too can spouses, adult children, and residential caregivers influence the experience of pain in older adults (Kerns et al. 2001). Health care providers are encouraged to be flexible in their definition of "family" because they may find it necessary at times to include individuals outside the nuclear family who possess high reinforcement potential, such as friends, neighbors, and other health care providers. This consideration is especially important when treating patients from different cultures who may reside with extended family members or in multifamily dwellings. For such patients, it may be clinically useful to include an extended family member (e.g., an aunt or grandparent) or a close friend in order to maximize treatment efficacy.

CULTURE AND PAIN

In today's multicultural health care system, the provision of quality care requires that clinicians understand how a patient's history and beliefs affect his or her presentation of medical symptoms. Given that patient satisfaction and compliance with medical recommendations are closely related to the effectiveness of communication between the health care provider and the patient (Novak 1995), it is essential for providers to learn the skills necessary to effectively communicate with patients of different cultures. Certainly, pain is affected by our own past experiences and the social world in which we live (Morris 1999). Culture is a shared system of values, beliefs, and learned patterns of behaviors and is not simply defined by ethnicity. Culture is also shaped by such factors as proximity, education, gender, age, and sexual preference (Low 1984).

CULTURE, BELIEFS, AND ATTRIBUTIONS

Research supports the notion that an individual's beliefs can have a significant impact on his or her experience of pain (DeGood and Shutty

1992). Especially important are beliefs about cause, control, duration, outcome, and blame (Williams and Thorn 1989; Jensen et al. 1991). Patients
function better if they believe that they have some control over their pain,
that medical services are helpful, and that they are not severely disabled
from their pain (Jensen and Karoly 1992). Studies exploring the influence of
cognitions on the experience of pain suggest that understanding patients'
idiosyncratic beliefs about pain can be beneficial in helping them to develop
adaptive coping skills (Turk 1996). An individual's pain beliefs may reflect
shared values and understandings that flow throughout a specific culture.
How our culture instructs and guides us, overtly or covertly, in conceptualizing pain can influence our ability to adapt to a chronic pain condition
(Morris 1999).

Cultural variations in symptom attribution affect the clinical presentation, course, and outcome of many disorders. Attributions may be thought of
as cognitive or conceptual links between an experience or event and knowledge structures that help us to interpret it (Kirmayer et al. 1994). An example of a causal attribution is: "my headache is caused by stress." Symptom attributions lead to specific predictions about the severity, likely course,
appropriate treatment, and wider social significance of symptoms (Kirmayer
et al. 1994). Once an illness schema is made salient by attribution, individuals tend to confirm the schema by seeking additional symptoms that fit it
(Pennebaker 1982). In addition, attributions influence the use of coping
strategies, patterns of self-care or help seeking, and the clinical presentation
of distress, which in turn influences diagnosis and treatment (Kirmayer et al.
1994). Cultural beliefs may influence these symptom attributions, which
can, in turn, influence the patient's perception of the severity of a disorder
such as chronic pain.

RESEARCH ON CULTURE AND PAIN

In our attempts to understand the experience of pain, we need to understand the individual. It is important to recognize that cultural background
can profoundly affect an individual's pain behavior (Streltzer 1997). Pain
depends not only on neural circuits, but also on the complex cognitive
processes by which we interpret specific stimuli in specific situations (Morris 1999). Pain beliefs reflect shared values and understandings that exist
within a specific culture or subculture (Morris 1999). The source of pain
may also be significant in terms of the varying meanings conveyed. For
instance, cancer pain may be viewed differently than benign pain by various
cultural groups. At the 7th World Congress on Pain in Paris, France, in
1993, pain was reported to be a common experience for cancer patients in

Denmark, Norway, France, and Germany (Streltzer 1997). Pain experts in those countries believed that this type of pain was frequently undertreated. However, in China, cancer pain was considered to be less of a problem, leading to fewer prescriptions of opioids (Streltzer 1997). The Chinese perspective stands in contrast to that of European physicians, who concluded that there was a great need for opioid analgesics and that these medications were greatly underutilized.

The effects of culture on pain report were investigated in a study by Bates (1996), who compared patients treated at a pain center in New England to those at an outpatient medical facility in Puerto Rico. The results indicated lower pain intensity ratings among New Englanders when compared to patients in Puerto Rico. When comparing Puerto Rican immigrants living in New England to residents of Puerto Rico, Bates determined that the pain response of immigrants living in New England more closely resembled the non-Latino New England group. The results of the study suggest that the pain response of members of this ethnic group was shaped by the culture and social context in which they lived. A study by Rosmus et al. (2000) examined the behavioral response of 2-month-old Canadian-born Chinese babies receiving a routine immunization to those of non-Chinese infants in similar situations. Facial expressions and crying were used as measures of pain response. The results indicated that Chinese babies demonstrated a significantly different pain response when compared to the non-Chinese infants. These results suggest the influence of culture on acute pain response by at least 2 months of age.

RESEARCH ON ETHNICITY AND PAIN

In contrast to the relative dearth of research on the interaction of culture and pain, studies on ethnicity and pain management are quite abundant. Ethnic groups often have unique cultural experiences and attitudes that may influence nociception as well as psychological and behavioral responses to pain (Juarez et al. 1998). Several experimental pain studies have documented differences in the report of pain across ethnic groups. For example, Woodrow et al. (1972) investigated ethnic differences in pain tolerance to mechanical pressure on the Achilles tendon in more than 40,000 study participants. Their results indicated that Caucasians showed the highest, African-Americans the second-highest, and Asian-Americans the lowest pain tolerance. A study by Edwards et al. (2001) compared 337 African-Americans and Caucasians on an experimental pain procedure to assess pain tolerance and self-reported disability. The results indicated that African-Americans reported higher levels of clinical pain, less pain tolerance during the procedure, and higher levels of disability. Similar results with respect to pain threshold and unpleasantness have emerged from other experimental pain studies (Edwards and Fillingim 1999; Sheffield et al. 2000).

Clinical studies also report ethnic differences in pain perception and response to pain. For example, studies have documented differences between African-Americans and Caucasians in the experience of pain associated with glaucoma and AIDS, as well as various other forms of clinical pain including migraine headaches, jaw pain, postoperative pain, and myofascial pain (Faucett et al. 1994; Widmalm et al. 1995; Breitbart et al. 1996; Nelson et al. 1996; Stewart et al. 1996; Sherwood et al. 1998). In a study of patients attending a chronic pain clinic, Bates and Edwards (1993) found that Hispanics showed the clearest differences when compared to Caucasians, Anglo-Saxon Protestants, French Canadians, and those of Irish, Italian, or Polish background. Hispanics complained of more pain, were less likely to be working, were more expressive of their pain, sought more advice about their pain, felt more unhealthy in general, and believed more strongly that the presence of pain meant that an unhappy life was inevitable. In contrast, studies on the use of patient-controlled analgesia for postoperative pain report no significant difference by ethnic group in the amount of self-administered pain medication (Ng et al. 1996a,b).

Research suggests that belonging to an ethnic group can also affect the provision of pain medication. A study by Streltzer and Wade (1981) found that Caucasians and Hawaiian patients were prescribed significantly more analgesics than were Filipino, Japanese, or Chinese patients. A study examining the treatment of 139 adults with isolated long bone fractures found that Hispanics were twice as likely as African-Americans to receive no pain medication in the emergency department (Todd et al. 1993). A retrospective cohort study in an urban emergency department found that Caucasian patients were significantly more likely than African-American patients to receive analgesics, despite similar medical records of pain complaints (Todd et al. 2000). The risk of receiving no analgesics while in the emergency department was 66% greater for African-American patients than for Caucasian patients. A series of studies of clinics that served ethnic and racial minorities found that outpatients with cancer were three times more likely to be undermedicated with analgesics than were patients in other settings (Cleeland et al. 1994, 1997). The percentage of patients indicating inadequate analgesia was significantly higher in community oncology programs that treated predominantly African-American and Hispanic patients than in university cancer centers and community-based hospitals. In addition, African-American and Hispanic patients were more likely than nonminority patients to have been prescribed inadequate analgesia, regardless of the setting. Overall, these studies suggest that ethnicity can have a significant impact on the self-report of experimental and clinical pain, and that it can influence the provision of analgesic medication across a variety of treatment settings. However, very little research has investigated the mechanisms by which this phenomenon occurs.

HYPOTHESIZED SOURCES OF DISPARITY IN PAIN TREATMENT

The disparity observed among ethnic groups in the treatment of pain has several possible causes (Bonham 2001). First, health care providers' perceptions of patients' race, which are not necessarily based on communication with the patient, may be recorded and used by the health care team to make clinical decisions, predict behaviors, and to make medical and social judgments about the patient (Schulman et al. 1999). Therefore, it is important to understand how information about race and ethnicity is collected and how clinicians' preconceptions may bias treatment of pain.

The health care provider's level of fluency in a patient's primary language is an important factor in effective communication about pain (Perez-Stable et al. 1997). Providers who are unfamiliar with a patient's language or culture may not understand his or her verbal expression of pain. In addition, patients might contribute less to participatory medical visits because of factors such as language barriers, low health literacy, little education, and minimal capacity to advocate for one's health (Cooper-Patrick et al. 1999). For example, members of some cultures may be reluctant to report pain because they find it important to be viewed as "good patients" (Ramer et al. 1999).

Race, ethnicity, and socioeconomic status are often interconnected in the United States (Bonham 2001). Socioeconomic status includes both resource-based measures (e.g., income and wealth) and prestige-based measures (e.g., occupational status and educational level). The influence that a patient's socioeconomic status has on the treatment of pain should be studied further, and this variable should be separated from the patient's race and ethnicity to allow investigators to clarify its relationship to disparities in pain treatment. Research should consider patients' resources as well as the type of medical facility where they receive care as possible contributing factors to pain treatment disparities.

A comprehensive pain assessment is the first step before creating a treatment plan; therefore, it is important to determine whether there are factors that might contribute to bias during this process. The reporting of pain is a social transaction between the health care provider and the patient (Dalton and McNaull 1998). Clinicians should consider that not all cultures will be equally able reduce the subjective sensation of pain to a number between 0 and 10 (Douglas 1999). Patients who may be culturally instructed to be either stoic or very expressive of pain might under- or overrate their pain when using a numeric scale. Some cultures may need to express a constellation of feelings, symptoms, and consequences of pain to convey the nature of the pain experience. Assigning adjectives to specific numbers on the scale may represent the prevailing culture's values of those adjectives, but those same adjectives may represent different numbers in another culture.

CLINICAL IMPLICATIONS AND RECOMMENDATIONS

In medical systems that serve multicultural populations, it is important for clinicians to be aware of patients' culturally based health care beliefs and behaviors. One step that should be taken is to educate and enhance cultural awareness among staff members. This effort could be accomplished through printed material, online education, or by providing periodic in-house services led by community representatives, local academics specializing in culture or sociology, or mental health providers with first-hand experience working with the specific ethnic groups and cultures serviced by that facility. The goals of these services should include providing health care providers with a fundamental understanding of the cultural beliefs and ethnic factors that could influence patient presentation in the medical setting, which ultimately should increase communication between the patient and the provider. Rather than attempting to learn an encyclopedia of culture-specific issues, a more practical approach would be to explore the various types of problems that are likely to occur in cross-cultural medical encounters and to learn to identify and deal with these as they arise. Providers should be encouraged to reflect on their own cultural biases and how they may influence provision of medical treatment. Professionals should raise awareness within their discipline of racial disparities in medical treatment decisions by engaging in open and broad discussions about the issue. Health care facilities should also have a plan in place for the availability of language translation by medically trained personnel when needed.

When performing a pain assessment interview with patients from different cultures, providers should ask questions that will facilitate opportunities for patients to express information about the experience of pain, such as their beliefs, feelings, and expectations about pain, sources of support, and a detailed description of their pain intensity and location. Table II presents a list of a few pain assessment questions that clinicians can ask patients from different cultures in an effort to obtain accurate information about their pain (Lasch 2000).

Table II
Pain assessment questions

1. Why do you think you have this pain?
2. What does your pain mean for your body?
3. How severe is your pain? How long do you think it will last?
4. Do you have any fears about your pain? If so, what do you fear most about your pain?
5. What are the biggest problems that your pain causes for you?
6. What kind of treatment do you think you should receive? What are the most important results that you hope to receive from treatment?
7. What cultural remedies have you tried to help you with your pain?
8. Have you seen a traditional healer for your pain? Do you want to?
9. Who, if anyone, in your family do you talk to about your pain? What do they know? What do you want them to know? Do you have family and friends who help you because of your pain? Who helps you?

Self-report pain assessment questionnaires can be useful tools for supplementing the clinical pain interview. Research on the cross-cultural validation and translation of pain assessment measures is encouraged and would be particularly useful in medical centers that provide services in culturally diverse areas. One example of a measure that has been validated for use by several languages is the West Haven-Yale Multidimensional Pain Inventory (WHYMPI). The WHYMPI is a widely used 52-item self-report questionnaire that is designed to provide a brief, psychometrically sound, and comprehensive assessment of the most important components of the chronic pain experience (Kerns et al. 1985). The WHYMPI has been validated and used cross-culturally and has been translated into nine different languages. This measure has been adapted to assess pain-relevant responses of significant others (Kerns and Rosenberg 1995).

CONCLUSIONS AND FUTURE DIRECTIONS

In sum, there is clearly a need for more comparative cultural studies in the area of chronic pain and for future lines of research to continue to follow up the existing assessment and treatment studies. While cultural differences in the expression and conceptualization of pain have been documented, relatively few studies have examined culture-specific symptoms of pain or cultural differences in ways of coping with pain. It is important for us to understand the ways persons of different cultures and ethnic backgrounds experience pain conditions and the coping skills they choose for dealing with the daily stress that accompanies chronic pain. Finally, culturally sensitive intervention approaches must be developed for families and must be implemented by clinicians who are aware of the unique needs of diverse populations. In effect, efforts to understand the role of culture and the family in the experience of chronic pain are in their earliest stages, yet promise to be important areas of future research.

Effective pain management requires that each patient be viewed as an individual with many characteristics including a particular cultural background. While the need for cultural research is great, it is important to remember that even within a defined culture, individual beliefs, expectations, and behaviors associated with the experience of pain will differ and should be considered throughout the treatment process.

ACKNOWLEDGMENTS

Preparation of this manuscript was supported by a Merit Review grant from the Veterans Health Administration Office of Research and Development, Medical Research Service.

REFERENCES

Ahern D, Adams A, Follick M. Emotional and marital disturbance in spouses of chronic low back pain patients. *Clin J Pain* 1985; 1:69–74.

Bates M. *Biocultural Dimensions of Chronic Pain: Implications for Treatment of Multiethnic Populations.* New York: SUNY Press, 1996.

Bates M, Edwards W. Ethnic variations in the chronic pain experience. *Ethn Dis* 1993; 2:63–83.

Block A, Kremer E, Gaylor M. Behavioral treatment of chronic pain: the spouse as a discriminative cue for pain behavior. *Pain* 1980; 9:243–252.

Bonham V. Race, ethnicity, and pain treatment: striving to understand the causes and solutions to disparities in pain treatment. *J Law Med Ethics* 2001; 29:52–68.

Breitbart W, McDonald M, Rosenfeld B, et al. Pain in ambulatory AIDS patients: pain characteristics and medical correlates. *Pain* 1996; 68:315–321.

Cleeland C, Gonin R, Hatfield A, et al. Pain and its treatment in outpatients with metastatic cancer. *N Engl J Med* 1994; 330:592–596.

Cleeland C, Gonin R, Baez L, Loehrer P, Pandya K. Pain and treatment of pain in minority patients with cancer. *Ann Intern Med* 1997; 127:813–816.

Cooper-Patrick L, Gallo J, Gonzales J, et al. Race, gender, and partnership in the patient-physician relationship. *JAMA* 1999; 282:583.

Dalton J, McNaull F. A call for standardizing the clinical rating of pain intensity using a 0 to 10 rating scale. *Cancer Nurs* 1998; 21:46–49.

DeGood D, Shutty M. Assessment of pain beliefs, coping, and self-efficacy. In: Turk DC, Melzack R (Eds). *Handbook of Pain Assessment.* New York: Guilford Press, 1992, pp 214–234.

Douglas M. Pain as the fifth vital sign: will cultural variations be considered? *J Transcultural Nurs* 1999; 10:285.

Edwards RR, Fillingim RB. Ethnic differences in thermal pain processes. *Psychosom Med* 1999; 61:346–354.

Edwards RR, Doleys DM, Fillingim RB, Lowery D. Ethnic differences in pain tolerance: clinical implications in a chronic pain population. *Psychosom Med* 2001; 63:316–323.

Faucett J, Gordon N, Levine J. Differences in postoperative pain severity among four ethnic groups. *J Pain Symptom Manage* 1994; 9:383–389.

Feuerstein M, Sult S, Houle M. Environmental stressors and chronic low back pain: life events, family and work environment. *Pain* 1985; 22:295–307.

Flor H, Turk DC, Scholz OB. Impact of chronic pain on the spouse: marital, emotional, and physical consequences. *J Psychosom Res* 1987; 31:63–71.

Flor H, Turk DC, Rudy TE. Relationship of pain impact and significant other reinforcement of pain behaviors: the mediating role of gender, marital status and marital satisfaction. *Pain* 1989; 38:45–50.

Fordyce WE. *Behavioral Methods for Chronic Pain and Illness.* St. Louis: C.V. Mosby, 1976.

Fox BH. Cancer survival and the family. In: Ramsey CN Jr (Ed). *Family Systems in Medicine.* New York: Guilford, 1989, pp 273–280.

Goldfried MR, Davidson GC. *Clinical Behavior Therapy.* New York: Wiley, 1994.

Jensen M, Karoly P. Pain-specific beliefs, perceived symptom severity, and adjustment to chronic pain. *Clin J Pain* 1992; 8(2):123–130.

Jensen M, Turner J, Romano J, Karoly P. Coping with chronic pain: a critical review of the literature. *Pain* 1991; 47(3):249–283.

Johnson SB. Family management of childhood diabetes. *J Clin Psychol Med Settings* 1998; 1:309–315.

Juarez G, Ferrell B, Borneman T. Influence of culture on cancer pain management in Hispanic patients. *Cancer Pract* 1998; 6:262–269.

Kerns RD. Family assessment and intervention in chronic illness. In: Nicassio P, Smith T (Eds). *Managing Chronic Illness: A Biopsychosocial Perspective.* Washington, DC: American Psychological Association, 1995.

Kerns RD, Otis JD. Family therapy with pain patients: evidence for its effectiveness. *Semin Pain Med;* in press.

Kerns RD, Rosenberg R. Pain-relevant responses from significant others: development of a significant other version of the WHYMPI scales. *Pain* 1995; 61:245–249.

Kerns RD, Weiss LH. Family influences on the course of chronic illness: a cognitive-behavioral transactional model. *Ann Behav Med* 1994; 16:116–130.

Kerns, RD, Turk DC, Rudy TE. The West Haven-Yale Multidimensional Pain Inventory (WHYMPI). *Pain* 1985; 23:345–356.

Kerns RD, Haythornthwaite J, Southwick S, Giller EL. The role of marital interaction in chronic pain and depressive symptom severity. *J Psychosom Res* 1990; 34:401–408.

Kerns RD, Southwick S, Giller EL, et al. The relationship between reports of pain-related social interactions and expressions of pain and affective distress. *Behav Ther* 1991; 22:101–111.

Kerns RD, Otis JD, Stein K. Cognitive-behavioral treatment for geriatric pain. *Clin Geriatr Med* 2001; 17(3):503–523.

Kerns RD, Otis JD, Wise E. Treating families of chronic pain patients: application of a cognitive-behavioral transactional model. In: Gatchel RJ, Turk DC (Eds). *Psychological Approaches to Pain Management,* 2nd ed. New York: Guilford Press, 2002.

Kirmayer L, Young A, Robbins J. Symptom attribution in cultural perspective. *Can J Psychiatry* 1994; 39:584–595.

Lasch K. Culture, pain, and culturally sensitive pain care. *Pain Manage Nurs* 2000; 1:16–22.

Lousberg R, Schmidt AJM, Groenman NH. The relationship between spouse solicitousness and pain behavior: searching for more experimental evidence. *Pain* 1992; 51:75–79.

Low SM. The cultural basis of health, illness and disease. *Soc Work Health Care* 1984; 9:13–23.

Marriott A, Donaldson C, Tarrier N, Burns A. Effectiveness of cognitive-behavioral family intervention in reducing the burden of care in carers of patients with Alzheimer's disease. *Br J Psychiatry* 2000; 176:557–562.

Maruta T, Osborne D, Swenson DW, Holling JM. Chronic pain patients and spouses: marital and sexual adjustment. *Mayo Clin Proc* 1981; 56:307–310.

Morris D. Sociocultural and religious meanings of pain. In: Gatchel R (Ed). *Psychosocial Factors in Pain: Critical Perspective.* New York: Guilford Press, 1999, pp 118–131.

Nelson D, Novy D, Averilla P, Berry L. Ethnic comparability of the MMPI in pain patients. *J Clin Psychol* 1996; 52:485–497.

Ng B, Dimsdale J, Shragg G, Deutsch R. Ethnic differences in analgesic consumption for post-operative pain. *Psychosom Med* 1996a; 58:125–129.

Ng B, Dimsdale J, Rolink J, Shapiro H. The effect of ethnicity on prescriptions for PCA for post-operative pain. *Pain* 1996b; 66:9–12.

Novak D. Therapeutic aspects of the clinical encounter. In: Lipkin M Jr, Putnam SM, Lazare A (Eds). *The Medical Interview: Clinical Care, Education, and Research.* New York: Springer-Verlag, 1995, pp 32–49.

Patterson JM, Garwick AW. The impact of chronic illness on families: a family systems perspective. *Ann Behav Med* 1994; 16:131–142.

Paulsen JS, Altmaier EM. The effects of perceived versus enacted social support on the discriminative cue function of spouses for pain behaviors. *Pain* 1995; 60:103–110.

Pennebaker J. *The Psychology of Physical Symptoms.* New York: Springer-Verlag, 1982.

Perez-Stable E, Napoles-Springer A, Miramontes J. The effects of ethnicity and language on medical outcomes of patients with hypertension or diabetes. *Med Care* 1997; 35:1212–1219.

Ramer L, Richardson J, Cohen M, et al. Multimeasure pain assessment in an ethnically diverse group of patients with cancer. *J Transcult Nurs* 1999; 10:94–101.

Ramsey CN. *Family Systems in Medicine.* New York: Guilford Press, 1989.

Robinson ME, Riley JL. Role of emotion in pain. In: Gatchel R, Turk DC (Eds). *Psychosocial Factors in Pain.* New York: Guilford Press, 1998.

Rodrigue JR, Pearman TP, Moreb J. Morbidity and mortality following bone marrow transplantation: predictive utility of pre-BMT affective functioning, compliance, and social support stability. *Int J Behav Med* 1999; 6:241–254.

Romano JM, Turner JA, Friedman LS, et al. Sequential analysis of chronic pain behaviors and spouse responses. *J Consult Clin Psychol* 1992; 60:777–782.

Romano JM, Turner JA, Jensen MP, et al. Chronic pain patient-spouse behavioral interactions predict patient disability. *Pain* 1995; 63:353–360.

Rosmus C, Johnson CC, Chan-Yip A, Yang F. Pain response in Chinese and non-Chinese Canadian infants: is there a difference? *Soc Sci Med* 2000; 51:175–184.

Roy R (Ed). *Social Relations and Chronic Pain.* New York: Plenum, 2001.

Sanders SH. The role of learning in chronic pain states. In: Brena SF, Chapman S (Eds). *Clinics and Anesthesiology: Pain Control.* Philadelphia: Saunders, 1985, pp 57–73.

Schulman K, Berlin J, Harless W, et al. The effect of race and sex on physicians' recommendations for cardiac catheterization. *N Engl J Med* 1999; 340:618–626.

Sheffield D, Biles PL, Orom H, Maxiner W, Sheps DS. Race and sex differences in cutaneous pain perception. *Psychosom Med* 2000; 62:517–523.

Sherwood M, Garcia-Siekavizza A, Meltzer M, et al. Glaucoma's impact on quality of life and its relation to clinical indicators. *Ophthalmology* 1998; 105:561–566.

Stewart W, Lipton R, Liberman J. Variations in migraine prevalence by race. *Neurology* 1996; 47:52–59.

Streltzer J. Pain. In: Tseng W, Streltzer J (Eds). *Culture and Psychopathology: A Guide to Clinical Assessment.* New York: Brunner/Mazel, pp 87–100.

Streltzer J, Wade T. The influence of cultural group on the undertreatment of postoperative pain. *Psychosom Med* 1981; 43:396–403.

Todd K, Samaroo N, Hoffman J. Ethnicity as a risk factor for inadequate emergency department analgesia. *JAMA* 1993; 269:1537–1539.

Todd KH, Deaton C, D'Amo AP, Goe L. Ethnicity and analgesic practice. *Ann Emerg Med* 2000; 35:77–92.

Turk DC. Biopsychosocial perspective on chronic pain. In: Gatchel RJ, Turk DC (Eds). *Psychological Approaches to Pain Management: A Practitioner's Handbook.* New York: Guilford Press, 1996, pp 3–32.

Turk DC, Kerns RD. *Health, Illness and Families: A Life-Span Perspective.* New York: Wiley Interscience, 1985.

Turk DC, Meichenbaum D, Genest M. (Eds). *Pain and Behavioral Medicine: A Cognitive-Behavioral Perspective.* New York: Guilford Press, 1983.

Turk DC, Kerns RD, Rosenberg R. Effects of marital interaction on chronic pain and disability: examining the down side of social support. *Rehabil Psychol* 1992; 37:259–274.

Weiss LH, Kerns RD. Patterns of pain-relevant social interactions. *Int J Behav Med* 1995; 2:157–171.

Widmalm S, Gunn S, Christiansen R, Hawley L. Association between CMD signs and symptoms, oral parafunctions, race, and sex, in 4–6 year-old African-American and white children. *J Oral Rehabil* 1995; 22:95–100.

Williams DA, Thorn BE. An empirical assessment of pain beliefs. *Pain* 1989; 36:351–358.

Woodrow K, Friedman G, Siegelaub A, Collen M. Pain tolerance: differences according to age, sex, and race. *Psychosom Med* 1972; 34:548–556.

Correspondence to: Robert D. Kerns, PhD, Psychology Service (116B), VA Connecticut Healthcare System, West Haven, CT 06516, USA. Tel: 203-937-3841; Fax: 203-937-4951; email: robert.kerns@med.va.gov.

Psychosocial Aspects of Pain: A Handbook for Health Care Providers, Progress in Pain Research and Management, Vol. 27, edited by Robert H. Dworkin and William S. Breitbart, IASP Press, Seattle, © 2004.

3

Biopsychosocial Models of Pain

Herta Flor and Christiane Hermann

Department of Clinical and Cognitive Neuroscience at the University of Heidelberg, Central Institute of Mental Health, Mannheim, Germany

Chronic pain has many physiological and psychological aspects. It is important to examine how these factors interact, and specifically, to determine how psychological mechanisms may translate into physiological changes. Several authors (e.g., Feuerstein et al. 1987) have acknowledged the importance of behavioral and biological factors in chronic pain states, but none of their models has specifically addressed biobehavioral interactions or the role of learning in chronic pain.

We have proposed a multifactorial psychobiological model of chronic pain that incorporates the dynamic interrelationship of physiological and psychological factors (e.g., Flor et al. 1990; Turk and Flor 1999). We view pain as a response with physiological, behavioral-motor, and subjective-verbal components that may or may not have an underlying pathological basis in the sense of a structural change, but will always have physiological antecedents and consequences. The physiological component comprises ascending and descending neuronal connections, spinal and supraspinal mechanisms, and biochemical processes. The behavioral-motor component involves pain behaviors ranging from medication intake to grimacing, limping, and use of the health care system. The subjective-verbal component consists of thoughts, feelings, and images that can be verbally represented and expressed. In our model, interactions are continuous: learning occurs in physiological mechanisms, and physiological mechanisms are modified by behavioral and subjective changes (Flor and Birbaumer 1994a; Flor 2000). This view is consistent with the International Association for the Study of Pain's definition of pain as an "unpleasant sensory and emotional experience associated with actual or potential tissue damage, or described in terms of such damage" (Merskey 1986). In addition, the psychobiological model emphasizes that cognitive and learning parameters are integral to the experience of pain as a dynamic process.

BASIC COMPONENTS IN THE DEVELOPMENT OF CHRONIC PAIN

This section focuses on the development of chronic pain states. Although everyone experiences acute pain, only a small percentage of the population develops chronic pain syndromes. We suggest that the preconditions for chronic pain include predisposing factors, eliciting stimuli, eliciting responses, and maintaining processes. These preconditions are illustrated in Fig. 1.

PREDISPOSING FACTORS

The existence of a physiological predisposition or *diathesis* involving a specific body system is one important precondition for the development of chronic pain syndromes. This predisposition consists of a reduced threshold for nociceptive activation that may be related to genetic variables, previous trauma, or social learning experiences and results in a stereotypical pattern of physiological responses within the specific body system.

ELICITING STIMULI

Pain-related stimuli or other stressors with a negative subjective meaning, such as familial conflicts or job-related pressures, can activate the sympathetic nervous system and induce muscular tension or other nociception-inducing processes. These stressors, which can function as unconditioned or conditioned stimuli, motivate avoidance responses and thus are important triggers of pain and pain behavior.

ELICITING RESPONSES

An *inadequate* or *maladaptive* behavioral, cognitive, or physiological repertoire will exacerbate the impact of these aversive environmental or internal stimuli. An important role is played by the cognitive processing of external or internal stimuli related to the experience of stress and pain. An increased perception of, preoccupation with, and overinterpretation of physical symptoms are examples of such maladaptive cognitive processes related to physical symptoms. Their detrimental effect may further be enhanced by an inadequate perception of internal stimuli such as muscle tension levels, as

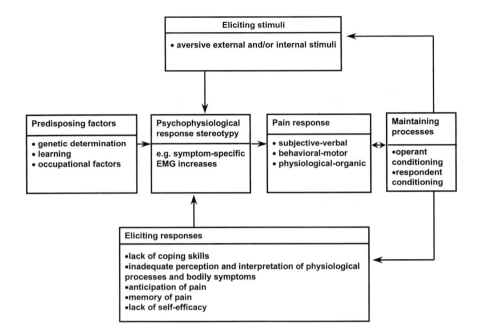

Fig. 1. Psychobiological model of chronic pain.

has been demonstrated in chronic pain patients. Moreover, the nature of the coping response may contribute to the development of chronic pain problems and influence their course. Subsequent maladaptive physiological responses such as increased sympathetic arousal or muscular reactivity as well as overactivation of the nociceptive system may induce, exacerbate, or maintain pain episodes.

MAINTAINING PROCESSES

Learning processes can take the form of respondent conditioning of fear of activity or pain-related overt and covert social, motor, and cognitive responses as well as physiological responses, observational learning of responses to injury and illness, and operant learning of pain behaviors. These learning processes make important contributions to the maintenance of chronicity by interacting with unconditioned physiological processes to form powerful *pain memories* at all levels of the nervous system. Over time, such memories can maintain pain in the absence of peripheral nociceptive input.

The psychobiological model deals primarily with typical musculoskeletal pain syndromes such as headaches, back pain, temporomandibular disorders, pain in the rheumatic disorders, and fibromyalgia syndrome or chronic widespread pain, which are by far the most common chronic pain syndromes (Rasmussen and Olesen 1994; Waddell 1996; Volinn 1997). However, this model can be extended to other types of pain such as phantom pain or neuropathic pain. In the following section we will describe these factors and their interactions. We will focus separately on these factors for reasons of simplicity, although they do not necessarily act in a linear fashion and are not mutually exclusive.

PREDISPOSING FACTORS

GENETIC FACTORS

Genetic predisposition has been implicated in several chronic pain syndromes, although empirical evidence for the role of genetic factors is still scarce. In pain states that are unrelated to acute trauma, genetic predisposition may play a significant role in the location and type of the pain (e.g., migraine; Merikangas 1996; Nyholt et al. 1998).

Congenital insensitivity to pain has been described in humans (see Nagasako et al. 2003 for a review). In one variant of the disease a specific gene defect at loci that express the trkA receptor prevents the development of an intact nociceptive system (Indo et al. 1996). The converse phenomenon, congenital hypersensitivity to pain, has not been observed, although different strains of rats and mice have variable tolerances for noxious stimulation (Mogil et al. 2000). Interindividual differences in pain-inhibiting mechanisms (e.g., endorphinergic mechanisms) may also account for differential pain sensitivity (Droste et al. 1986; Mogil et al. 1996).

PRIOR LEARNING AS A PREDISPOSING FACTOR

Children acquire attitudes about health and health care, gather information about the perception and interpretation of physical symptoms and physiological processes, and learn appropriate responses to injury from their parents and by observing others (Baranowski and Nader 1985). Thus, based on prior experience children may be more or less likely to ignore or overemphasize symptoms, and these learned behaviors will greatly influence how they cope with and adapt to illness later in life (see Nerenz and Leventhal 1983; Leventhal et al. 1998). How others respond to pain episodes is an important source of information. In a recent study, children reported more or less pain in a cold pressor test when their mothers interacted with them in a pain-promoting or pain-reducing manner, respectively (Chambers et al. 2002). Like children, adults also learn by observing the responses of others. Craig

and colleagues have reported a large body of evidence to support the importance of observational learning in modulating pain threshold, pain tolerance,
and pain ratings (see Craig 1986 for a review). In an observational study,
Fagerhaugh (1974) noted that the stoic behavior of some patients in a burn
unit appeared to produce similar behavioral expression by others, whereas
the presence of a more demonstrative patient elicited a greater amount of
overt distress. Controlled laboratory studies also suggest that responses to
pain such as avoidance behavior can be acquired by vicarious experiences
(Turkat and Guise 1983). Vaughan and Lanzetta (1980, 1981) demonstrated
that physiological responses to pain stimuli can also be vicariously conditioned by observation of others in pain. Studying patients with low back
pain, Block (1981) showed that spouses of pain patients respond with elevated physiological activation to viewing their spouses in pain. This physiological activation may later result in symptoms in the spouses (Flor et al.
1987). Evidence indicates that observing pain in other family members may
predispose individuals to similar pain problems (see Apley and Hale 1973;
Christensen and Mortensen 1975; Turkat et al. 1984). This finding implicates a learning process in the development of a diathesis that will serve as a
template through which future stressful and painful circumstances will be
filtered.

Pain experiences, especially early in life, may exert a priming effect on
pain sensitivity. In rat pups as well as human neonates, the early experience
of pain leads to lasting alterations of the nociceptive system in both the
peripheral and central nervous systems (see Fitzgerald and Walker 2003 for
a review). These findings are in accordance with the vast literature on cortical reorganization related to injury and environmental changes (cf. Flor and
Elbert 1998; Kaas 2000). Natural observation of 3–7-year-old children in a
day care center revealed that children who experienced the highest rate of
everyday pain incidents also demonstrated the strongest response to pain
(Fearon et al. 1996). This finding suggests that increased exposure to acute
pain may sensitize children to pain and thereby reduce their threshold for
labeling noxious stimuli as painful. Whether these alterations are associated
with a heightened vulnerability to chronic pain in the long run awaits empirical testing.

The occurrence of pain-related traumatic events may also increase the
likelihood of physiological overreactivity in a certain body part. For example, Harvey and Greer (1982) noted that unpredictable shock to a limb
leads to an anticipatory stiffening of the limb to reduce the impact of the
aversive stimulus. Similar responses could occur in children exposed to
physical or sexual abuse and might later lead to tension-induced musculoskeletal pain. A higher prevalence of physical abuse in childhood has been

reported in certain types of chronic pain (Linton 1997; Goldberg et al. 1999). Several reports have described a specific relationship between sexual abuse and chronic pelvic pain in women (Walling et al. 1994; Heim et al. 1998). Aside from the excessive stimulation of certain body parts, physical and sexual abuse may lead to excessive attentiveness to and overinterpretation of bodily symptoms (Riley et al. 1998).

Ethnomedical observations suggest that early exposure to traumatic injury, for example through rituals such as piercing the ear lobes or the nose, may reduce susceptibility to pain later in life (e.g., Schiefenhövel 1980; Sargent 1984) and may help children learn adequate responses to pain. These assumptions seemingly contradict the results on neonatal pain exposure and physical abuse. The controllability and intensity of the noxious stimulation as well as psychological factors such as attention, learning, and the psychosocial context (including responses of others to the expression of pain and the personal meaning of the experience) are likely to account for the discrepant findings. For example, Buchner et al. (1999) recently demonstrated that reorganizational changes in the primary somatosensory cortex are modulated by attention. Focusing of attention leads to an expansion of the cortical representation of anesthetized fingers in the primary somatosensory cortex, while distraction leads to the opposite effect—a reduced interdigital distance.

OCCUPATIONAL FACTORS

Workplace design (ergonomic factors), body postures, repetitive motion, vibration, lifting, and twisting have all been considered to be predisposing occupational factors for the subsequent development of musculoskeletal pain. For example, excessive use of a specific body part may make the musculature and joints more susceptible to nociceptive responding (Schüldt et al. 1987). Musicians are known to develop instrument-specific pain syndromes (e.g., Moulton and Spence 1992), and keyboard operators often complain about strain-related upper back and shoulder problems (Kiesler and Finholt 1988). Overuse combined with disregard of tension (because stopping work might result in negative consequences) may lead to chronic muscular tension and pain. Constant hyperactivity of muscles exerts pressure on adjacent joints and disks that can cause damage (Andersson et al. 1977).

Strain related to occupational factors may also induce changes in the cortical map in the primary somatosensory cortex. Several studies with monkeys have shown that repetitive movements of the hand may, over time, lead to a degradation of the representation of the hand in the primary somatosensory cortex so that the individual digits are no longer represented separately (for a summary see Byl and Melnick 1997). This learning-induced cortical reorganization leads to problems in motor control and eventually causes pain. Similar data have been reported for musicians with focal hand dystonia (Elbert et al. 1998).

We should not overlook the role of observational learning and expectation in overuse syndromes. A contagion effect has been observed where the presence of a few individuals with overuse syndromes increases the prevalence of symptoms in the workplace even in the absence of objective findings (Hadler 1992). Job dissatisfaction is another factor known to affect the likelihood of reporting overuse symptoms. Several epidemiological studies have reported the highest incidence of pain syndromes in workers who are under physical strain related to the affected body part, but who also report job dissatisfaction and other life stressors (e.g., Buckle 1997).

While there is little doubt about a physiological diathesis to nociceptive stimulation that is related to a range of genetic factors, learning experiences, and exposure to physical demands, the underlying mechanisms have yet to be elucidated. A final common pathway to chronicity may be the development of a *response stereotypy*, a consistent pattern of physiological responses to stimulation that is specific to each individual and is based on the acquired diathesis (Lacey and Lacey 1958). A predisposition may be necessary for the development of chronic pain, but is unlikely to be sufficient.

ELICITING STIMULI

Aversive internal or external stimuli, usually labeled *stressors,* may act as precipitating factors in the development of chronic pain syndromes. Stress is an elusive concept. We use the term *stress* in accordance with Lazarus and Folkman (1984) to denote the ongoing transaction of potentially aversive stimulation with the individual's appraisal and coping efforts. Stress may originally be viewed as resulting from *unconditioned stimuli* that lead to a multitude of physiological, biochemical, and psychological responses but may become associated with conditioned stimuli through learning processes.

ACUTE-ONSET PAIN

Many activities that are neutral or pleasurable may elicit or exacerbate acute pain (e.g., injury-related pain) and thus are experienced as aversive. Over time, an individual with an acute pain condition may associate an increasing set of activities with the anticipation of pain and consequently will avoid them. As fear of pain becomes associated with an expanding number of situations, simple physical activities may be avoided including work, leisure activities, and sex. Pain-related fear and avoidance may result in physical disuse, muscular reactivity, and hypervigilance to internal and external illness information (see Vlaeyen and Linton 2000 for a review). For example, observation of activities that are anticipated to be painful can induce site-specific muscular activation in chronic back pain patients (Vlaeyen et al. 1999). When these patients are confronted with potentially pain-eliciting situations, their pain may be exacerbated and maintained due to anxiety-related sympathetic activation, and their muscle tension may increase. These increases in nociceptive excitability may be site-specific. It has long been known that nociceptors start to express adrenoceptors and become responsive to catecholamines following nerve injury. This mechanism may partially explain the increase in nociceptive excitability of body parts affected by nerve injury (Devor and Jänig 1981). Moreover, repeated nociceptive input such as occurs during injury induces central sensitization, which is characterized by long-term enhanced sensitivity to potentially painful stimuli and is considered an important mechanism of pain memory (Sandkühler 2000).

Over time, additional physiological changes occur due to the increasing inactivity and immobility related to avoidance behavior. These changes may be quite specific, such as immobilization of a finger or a leg. The tendency may develop to react to stressful stimulation with stereotypic hyperactivity of the affected body part. For example, our own research on chronic back pain and temporomandibular disorders (e.g., Flor et al. 1992) suggests that hyperreactivity to stressful stimulation and delayed return to baseline levels of reactivity in the affected muscle group are characteristic for many of these chronic pain patients (see Flor and Turk 1989 for a review).

Taken together, the evidence suggests a direct effect of learning processes on physiology that may result from increased physiological activation, which may be especially marked at the site of an injury. The subsequent avoidance behaviors may be reinforced by significant others, but also by the successful evasion of undesirable activities. The health care system may also play a role in this process by its emphasis on bed rest and sick leave from work, which may be appropriate in early stages of an acute problem but can be detrimental later on.

PAIN UNRELATED TO TRAUMA

Hagberg (1984) suggested that prolonged activity in a tension-producing body position without relief may increase the likelihood that the affected body part will overreact to stressful stimulation. This or some other physiological vulnerability may be the basis for the gradual development of stress-related pain in many cases of temporomandibular pain, certain types of back pain, headaches, and cumulative trauma (repetitive strain injuries). The acute increase in muscle tension and vasoconstriction related to stress episodes may be interpreted as an anticipated fight-or-flight response that once may have served adaptive purposes (Hollis 1982). In other patients withdrawal reactions might be more dominant, leading to depression and inactivity in response to stress and pain (Henry and Stephens 1981).

If muscle strain is of sufficient intensity, frequency, and duration, ischemia and hypoxia may develop in the affected muscle, and algogenic substances such as bradykinin are released (e.g., Graven-Nielsen and Mense 2001). Subsequently, chemosensitive nociceptors are activated and the thresholds of mechanosensitive receptors are reduced (Mense 1993). The ensuing pain experience increases muscular hyperactivity and sympathetic activity, thus leading to a *vicious circle* of pain, muscle tension, sympathetic activation, and more pain (Wiesenfeld-Hallin and Hallin 1984).

In chronic pain patients, pain episodes may represent a constant stressor. Having a chronic pain syndrome may increase the stressfulness of many everyday stimuli. For example, chronic pain patients often report negative consequences of chronic pain on mood, marital and sexual functioning, employment, and financial status (e.g., Turner et al. 1987). Moreover, increased daily hassles, greater marital and work-related conflicts, a perception of decreased social support, and reduced problem-solving abilities have been observed in chronic pain patients compared to healthy controls (e.g., Feuerstein et al.1985; Kearney et al.1987; Flor and Birbaumer 1994b). Patients suffering from chronic back pain respond with increased paravertebral EMG levels to discussions or imagery of pain or stress episodes (Flor et al. 1985; Moulton and Spence 1992).

Numerous additional physiological and psychological factors are involved in acute stress responses. Stressors usually produce decreased sensitivity to painful stimuli, which is known as *stress-induced analgesia* (SIA) or *hypoalgesia* and has been demonstrated both in animals (e.g., Grau et al. 1981) and in humans (Flor and Grüsser 1999; Flor et al. 2002a). Pharmacological blockades and behavioral observations have revealed two types of SIA: one is opioid mediated and depends on the pituitary-adrenal system, and the other is nonhormonal (Watkins and Mayer 1982). The opioid-mediated type depends on more frequent stress exposure and on learning that the stressor is inescapable (Maier et al. 1984; Maier and Keith 1987). It has been suggested that *memory activation* may play a significant role in stress-related hypoalgesia and that the memory of an aversive event may elicit opioid release. Consistent with this view, initial evidence suggests that the release of endogenous opioids is much more closely related to the cognitive processing of aversive stimulation than to pain intensity and duration per se (Grau 1981, 1987).

Uncontrollability of stressors is likely to play a major role in intractable chronic pain states. A lack of self-efficacy and of perceived control is characteristic of chronic pain patients (Dolce 1987; Flor and Turk 1988; Jensen and Karoly 1991, 1992). We hypothesize that prolonged stress leads to excessive activation of the opioid system, which may induce hypoalgesia in the short term, but will over time cause opioid depletion. This situation may contribute to a progressive lack of stress-related analgesia and increase the patient's susceptibility to pain and stress. Reduced levels of endogenous opioids have been observed in the cerebrospinal fluid of chronic pain patients (see Bruehl et al. 1999 for a review).

Conversely, increased levels of self-efficacy should increase the efficacy of the opioid system. Consistent with this assumption, Bandura et al. (1987) demonstrated in healthy subjects that training in pain-coping skills increased self-efficacy, which in turn predicted pain tolerance in the cold pressure test. Most interestingly, naloxone (an opioid antagonist) blocked the effects of cognitive coping attempts. This result implies that cognitions may have a direct effect on pain tolerance and that this influence is at least partially mediated by the endogenous opioid system. It also suggests that effective coping with pain and stress may preserve the functioning of the endogenous opioid system.

Immunological processes also exert important influences on nociceptive processing. Growing evidence indicates that the nociceptive system and the immunological system interact and that these influences are especially strong in inflammatory states such as rheumatoid arthritis (see Stein 1996). For example, nerve growth factor, which has been implicated in the sensitization of nociceptors, is synthesized, stored, and released from immune system cells such as T lymphocytes (Ehrhard et al. 1993). On the other hand, nociceptors can influence immune responses. For example, substance P, which is released from nociceptors, can enhance inflammatory processes. Immune system cells are also capable of synthesizing peripheral opioids that can reduce the sensitivity of nociceptors (Stein et al. 1995). Given that immunological processes are highly susceptible to psychological influences (e.g., Kiecolt-Glaser 1999), this neuroimmunological interaction offers an additional route for the influence of psychological factors on pain processing. An illustration of these interactions is the psychological treatment of rheumatoid arthritis, an autoimmune disease that may result from impaired functioning of the suppressor T-cell system. For example, O'Leary et al.

(1988) provided stress management treatment to patients with rheumatoid arthritis and found a significant correlation between self-efficacy beliefs regarding the ability to control pain and disability and treatment effectiveness. Even more importantly, patients with the greatest gains in self-efficacy displayed more suppressor T cells.

Chronic pain may lead to alterations on spinal and supraspinal levels that can increase an individual's susceptibility for all somatosensory input. The chronicity-related expansion of the back representation in the cortex of chronic back pain patients (Flor et al. 1997a)—termed *cortical reorganization*—should have perceptual consequences. It has long been known that the size of the representation of a body part in the primary somatosensory cortex is directly proportional to the sensitivity of this body region. For example, the mouth and the fingertips have much larger representation than the upper arm or thigh, reflecting the fact that they are much more sensitive. It is assumed that this representational size is acquired by behaviorally significant inputs from these regions over extended periods of time (Kaas 1995). Pain is a highly significant event and can be expected to lead to reorganizational changes, even in adults. The expanded representation of the affected body part will lead to heightened sensitivity of the pain-affected region and of adjacent regions that are involved in the reorganizational process and which may additionally be affected by stress-induced hyperreactivity.

Longitudinal studies following patients from an acute to a chronic pain state or assessing high-risk populations (e.g., children of chronic pain patients) would be helpful to determine to what extent stress responses are a cause or a consequence of chronic pain. Dworkin et al. (1992) followed patients with herpes zoster for 1 year to identify the factors that predict who will develop postherpetic neuralgia. Consistent with the psychobiological model, the study revealed an important role of both initial pain severity and level of emotional distress at disease onset in the development of chronic postherpetic neuralgia.

ELICITING RESPONSES

PERCEPTION OF PHYSIOLOGICAL PROCESSES AND BODILY SYMPTOMS

The reaction to stressful stimulation is determined by the degree to which the stressor is perceived to be threatening; by the available resources by which to respond; and by the cognitive or behavioral efforts expended to meet environmental and internal demands, or conversely, the degree of helplessness the stressor induces (Lazarus and Folkman 1984). The perception and interpretation of physical symptoms and physiological processes is important in all psychophysiological disorders (Pennebaker 1982).

The perception of bodily symptoms and stimuli leads to specific interpretations, both conscious and subconscious, and serves as an impetus for action (Nerenz and Leventhal 1983; Leventhal et al. 1998; Pennebaker 2000). Chronic illness poses a special problem because patients often adhere to the acute disease model with which they are most familiar. They therefore continue to seek a tangible physical cause of the symptom even if they have received evidence that the original injury has resolved. Moreover, they may interpret pain symptoms as indicative of an underlying disease process that, if the pain persists, could signify progressive disease. In acute back pain, bed rest is often prescribed to relieve pressure on the spine. People who believe that any movement of the back may worsen their condition may maintain this belief in the chronic pain stage, when prolonged inactivity is not only unnecessary but detrimental. Once cognitive structures form involving memories of a disease and beliefs about its meaning, they become stable and are difficult to modify (Pennebaker et al. 1985). Patients tend to avoid experiences that could invalidate their beliefs. They behave in accordance with these beliefs even in situations where the beliefs are no longer valid. Consequently, they do not receive corrective feedback, and this situation further perpetuates inactivity and fosters the maladaptive beliefs. In the case of musculoskeletal pain syndromes such as chronic low back pain, avoidance of activity may exacerbate the problem due to disuse and ensuing atrophy of the muscles.

An important factor contributing to the maintenance of chronic pain is the *misinterpretation* of physical sensations as painful symptoms. For example, Anderson and Pennebaker (1980) reported that healthy subjects rated an ambiguous but affectively neutral vibrating sensation as painful or pleasant depending on information they received about whether it would be painful or pleasant. In fact, they insisted later after debriefing that the sensation they had felt was exactly what they had reported. A recent study showed that the perceived intensity and aversiveness of nonpainful and painful stimuli can be modified by systematically pairing them with an unpleasant or pleasant slide, respectively. This change in stimulus perception occurred even though the subjects were unaware of the contingency between the stimuli and the slides (Wunsch et al. 2003). Thus, it is quite possible that patients will interpret symptoms that normally are not considered painful as painful if they have learned to do so and if their expressions of pain are subsequently reinforced, at least within certain limits of nociceptive input intensity.

Increasing evidence demonstrates that irritable bowel syndrome (IBS) may be associated with altered visceral perception. IBS patients report pain at very low levels of bowel distension compared to healthy controls (e.g., Ritchie 1973). Most interestingly, these thresholds are also lower when sham distension is used, and are normalized when the influence of psychological factors is minimized (Whitehead and Palsson 1998). Consistent with the hypothesis that selective attention to gastrointestinal sensations and disease attribution account for the enhanced pain sensitivity, a recent study demonstrated that IBS patients show an altered brain response to actual or simply anticipated rectal distension, especially in regions such as the anterior cingulate cortex that are important for attention to and perception of sensory and emotional information (Naliboff et al. 2001).

Physiological responses with a lower threshold for conscious perception might be more likely to be reinforced than those that are difficult to perceive (Whitehead et al. 1979). Proprioception, which includes the perception of muscle tension, is a better developed skill than visceral perception (Hefferline 1958) and may thus be especially susceptible to learning processes. We must recall that the detection of ongoing physiological responses and the perception of physical symptoms are two processes that are not highly correlated (Pennebaker 1982; Pennebaker and Epstein 1983).

Ambiguous symptoms are reported by the majority of patients seeking medical attention. For example, no physical basis for the symptoms is found in 10–30% of all patients reporting with what has come to be called "noncardiac" chest pain (Serlie et al. 1996). In approximately 50% of these cases, the pain will persist despite the absence of identifiable physical pathology. The case for noncardiac chest pain is not an isolated instance. The two most common symptoms that bring patients to doctors, other than upper respiratory infections, are back pain and headaches. In most cases, no physical cause for headaches can be identified, and in up to 85% of cases of back pain little objective pathology can be detected (Deyo 1988).

Patients with unexplained chest, back, and head pain feel anxious, misunderstood, and abandoned by their doctors. The failure of physicians to identify the cause of their pain implicitly leads patients to feel that their complaints are no longer taken seriously, and these feelings of rejection may be accurate. In the absence of physical findings to substantiate patients' complaints of pain, some health care professionals do believe that pain is caused primarily by psychological factors—that it is *psychogenic*. Alternatively, they may believe that complaints in the absence of pathology are motivated by the desire for attention, time off from work, avoidance of undesirable activities, or financial gain in the form of disability compensation.

It is possible that chronic pain patients become preoccupied with and overemphasize physical symptoms related to increases in muscle tension and other physiological processes and interpret them as painful stimulation. They also may be less able than healthy controls to differentiate tension levels. We have examined the perception of physical symptoms and of muscle tension in chronic back pain patients and patients suffering from temporomandibular pain (Flor et al. 1999). Chronic pain patients were less able to correctly perceive muscle tension levels, not only at the affected muscle but also at a muscle unrelated to the pain problem (see Fig. 2). On the other hand, they greatly *over*estimated physical symptoms related to tension-producing tasks, rated the tasks as more aversive, and experienced more pain upon tensing their muscles.

Numerous studies have demonstrated that objective physical impairments are only modestly related to disability (e.g., Flor and Birbaumer 1993; Hidding et al. 1994; Turk et al. 1996). Chronic pain patients have a tendency to overemphasize physical symptoms. This tendency is especially likely in the case of patients with few organic findings who are "in need" of demonstrable signs to justify their pain complaints. It is possible that preoccupation with painful stimuli and a high probability of familial reinforcement for reporting pain (Turk and Flor 1987b) increase the probability with which

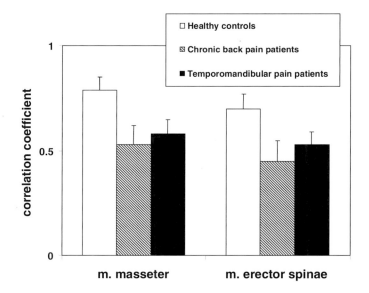

Fig. 2. Ability to discriminate muscle tension levels in patients with chronic back pain, patients with temporomandibular pain, and matched healthy controls. Data are based on correlation coefficients between the muscle tension levels the participants were requested to produce and those that were actually obtained (Flor et al. 1999).

patients label symptoms as painful. However, it is not clear whether this labeling of muscle tension as painful is related to altered physiological processes or if patients are more likely to perceive any sensation as painful, thus indicating a generalized hypervigilance and lowering of pain perception threshold (Tunks et al. 1988). This issue warrants more careful experimental investigation.

ANTICIPATION AND PREDICTABILITY OF PAIN

In acute pain states induced in the laboratory, forewarning of the impending painful stimulation may reduce its aversive impact, especially if there is some form of control over the stimulation (Averill 1973). However, ample evidence also shows that the explicit expectation of uncontrollable painful stimulation may make the following nociceptive input more noxious (Leventhal and Everhart 1979). Thus, patients who have associated activity with pain may expect heightened levels of pain when they attempt to become involved in activity and then perceive higher levels of pain, which in turn may lead them to avoid activity altogether. For example, chronic back pain patients performed more poorly on a treadmill task and in the cold pressor test (Schmidt 1985; Schmidt and Brand 1986). Interestingly, their performance was best predicted by prior beliefs in their ability to perform well in the task and by previous pain levels rather than by the amount of pain or physical exertion experienced during the task itself.

The presence of pain may change the way individuals process pain-related and other information. Pain is disruptive and difficult to disengage from, especially when somatic information is perceived as threatening (Crombez et al. 1997, 1998). Hence, having chronic pain may focus one's attention on all types of bodily signals. Chronic pain patients are known to report a multitude of bodily symptoms in addition to pain (e.g., Turk and Flor 1987a). Conversely, the expectation of pain reduction can reduce pain perception and avoidance of activity (e.g., Price et al. 1999). Medication, avoidance of activity, and bed rest thus may obtain additional reinforcing properties by the associated positive effects of the anticipation of pain reduction.

MEMORY OF PAIN

The expectation of painful stimulation may also be enhanced by the fact that patients tend to be more likely to remember pain when they are in a pain state than when they are not (e.g., Eich et al. 1985). Thus, they may selectively focus on stimuli that predict pain and become overavoidant.

Moreover, images and thoughts of impending pain or exacerbation of pain instigate sympathetic activation and muscular activity and may themselves become stimuli for the activation of nociceptive input. For example, Rimm and Litvak (1969) demonstrated that subjects exhibit physiological arousal when they merely *think* about or imagine painful experiences. Moreover, pain-associated words elicit an enhanced early negative evoked potential (N150) in chronic and subacute pain patients (Flor et al. 1997b; Knost et al. 1997). Several studies have also shown that chronic pain patients selectively focus on negative and painful life events when they are asked to report experiences from their lives in autobiographical memory tasks (Eich et al. 1990; Wright and Morley 1995).

SOMATOSENSORY PAIN MEMORIES

Somatosensory pain memories that manifest themselves in an altered representation of pain-affected body parts may play an important pain-enhancing and pain-maintaining role (see Melzack 1993). Somatosensory pain memories may also affect the processing of painful and nonpainful somatosensory stimulation in chronic pain patients. For example, not only do chronic back pain patients show an enhanced cortical response to painful stimulation of the back, but the cortical representation of the back is also shifted toward the leg area (Flor et al. 1997a). Moreover, the longer the duration of the pain, the more pronounced is the cortical hyperreactivity. The role of somatosensory pain memories has been studied most extensively in phantom limb pain. Such pain differs from stump pain and is paradoxically localized in the limb that has been amputated. Approximately 60–80% of amputees are affected by phantom limb pain (Sherman 1997). Both peripheral and central factors have been discussed as important in its development, but the cause of phantom sensations and phantom limb pain remains elusive. Consistent evidence has demonstrated that phantom limb pain patients show reorganization of the primary somatosensory cortex (Elbert et al. 1994; Yang et al. 1994), and this reorganization is similar to the cortical changes previously observed in amputated animals (e.g., Merzenich et al. 1984). In a number of studies we found that phantom limb *pain* rather than phantom sensations or referred sensations was related to an altered somatosensory and motor cortical representation of the mouth and hand zone in upper-extremity amputees (e.g., Flor et al. 1995, 1998; Lotze et al. 1999; Grüsser et al. 2001; Karl et al. 2001; Flor 2002). Nonpainful phantoms seem to be more closely related to activation of the posterior parietal and the secondary somatosensory cortex, similar to the phenomena of neglect or supernumerary limbs (Hari et al. 1998), than to reorganization in the primary somatosensory cortex (Flor 2000).

An interesting feature of phantom limb pain is that it is often similar to pain experienced prior to the amputation, suggesting a role of somatosensory pain memories (Katz and Melzack 1990; Melzack 1992; see also Flor et al. 2000). Consistent with this view, we found that both longstanding preamputation pain and pain just prior to the amputation are highly correlated with both phantom limb pain and cortical reorganization (Huse et al., in press). When a shift of adjacent cortical areas into the amputation zone occurs, the nociceptive neurons of the amputation zone now respond to input from neighboring regions, but the sensation is perceived as coming from the amputated body part, and phantom limb pain ensues. Peripheral mechanisms may play a significant role in maintaining this reorganizational shift (see Devor 1997).

COPING WITH PAIN

The evolution of chronic pain as described in the previous sections will be facilitated in those with few resources to cope with stress and especially pain. A more active type of coping may be differentiated from rather passive, contemplative modes (see Lazarus and Folkman 1984; Brown and Nicassio 1987). Abundant evidence shows that passive coping is associated with greater pain-related distress and disability, while active coping is related to greater activity and lower levels of psychosocial distress (e.g., Turner et al. 1987; Martin et al. 1996; Snow-Turek et al. 1996). Moreover, decreases in catastrophizing and increases in perceived control over pain are associated with a decrease in subjective disability, pain intensity, and depression in chronic pain patients participating in a pain management training (Flor and Birbaumer 1993; Jensen et al. 2001; Burns et al. 2003). It is possible that chronic pain patients respond habitually to stress with overactivity and frequent increases in muscle tension as well as sympathetic activation. The alternative response pattern, that of giving up and withdrawing to conserve energy, leads to increasing inactivity and immobilization with increasing tonic muscle tension and can thus also involve the muscular system. As described earlier, peripheral hyperreactivity may result in changes in nociceptive input, thus contributing to the development of chronic pain.

**MAINTAINING VARIABLES: THE ROLE
OF LEARNING PROCESSES**

Thus far, we have emphasized the role of learning in the development of chronic pain. This section discusses how learning processes are relevant to the maintenance of chronic pain.

OPERANT LEARNING

One of the earliest psychological models of chronic pain is Fordyce's (1976) influential operant conditioning approach to pain. This model postulates that verbal expression of pain and nonverbal pain behaviors (e.g., grimacing, guarding) may be maintained by contingencies of reinforcement. Pain behaviors may be positively reinforced if they are followed by positive consequences such as attention from others. Pain behaviors may also be maintained by negative reinforcement, that is, the nonoccurrence of aversive stimuli. An insufficient reinforcement of healthy behaviors including physical activity may also contribute to the maintenance of pain. Pain behaviors may persist even though the original source of the pain may no longer be existent or may have been substantially reduced. The pain behaviors will, over time, be maintained by specific environmental or internal contingencies.

Linton et al. (1985) have further characterized some aspects of the process of chronicity related to operant learning. They describe the acquisition of pain behaviors as a process that is originally determined by *avoidance behavior*. In the acute phase, pain presumably becomes a discriminative stimulus for actions that are pain-reducing, for example bed rest, changes in posture, or the consumption of analgesics. Over time, avoidance behavior develops. Certain pain-eliciting situations will cause anticipatory fear and will be avoided from the very beginning (Vlaeyen et al. 1999). The pain sufferer learns to completely avoid anticipated pain-eliciting situations such as movements, with the result that noxious stimuli no longer occur in this situation. Avoidance learning is especially resistant to extinction because the nonoccurrence of the negative stimulus—pain—is not experienced.

Discriminative stimuli for avoidance behavior are often conditioned stimuli, and avoidance behavior may be additionally reinforced by the reduction of fear. Over time specific avoidance behaviors may generalize to many potentially pain-eliciting stimuli, and the behavioral repertoire of the pain sufferer may be reduced even further. Linton et al. (1985) discuss the reinforcement of passive behavior and an inactive lifestyle as important factors of the increasing interference of pain with the patient's life. They point out that a large portion of the daily behavior of pain sufferers may be avoidance behavior guided by specific discriminative stimuli and that positive consequences for passive and inactive behavior may play an increasingly important role. For example, inactivity and a sick status may lead to greater time for leisure, interaction with one's spouse, and so forth.

Increases in muscle tension may also be subject to operant conditioning. In persons with chronic pain, as well as those at high risk for chronic pain, but not in healthy controls, increased levels of muscle tension both relieved pain and reduced the amplitude of pain-evoked brain potentials (Knost et al.

1999b). Increases in muscle tension can obviously be negatively reinforced by pain reduction. In a related study, both healthy controls and pain patients learned to increase or decrease pain ratings depending on whether a higher or lower level of reported pain was positively reinforced (Flor et al. 2002c). The chronic pain patients maintained the learned pain response even when it was no longer reinforced, whereas the response extinguished completely in the healthy controls. This effect was most pronounced in the early negative component of the pain-evoked brain potential (N150), a physiological correlate of pain.

Several studies (e.g., Rosenfeld et al. 1984; Miltner et al. 1988; Dowman 1996) used operant conditioning to modify the somatosensory evoked potential of the EEG. Subjects were either taught to increase or to decrease the N150 and P260 components of the pain-evoked potential. Subjects are capable of successfully modifying their brain wave potentials and as a consequence, they experience more or less pain depending on the level of the brain response. These data illustrate the important role of learning on physiological changes that have been associated with pain, and indicate that operant conditioning of pain behaviors may also generalize to the physiological level and may be maintained long after the immediate learning process has taken place.

We assume that operant conditioning processes may lead to the establishment of both explicit (conscious) and implicit (subconscious and automatic) memories for pain that lead to the formation of cortical and subcortical cell assemblies with a large pain-related associative network. Even minor pain-associated discriminative and conditioned stimuli may later—once the network is established—lead to the activation of the entire network. Thus, such memories increase the likelihood that a chronic pain sufferer will maintain a host of learned pain repsonses on the subjective-verbal, the physiological, and the motor-behavioral level and on all levels of the nervous system. Many of these learned pain memories are implicit, so that the pain sufferer may not be aware that his or her responses are triggered by conditioned or discriminative stimuli.

Preliminary data confirm that implicit pain memories, presumably acquired through operant conditioning, may be important. These data also reveal that the presence of a significant other can alter the brain's response to painful stimulation. In a sample of chronic back pain patients with solicitous spouses, the global field power of the EEG (a general measure of the overall response of the brain to an external event) elicited by a painful stimulus to the back was substantially increased when the spouse was present during the EEG recording (Knost et al. 1999a; Flor et al. 2002b). A painful stimulus applied to the finger had no such effect.

RESPONDENT LEARNING

As described earlier, respondent conditioning of pain and stress responses such as fear of activity contributes to the development of chronic pain. Its role has so far not been sufficiently addressed in the chronic pain literature, although respondent conditioning is a learning process that often occurs before instrumental conditioning takes place. Although for chronic pain of acute onset the role of respondent learning has been discussed (e.g., Lethem et al. 1983; Vlaeyen and Linton 2000), very little is known about this phenomenon in gradually developing chronic pain states.

Chronicity can be related to respondent conditioning processes. For example, it may be very useful during acute pain states to reduce any type of movement in order to facilitate the healing process. As noted above, over time an anticipatory anxiety of movement may develop that leads to a conditioned avoidance response. Pain-related fears are better predictors for disability than pain itself (Crombez et al. 1999; Vlaeyen et al. 2002). The anticipation of pain related to movement may lead, as previously mentioned, to immobility and inactivity and to an increased deconditioning of the muscles as well as to increasing difficulties with posture and gait. These findings have important implications for treatment because patients with high levels of anticipatory fear may require a specifically tailored treatment protocol. In a preliminary study, Vlaeyen et al. (2002) demonstrated that in patients with substantial pain-related fears, exposure to a set of individually determined physical movements rather than a simple regimen of graded activity may be more effective in reducing pain-related fears and catastrophizing as well as in improving activity levels. It is very important for the therapist to realize that many of the observable pain behaviors a patient displays, such as altered gait or maladaptive postures, are not necessarily instigated by an underlying degenerative process but may be entirely or to a large degree motivated by anticipatory anxiety and fear and by subsequent corrective (i.e., escape or avoidance) behaviors as well as by operant reinforcement. The anticipation of pain and the expectancy that further pain may be prevented may lead to long-lasting maladaptive avoidance behaviors.

In cases where no dramatic onset of chronic pain can be determined, muscle tension and sympathetic activation may be viewed as unconditioned stimuli that lead over time to intense pain, if they occur frequently and with high intensity (see Christensen 1986a,b). These unconditioned stimuli can be associated with a number of neutral (conditioned) stimuli leading to the induction of tension and pain in a large number of situations. An important factor in this process may be small alterations in bodily symptoms or certain postures. Such changes in muscle tension level or in posture may over time serve as conditioned stimuli and lead to conditioned muscle tension increase and conditioned sympathetic activation.

The consumption of analgesic medication may also be guided by the anticipation of pain and may be viewed as avoidance behavior. For example, the frequent experience that initial minor pain states may quickly escalate into very severe pain episodes may teach the pain sufferer that even minor fluctuations in pain level should be viewed as warning signals of imminent unbearable pain. Slight increases in pain thus may motivate the pain sufferer to take analgesic medication to prevent the onset of pain that is difficult to control. Pain-contingent consumption of analgesic medication may thus negatively reinforce pain and thereby maintain it. Over time, analgesic medication may be taken earlier in the development of a pain episode and also more frequently. As a consequence, analgesic medication may lose its efficacy, and in some pain conditions such as headaches, it may lead to additional medication-induced pain that can be eliminated by tapering off the medication (e.g., Diener et al. 1989).

As noted earlier, plasma endorphin levels increase dramatically during high stress and pain conditions and can induce hypoalgesia. This stress-induced analgesia (SIA) is also subject to respondent conditioning. Maier and colleagues (e.g., Maier et al. 1984) have conduced extensive studies on the conditionability of stress hypoalgesia (or analgesia) in animals. We examined the conditionability of SIA in humans as well as the mechanisms of this conditioning process (e.g., Flor and Grüsser 1999). In one study (Flor et al. 2002a), subjects first underwent differential conditioning using two neutral stimuli as conditioned stimuli, one of which (CS+) was followed by a stressful cognitive task (mental arithmetic and noise) as the unconditioned stimulus, while the other conditioned stimulus (CS–) was presented by itself. After conditioning, the subjects were exposed to the CS+ and CS– stimuli after receiving an infusion of placebo or naloxone. Naloxone, but not placebo, reversed the conditioned SIA associated with CS+ presentation, as assessed by increased pain tolerance and pain threshold to electric stimulation. These data suggest that learning processes influence not only pain-inducing but also pain-inhibiting mechanisms and also act on biochemical processes.

Circumstances that are appraised as potentially threatening to safety or comfort are also subject to respondent conditioning and are likely to generate strong physiological reactions. Earlier we described the importance of nondeclarative and declarative pain memories. Respondent conditioning is one important mechanism that can explain how stimuli can acquire the status of cues for pain that elicit pain-related peripheral and central responses.

For example, the enhanced cortical response to pain-related words observed in chronic and subacute pain patients (Flor et al. 1997b; Knost et al. 1997) may reflect previous conditioning experiences. Montoya et al. (1996) confirmed this assumption by demonstrating that neutral words (conditioned stimuli) can acquire characteristics of a pain stimulus (unconditioned stimuli) with which they were paired. In particular, similar to the Flor et al. (1997b) study, they observed an enhanced early negative evoked potential (N150) to the word stimuli that had previously been paired with painful electric shock.

SUMMARY AND CONCLUSIONS

The psychobiological perspective of pain constitutes a comprehensive diathesis-stress model that focuses on the interplay between a genetic or acquired predisposition and eliciting stimuli and responses. It not only takes into account the subjective-verbal, motor-behavioral, and physiological dimensions of pain as well as their interaction, but also specifically delineates how learning processes such as respondent and operant conditioning contribute on all levels to the development and maintenance of pain. A specific emphasis is given to semantic and neuronal pain memories and their importance for pain chronicity. Substantial evidence for the role of learning processes has accrued for chronic pain with acute onset. More systematic research is needed to gain a better understanding for its role in chronic pain with a gradual onset. The psychobiological model provides a theoretical framework for a multidimensional approach to the assessment and treatment of chronic pain.

ACKNOWLEDGMENTS

This work was supported by grants from the Deutsche Forschungsgemeinschaft to H. Flor and C. Hermann and by the Max Planck Research Award for International Cooperation to H. Flor.

REFERENCES

Anderson DB, Pennebaker JW. Pain and pleasure: alternative interpretations for identical stimulation. *Eur J Soc Psychol* 1980; 10:207–212.
Andersson G, Örtengren R, Nachemson A. Intradiscal pressure, intraabdominal pressure and myoelectric back muscle activity related to posture and loading. *Clin Orthop* 1977; 129:156–164.

Apley J, Hale B. Children with recurrent abdominal pain: how do they grow up? *BMJ* 1973; 3:7–9.

Averill JR. Personal control over aversive stimuli and its relationship to stress. *Psychol Bull* 1973; 80:286–303.

Bandura A, O'Leary A, Taylor BC, Gauthier J, Gossard D. Perceived self-efficacy and pain control: opioid and nonopioid mechanisms. *J Pers Soc Psychol* 1987; 53:563–571.

Baranowski T, Nader PR. Family health behavior. In: Turk DC, Kerns RD (Eds). *Health, Illness, and Families: A Lifespan Perspective*. New York: Wiley-Interscience, 1985, pp 51–80.

Block AR. Investigation of the response of the spouse to chronic pain behavior. *Psychosom Med* 1981; 43:415–422.

Brown GK, Nicassio PM. Development of a questionnaire for the assessment of active and passive coping strategies in chronic pain patients. *Pain* 1987; 31:53–64.

Bruehl S, McCubbin JA, Harden RN. Theoretical review: altered pain regulatory systems in chronic pain. *Neurosci Biobehav Rev* 1999; 23:877–890.

Buchner H, Reinartz U, Waberski TD, et al. Sustained attention modulates the immediate effect of de-afferentation on the cortical representation of the digits: source localization of somatosensory evoked potentials in humans. *Neurosci Lett* 1999; 260:57–60.

Buckle P. Upper limb disorders and work: the importance of physical and psychosocial factors. *J Psychosom Res* 1997; 43:17–25.

Burns JW, Kubilus A, Bruehl S, Harden RN, Lofland K. Do changes in cognitive factors influence outcome following multidisciplinary treatment for chronic pain? A cross-lagged panel analysis. *J Consult Clin Psychol* 2003; 71:81–91.

Byl NN, Melnick M. The neural consequences of repetition: clinical implications of a learning hypothesis. *J Hand Ther* 1997; 10:160–174.

Chambers CT, Craig KD, Bennett SM. The impact of maternal behavior on children's pain experiences: an experimental analysis. *J Pediatr Psychol* 2002; 27:293–301.

Christensen LV. Physiology and pathophysiology of skeletal muscle contraction. Part I. Dynamic activity. *J Oral Rehabil* 1986a; 13:451–461.

Christensen LV. Physiology and pathophysiology of skeletal muscle contraction. Part II. Static activity. *J Oral Rehabil* 1986b; 13:463–477.

Christensen MF, Mortensen O. Long-term prognosis in children with recurrent abdominal pain. *Arch Dis Child* 1975; 50:110–114.

Craig KD. Social modeling influences: pain in context. In: Sternbach RA (Ed). *The Psychology of Pain*. New York: Raven Press, 1986, pp 67–95.

Crombez G, Eccleston C, Baeyens F, Eelen P. Habituation and the interference of pain with task performance. *Pain* 1997; 70:149–154.

Crombez G, Eccleston C, Baeyens F, Eelen P. When somatic information threatens, catastrophic thinking enhances attentional interference. *Pain* 1998; 75:187–198.

Crombez G, Vlaeyen JW, Heuts PH, Lysens R. Pain-related fear is more disabling than pain itself: evidence on the role of pain-related fear in chronic back pain disability. *Pain* 1999; 80:329–339.

Devor M. Phantom pain as an expression of referred and neuropathic pain. In: Sherman RA (Ed). *Phantom Pain*. New York: Plenum Press, 1997, pp 33–57.

Devor M, Jänig W. Activation of myelinated afferents ending in a neuroma by stimulation of the sympathetic supply in the rat. *Neurosci Lett* 1981; 24:43–47.

Deyo R. Measuring the functional status of patients with low back pain. *Arch Phys Med Rehabil* 1988; 69:1044–1053.

Diener HC, Dichgans J, Scholz E, et al. Analgesic-induced chronic headache: long-term results of withdrawal therapy. *J Neurol* 1989; 236:9–14.

Dolce JJ. Self-efficacy and disability beliefs in behavioral treatment of pain. *Behav Res Ther* 1987; 25:289–299.

Dowman R. Effects of operantly conditioning the amplitude of the P200 peak of the SEP on pain sensitivity and the spinal nociceptive withdrawal reflex in humans. *Psychophysiology* 1996; 33:252–261.

Droste C, Greenlee MW, Roskamm H. A defective angina pectoris pain warning system: experimental findings of ischemic and electrical pain test. *Pain* 1986; 26:199–209.

Dworkin RH, Hartstein G, Rosner HL, et al. A high-risk method for studying psychosocial antecedents of chronic pain: the prospective investigation of herpes zoster. *J Abnorm Psychol* 1992; 101:200–205.

Ehrhard PB, Erb P, Graumann U, Otten U. Expression of nerve growth factor and nerve growth factor receptor tyrosine kinase Trk in activated CD4-positive T-cell clones. *Proc Natl Acad Sci USA* 1993; 90:10984–10988.

Eich E, Reeves JL, Jaeger B, Graff-Radford SB. Memory for pain: relation between past and present pain intensity. *Pain* 1985; 23:375–380.

Eich E, Rachman S, Lopatka C. Affect, pain, and autobiographical memory. *J Abnorm Psychol* 1990; 99:174–178.

Elbert TR, Flor H, Birbaumer N, et al. Extensive reorganization of the somatosensory cortex in adult humans after nervous system injury. *Neuroreport* 1994; 5:2593–2597.

Elbert T, Candia V, Altenmuller E, et al. Alteration of digital representations in somatosensory cortex in focal hand dystonia. *Neuroreport* 1998; 9:3571–3575.

Fagerhaugh SY. Pain expression and control on a burn care unit. *Nurs Outlook* 1974; 22:645–650.

Fearon I, McGrath PJ, Achat H. 'Booboos': the study of everyday pain among young children. *Pain* 1996; 68:55–62.

Feuerstein M, Sult S, Houle M. Environmental stressors and chronic low back pain: live events, family and work environment. *Pain* 1985; 22:295–307.

Feuerstein M, Papciak AS, Hoon PE. Biobehavioral mechanisms of chronic low back pain. *Clin Psychol Rev* 1987; 7:243–273.

Fitzgerald M, Walker S. The role of activity in developing pain pathways. In: Dostrovsky JO, Carr DB, Koltzenburg M (Eds). *Proceedings of the 10th World Congress on Pain,* Progress in Pain Research and Management, Vol. 24. Seattle: IASP Press, 2003, pp 1–46.

Flor H. The functional organization of the brain in chronic pain. *Prog Brain Res* 2000; 129:313–322.

Flor H. Phantom limb pain: characteristics, causes and treatment. *Lancet Neurol* 2002;1:82–89.

Flor H, Birbaumer N. Comparison of the efficacy of electromyographic biofeedback, cognitive-behavioral therapy, and conservative medical interventions in the treatment of chronic musculoskeletal pain. *J Consult Clin Psychol* 1993; 61:653–658.

Flor H, Birbaumer N. Acquisition of chronic pain: Psychophysiological mechanisms. *Am Pain Soc J* 1994a; 32:119–127.

Flor H, Birbaumer N. Basic issues in the psychobiology of pain. In: Gebhart GF, Hammond DL, Jensen TS (Eds). *Proceedings of the 7th World Congress on Pain,* Progress in Pain Research and Management, Vol. 2. Seattle: IASP Press, 1994b, pp 113–125.

Flor H, Elbert T. Maladaptive consequences of cortical reorganisation in humans. *Neurosci News* 1998; 1:4–11.

Flor H, Grüsser SM. Conditioned stress-induced analgesia in humans. *Eur J Pain* 1999; 3:317–324.

Flor H, Turk DC. Chronic back pain and rheumatoid arthritis: predicting pain and disability from cognitive variables. *J Behav Med* 1988; 11:251–265.

Flor H, Turk DC. Psychophysiology of chronic pain: do chronic pain patients exhibit symptom-specific psychophysiological responses? *Psychol Bull* 1989; 105:215–259.

Flor H, Turk DC, Birbaumer N. Assessment of stress-related psychophysiological reactions in chronic back pain patients. *J Consult Clin Psychol* 1985; 53:354–364.

Flor H, Turk DC, Scholz OB. Impact of chronic pain on the spouse: marital, emotional and physical consequences. *J Psychosom Res* 1987; 31:63–71.

Flor H, Birbaumer N, Turk DC. The psychobiology of chronic pain. *Adv Behav Res Ther* 1990; 12:47–84.

Flor H, Birbaumer N, Schugens MM, Lutzenberger W. Symptom-specific psychophysiological responses in chronic pain patients. *Psychophysiology* 1992; 29:452–460.

Flor H, Elbert T, Knecht S, et al. Phantom-limb pain as a perceptual correlate of cortical reorganization following arm amputation. *Nature* 1995; 375:482–484.

Flor H, Braun C, Elbert T, Birbaumer N. Extensive reorganization of primary somatosensory cortex in chronic back pain patients. *Neurosci Lett* 1997a; 224:5–8.

Flor H, Knost B, Birbaumer N. Processing of pain- and body-related verbal material in chronic pain patients: central and peripheral correlates. *Pain* 1997b; 73:413–421.

Flor H, Elbert T, Mühlnickel W, et al. Cortical reorganization and phantom phenomena in congenital and traumatic upper-extremity amputees. *Exp Brain Res* 1998; 119:205–212.

Flor H, Fürst M, Birbaumer N. Deficient discrimination of EMG levels and overestimation of perceived tension in chronic pain patients. *Appl Psychophysiol Biofeedback* 1999; 24:55–66.

Flor H, Birbaumer N, Sherman RA. Phantom limb pain. *Pain Clinical Updates* 2000; 8(3):1–4.

Flor H, Birbaumer N, Schulz R, Grüsser SM, Mucha RF. Pavlovian conditioning of opioid and nonopioid pain inhibitory mechanisms in humans. *Eur J Pain* 2002a; 6:395–402.

Flor H, Lutzenberger W, Knost B, Diesch E, Birbaumer N. Spouse presence alters brain response to pain. *Online Abstract Viewer/Itinerary Planner*. Washington, DC: Society for Neuroscience, 2002b.

Flor H, Knost B, Birbaumer N. The role of operant conditioning in chronic pain: an experimental investigation. *Pain* 2002c; 95:111–118.

Fordyce WE. *Behavioral Methods for Chronic Pain and Illness*. St. Louis: Mosby, 1976.

Goldberg RT, Pachas WN, Keith D. Relationship between traumatic events in childhood and chronic pain. *Disabil Rehabil* 1999; 21:23–30.

Grau JW. Activation of the opioid and nonopioid analgesic systems: evidence for a memory hypothesis and against the coulometric hypothesis. *J Exp Psychol Anim Behav Process* 1987; 13:215–225.

Grau JW, Hyson RL, Maier SF, Madden J, Barchas JD. Long-term stress-induced analgesia and activation of the opiate system. *Science* 1981; 213:1409–1411.

Graven-Nielsen T, Mense S. The peripheral apparatus of muscle pain: evidence from animal and human studies. *Clin J Pain* 2001; 17:2–10.

Grüsser SM, Winter C, Mühlnickel W, et al. The relationship of perceptual phenomena and cortical reorganization in upper extremity amputees. *Neuroscience* 2001; 102:263–272.

Hadler NM. Arm pain in the workplace. A small area analysis. *J Occup Med* 1992; 34:113–119.

Hagberg M. Occupational musculoskeletal stress and disorders of the neck and shoulders: a review of possible pathophysiology. *Int Arch Occup Environ Health* 1984; 53:269–278.

Hari R, Hanninen R, Makinen T, et al. Three hands: fragmentation of human bodily awareness. *Neurosci Lett* 1998; 240:131–134.

Harvey N, Greer K. Force and stiffness: further considerations. *Behav Brain Sci* 1982; 5:547–548.

Hefferline RF. The role of proprioception in the control of behavior. *Trans NY Acad Sci* 1958; 20:739–764.

Heim C, Ehlert U, Hanker JP, Hellhammer DH. Abuse-related posttraumatic stress disorder and alterations of the hypothalamic-pituitary-adrenal axis in women with chronic pelvic pain. *Psychosom Med* 1998; 60:309–318.

Henry JP, Stephens PM. *Stress, Health and the Social Environment: A Sociobiologic Approach to Medicine*. New York: Springer-Verlag, 1981.

Hidding A, van Santen M, De Klerk E, et al. Comparison between self-report measures and clinical observations of functional disability in ankylosing spondylitis, rheumatoid arthritis and fibromyalgia. *J Rheumatol* 1994; 21:818–823.

Hollis CL. Pavlovian conditioning of signal-centered action patterns and autonomic behavior: a biological analysis of function. *Adv Study Behav* 1982; 12:1–64.

Huse E, Larbig W, Gerstein J, et al. Pain-related and psychological predictors of phantom limb and residual limb pain and non-painful phantom phenomena. *Pain*; in press.

Indo Y, Tsuruta M, Hayashida Y, et al. Mutations in the TRKa/NGF receptor gene in patients with congenital insensitivity to pain with anhidrosis. *Nat Genet* 1996; 13:485–488.

Jensen MP, Karoly P. Control beliefs, coping efforts, and adjustment to chronic pain. *J Consult Clin Psychol* 1991; 59:431–438.

Jensen MP, Karoly P. Pain-specific beliefs, perceived symptom severity, and adjustment to chronic pain. *Clin J Pain* 1992; 8:123–130.

Jensen MP, Turner JA, Romano JM. Changes in beliefs, catastrophizing, and coping are associated with improvement in multidisciplinary pain treatment. *J Consult Clin Psychol* 2001; 69:655–662.

Kaas JH. How cortex reorganizes. *Nature* 1995; 375:735–736.

Kaas JH. The reorganization of sensory and motor maps after injury in adult mammals. In: Gazzangia MS (Ed). *The New Cognitive Neurosciences,* 2nd ed. Boston: MIT Press, 2000, pp 223–236.

Karl A, Birbaumer N, Lutzenberger W, Cohen LG, Flor H. Reorganization of motor and somatosensory cortex in upper extremity amputees with phantom limb pain. *J Neurosci* 2001; 21:3609–3618.

Katz J, Melzack R. Pain 'memories' in phantom limbs: review and clinical observations. *Pain* 1990; 43:319–336.

Kearney BG, Wilson PH, Haralambous G. Stress appraisal and personality characteristics of headache patients: Comparisons with tinnitus and normal control groups. *Behav Change* 1987; 4:25–32.

Kiecolt-Glaser JK. Norman Cousins Memorial Lecture 1998. Stress, personal relationships, and immune function: health implications. *Brain Behav Immun* 1999; 13:61–72.

Kiesler S, Finholt T. The mystery of RSI. *Am Psychol* 1988; 43:1004–1015.

Knost B, Flor H, Braun C, Birbaumer N. Cerebral processing of words and the development of chronic pain. *Psychophysiology* 1997; 34:474–481.

Knost B, Flor H, Birbaumer N. Schmerzverhalten, Partnerreaktion und schmerzevozierte Potentiale bei chronischen Schmerzpatienten während eines akuten Schmerztests [Pain behaviors, spouse responses and pain-evoked potentials in chronic pain patients during an acute pain test]. *Z Klin Psychol* 1999a; 28:242–247.

Knost B, Flor H, Birbaumer N, Schugens MM. Learned maintenance of pain: muscle tension reduces central nervous system processing of painful stimulation in chronic and subchronic pain patients. *Psychophysiology* 1999b; 36:755–764.

Lacey JI, Lacey BC. Verification and extension of the principle of autonomic response stereotypy. *Am J Psychol* 1958; 71:50–73.

Lazarus RS, Folkman S. *Stress, Appraisal, and Coping.* New York: Springer, 1984.

Lethem J, Slade PD, Troup JDG, Bentley G. Outline of a fear-avoidance model of exaggerated pain perception. *Behav Res Ther* 1983; 21:401–408.

Leventhal H, Everhart D. Emotion, pain and physical illness. In: Izard CE (Ed). *Emotion and Psychopathology.* New York: Plenum, 1979, pp 263–299.

Leventhal H, Leventhal EA, Contrada RJ. Self-regulation, health, and behavior: a perceptual-cognitive approach. *Psychol Health* 1998; 13:717–733.

Linton SJ. A population-based study of the relationship between sexual abuse and back pain: establishing a link. *Pain* 1997; 73:47–53.

Linton SJ, Melin L, Götestam KG. Behavioral analysis of chronic pain and its management. In: Hersen ABM, Eisler M (Eds). *Progress in Behavior Modification.* New York: Academic Press, 1985, pp 1–42.

Lotze M, Grodd W, Birbaumer N, et al. Does use of a myoelectric prosthesis prevent cortical reorganization and phantom limb pain? *Nature Neurosci* 1999; 2:501–502.

Maier SF, Keith JR. Shock signals and the development of stress-induced analgesia. *J Exp Psychol Anim Behav Process* 1987; 13:226–238.

Maier SF, Dugan JW, Grau R, Hyson AS. Learned helplessness, pain inhibition and the endogenous opioids. In: Zeiler M, Harzem P (Eds). *Advances in the Analysis of Behavior*. New York: Wiley, 1984, pp 102–114.

Martin MY, Bradley LA, Alexander RW, et al. Coping strategies predict disability in patients with primary fibromyalgia. *Pain* 1996; 68:45–53.

Melzack R. Phantom limbs. *Sci Am* 1992; 266:120–126.

Melzack R. Pain: past, present, and future. *Can J Exp Psychol* 1993; 47:615–629.

Mense S. Nociception from skeletal muscle in relation to clinical muscle pain. *Pain* 1993; 54:241–289.

Merikangas KR. Genetics of migraine and other headache. *Curr Opin Neurol* 1996; 9:202–205.

Merskey H. Classification of chronic pain: descriptions of chronic pain syndromes and definitions of pain terms. *Pain Suppl* 1986; 3:1–226.

Merzenich MM, Nelson RJ, Stryker MP, et al. Somatosensory cortical map changes following digit amputation in adult monkeys. *J Comp Neurol* 1984; 224:591–605.

Miltner W, Larbig W, Braun C. Biofeedback of somatosensory event-related potentials: can individual pain sensations be modified by biofeedback-induced self-control of event-related potentials? *Pain* 1988; 35:205–213.

Mogil JS, Sternberg WF, Marek P, et al. The genetics of pain and pain inhibition. *Proc Natl Acad Sci USA* 1996; 93:3048–3055.

Mogil JS, Yu L, Basbaum AI. Pain genes?: natural variation and transgenic mutants. *Annu Rev Neurosci* 2000; 23:777–811.

Montoya P, Larbig, Pulvermüller, et al. Cortical correlates of semantic classical conditioning. *Psychophysiology* 1996; 33:644–649.

Moulton B, Spence SH. Site-specific muscle hyper-reactivity in musicians with occupational upper limb pain. *Behav Res Ther* 1992; 30:375–386.

Nagasako EM, Oaklander AL, Dworkin RH. Congenital insensitivity to pain: an update. *Pain* 2003; 101:213–219.

Naliboff BD, Derbyshire SW, Munakata J, et al. Cerebral activation in patients with irritable bowel syndrome and control subjects during rectosigmoid stimulation. *Psychosom Med* 2001; 63:365–375.

Nerenz DR, Leventhal H. Self regulation theory in chronic illness. In: Meichenbaum DH, Jaremko JE (Eds). *Stress Reduction and Prevention*. New York: Plenum, 1983, pp 5–38.

Nyholt DR, Dawkins JL, Brimage PJ, et al. Evidence for an X-linked genetic component in familial typical migraine. *Hum Mol Genet* 1998; 7:459–463.

O'Leary A, Shoor S, Loring K, Holman HR. A cognitive-behavioral treatment for rheumatoid arthritis. *Health Psychol* 1988; 7:527–544.

Pennebaker JW. *The Psychology of Physical Symptoms*. New York: Springer, 1982.

Pennebaker JW. Psychological factors influencing the reporting of physical symptoms. In: Stone AA, Turkkan JS, Bachrach CA et al. (Eds). *The Science of Self-Report: Implications for Research and Practice*. Hillsdale, NJ: Erlbaum, 2000, pp 299–315.

Pennebaker JW, Epstein D. Implicit psychophysiology: effects of common beliefs and idiosyncratic physiological responses on symptom reporting. *J Pers* 1983; 51:468–496.

Pennebaker JW, Gonder-Frederick LA, Cox DJ, Hoover CW. The perception of general vs. specific visceral activity and the regulation of health-related behavior. In: Katkin ES, Manuck SB (Eds). *Advances in Behavioral Medicine*. Greenwich, CT: JAI Press, 1985, pp 165–198.

Price DD, Milling LS, Kirsch I, et al. An analysis of factors that contribute to the magnitude of placebo analgesia in an experimental paradigm. *Pain* 1999; 83:147–156.

Rasmussen BK, Olesen J. Epidemiology of migraine and tension-type headache. *Curr Opin Neurol* 1994; 7:264–271.

Riley JL III, Robinson ME, Kvaal SA, Gremillion HA. Effects of physical and sexual abuse in facial pain: direct or mediated? *Cranio* 1998; 16:259–266.

Rimm OL, Litvak SB. Self-verbalization and emotional arousal. *J Abnorm Psychol* 1969; 74:181–187.

Ritchie J. Pain from distension of the pelvic colon by inflating a balloon in the irritable colon syndrome. *Gut* 1973; 14:125–132.

Rosenfeld JP, Dowman R, Silvia R, Heinricher M. Operantly controlled somatosensory brain potentials: specific effects on pain processes. In: Elbert T, Rockstroh B, Lutzenberger W, Birbaumer N (Eds). *Self-Regulation of the Brain and Behavior.* Berlin: Springer-Verlag, 1984, pp 164–179.

Sandkühler J. Learning and memory in pain pathways. *Pain* 2000; 88:113–118.

Sargent C. Between death and shame: dimensions of pain in Bariba culture. *Soc Sci Med* 1984; 19:1299–1304.

Schiefenhövel W. Verarbeitung von Schmerz und Krankheit bei den Eipo, Hochland West-Neuguinea [Responses to pain and illness in the Eipo tribe, West New Guinea]. *Med Psychol* 1980; 6:219–234.

Schmidt AJM. Cognitive factors in the performance level of chronic low back pain patients. *J Psychosom Res* 1985; 29:183–189.

Schmidt AJM, Brand A. Resistance behavior of CLBP patients in an acute pain situation. *J Psychosom Res* 1986; 30:339–346.

Schüldt K, Ekholm J, Harms-Ringdahl K, Arborelius U, Nemeth G. Influences of sitting postures on neck and shoulder EMG during arm-hand work movements. *Clin Biomech* 1987; 2:126–139.

Serlie AW, Duivenvoorden HJ, Passchier J, et al. Empirical psychological modeling of chest pain: a comparative study. *J Psychosom Res* 1996; 40:625–635.

Sherman RA. *Phantom Pain.* New York: Plenum Press, 1997.

Snow-Turek AL, Norris MP, Tan G. Active and passive coping strategies in chronic pain patients. *Pain* 1996; 64:455–462.

Stein C. Nociceptors and neuroimmune interactions. In: Belmonte C, Cervero F (Eds). *Neurobiology of Nociceptors.* Oxford: Oxford University Press, 1996, pp 439–454.

Stein C, Schafer M, Hassan AH. Peripheral opioid receptors. *Ann Med* 1995; 27:219–221.

Tunks E, Crook J, Norman J, Kalaher S. Tender points in fibromyalgia. *Pain* 1988; 34:11–19.

Turk DC, Flor H. Pain behaviors: The utility and limitations of the pain behavior. *Pain* 1987a; 31:277–295.

Turk DC, Flor H. Pain > pain behaviors: the utility and limitations of the pain behavior construct. *Pain* 1987b; 31:277–295.

Turk DC, Flor H. Chronic pain: a biobehavioral perspective. In: Gatchel RJ, Turk DC (Eds). *Psychosocial Factors in Pain: Critical Perspectives.* New York: Guilford Press, 1999, pp 18–34.

Turk DC, Okifuji A, Starz TW, Skinar GS. Pain, disability, and physical functioning in subgroups of patients with fibromyalgia. *J Rheumatol* 1996; 23:1255–1262.

Turkat ID, Guise BJ. The effects of vicarious experience and stimulus intensity on pain termination and work avoidance. *Behav Res Ther* 1983; 21:241–245.

Turkat ID, Kuczmierczyk AR, Adams HE. An investigation of the etiology of chronic headache: the role of headache models. *Br J Psychiatry* 1984; 145:665–666.

Turner JA, Clancy S, Vitaliano PP. Relationships of stress, appraisal and coping, to chronic low back pain. *Behav Res Ther* 1987; 25:281–288.

Vaughan KB, Lanzetta JT. Vicarious instigation and conditioning of facial expressive and autonomic responses to a model's expressive display of pain. *J Pers Soc Psychol* 1980; 38:909–923.

Vaughan KB, Lanzetta JT. The effect of modification of expressive displays on vicarious emotional arousal. *J Exp Soc Psychol* 1981; 17:16–30.

Vlaeyen JW, Linton SJ. Fear-avoidance and its consequences in chronic musculoskeletal pain: a state of the art. *Pain* 2000; 85:317–332.

Vlaeyen JW, Seelen HA, Peters M, et al. Fear of movement/(re)injury and muscular reactivity in chronic low back pain patients: an experimental investigation. *Pain* 1999; 82:297–304.

Vlaeyen JW, de Jong J, Geilen M, Heuts PH, van Breukelen G. The treatment of fear of movement/(re)injury in chronic low back pain: further evidence on the effectiveness of exposure in vivo. *Clin J Pain* 2002; 18:251–261.

Volinn E. The epidemiology of low back pain in the rest of the world. A review of surveys in low- and middle-income countries. *Spine* 1997; 22:1747–1754.

Waddell G. Low back pain: a twentieth century health care enigma. *Spine* 1996; 21:2820–2825.

Walling MK, Reiter RC, O'Hara MW, et al. Abuse history and chronic pain in women: I. Prevalences of sexual abuse and physical abuse. *Obstet Gynecol* 1994; 84:193–199.

Watkins LR, Mayer DJ. Organization of endogeneous opiate and nonopiate pain control systems. *Science* 1982; 216:1185–1192.

Whitehead WE, Palsson OS. Is rectal pain sensitivity a biological marker for irritable bowel syndrome: psychological influences on pain perception. *Gastroenterology* 1998; 115:1263–1271.

Whitehead WE, Fedoravicious AS, Blackwell B, Wooley S. A behavioral conceptualization of psychosomatic illness: psychosomatic illness as a learned response. In: McNamara JR (Ed). *Behavioral Approaches to Medicine: Application and Analysis.* New York: Plenum Press, 1979.

Wiesenfeld-Hallin Z, Hallin RG. The influence of the sympathetic system on mechanoreception and nociception: a review. *Hum Neurobiol* 1984; 3:41–46.

Wright J, Morley S. Autobiographical memory and chronic pain. *Br J Clin Psychol* 1995; 34:255–265.

Wunsch A, Philippot P, Plaghki L. Affective associative learning modifies the sensory perception of nociceptive stimuli without participant's awareness. *Pain* 2003; 102:27–38.

Yang TT, Schwartz B, Gallen C, et al. Sensory maps in the human brain. *Nature* 1994; 368:592–593.

Correspondence to: Herta Flor, PhD, Department of Clinical and Cognitive Neuroscience at the University of Heidelberg, Central Institute of Mental Health, Mannheim 68072, Germany. Tel: 49-621-170-3918; Fax: 49-621-170-3932; email: flor@zi-mannheim.de.

Part II

Evaluating Pain Patients

Psychosocial Aspects of Pain: A Handbook for Health
Care Providers, Progress in Pain Research and
Management, Vol. 27, edited by Robert H. Dworkin
and William S. Breitbart, IASP Press, Seattle, © 2004.

4

Evaluating Acute Pain

David A. Williams

Division of Rheumatology, Department of Medicine,
University of Michigan, Ann Arbor, Michigan, USA

Pain is amongst the most common complaints for which people seek medical attention. In any given year, more than 70% of the adult U.S. population experiences some form of pain (Sternbach 1986). Some of this pain will be associated with injury or trauma, some will involve chronic diseases or acute exacerbations of preexisting painful conditions, some will be associated with medical procedures such as surgery, and some will be of unknown origin. Despite extraordinary advances in our understanding of the underlying sensory mechanisms, the complete phenomenon of pain, which includes biological, psychological, and social components, is still poorly understood. Incomplete understanding of these areas has hampered the assessment of acute pain. This chapter explores strategies for assessing acute pain and highlights the important role of patients' psychosocial factors in providing clinicians with an accurate impression of their pain.

ACUTE CLINICAL PAIN ASSESSMENT

At the present time there is no machine capable of objectively measuring clinical pain in patients. Any assessment of pain through verbal report, behavioral observation, or physiological measurement will be at best an indirect corollary of the patient's private experience of pain. The most common method of assessing acute clinical pain is to have patients complete a quantitative pain scale where one end of the scale represents no pain and the other end represents extreme pain (Agency for Health Care Policy and Research 1992). Despite its apparent simplicity, this strategy has many variations that can lead to differing clinical impressions in a given patient. The following is a description of several common approaches to acute clinical pain assessment.

QUANTITATIVE PAIN ASSESSMENT TOOLS

Quantitative self-reported clinical pain assessment most commonly occurs in one of three forms: numeric rating scales, verbal rating scales, and visual analogue scales. This section reviews these methods and provides an overview of their advantages and disadvantages.

Numeric rating scales. Of the quantitative methods, the numeric rating scale (NRS) is the most commonly used form of pain assessment in clinical settings. It asks patients to rate the intensity of their pain along a single numeric dimension (e.g., 0–10 or 0–100). The end points typically have verbal descriptors such as "no pain" and "worst pain" and can be administered on paper or orally, either in person or over the telephone. The patient simply needs to indicate which number best describes the intensity of the pain being assessed. Scoring is equally simple because the patient's response requires no further interpretation. In addition to the ease of administration and scoring, the NRS can be completed in less than 10 seconds and can be given repeatedly over time with little inconvenience to the patient.

Historically the 101-point scale (i.e., 0–100) was considered the most desirable because it more closely approximated a continuous distribution and provided more response categories (Karoly and Jensen 1987). The 21-point scale (i.e., 0–20) is a briefer option with fewer response options, yet there appears to be no loss of information or sensitivity when a 0–100 point scale is converted to this briefer metric (Jensen et al. 1994a). Studies have found the NRS to be sensitive to treatment effects (e.g., Paice and Cohen 1997), and recent studies have developed criteria for identifying clinically meaningful changes on these scales (Farrar et al. 2000).

Disadvantages of the NRS stem mainly from the inability of some patients, such as older adults and some cultural groups, to conceptualize a bodily sensation such as pain as a number. Confusion about how to use the scale can introduce errors into pain assessment that are related to the measurement strategy and have little to do with the amount of pain being experienced. A second disadvantage is that the NRS does not demonstrate ratio scale properties; despite the numbers being spaced equally, patients perceive the intensity of pain between some numbers as being greater than between others. Thus, interpretation of changes in pain using an NRS may be limited to relative changes (increases or decreases) rather than percentages (Price et al. 1994).

Verbal rating scales. Verbal rating scales (VRS) comprise a list of adjectives arranged along a linear dimension with words describing low levels of pain at one end and extreme pain at the other. The number of adjectives along the dimension has varied across different instruments, with some having as few as four adjectives (Seymour 1982) and others as many as 15 (Gracely et al. 1978). Each adjective is arranged semantically to represent increasing intensity along a line and is assigned a numeric value as a function of its rank order.

An advantage of this approach compared to numerical scales is that the linguistic descriptors of pain might more accurately represent the experience of pain for patients than do numbers. Disadvantages include the criticism that the amount of pain represented by adjacent adjectives may not represent equal intervals of intensity, thus limiting this scale, like the NRS, to descriptions of increases or decreases in pain. A second disadvantage of this method is that it is limited to written administration because the difficulty of committing multiple adjectives to memory (as would be done over the telephone or in an interview) might compromise the reliability and validity of the assessment.

There are, however, ways of improving on the VRS that take advantage of sophisticated cross-modality matching procedures. These scales, known as verbal descriptor scales (VDS), utilize empirical placement of the adjectives on the line and thus may not have adjectives spaced evenly across the intensity dimension. An example of such a scale would be the Gracely Box Scale (GBS; Gracely et al. 1979). This scale consists of 21 sequentially numbered boxes arranged vertically with "0" as the lowest box and "20" as the highest. Beside the column of numbered boxes are verbal descriptors (such as "faint," "mild," or "strong") that convey degrees of pain intensity. The positions of the verbal descriptors relative to the numbers are consistent with previous cross-modality matching procedures for the word descriptors—a process by which a sample of subjects rated the attributes of various sensory calibration stimuli (line lengths, sounds, odors, etc.) and matched them to the amount of pain intensity implied by the verbal descriptors (Gracely et al. 1978). A number may not have a verbal descriptor if empirical evidence did not show that number to be related to a known verbal descriptor of pain. The GBS is a logarithmic pain scale (as opposed to the linear categorical scaling of the NRS), with ratio scale properties to better reflect the psychophysiological properties of how patients are thought to experience pain. On a logarithmic scale, relatively small changes will reflect rather large changes in the pain experienced by patients. A disadvantage of the VDS is that, like the VRS, it must be administered in writing rather than orally.

Visual analogue scales. The visual analogue scale (VAS) is a straight line, usually 10 cm in length, with verbal descriptors only at the ends. The patient is asked to simply place a mark on the line that indicates the intensity of pain. Scoring of the VAS requires measuring where the mark occurred on the paper and translating the value into a quantitative rating of pain. The VAS is especially useful when working with children who may not be able to conceptualize pain as a number, or when working with cognitively impaired populations who are unable to make the fine verbal discriminations of pain intensity required by the verbal scales (Varni et al. 1986). As in the case of the VDS, evidence indicates that the VAS may possess ratio-scaling properties, which would permit the calculation of percentages associated with change (Price et al. 1994). Disadvantages of the VAS include inconsistencies in how it is scored by different clinicians, and variation in the length of the line being measured (e.g., a 10-cm line that is photocopied many times in a clinic setting will tend to grow in length). A further difficulty is that not all patients understand how to translate their pain experience into a mark on a line. The method is also not recommended for individuals with injuries to their writing hand. A study of 218 physicians found that 56% preferred NRS, 19.5% preferred VRS, and only 7% preferred VAS (Price et al. 1994).

QUALITATIVE AND PICTORIAL METHODS
OF ACUTE PAIN ASSESSMENT

Qualitative methods. Alternatives to quantitative measures of pain are instruments that assess qualitative aspects of the pain experience. Given that many individuals have difficulty transforming their pain experience into a number or a mark on a line, some assessment instruments attempt to capture the complexity of pain by identifying various qualities of the experience. Once such measure is the McGill Pain Questionnaire (MPQ; Melzack 1975). This instrument has been used in hundreds of acute pain studies, has been translated into over 20 languages, and has a validated short-form version for pain assessment when time is limited (Melzack 1987). The full version of the MPQ consists of 78 pain descriptors (adjectives) grouped into 20 categories, each representing a different quality of the pain experience (e.g., pressure sensations, burning sensations, and tearing sensations). The 20 categories may be consolidated into sensory descriptors, affective descriptors, and evaluative descriptors.

An advantage of the MPQ is its ability to discriminate between different pain conditions based upon how patients reported experiencing the pain (e.g., Grushka and Sessle 1984; Melzack et al. 1986; Masson et al. 1989). For example, arthritic pain has been characterized by descriptors such as gnawing, aching, exhausting, and annoying, whereas tooth pain has been described as throbbing, boring, sharp, sickening, and annoying (Dubuisson and Melzack 1976). Disadvantages of qualitative assessments include less familiarity on the part of clinicians with how to score and utilize the information obtained in this fashion, and a slightly greater burden on the patient (in terms of time) to complete this type of questionnaire compared to an NRS. The full version of the MPQ also includes an intensity measure on a scale of 1–5 and a body map upon which patients can draw the anatomical distribution of pain.

Pictorial methods. Picture or face scales use series of photographs or drawings that illustrate increasing amounts of pain. Patients are asked to choose the face that best depicts the expression representing the amount of pain they are experiencing (Keck et al. 1996). As for the VRS, rank-ordered numeric values can be attached to faces for scoring purposes, but typically patients are not asked to translate their pain into a numeric value. This method is particularly useful when assessing pain in pediatric populations or with populations of questionable literacy, and may be a preferred alternative for assessing pain in adults in general (Stuppy 1998). Like many of the quantitative methods, however, this approach still requires some explanation to patients that they are being asked to translate their personal pain experience into the facial expression of another individual (an exercise that might require the capacity to detect and comprehend suffering in the facial expressions of others). Like the NRS and VRS, this scale does not possess the ratio scale properties needed to make statements that go beyond simple increases or decreases in pain.

PSYCHOSOCIAL FACTORS AND ACUTE PAIN

Psychological factors need not be considered pathological to influence pain perception. In fact, brain imaging data suggest that the afferent central processing of pain is highly dependent upon psychological factors to produce what is commonly considered to be the experience of pain. In a model of pain processing by Price (2000), afferent nociceptive signals serially recruited both cognitive and affective brain regions to produce an integrated pain experience. These regions included areas associated with fear and arousal; evaluative centers for intensity, pain quality, and threat to self; areas associated with learning and memory of previous pain; and finally, integrative areas that combined affective, sensory, and evaluative components.

The private experience of pain, however, is very different from the behavior of communicating that experience to others. Translating the pain experience into something others can understand, such as an oral or written report of pain, is vulnerable to conscious censorship or augmentation on the part of the patient. Memory, emotions, cognitive/evaluative processes, and demands from the social environment, such as cultural norms and interpersonal relationships between the patient and the individual asking for the pain rating, all influence how pain is reported. The remainder of this chapter explores many of the psychosocial factors that influence the behavior of reporting acute pain in the clinic setting.

MEMORY AND AFFECT IN ACUTE PAIN REPORTING

Many of the acute pain assessment instruments described in the previous section include instructions for recalling pain over a given time period (e.g., "What was your average pain in the last 24 hours?" "... in the past week?" "... since your initial visit?"). Depending upon the time frame, different information will be obtained because memory for pain is often imperfect and is made worse by affective factors.

For the patient, recall of pain is a complex process that involves (a) the active mental reconstruction of the pain experience for a defined time period, (b) the mental summarization of the pain experience into a single global impression, and (c) the translation of that summary impression into a quantifiable pain rating that can be communicated to the clinician. Although not all agree (e.g., Hunter et al. 1979; Smith et al. 1993), many researchers have challenged the accuracy of this approach for both research and clinical practice, due to the complexity of the cognitive process involved in reporting pain over time (Feine et al. 1998; Price et al. 1999; Hufford and Shiffman 2002).

Emotions may be largely responsible for disrupting the accurate reconstruction of the pain experience. Several studies have found that when pain is assessed at the time of a painful event, such as a painful medical procedure, and then later the patient is asked to recall the amount of pain that was experienced, the recalled rating of pain is usually higher than what was originally reported (Linton and Melin 1982; Linton and Gotestam 1983). The recalling of higher pain may be due in part to a telescoping effect of negative affect on recalled pain. In one study where the pain of a medical procedure was being recalled, only the moment of worst pain and the final 3 minutes of the procedure were reflected in recalled pain (Redelmeier and Kahneman 1996). The inflated pain report failed to reflect the lower pain intensities that accompanied most of the procedure.

The amount of pain being experienced by patients when they try to reconstruct a memory for previously experienced pain also appears to be a biasing factor. Several studies suggest that regardless of the amount of pain that was experienced in the defined period of recall, if pain is high at the time a patient is being asked to recall this period, the memory of pain is likely to be overestimated (Eich et al. 1985; Smith and Safer 1993). Similar findings have been reported for the recall of pain relief following interventions such as nerve blocks. In one study, patients reported relief at the time of the nerve block, but several weeks later, when its effects had diminished, patients recalled receiving much less relief than they had previously reported (Porzelius 1995). Inflated memories of pain for previous medical procedures or memories of minimal pain relief from pain management strategies is problematic because such memory biases can lead patients to avoid needed medical care or may diminish the perceived effectiveness of pain management procedures.

In contrast to studies in which negative emotions lead to inflated memories of pain, several studies have examined recall of pain associated with a potentially positive event such as childbirth. One such study found deflated pain recall in a group of postpartum mothers who recalled the intensity of the pain of childbirth as being lower than they had reported during the delivery itself (Norvell et al. 1987). Positive affect may also lead to underestimation of anticipated pain, even in individuals with previous pain experience. In a study of expectant mothers, both primiparas and multiparas tended to underestimate their pain during labor, regardless of their prior labor experience (Fridh and Gaston-Johansson 1990).

Experimental studies of the effects of inaccurate pain expectations have suggested that the underprediction of pain can leave patients vulnerable to an unpleasant surprise when a procedure is more noxious than anticipated. Such a discrepancy between prediction and experience can create negative emotions such as anxiety or fear that can interfere with the body's own natural means of pain habituation (Arntz et al. 1991). Such underprediction of pain based on inaccurate memories could theoretically lead to inadequate preparation on the part of the patient and clinical staff, or to underutilization of available pain management resources.

ANXIETY AND ACUTE PAIN REPORTING

Anxiety, depression, and anger are perhaps the three most prominent emotions that influence pain. Of these emotions, anxiety remains the best studied for acute pain (Chapman and Turner 1990). A recent study determined that anxiety was a prominent predictor of acute pain intensity, whether measured by the VAS, VRS, or the MPQ (Lazaro et al. 2002). Anxiety associated with the anticipation of pain also plays one of greatest roles in distorting pain reports and influencing attempts to manage pain successfully. In a sample of children undergoing surgery, presurgical ratings of anticipatory anxiety were significant predictors of postoperative pain. In this study, greater anticipatory anxiety was associated with greater pain at the time of the procedure (Palermo and Drotar 1996). Anticipatory anxiety surrounding pain for dental procedures can transform benign procedures into traumatic experiences associated with great pain and difficult management (Klepac et al. 1980; Litt 1996). Such studies from the dental literature highlight the importance of not only controlling the sensory component of pain but also assessing and managing the anticipatory fear of pain prior to beginning a procedure (Ploghaus et al. 1999).

In addition to being associated with increased pain perception, anxiety has been linked to increased risks to physical health and to prolongation of the pain experience (Bonica and Procacci 1990; Krauss 2001). In one sample of 27 patients with acute burn injuries, a patient's level of anxiety not only predicted future procedural pain but was also one of the best predictors of medication use and functional ability at discharge (Aaron et al. 2001). In a larger sample of over 700 women who gave birth in the United Kingdom, preoperative anxiety about labor pain was one of the strongest predictors of negative experiences such as pain during labor, lack of satisfaction with the birth, and poor emotional well-being postnatally (Green 1993). In one of the few prospective studies to examine the impact of anxiety on the development of pain, a sample of initially pain-free individuals were followed over 2.5 years for the development of temporomandibular disorders (TMD). Individuals who developed TMD had significantly higher baseline anxiety values than did those who remained free of TMD symptoms (Bhalang et al. 2002). These findings support the notion that anxiety plays an important role in both the reporting and chronicity of pain.

Not all researchers agree, however, that anxiety universally elevates acute pain sensitivity. To date, several studies have suggested that males, either in the laboratory (Fillingim et al. 1996) or in clinical settings (Edwards et al. 2000), are much more likely to have their pain report influenced by anxiety than are females. In a sample of healthy volunteers exposed to a cold pressor paradigm, male participants scoring above the median on trait anxiety reported significantly greater pain intensity, unpleasantness, and lower pain tolerances than did males scoring below the median on trait anxiety. Females, on the other hand, showed no relationship between trait anxiety and these measures of pain (Jones et al. 2002). Future studies will need to further clarify the precise relationship between affect and pain reporting, because many clinicians assume this relationship to be far more precise than laboratory studies are suggesting.

COGNITIVE/EVALUATIVE FACTORS
AND ACUTE PAIN REPORTING

Cognitive factors can also influence how acute pain is reported. Two factors that have received relatively greater research efforts are (a) attention and discrimination and (b) appraisal and perceived control over pain.

Attention and discrimination. In humans, it has been assumed that nociceptive signals must be consciously recognized in order for pain to be experienced. Similarly, any process that permits those signals to be ignored, missed, or interpreted as something other than pain is likely to diminish pain. Focusing one's attention on pain is thought to increase pain intensity. In one study, when patients were encouraged to focus on and talk about pain-related content, they had higher pain intensity ratings than similar patients who were encouraged to talk about nonpain-related topics (White and Sanders 1986). The authors of the study concluded that differences in reported pain were attributable both to the focus of attention on pain by the one group and to the benefit of distraction occurring in the context of social conversation in the second group.

Either passive lack of attention or active distraction is likely to inhibit pain. Support for the utility of distraction as a suppressor of pain perception comes from the experimental pain literature, where distraction through cognitive tasks or through distracting imagery has been associated with increased tolerance to experimentally induced pain (Kanfer and Goldfoot 1966; Kanfer and Seidner 1973; Jaremko 1978; Worthington 1978; Hodes et al. 1990; Neumann et al. 1997). More recent studies have similarly demonstrated both auditory (Terkelsen et al. 2002) and visual (Valet et al. 2002) forms of distraction to be effective in reducing the intensity and unpleasantness of experimental painful stimuli. In Valet's study, which included functional imaging, the thalamus was postulated as being responsible for the modulatory effect of distraction on pain. Current nonpharmacological approaches to clinical pain management continue to highlight the importance of distraction techniques as one of the best tools for diminishing many forms of pain (Turk et al. 1983; Keefe 1996; ter Kuile et al. 1996).

Appraisal and perceived control over pain. Two individuals may be exposed to identical painful events and yet experience pain quite differently. This fascinating observation underlies why work on the appraisal process (Lazarus and Folkman 1984) is so often considered relevant when trying to understanding cognitive events that determine one's perception of pain. According to theory, once a nociceptive event occurs, individuals make an appraisal of the event. Primary appraisal typically determines whether the nociceptive event is harmful, threatening, or of some benefit. If it is judged harmful or threatening, a secondary appraisal process helps to determine whether the individual possesses the necessary resources for controlling and dealing with the nociceptive event. If resources are adequate, then appropriate coping can commence and the pain experience can diminish. If resources are inadequate, then affective responses such as anxiety or fear may further heighten the perception of pain until appropriate resources for relieving the pain are discovered. If adaptive resources for comfort are not identified, potentially maladaptive responses such as helplessness and illness behaviors begin to operate in the person's life. This response can result in acute pain becoming more chronic (Gatchel 1996).

Many beliefs have been identified that can profoundly affect how both primary and secondary appraisals of pain are determined (Williams and Thorn 1989; Shutty et al. 1990; Jensen et al. 1991, 1994b; Williams and Keefe 1991; Williams et al. 1994; Weisenberg 1999). Examples of such beliefs might include beliefs about the cause of pain, its future course, and its treatability, and about one's ability to function with pain. Several studies of chronic pain have explored the utility of pain beliefs in the prediction of treatment outcome. In one study, patient pain beliefs demonstrated utility in predicting social, psychological, and physiological adjustment 1–7 years after inpatient pain treatment (Jensen and Karoly 1991). A second study found that increases in perceived control over pain were associated with decreased disability, reduced pain intensity, and less depression (Jensen et al. 2001). A third study showed that beliefs about pain accounted for 44% of the variance in physical functional status and 29% of the variance in depressive symptoms (Turner et al. 2000). These findings were replicated in a related study on patients with TMD that found that 33% of the variance in functional limitations and 44% of the variance in depression was attributable to beliefs about pain (Turner et al. 2001).

Pain beliefs not only affect outcomes but also influence treatment adherence. In one study, greater endorsement of maladaptive pain beliefs was associated with poorer adherence to physical therapy and behavioral medicine treatment regimens (Williams and Thorn 1989). These findings supported earlier work (Becker and Maiman 1975; Schwartz et al. 1985) that suggested that treatment adherence would diminish if personal beliefs about the illness were discordant with the treatment offered.

Once primary appraisal has determined that nociception is harmful or threatening, secondary appraisal must evaluate the available coping resources. Beliefs regarding personal efficacy to cope with and to control pain have been discussed in numerous studies on reported pain (Jensen and Karoly 1991). An example of how the perception of control can influence the report of pain comes from an experimental cold pressor pain study that manipulated control by telling participants (a) that the pain stimulus would be limited to 3 minutes or (b) that the pain stimulus was open-ended and that they should remain in the water as long as possible. In this study, the pain stimulus and the duration of pain were identical for all subjects 2 minutes into the test, but the subjects who believed that the pain trial was fixed to a 3-minute duration reported significantly lower pain ratings than did those who were told the duration of the pain trial was open-ended (Williams and Thorn 1986). These findings were replicated in a second experimental pain study using an ischemic pain stimulus (Thorn and Williams 1989). Together, these two studies underscore the importance of secondary appraisal, which in these cases suggests that subjects believed they possessed sufficient resources to cope with pain for a limited duration, but not indefinitely. In the open-ended condition, affective factors associated with the secondary appraisal that coping resources were inadequate may have contributed to the significantly higher pain ratings at the 2-minute comparison point.

One additional pertinent study evaluated expectancies in a heterogeneous sample of 126 postsurgical patients in an attempt to identify which of a group of variables were most strongly associated with pain (Bachiocco et al. 1993). Variables included self-control expectancies, previous pain behavior, familial pain tolerance, personality, locus of control, and expected ability to cope with pain. Of these variables, the secondary appraisal, "expected ability to cope with pain," was the most strongly associated with the total pain experience (e.g., intensity and duration). Enhancement of the perception of control and of the ability to cope with pain continues to be the target of clinical investigations into improved acute pain management.

SOCIAL FACTORS AND ACUTE PAIN REPORTING

The previous sections have focused on factors that are largely internal to the individual experiencing the pain, such as memory, affect, and cognitions. However, the environment in which pain must be reported is equally influential. Three areas that can have profound effects on how pain is reported are social modeling of pain, cultural factors, and situational demand characteristics.

Social modeling. Individuals will learn how to communicate pain from other individuals in their environment. An example of this social modeling is that an individual receiving the same pain stimuli as another individual is likely to report the pain as more or less intense depending upon the pain report of the other person. In one such experimental study, pain thresholds were reduced in response to novel electric shock when the subject was in the presence of another person who was intolerant of the shock. Conversely, when subjects were in the presence of a model who was tolerant of the shock, pain thresholds were higher (Craig and Weiss 1971).

When faced with an unfamiliar clinical pain experience, patients will tend to utilize whatever information is available at the time to construct a framework or schema for evaluating the novel experience. For example, in a study of hospitalized patients receiving arteriotomies, patients were given one of two suggestions about the sensations associated with the procedure. One condition specifically mentioned pain whereas the other mentioned coolness and numbness. Significantly reduced pain levels were associated with the suggestions about coolness and numbness (Austan et al. 1997). Studies of children who were candidates for surgical and dental procedures viewed films of peers undergoing the procedure that they would be receiving. Those who viewed films showing peers responding to treatment in a competent fashion experienced decreased complications and anxiety with their own procedures (Melamed and Siegel 1975; Craig 1978; Melamed et al. 1978). Family members can also influence how pain is experienced and expressed. Patients coming from families who modeled good pain tolerance tended to show better tolerance for pain and less severe pain associated with their own medical procedures (Bachiocco et al. 1993).

Cultural factors. The term *race* is used to describe groups of individuals with a shared biological make-up, whereas the term *ethnicity* subsumes race but also describes groups of individuals with distinguishing behaviors and shared culture, history, ancestry, and beliefs (Edwards et al. 2001). *Cultural affiliation* is a term that has been used to describe the degree to which an individual identifies with a particular ethnic group.

Multiple studies have shown that cultural affiliation influences subjects' perception of and response to both experimental and acute pain (Zborowski 1952; Lipton and Marbach 1984; Greenwald 1991; Bates et al. 1993). Important factors include the culture's tendency to be emotionally expressive or stoic, beliefs about the meaning of pain and its controllability, and learned models for illness behaviors that influence how a patient should respond to pain. Cultural norms for the expression of pain appear to be learned at an early age and result in differences in pain expression between cultural groups in later life (Zborowski 1952).

Experimental pain studies have suggested that differences in the interpretation of the pain experience may play a larger role in determining cultural differences in pain report than do physiological factors. A study of healthy females compared responses to a standardized experimental stimulus in a U.S. sample representing four different cultural backgrounds including Anglo-Saxon, Irish, Italian, and Jewish women (Sternbach and Tursky 1965).

Pain thresholds did not differ among groups, but differences in pain tolerance emerged, with Italian women having the lowest tolerance. Attitudes toward pain were considered partially responsible for the differences in pain tolerance. Stoic or neutral responses were characteristic of the Irish and Anglo-Saxon groups, and diminished reactivity was found in the Jewish sample, who tended to minimize the significance of the experimental pain because it had no clinical relevance. The Italian women, demonstrating the lowest tolerance for pain, focused on the immediacy of the pain experience. A more recent mixed-gender study of 543 acute postoperative dental pain patients evaluated pain in Asian, African-American, European, and Latin American patients. In this study, the African-American and Latin American patients reported significantly greater pain than did the other groups (Faucett et al. 1994). Several other studies have also found that African-Americans report higher pain intensity ratings than do Caucasians undergoing similar acute medical procedures (Edwards and Fillingim 1999; White et al. 1999).

Differences among ethnic groups in the United States may be diminishing as assimilation and acculturation produce a blending of cultural influences on pain. While cultural assimilation may be obscuring sensory differences, affective differences may be more stable. In a study of individuals whose families were not recent immigrants to the United States and who had pain from cancer, no differences among ethnic groups were found on the sensory pain scores of the MPQ, but affective scores were significantly lower for individuals identifying themselves as being from the United Kingdom (including Scotland and Wales), Germany, Scandinavia, and Italy. Higher affective scores were associated with family origins in France or Eastern Europe or with Jewish heritage (Greenwald 1991).

In an attempt to identify the most salient factors that determine ethnic differences in pain perception, Bates and Edwards (1992) investigated clinical pain in 372 patients from six ethnic groups. The authors concluded that the most salient predictors of differing ethnic pain reports were heritage consistency (i.e., strength of cultural identification) and the perceived ability to control pain, surpassing genetic influences, behavioral factors, attitudinal and psychopathology, socioeconomic status, treatment history, clinical diagnosis, and medication intake.

Situational demand characteristics. Long recognized as a confound in experimental pain studies, the interaction between the subject and the experimenter can importantly influence the report of pain given by subjects. In a study supporting this relationship, subjects were asked to report cold pressor pain in front of either an attractive male or attractive female experimenter. The results of this study found that males reported significantly less pain in front of a female experimenter than in front of a male experimenter.

The difference for females was not as great, although the tendency was for females to report greater pain to the male experimenter (Levine and DeSimon 1991).

The perceived status of the individual requesting the pain rating may also partially affect the subject's intensity rating. Studies in which patients were asked to report the benefits of treatment by giving a rating of pain relief found that a physician was likely to elicit lower pain ratings from a patient than was a research assistant or disinterested third party asking about the same pain condition over the same time period (Long and Erickson 1975; North et al. 1991; Williams et al. 2003). This discrepancy has been discussed in the context of patients' fear that a higher pain rating might lead to additional painful procedures, fear of disappointing their physician, or fear of being referred to a different physician.

CONCLUSIONS

This chapter has highlighted the importance of both accurately assessing pain and being aware of the many factors that might bias information that clinicians obtain about pain. These issues are of particular importance given the increased use of pain assessment devices in clinical settings as mandated by the Joint Commission for Accreditation of Healthcare Organizations (2000) and supported by those promoting pain as the fifth vital sign (Veterans Health Administration Acute Care Strategic Healthcare Group 2001). These recommendations span postoperative care, procedural care, ambulatory care, and home health care. While some clinicians may consider psychosocial factors as contaminants of "accurate" pain assessment, it must be realized that cognition and affect are in fact integral parts of pain perception and cannot be separated from it (Price 2000). Where affect, cognitions, and social factors potentially "contaminate" the report of pain is in the secondary translation of the pain experience into a behavioral response that can be communicated orally or in writing to others. While these factors mean that clinicians must be careful of how they assess and interpret pain reports, it is in this arena that promise for new methods of acute pain assessment resides.

ACKNOWLEDGMENTS

Preparation of this manuscript was supported in part by Department of Army grant DAMD17-00-2-0018.

REFERENCES

Aaron LA, Patterson DR, Finch CP, Carrougher GJ, Heimbach DM. The utility of a burn specific measure of pain anxiety to prospectively predict pain and function: a comparative analysis. *Burns* 2001; 27:329–334.

Agency for Health Care Policy and Research. *Acute Pain Management: Operative or Medical Procedures and Trauma,* Clinical Practice Guideline No. 1, Publication No. 92–0032. Rockville, MD: U.S. Department of Health and Human Services, 1992.

Arntz A, Van den Hout MA, van den Berg G, Meijboom A. The effects of incorrect pain expectations on acquired fear and pain responses. *Behav Res Ther* 1991; 29:547–560.

Austan F, Polise M, Schultz TR. The use of verbal expectancy in reducing pain associated with arteriotomies. *Am J Clin Hypn* 1997; 39:182–186.

Bachiocco V, Scesi M, Morselli AM, Carli G. Individual pain history and familial pain tolerance models: relationships to post-surgical pain. *Clin J Pain* 1993; 9:266–271.

Bates MS, Edwards WT. Ethnic variations in the chronic pain experience. *Ethn Dis* 1992; 2:63–83.

Bates MS, Edwards WT, Anderson KO. Ethnocultural influences on variation in chronic pain perception. *Pain* 1993; 52:101–112.

Becker MH, Maiman LA. Sociobehavioral determinants of compliance with health and medical care recommendations. *Med Care* 1975; 13:10–24.

Bhalang K, Slade GD, Sigurdsson A, Maixner W. The roles of anxiety and somatization in the development of temporomandibular disorders. *Abstracts: 10th World Congress on Pain.* Seattle: IASP Press, 2002, p 179.

Bonica JJ, Procacci P. The general considerations of acute pain. In: Bonica JJ (Ed). *The Management of Pain,* Vol. 1. Philadelphia: Lea & Febiger, 1990, pp 159–179.

Chapman CR, Turner JA. Psychologic and psychosocial aspects of acute pain. In: Bonica JJ (Ed). *The Management of Pain,* Vol. 1. Philadelphia: Lea & Febiger, 1990, pp 122–132.

Craig KD. Social modelling influences on pain. In: Sternbach RA (Ed). *The Psychology of Pain.* New York: Raven Press, 1978, pp 73–109.

Craig KD, Weiss SM. Vicarious influences on pain-threshold determinations. *J Pers Soc Psychol* 1971; 19:53–59.

Dubuisson D, Melzack R. Classification of clinical pain descriptors by multiple group discriminant analysis. *Exp Neurol* 1976; 51:480–487.

Edwards CL, Fillingim RB, Keefe FJ. Race, ethnicity, and pain. *Pain* 2001; 94:133–137.

Edwards RR, Fillingim RB. Ethnic differences in thermal pain responses. *Psychosom Med* 1999; 61:346–354.

Edwards R, Auguston EM, Fillingim RB. Sex-specific effects of pain-related anxiety on adjustment to chronic pain. *Clin J Pain* 2000; 16:46–53.

Eich E, Reeves JL, Jaeger B, Graff-Radford SB. Memory for pain: relation between past and present pain intensity. *Pain* 1985; 23:375–380.

Farrar JT, Portenoy RK, Berlin JA, Kinman JL, Strom BL. Defining the clinically important difference in pain outcome measures. *Pain* 2000; 88:287–294.

Faucett J, Gordon N, Levine J. Differences in postoperative pain severity among four ethnic groups. *J Pain Symptom Manage* 1994; 9:383–389.

Feine JS, Lavigne GJ, Dao TT, Morin C, Lund JP. Memories of chronic pain and perceptions of relief. *Pain* 1998; 77:137–141.

Fillingim RB, Keefe FJ, Light KC, Booker DK, Maixner W. The influence of gender and psychological factors on pain perception. *J Gender, Culture, Health* 1996; 1:21–36.

Fridh G, Gaston-Johansson F. Do primiparas and multiparas have realistic expectations of labor? *Acta Obstet Gynecol Scand* 1990; 69:103–109.

Gatchel RJ. Psychological disorders and chronic pain: cause-and-effect relationships. In: Gatchel RJ, Turk DC (Eds). *Psychological Approaches to Pain Management: A Practitioner's Handbook.* New York: Guilford Press, 1996, pp 33–52.

Gracely RH, McGrath F, Dubner R. Ratio scales of sensory and affective verbal pain descriptors. *Pain* 1978; 5:5–18.

Gracely RH, Dubner R, McGrath PA. Narcotic analgesia: fentanyl reduces the intensity but not the unpleasantness of painful tooth pulp sensations. *Science* 1979; 203:1261–1263.

Green JM. Expectations and experiences of pain in labor: findings from a large prospective study. *Birth* 1993; 20:65–72.

Greenwald HP. Interethnic differences in pain perception. *Pain* 1991; 44:157–163.

Grushka M, Sessle BJ. Applicability of the McGill Pain Questionnaire to the differentiation of "toothache" pain. *Pain* 1984; 19:49–57.

Hodes RL, Howland EW, Lightfoot N, Cleeland CS. The effects of distraction on responses to cold pressor pain. *Pain* 1990; 41:109–114.

Hufford MR, Shiffman SS. Methodological issues affecting the value of patient-reported outcomes data. *Expert Rev Pharmacoeconomics Health Outcomes* 2002; 2:119–128.

Hunter M, Philips C, Rachman S. Memory for pain. *Pain* 1979; 6:35–46.

Jaremko ME. Cognitive strategies in the control of pain tolerance. *J Behav Ther Exp Psychiatry* 1978; 9:239–244.

Jensen MP, Karoly P. Control beliefs, coping efforts, and adjustment to chronic pain. *J Consult Clin Psychol* 1991; 59:431–438.

Jensen MP, Turner JA, Romano JM, Karoly P. Coping with chronic pain: a critical review of the literature. *Pain* 1991; 47:249–283.

Jensen MP, Turner JA, Romano JM. What is the maximum number of levels needed in pain intensity measurement? *Pain* 1994a; 58:387–392.

Jensen MP, Turner JA, Romano JM, Lawler BK. Relationship of pain-specific beliefs to chronic pain adjustment. *Pain* 1994b; 57:301–309.

Jensen MP, Turner JA, Romano JM. Changes in beliefs, catastrophizing, and coping are associated with improvement in multidisciplinary pain treatment. *J Consult Clin Psychol* 2001; 69:655–662.

Joint Commission on Accreditation of Health Care Organizations. *Background on the Development of the Joint Commission Standards on Pain Management.* Available via the Internet: www.jcaho.org. Accessed 2000.

Jones A, Zacharie R, Arendt-Nielsen L. Dispositional anxiety and the experience of pain: gender-specific effects. *Abstracts: 10th World Congress on Pain.* Seattle: IASP Press, 2002, pp 75–76.

Kanfer FH, Goldfoot DA. Self-control and tolerance of noxious stimulation. *Psychol Rep* 1966; 18:79–85.

Kanfer FH, Seidner ML. Self-control: factors enhancing tolerance of noxious stimulation. *J Pers Soc Psychol* 1973; 25:381–389.

Karoly P, Jensen MP. *Multimethod Assessment of Chronic Pain.* New York: Pergamon Press, 1987.

Keck JF, Gerkensmeyer JE, Joyce BA, Schade JG. Reliability and validity of the faces and word descriptor scales to measure procedural pain. *Pediatr Nurs* 1996; 11:368–374.

Keefe FJ. Cognitive behavioral therapy for managing pain. *Clin Psychol* 1996; 49:4–5.

Klepac RK, McDonald M, Hauge G, Dowling J. Reactions to pain among subjects high and low in dental fear. *J Behav Med* 1980; 3:373–384.

Krauss B. Managing acute pain and anxiety in children undergoing procedures in the emergency department. *Emerg Med* 2001; 13:293–304.

Lazaro C, Torrubia R, Caseras X, Canellas M, Banos JE. Impact of anxiety and depression on pain assessment in acute and chronic pain patients. *Abstracts: 10th World Congress on Pain.* Seattle: IASP Press, 2002, p 576.

Lazarus RS, Folkman S. *Stress, Appraisal, and Coping.* New York: Springer, 1984, pp 445.

Levine FM, DeSimon LL. The effects of experimenter gender on pain report in male and female subjects. *Pain* 1991; 44:69–72.

Linton SJ, Gotestam KG. A clinical comparison of two pain scales: correlation, remembering chronic pain, and a measure of compliance. *Pain* 1983; 17:57–65.

Linton SJ, Melin L. The accuracy of remembering chronic pain. *Pain* 1982; 13:281–285.

Lipton JA, Marbach JJ. Ethnicity and the pain experience. *Soc Sci Med* 1984; 19:1279–1298.

Litt MD. A model of pain and anxiety associated with acute stressors: distress in dental procedures. *Behav Res Ther* 1996; 34:459–476.

Long DM, Erickson DE. Stimulation of the posterior columns of the spinal cord for relief of intractable pain. *Surg Neurol* 1975; 4:134–141.

Masson EA, Hunt L, Gem JM, Boulton AJM. A novel approach to the diagnosis and assessment of symptomatic diabetic neuropathy. *Pain* 1989; 38:25–28.

Melamed BG, Siegel LJ. Reduction of anxiety in children facing hospitalization and surgery by use of filmed modeling. *J Consult Clin Psychol* 1975; 43:511–521.

Melamed BG, Yurcheson R, Fleece EL, Hutchinson S, Hawes R. Effects of film modeling on the reduction of anxiety-related behaviors in individuals varying in level of previous experience in the stress situation. *J Consult Clin Psychol* 1978; 46:1357–1367.

Melzack R. The McGill Pain Questionnaire: major properties and scoring methods. *Pain* 1975; 1:277–299.

Melzack R. The short-form McGill Pain Questionnaire. *Pain* 1987; 30:191–197.

Melzack R, Terrence C, Fromm G, Amsel R. Trigeminal neuralgia and atypical facial pain: use of the McGill Pain Questionnaire for discrimination and diagnosis. *Pain* 1986; 27:297–302.

Neumann W, Kugler J, Pfand-Neumann P, et al. Effects of pain-incompatible imagery on tolerance of pain, heart rate, and skin resistance. *Percept Mot Skills* 1997; 84:939–943.

North RB, Ewend MG, Lawton MT, Kidd DH, Piantadosi S. Failed back surgery syndrome: 5-year follow-up after spinal cord stimulator implantation. *Neurosurgery* 1991; 28:692–699.

Norvell KT, Gaston-Johnsson F, Fridh G. Remembrance of labour pain: how valid are retro-spective pain measures? *Pain* 1987; 31:77–86.

Paice JA, Cohen FA. Validity of a verbally administered numeric rating scale to measure cancer pain intensity. *Cancer Nurs* 1997; 20:88–93.

Palermo TM, Drotar D. Prediction of children's postoperative pain: the role of presurgical expectations and anticipatory emotions. *J Pediatric Psychol* 1996; 21:683–698.

Ploghaus A, Tracey I, Gati JS, et al. Dissociating pain from its anticipation in the human brain. *Science* 1999; 284:1979–1981.

Porzelius J. Memory for pain after nerve-block injections. *Clin J Pain* 1995; 11:112–120.

Price DD. Psychological and neural mechanism of the affective dimension of pain. *Science* 2000; 28:1769–1772.

Price DD, Bush FM, Long S, Harkins SW. A comparison of pain measurement characteristics of mechanical visual analogue and simple numerical rating scales. *Pain* 1994; 56:217–226.

Price DD, Milling LS, Kirsch I, et al. An analysis of factors that contribute to the magnitude of placebo analgesia in an experimental paradigm. *Pain* 1999; 83:147–156.

Redelmeier DA, Kahneman D. Patients' memories of painful medical treatments: real-time and retrospective evaluations of two minimally invasive procedures. *Pain* 1996; 66:3–8.

Schwartz DP, DeGood DE, Shutty MS. Direct assessment of beliefs and attitudes of chronic pain patients. *Arch Phys Med Rehabil* 1985; 66:806–809.

Seymour RA. The use of pain scales in assessing the efficacy of analgesics in post-operative dental pain. *Eur J Clin Pharmacol* 1982; 23:441–444.

Shutty MSJ, DeGood DE, Tuttle DH. Chronic pain patients' beliefs about their pain and treatment outcomes. *Arch Phys Med Rehabil* 1990; 71:128–132.

Smith AF, Salovey P, Turk DC, Jobe JB, Willis GB. Theoretical and methodological issues in assessing memory for pain: a reply. *Am Pain Soc J* 1993; 2:203–206.

Smith WB, Safer MA. Effects of present pain level on recall of chronic pain and medication use. *Pain* 1993; 55:355–361.

Sternbach RA. Survey of pain in the United States: the Nuprin pain report. *Clin J Pain* 1986; 2:49–53.

Sternbach RA, Tursky B. Ethnic differences among housewives in psychosocial and skin potential responses to electric shock. *Psychophysiology* 1965; 1:241–246.

Stuppy DJ. The Faces Pain Scale: reliability and validity with mature adults. *Appl Nurs Res* 1998; 11:89.

ter Kuile MM, Spinhoven P, Linssen AC, van Houwelingen HC. Cognitive coping and appraisal processes in the treatment of chronic headaches. *Pain* 1996; 64:257–264.

Terkelsen AJ, Andersen O, Jensen TS. Effect of attention and distraction on pain, unpleasantness and the nociceptive withdrawal reflex. *Abstracts: 10th World Congress on Pain.* Seattle: IASP Press, 2002, p 516.

Thorn BE, Williams GA. Goal specification alters perceived pain intensity and tolerance latency. *Cognit Ther Res* 1989; 13:171–183.

Turk DC, Meichenbaum D, Genest M. *Pain and Behavioral Medicine: A Cognitive-Behavioral Perspective.* New York: Guilford Press, 1983, p 452.

Turner JA, Jensen MP, Romano JM. Do beliefs, coping, and catastrophizing independently predict functioning in patients with chronic pain? *Pain* 2000; 85:115–125.

Turner JA, Dworkin SF, Mancl L, Huggins KH, Truelove EL. The roles of beliefs, catastrophizing, and coping in the functioning of patients with temporomandibular disorders. *Pain* 2001; 92:41–51.

Valet M, Willoch F, Erhard P, et al. Pain inhibiting mechanisms of distraction on pain processing—a fMRI study. *Abstracts: 10th World Congress on Pain.* Seattle: IASP Press, 2002, p 375.

Varni JW, Jay SM, Masek BJ, Thompson KL. Cognitive-behavioral assessment and management of pediatric pain. In: Holzman AD, Turk DC (Eds). *Pain Management: A Handbook of Psychological Treatment Approaches.* New York: Pergamon, 1986.

Veterans Health Administration Acute Care Strategic Healthcare Group. *Pain as the 5th Vital Sign: Take 5.* Available via the Internet: www.va.gov/oaa/pocketcard/pain.asp. Accessed 2001.

Weisenberg M. Cognitive aspects of pain. In: Wall PD, Melzack R (Eds). *Textbook of Pain.* Edinburgh: Churchill Livingstone, 1999, pp 345–358.

White B, Sanders SH. The influence on patients' pain intensity ratings of antecedent reinforcement of pain talk or well talk. *J Behav Ther Exp Psychiatry* 1986; 17:155–159.

White SF, Asher MA, Lai SM, Burton DC. Patients' perceptions of overall function, pain, and appearance after primary posterior instrumentation and fusion for idiopathic scoliosis. *Spine* 1999; 24:1693–1699.

Williams DA, Keefe FJ. Pain beliefs and the use of cognitive-behavioral coping strategies. *Pain* 1991; 46:185–190.

Williams DA, Thorn BE. Can research methodology affect treatment outcome? A comparison of two cold pressor test paradigms. *Cognit Res Ther* 1986; 10:539–546.

Williams DA, Thorn BE. An empirical assessment of pain beliefs. *Pain* 1989; 36:351–358.

Williams DA, Robinson ME, Geisser ME. Pain beliefs: assessment and utility. *Pain* 1994; 59:71–78.

Williams DA, Park KM, Clauw DJ. Outcomes assessment for procedural pain relief: results depend upon who is asking. *Abstracts: 22nd Annual Meeting of the American Pain Society.* Glenview, IL: American Pain Society, 2003.

Worthington EI. The effect of imagery content, choice of imagery content, and self-verbalization on the self-control of pain. *Cognit Ther Res* 1978; 2:225–240.

Zborowski M. Cultural components in responses to pain. *J Soc Issues* 1952; 8:16–30.

Correspondence to: David A. Williams, PhD, Department of Medicine/Rheumatology, University of Michigan, 24 Frank Lloyd Wright Drive, P.O. Box 385, Lobby M, Ann Arbor, MI 48106, USA. Tel: 734-998-6961; Fax: 734-998-6900; email: daveawms@umich.edu.

Psychosocial Aspects of Pain: A Handbook for Health Care Providers, Progress in Pain Research and Management, Vol. 27, edited by Robert H. Dworkin and William S. Breitbart, IASP Press, Seattle, © 2004.

5

Assessing Chronic Pain and Its Impact

Amanda C. de C. Williams

INPUT Pain Management Unit, Guy's and St. Thomas' Hospital, London, United Kingdom

An informed choice of assessment measures for a trial or study of individuals with pain problems requires knowledge about the requirements and assumptions and the potential pitfalls and compromises of the assessment of chronic pain and its impact. This chapter discusses these aspects of pain measurement and describes some widely used assessment measures. Assessment measures are required for diagnosis, decisions about treatment, predictions of response to treatment, and evaluation of treatment effects (Turk and Okifuji 2003). Increasing appreciation of accountability, both to those who receive care and to those who fund it, demands evidence of treatment efficacy. Persistent pain has a pervasive impact on the lives of those affected, but psychological aspects are covered in other chapters in this volume. This chapter thus focuses on treatment evaluation and on assessing the impact of pain on the patient's function. Most comments apply to adult patients who are cognitively intact and therefore can be assessed by self-report, although some observational and proxy measures are described. Hadjistavropoulos et al. (2001) have described the particular issues surrounding pain assessment in those with compromised or underdeveloped communication.

TARGETS OF ASSESSMENT

The proliferation of research on chronic pain treatment has generated numerous assessment measures, some developed specifically for pain and others adopted or adapted from related fields in health studies. While this apparent wealth should facilitate the selection of suitable measures, in fact many appear in print only once, and data on their performance are thus restricted to the original authors' own study population and setting. In addition, the measures do not fall neatly into domains but instead describe related constructs in different ways, or combine apparently unrelated constructs. Grouping diverse measures into domains can help to provide a checklist of possible targets for clinicians and researchers. It is still far too common to read reports of large-scale trials of analgesics that employ several measures of pain but none of function, mood, or sleep, which may be affected by pain and by treatment and are often of concern to patients with chronic pain and to those who treat them.

While other chapters in this volume review psychological measures, this chapter describes psychological influences on measures of pain and its impact—an underaddressed area that is ripe for further research. It is becoming increasingly clear that cognitive and behavioral variables are important in their own right through their influence on pain persistence and on the extent of disability (Pincus et al. 2002). Recognition of the complex interrelationships of pain with cognitive, emotional, and behavioral factors effectively dismantles the traditional view of pain and pain relief as the determinants of behavioral and psychological impact.

MEASURING CHANGE

A more difficult issue than covering domains is that of deciding what, in terms of threshold of pain or amount of change, is clinically significant. Fifty percent pain relief was and is a common aim and outcome of analgesic treatment, although no one has demonstrated that 50% is sufficient for recovery of function and adequate reduction of pain impact on everyday life. Days of work lost through pain is another common outcome, but more detailed investigation shows that even where the number of workdays is unaffected, patients may report extensive effects on quality of work (Blyth et al. 2003). Clinicians will be familiar with accounts of patients who are held back from career progression or promotion by limitations related to pain; being back at work and rarely off sick (commonly identified as desirable outcomes) may still leave the patient disappointed and with his or her life plans derailed. Setting an adequate threshold or percentage of change is enormously difficult in the pain field because of the subjective nature of the targets of treatment and the absence of external referents. If, for instance, almost all patients who attained 50% pain relief also declined offers of further attempts at treatment, declared themselves satisfied, and reported significantly improved everyday function, then a minimum of 50% pain relief would be an obvious aim of treatment. Even in the thoughtful studies showing that around 30% relief is sufficient for cancer patients to refrain from requesting additional analgesics (Farrar et al. 2000), the authors acknowledge that factors other than satisfactory analgesia (such as patients' dislike of taking drugs, or unfounded fears about their use) can account for patients' decisions.

Careful data exploration before applying statistical tests offers the clinician or researcher the opportunity to address more specific hypotheses than the general ones about treatment efficacy, and to test for particular effects or interactions (Cohen 1994). Consideration of what is "good enough change" at an earlier stage than interpretation of statistical findings is highly recommended, and can be defined in terms of percentage change, or in terms of thresholds or healthy norms where available, or of absolute scores (e.g., absence of symptoms). Alternative statistical methods can be used to test for mean change in relation to standard deviation of scores (effect size; see Rosenthal 1994) and in relation to reliability of the measure (reliable change index; see Jacobson et al. 1999); see also Hsu (1999). More common in medical trials is the use of probability in relation to categorical outcomes, in particular odds and likelihood ratios, risk indices, and number needed to treat (see Sackett et al. 1991; Crombie and Davies 1996). Morley and Williams (2002) and Kendall et al. (1999) provide a fuller discussion of the options for defining clinical significance rather than substituting statistical significance values, as is common practice.

SELECTION OF MEASURES

The tasks expected of pain assessment measures are considerable and cannot all be met; a particular strength may be counterbalanced by relative weakness in an aspect of more importance for the specific task at hand. The clinician or researcher must consider the following: Are the theoretical constructs that are implied or instantiated in the measure consistent with his or her own outlook? Does the content include issues of prime concern and not too many irrelevant items? Is the output in continuous dimensions or is it categorical, and is that output therefore suitable for the task and the planned analyses? For children and adolescents, the context of cognitive and emotional development is also relevant. If the answers to these questions are positive, then psychometric properties and previous performance should be examined against the tasks to be addressed in the particular population and sample size of concern. Skipping the conceptual issues and checking only psychometric properties often results in considerable confusion when we try to interpret the measures that have fallen short of task expectations.

Assessment may serve a variety of purposes, not all of which can necessarily be anticipated when selecting measurement devices. Of the common purposes, some measures have more obvious clinical use in tracking progress or deterioration in a patient's condition or performance, in conveying that information to the patient or to other interested parties, and in enabling clinicians to test and disconfirm the working hypotheses that underpin treatment. Other measures are better for describing populations and for making broad comparisons across patients with the same condition, or may even, as with quality of life measures, be designed for comparison across all states of health and all conditions. Assessment can make substantial demands on the time of patients, assessors, and those who manage the database; thus, selection usually aims to identify measures that are able to serve multiple purposes. Measures are designed and even sometimes described by their proponents as suitable for all purposes. However, all measures are developed through iteration of costs (such as length) against benefits (such as extent of coverage), and compromises between these factors inevitably restrict their utility. Brevity is obtained at the cost of breadth or depth of content, and breadth and depth are attained at the cost of demands made on the respondent, demands that may exhaust the respondent's desire to answer as accurately as possible. A further cost, although for some purposes it could be a benefit, is that breadth of a measure makes a single summary score harder to interpret, although in some circumstances it will still represent the best compromise to be made. These comments are equally applicable to measures of pain and of its impact, although they are more usually made of the latter.

Arguably, these considerations still receive too little weight in the choice of outcome measures in many studies, and it is widely regarded as akin to train-spotting to show interest in the details of measurements. Fitzpatrick et al. (1998) listed the criteria for selection as appropriateness to purpose, reliability, validity, sensitivity to change, precision in making distinctions, interpretability, acceptability, and feasibility in practical terms. They deplored the failure to systematically assess and report these criteria and the consequent impossibility of creating a league table of measures. Data on reliability and validity are available for most measures, but while it would be enormously helpful if a measure could be described unconditionally as reliable and valid, this ideal is no more realistic than claiming to have found a universally effective and harm-free analgesic. Every measure originates in a population from which some individuals have inevitably been excluded by age, by pathology, by language or culture, or by state of health or illness. If it is clear why they have been excluded, then the limitations of straightforward interpretation of the measure are also clear. If the exclusions are inadvertent, unrecognized, or not described (perhaps because the measure was developed on a clinical population preselected by criteria obscure to the assessors), then those limitations are covert but may significantly affect interpretation.

Any attempt to identify reliability and validity is in a sense an exercise in separating systematic variation from random effects (see Dworkin and Sherman 2001). Systematic variation can be identified, and in some circumstances even manipulated, to improve interpretability of a measure; as clinicians we are quick to spot patterns (including illusory ones) and to attribute improvement to treatment rather than to random effects. The details of reliability and validity are well described in many texts on measurement (e.g., McDowell and Newell 1996), including an excellent source specific to the pain field (Turk and Melzack 2001a), and in less depth in chapters in pain textbooks (Williams 1999; Turk and Okifuji 2003). Becoming familiar with those details is a wise investment for any researcher. For the clinician, the more immediate concern is to read sufficient background on selected measures so as to be able to identify those that best meet the purposes of assessment. Measures described here have at least adequate published reports of their reliability and validity, although excluded measures are not necessarily inadequate. A complete guide is impossible within the confines of this chapter, which gives priority to measures in reasonably wide use in the pain field.

ASSESSMENT OF PAIN EXPERIENCE

The broadest dimensions in which pain can reasonably be described are sensory intensity, emotional and cognitive aspects, and interference with everyday life (Price 1999). Even pain-free subjects can distinguish intensity and unpleasantness of common pain events from memory (Kee et al. 2001). Each of these dimensions can be measured in a variety of ways: intensity can be described at its worst, at its least, on average, and at the moment of rating; interference can be subdivided into interference with domestic life, social life, employment, education or training, and so on. The effect of combining those different dimensions of pain into a single assessment tool can be problematic, whether by presenting the patient with a unidimensional measure or by recombining separate measures, as is common in headache. For instance, Clark and Yang (2001) found that emotional rather than sensory qualities of pain predicted pain ratings on a unidimensional scale, and concluded that such unidimensional scores are poor as measures. Although multidimensionality is thoroughly theorized (Holroyd et al. 1999; see Price 1999) and repeatedly demonstrated, unidimensional measures of pain remain the norm in clinical research and practice. Work on measurement of pain by Jensen and colleagues (2001) showed nonlinear relationships between numerically rated pain and its impact on function. Instead, this work showed thresholds for effects on function. In another study, some patients quantified their pain by reference to both function and mood (Williams et al. 2000). Of course, distinctions between dimensions of pain are conceptually difficult to investigate because sensory qualities can increase unpleasantness, and emotional and motivational variables can affect perceptual and memory processes necessitated by the act of rating pain (Kihlstrom et al. 1999; Price 1999).

SPATIAL, NUMERICAL, AND VERBAL SCALES

The visual analogue scale (VAS) remains one of the most popular measures, despite the slightly superior reliability and greater practicality of the numerical rating scale (NRS) (Jensen et al. 1999; Williams et al. 2000; Jensen and Karoly 2001; Turk and Okifuji 2003). Any expression of pain is effectively an exercise in cross-modality matching: a VAS or NRS expresses pain spatially or arithmetically. The more familiar the modality is to respondents, the less error may be introduced into the matching process; hence the decline in use of unfamiliar modalities such as squeeze against resistance. A 0–10-point rating scale with half integers marked offers a 21-point scale, the most that respondents appear to need or use (Williams et al. 2000). Jensen and Karoly (2001) discuss measurement of other important aspects of pain, including spatial aspects such as locations and body systems where pain is felt, and temporal aspects such as frequency, constancy, and pain-free periods. Surprisingly, patients' own descriptions of pain quantity such as "good/bad days" are not commonly used. Two-thirds of the graduates of a pain management program recorded an increase in "good days" and a decrease in "bad days," a result only in small part accounted for by average pain intensity and interference scores (personal observation).

Various scales have been proposed for children and adolescents, including cartoon and photographed faces for children under 5 years old, and adapted or adult spatial, verbal, and numerical scales for older children. These scales have been developed and tested almost exclusively in acute pain events rather than in persistent pain problems (e.g., Hicks et al. 2001; see also McGrath and Unruh 1999). The predominance of episodic pain such as headache in chronic pain treatment trials has established the use of diary forms that record (on numerical or verbal scales) intensity, duration, and frequency of pain or pain-free days (e.g., McGrath et al. 1992).

Another popular measure of pain is the McGill Pain Questionnaire (MPQ: Melzack 1975), developed partly for differential diagnosis but widely used in outcome evaluation. Although the structure varies somewhat across studies, doubtless because of differences in populations and in statistical methods, overall the questionnaire reliably provides scores of sensory, affective, and evaluative components of pain (Melzack and Katz 1999). While the search for robust factors is important, as are the implications of substantial correlations between factors, the major strength of the MPQ in separating these components of pain, if only partially, is lost in the use of its single summary measure—number of words chosen. Verbal scales, although generally easy to administer and high on face validity, present problems for scaling and scoring that compromise their usefulness for many purposes (Jensen and Karoly 2001).

The frequency and timing of ratings have been investigated more extensively. Jensen and Karoly (2001) recommend that an average of multiple recordings should be used whenever possible in preference to a single retrospective rating of average pain. Patients' preference for using electronic diaries rather than paper diaries (Jamison et al. 2001; Stone et al. 2003), their better adherence to electronic diaries, and the opportunity such diaries provide for random sampling that detects the considerable variability across the day (Peters et al. 2000) make electronic diaries the best option if funds permit. Mean pain levels obscure systematic and potentially important differences between, for instance, pain at rest and on activities that may provoke pain (such as walking or coughing), and specifically sampling these activities can be informative. Retrospective ratings differ from averaged diary ratings (Bolton 1999; Peters et al. 2000), and retrospective ratings of change are distinct from the difference between pre- and post-treatment pain ratings (Fischer et al. 1999). One claim (Fischer et al. 1999) of greater sensitivity of retrospective rating to change is based on its stronger association with satisfaction, but as satisfaction was assessed at the same time as the retrospective rating, the two measures are not sufficiently independent for this argument to stand. In addition, Haas et al. (2002) found a strong relationship between present pain and recalled relief; because the latter was higher for those with greater present pain, they recommended the use of calculated rather than recalled relief.

Surprisingly few studies compare measures of pain (Jensen and Karoly 2001 is an exception), but many papers that report the use of more than one measure for the same dimension of pain find good agreement to the extent that one or more measures are effectively redundant. These papers are the nearest we have to studies of reliability and validity; both concepts are hard to apply to fluctuating subjective experiences with no "gold standard" against which to compare patients' reports. The use of multiple unidimensional measures of pain is wasteful, although the pain scales included in measures of broad scope, such as that in the Short Form 36 (SF-36) of the Medical Outcomes Study (Ware et al. 1993) or the Nottingham Health Profile (Hunt et al. 1985), are usually unsatisfactory and require supplementing or extending if pain is a major focus of assessment (Wagner et al. 1996).

BEHAVIORAL MEASURES OF PAIN

Behavioral measures of pain, including facial expression, offer rich information where resources allow detailed observation and analysis. Behavioral measures are most suited to small-scale studies. Keefe and colleagues (2001) provide a rationale for the observation of pain behavior in clinical settings. Real-time assessments are now being developed that will make it easier to measure relevant behaviors and that will be preferable to self-report schedules of questionable reliability and validity. However, behavior is a broad category, and we have good arguments for distinguishing behaviors with little or incomplete voluntary control, such as facial expression, posture, and gait, from those resulting more from conscious decision, such as seeking help, taking analgesics, or taking time off from work (Williams 2003a). Of course, all behaviors are influenced by a range of social and contextual variables. Standard observational procedures are preferable for recording and controlling these variables; checklists inevitably convey pain behavior as entirely the property of the individual. With refinement and wider use of new observational measures, we should begin to understand the variables that determine frequency and intensity of pain behaviors, from medical variables (Keefe et al. 1984) to spouse behavior (Romano et al. 1992). Facial expression is particularly important for measuring pain in infants and small children (Craig et al. 2001); the Child Facial Coding System (Chambers et al. 1996) offers reliable real-time measurement protocols for clinicians and parents.

Facial expression of pain is well described by Craig et al. (2001); more recently, Prkachin et al. (2002) developed a promising real-time in vivo assessment tool for use during standard physical examination of patients with low back pain. It includes facial expression, defined by muscle actions; guarding (including stiff movement, limping, and flinching); and non-word sounds (such as moaning or sighing). This tool in turn built on the standard assessment developed by Keefe and Block (1982), usually recorded on videotape for later coding of samples. These methods offer tools for examining clinical interactions around pain problems, a relatively neglected area, although decisions resulting from these interactions determine how patients progress through the health care system.

IMPACT OF PAIN, DISABILITY, AND QUALITY OF LIFE

Any instrument has built-in definitions, values, and assumptions that may differ considerably among measures with the same title (such as quality of life). Publications on the development of disability and quality of life measures usually show that item content is drawn not from the population under study but from health professionals (Bowling 1997). Other definitions, even those as widely adopted as the World Health Organization's definition of health as total well-being, are not easy to operationalize in measurement tools. The issue of social validity—the demonstration that the goals of treatment are important to the patient—is rarely addressed (Foster and Mash 1999). Diverse individuals and groups with a stake in treatment outcome (such as family members, employers, colleagues, health care professionals, health care funders, taxpayers, and lawyers) may have goals that are incompatible or only partially compatible. Social validity is a particularly important quality in measures used for health comparisons or economic calculations.

The issue of definition is crucial: definitions of normality and health are built into scales of disability and quality of life, particularly in areas such as employment and sexual activity. Questions about employment do not always reflect the activities of the self-employed, of seasonal or casual or contract workers, or of homemakers. Questions about sex often imply heterosexual sexual activity and ignore the quality of the dyadic relationship and often of other social relationships. In addition to these obvious examples, other activities may encompass variables, including choice and opportunity, that may interact with pain to determine the response. Social goals, often of high importance to the patient, are generally underrepresented in favor of goals with implications for health and welfare services (Batterham et al. 1996). Surprisingly little research aims to identify what contributes to quality of life (Bowling 1997; Fitzpatrick et al. 1998) and how its determinants may change with age (Gagliese 2001). This situation leads to considerable difficulty in determining clinical significance of change.

The narrower the definition and scope of the content of a measure (the narrowest focusing on self-care and mobility, the broadest including social and spiritual well-being), the easier it is to operationalize in a questionnaire. Hyland (1992) and Batterham et al. (1996) drew attention to the lack of understanding of processes of change and improvement and emphasized that it is unknown how the respondent evaluates aspects of his or her life. Hyland particularly criticized the loss of information when domains are added to produce a single total, and also challenged assumptions of comparability of positive and negative quality of life. Content varies considerably for putatively equivalent questionnaires used in the health field (Williams 2003b), yet even the broadest is unlikely to be sufficient alone. Subscales commonly require supplementing with disease-specific measures to achieve adequate sensitivity (Bowling 1997; Fitzpatrick and Dawson 1997). Overall, quality of life measures lack theories and definitions (Bowling 1997; Gladis et al. 1999). Ideally, conceptual discussion would precede the development and marketing of yet more measures that instantiate particular cultural values, represent only patchily the goals closest to patients' hearts, and foster the illusion that a patient's life can be represented by a single score. However, shorter measures that focus on impact of pain on function tend not to include items describing positive well-being; such items are more commonly included in measures looking at the full scope of quality of life and may be highly relevant in the overall outcome of pain treatments.

As in pain ratings, emotional state can influence report of activity and activity limitations (Hyland 1992) and disability scores (Mannion et al. 2001; Turk and Melzack 2001b). Cognitive variables also influence reports of activity: events that respondents consider to be regular are retrieved as a rate of occurrence, while episodic and irregular events are more likely to be estimated with varying degrees of accuracy (Menon and Yorkston 1999). The implication of this finding is that categories for retrieval should match respondents' categories as well as possible, yet almost all measures of function and disability are derived from professionals' categories (Bowling 1997).

More directly, psychological variables can be major predictors of physical performance measures (Simmonds et al. 1998; Watson 1999; Rudy et al. 2003). Simmonds recommends the abandonment of impairment measures from which function is inferred, and is critical of self-report measures that are subject to cognitive bias. However, whether her aim of developing functional performance measures free of these influences is possible is a moot point. The field is moving from a simple position of using performance measures as a proxy for impairment to a more integrated understanding of the multiple influences on patients' behavior, some of which are inaccessible to self-report. One influence is the sense of safety that the attendance of a qualified health professional (supposedly as a "neutral observer") may convey in the test setting. This sense of safety gives a context to self-report in measures such as those reviewed below: they may tell us less about the ideal maximum performances the patient can achieve than about his or her beliefs about which activities it is safe to perform regularly.

Measures with acceptable psychometric properties (many reviewed by Gladis et al. 1999) are discussed briefly below; for more detail refer to Turk and Melzack (2001a), Williams (1999), and McDowell and Newell (1996).

IMPACT OF PAIN

Epidemiological studies are increasingly recognizing the influence of pain as an important variable in restricting usual activity (Blyth et al. 2001; Reyes-Gibby et al. 2002; see Von Korff 2001 for review). These studies may assess such influence by using a few carefully worded questions and a rating scale. Work records, if available, can usefully supplement patients' subjective ratings of impact of pain on work and recalled estimates of time lost from work. However, studies cannot justifiably use work alone to measure treatment outcome (Dionne et al. 1999), since work is related rather variably to broader functional status. A rarely used but telling statistic is the proportion by which household income has fallen as a result of pain in a wage-earner. In a study in The Netherlands (which has relatively generous disability rates), Kemler and Furnee (2002) discovered a 47% reduction in household income for male patients and a 29% reduction for females, with additional extra expenses of U.S.$1,350 yearly. Another important and underassessed area is the impact of pain on health service use. Ideally, health records are available and accessible; when they are not, patients' recall of inpatient and outpatient visits and procedures can provide some approximate measures of demands on the health system.

The Brief Pain Inventory (BPI), the Pain Disability Index (PDI), and the Chronic Pain Grade Scale (CPGS) are three short but useful measures of the impact of pain. The three measures sample from domains of interest in different ways: the BPI and CPGS are divided between pain and its impact on everyday activities. The BPI (Daut et al. 1983; Cleeland and Ryan 1994) also assesses the influence of pain on mood. It is mainly used for cancer patients but apparently performs well in chronic pain populations (Breitbart et al. 1996; Reyes-Gibby et al. 2002; C. Price et al.). The PDI (Tait et al. 1987, 1990) does not include pain items but samples seven aspects of function, including social activity, and normally gives a single measure of pain impact on function (Jacobs and Kerns 2001). However, the items may be too nonspecific to reflect the effect of pain on elderly people (Gagliese 2001). Both the BPI and PDI provide simple sums of unweighted scores of pain impact, making interpretation relatively straightforward. The CPGS (Von Korff et al. 1992; Von Korff 2001) also assesses the impact of pain on everyday activities and was developed in community and primary care settings. It includes eight questions that provide four categories or grades, the

lower two describing low and high pain intensity accompanied by low interference with usual, daily, social and recreational, and work activities, and
the higher two describing moderate and high interference of pain (of any
severity) with those activities. The measure is supplemented by an estimate
of days of pain in the preceding 6 months. The CPGS was designed primarily for cross-sectional rather than longitudinal research questions. Its brevity and acceptability recommend it for wide use in primary care settings, but
a ceiling effect is likely in hospitalized patients with chronic pain.

DISABILITY AND FUNCTION

Three shorter measures of disability or pain impact with narrower scope
than quality of life are in common use. The Roland and Morris short version
of the Sickness Impact Profile (Roland and Morris 1983) is the most biased
toward the physical domain, with 21 of its 24 questions concerned with
physical function, and the remaining three addressing impact of pain on
sleep, temper, and appetite. Although the yes/no response options may make
questions easy to answer, they may also blunt sensitivity to change. The
Oswestry Low Back Pain Disability Questionnaire (Fairbank et al. 1980),
most commonly used in the United Kingdom, is also predominantly physical
in content. One section concerns pain, six sections concern functions ranging from lifting to traveling, and the remainder concern sex life, social life,
and sleep. Respondents select the most appropriate statement from the six in
each section, which are graded in severity, and the total score is divided by
the possible maximum for a percentage. The Oswestry scale has largely
unknown psychometric properties, but offers varied data. An international
meeting of back pain researchers (Deyo et al. 1998) recommended the
Oswestry and Roland and Morris scales for standard use in patients with
back pain. They would make less sense for patients with predominantly
upper body pain: psychometric properties must be re-established for mixed
groups. The Multidimensional Pain Inventory (WHYMPI/MPI: Kerns et al.
1985; Jacobs and Kerns 2001) covers psychosocial and physical activity
more evenly and with superior content. It includes 3 questions on pain
severity, 9 on interference, 5 on cognitive and affective matters, 3 on social
support in general, 14 on a significant other person's response to pain, and
22 on frequency of a range of activities. It appears to perform well as an
outcome measure (Jacobs and Kerns 2001).

QUALITY OF LIFE

One of the broadest in scope and most widely used quality of life measures is the SF-36 (Ware et al. 1993; Ruta et al. 1994), covering physical functioning, role limitations (physical), pain, mental health, social functioning, role limitations (emotional), general health, and vitality domains in 36 items with varied response categories. The measure compensates for different numbers of items and response categories in subscales by weighting to give 0–100-point scales, but is potentially misleading. Its strengths include thorough development and the availability of norms from many populations and states of health and illness. Its weaknesses include low test-retest reliability of some subscales (Ware et al. 1993), floor effects for severely ill or disabled people, and ceiling effects for healthy people, all of which reduce its sensitivity to change and indicate poor construct validity. Physical function, for example, is heavily influenced by mobility problems (Bowling 1997). Details of the SF-36 and of a shorter version, the SF-12, are available on the Internet (www.sf36.com).

A quality of life measure of even broader scope that was developed for cross-cultural use is the WHOQOL-100 (WHOQOL Group 1995). It covers 25 dimensions (including pain and discomfort) grouped into six domains: physical, psychological, social, levels of independence (function), environment, and spirituality. The WHOQOL-100 has been tested in the pain field (Skevington 1998) and appears to be sensitive to change with treatment (Skevington et al. 2001). However, 100 questions is excessive for many patients. In addition, some questions (e.g., on environmental factors) deal with areas that are not expected to change with treatment but are more useful for comparing populations. A 16-item version, the WHOQOL-BREF assessment (WHOQOL Group 1998), is promising but has no track record in pain populations; details can be found on the Internet (www.who.int/msa/qol).

People close to the patient may also be asked for their estimates and opinions on the effect of pain on function and quality of life, for the patient and themselves. Surprisingly few well-developed measures address these issues; a review by Sharp and Nicholas (2000) commends the "significant other" version of the MPI (Kerns and Rosenberg 1995) for its content and psychometric properties. These questions, many parallel to the patient version, assess interference of pain with the patient's life and with that of the significant other, including emotional effects, social support, and responses of the significant other to the patient's pain. Clarifying the significant other as "the person with whom you feel closest" improves the response rate (Jacob and Kerns 2001). It is important, of course, to recognize that the proxy gives not an objective account but an alternative subjective account of the subject.

Adults can assess or rate the effect of pain on children's behavior at home, in the classroom, and among peers through scales widely used in pediatric psychology, which are beyond the scope of this chapter. Attribution of findings to pain itself may be difficult in persistent pain due to the lack of a pain-free baseline for comparison. Adolescent chronic pain studies report on several disability and quality of life scales, but the paucity of child and adolescent pain trials and the relative neglect of measures other than of pain (Eccleston and Malleson 2003) mean that none of these measures have yet acquired a track record that permits estimation of usefulness for research or clinical practice.

Another use for broad measures, but particularly for the MPI, is patient profiling to select for or predict the outcome of treatment. However, establishing their validity would require empirical testing incompatible with clinical practice, namely, assessing and treating all potential patients without selection (or randomly assigning them across treatments), then comparing the outcome to pretreatment scores. Even such data, if ever available, would warrant cautious analysis (see Morley and Williams 2002) because the multivariate determination of treatment outcome means that prediction will never be exact, and could result in unethical rejection of patients who would benefit from treatment. An alternative approach is to formulate problems in secure theory and to apply tested treatments individualized to the patient's goals and current performance, as in the work on fear-based avoidance of activity by Vlaeyen and colleagues (see Vlaeyen and Linton 2000; Vlaeyen 2003). Allowing patients to self-select for treatment components may result in their further avoidance of physical rehabilitation (Evers et al. 2002), and there is no a priori reason to expect that patients will select the most effective approach for their problems.

CONCLUSIONS

This chapter has largely taken the patient's perspective for assessment. Delivery of health care places greater weight than formerly on the patient's priorities and preferences in selecting and delivering treatments, and it is the patient who is, ultimately, sufficiently satisfied with treatment gains to return to a (more) normal life, to consider himself or herself reasonably healthy and no longer in need of health care, and to cease to be a patient. In many texts discussing pain as a major complaint, puzzled comments address the patient's dissatisfaction with the effect of a "successful" treatment. Such a comment points to the measure of "success" as the problem, rather than the patient's obduracy.

Neglected areas of measurement in published studies, and therefore unavailable to other researchers, include changes in work quality and quantity, in income and time available for social and leisure pursuits, and in health care use. A lack of models of interrelationship of measures leads to false assumptions of the domains sampled and invalid conclusions about statistical relationships discovered. For instance, poorer outcome of treatment in patients with compensation claims may be mediated by pain level and previous treatment (Burns et al. 1995) or by work status (Mendelson 1994), but if these factors are not assessed, the tendency is to attribute poor outcome simply to the compensation factor. In addition, measures are lacking in certain areas, particularly in assessing the impact of the pain on those close to the patient. More broadly, many measures are developed on a population base that is narrow in age and culture. Gender differences in a mixed population are often not investigated, although they may exist and be important to those proposing to use the measure. More thoughtful use of existing measures offers as much benefit as the development of new ones, and the researcher or clinician who can interpret and disseminate results with confidence in the tools used is on strong ground indeed.

REFERENCES

Batterham RW, Dunt DR, Disler PB. Can we achieve accountability for long-term outcomes? *Arch Phys Med Rehab* 1996; 77:1219–1225.

Blyth FM, March LM, Brnabic AJM, et al. Chronic pain in Australia: a prevalence study. *Pain* 2001; 89:127–134.

Blyth FM, March LM, Nicholas MK, Cousins MJ. Chronic pain, work performance and litigation. *Pain* 2003; 103:41–47.

Bolton JE. Accuracy of recall of usual pain intensity in back pain patients. *Pain* 1999; 83:533–539.

Bowling A. *Measuring Health,* 2nd ed. Buckingham: Open University Press, 1997.

Breitbart W, McDonald MV, Rosenfeld B, et al. Pain in ambulatory AIDS patients. I: Pain characteristics and medical correlates. *Pain* 1996; 68:315–321.

Burns JW, Sherman ML, Devine J, Mahoney N, Pawl R. Association between workers' compensation and outcome following multidisciplinary treatment for chronic pain: roles of mediators and moderators. *Clin J Pain* 1995; 11:94–102.

Chambers CT, Cassidy KL, McGrath PJ, Gilbert CA, Craig KD. *Child Facial Coding System: A Manual.* Halifax and Vancouver: Dalhousie University/University of British Columbia, 1996.

Clark WC, Yang JC. What do simple unidimensional pain scales really measure? *J Pain* 2001; 2(Suppl 1):6.

Cleeland CS, Ryan KM. Pain assessment: global use of the Brief Pain Inventory. *Ann Acad Med* 1994; 23:129–138.

Cohen J. The earth is round (p < .05). *Am Psychol* 1994; 49:997–1003.

Craig KD, Prkachin KM, Grunau RE. The facial expression of pain. In: Turk DC, Melzack R (Eds). *Handbook of Pain Assessment,* 2nd ed. New York: Guilford Press, 2001, pp 153–169.

Crombie IK, Davies HTO. *Research in Health Care: Design, Conduct and Interpretation of Health Services Research.* Chichester: John Wiley and Sons, 1996.

Daut RL, Cleeland CS, Flaner RC. Development of the Wisconsin Brief Pain Questionnaire to assess pain in cancer and other diseases. *Pain* 1983; 17:197–210.

Dionne CE, Von Korff M, Koepsell TD, et al. A comparison of pain, functional limitations, and work status indices as outcome measures in back pain research. *Spine* 1999; 24:2339–2345.

Deyo RA, Battie M, Beurskens AJHM, et al. Outcome measures for low back pain research: a proposal for standardized use. *Spine* 1998; 23:2003–2013.

Dworkin SF, Sherman JJ. Relying on objective and subjective measures of chronic pain: guidelines for use and interpretation. In: Turk DC, Melzack R (Eds). *Handbook of Pain Assessment,* 2nd ed. New York: Guilford Press, 2001, pp 619–638.

Eccleston C, Malleson P. Managing chronic pain in children and adolescents. *BMJ* 2003; 326:1408–1409.

Evers AWM, Kraaimaat FW, van Riel PLCM, de Jong AJL. Tailored cognitive-behavioral therapy in early rheumatoid arthritis for patients at risk: a randomized controlled trial. *Pain* 2002; 100:141–153.

Fairbank JCT, Couper J, Davies JB, O'Brien JP. The Oswestry low back pain Disability Questionnaire. *Physiotherapy* 1980; 66:271–273.

Farrar JT, Portenoy RK, Berlin JA, Kinman JL, Strom BL. Defining the clinically important difference in pain outcome measures. *Pain* 2000; 88:287–294.

Fischer D, Stewart AL, Bloch DA, et al. Capturing the patient's view of change as a clinical outcome measure. *JAMA* 1999; 282:1157–1162.

Fitzpatrick R, Dawson J. Health-related quality of life and the assessment of outcomes of total hip replacement surgery. *Psychol Health* 1997; 12:793–803.

Fitzpatrick R, Davey C, Buxton MJ, Jones DR. Evaluating patient-based outcome measures for use in clinical trials. *Health Technol Assess* 1998; 2:14.

Foster SL, Mash EJ. Assessing social validity in clinical treatment research: issues and procedures. *J Consult Clin Psychol* 1999; 67:308–319.

Gagliese L. Assessment of pain in elderly people. In: Turk DC, Melzack R (Eds). *Handbook of Pain Assessment,* 2nd ed. New York: Guilford Press, 2001, pp 119–133.

Gladis MM, Gosch EA, Dishuk NM, Crits-Cristoph P. Quality of life: expanding the scope of clinical significance. *J Consult Clin Psychol* 1999; 67:320–331.

Haas M, Nyiendo J, Aickin M. One-year trend in pain and disability relief in acute and chronic ambulatory low back pain patients. *Pain* 2002; 95:83–91.

Hadjistavropoulos T, von Baeyer C, Craig KD. Pain assessment in persons with limited ability to communicate. In: Turk DC, Melzack R (Eds). *Handbook of Pain Assessment,* 2nd ed. New York: Guilford Press, 2001, pp 134–149.

Hicks CL, von Baeyer CL, Spafford PA, van Korlaar I, Goodenough B. The Faces Pain Scale-Revised: toward a common metric in pediatric pain measurement. *Pain* 2001; 93:173–183.

Holroyd KA, Malinoski P, Davis MK, Lipchik GL. The three dimensions of headache impact: pain, disability and affective distress. *Pain* 1999; 83:571–578.

Hsu LM. Caveats concerning comparisons of change rates obtained with five methods of identifying significant client changes: comment on Speer and Greenbaum (1995). *J Consult Clin Psychol* 1999; 67:594–598.

Hunt SM, McEwen J, McKenna SP. Measuring health status: a new tool for clinicians and epidemiologists. *J R Coll Gen Pract* 1985; 35:185–188.

Hyland ME. A reformulation of quality of life for medical science. *Qual Life Res* 1992; 1:267–272.

Jacobs MC, Kerns RD. Assessment of the psychosocial context of the experience of chronic pain. In: Turk DC, Melzack R (Eds). *Handbook of Pain Assessment,* 2nd ed. New York: Guilford Press, 2001, pp 362–384.

Jacobson NS, Roberts LJ, Berns SB, McGlinchey JB. Methods for defining and determining the clinical significance of treatment effects: description, application, and alternatives. *J Consult Clin Psychol* 1999; 67:300–307.

Jamison RN, Raymond SA, Levine JG, et al. Electronic diaries for monitoring chronic pain: 1-year validation study. *Pain* 2001; 91:277–285.

Jensen MP, Karoly P. Self-report scales and procedures for assessing pain in adults. In: Turk DC, Melzack R (Eds). *Handbook of Pain Assessment,* 2nd ed. New York: Guilford Press, 2001, pp 15–34.

Jensen MP, Turner JA, Romano JM, Fisher LD. Comparative reliability and validity of chronic pain intensity measures. *Pain* 1999; 83:157–162.

Jensen MP, Smith DG, Ehde DM, Robinson LR. Pain site and the effects of amputation pain: further clarification of the meaning of mild, moderate and severe pain. *Pain* 2001; 91:317–322.

Kee WG, Manning EL, Wallsten TS. Do intensity and unpleasantness function independently in predicting the aversiveness of pain events? *J Pain* 2001; 2(Suppl 1):7.

Keefe FJ, Block AR. Development of an observation method for assessing pain behavior in chronic low back pain patients. *Behav Ther* 1982; 13:363–375.

Keefe FJ, Wilkins RH, Cook WA. Direct observation of pain behavior in low back pain patients during physical examination. *Pain* 1984; 20:59–68.

Keefe FJ, Williams DA, Smith SJ. Assessment of pain behaviors. In: Turk DC, Melzack R (Eds). *Handbook of Pain Assessment,* 2nd ed. New York: Guilford Press, 2001, pp 170–187.

Kemler MA, Furnee CA. The impact of chronic pain on life in the household. *J Pain Symptom Manage* 2002; 23:433–441.

Kendall PC, Marrs-Garcia A, Nath SR, Sheldrick RC. Normative comparisons for the evaluation of clinical significance. *J Consult Clin Psychol* 1999; 47:285–299.

Kerns RD, Rosenberg R. Pain relevant responses from significant others: development of a significant-other version of the WHYMPI scales. *Pain* 1995; 61:245–259.

Kerns RD, Turk DC, Rudy TE. The West Haven-Yale Multidimensional Pain Inventory (WHYMPI). *Pain* 1985; 23:345–356.

Kihlstrom JF, Eich E, Sandbrand D, Tobias BA. Emotion and memory: implications for self-report. In: Stone AA, Turkkan JS, Bachrach CA, et al. (Eds). *The Science of Self-Report: Implications for Research and Practice*. Mahwah, NJ: Lawrence Erlbaum, 1999, pp 81–99.

Mannion AF, Junge A, Taimela S, et al. Active therapy for chronic low back pain: Part 3. Factors influencing self-rated disability and its change following therapy. *Spine* 2001; 26:920–929.

McDowell I, Newell C. *Measuring Health: A Guide to Rating Scales and Questionnaires,* 2nd ed. New York: Oxford University Press, 1996.

McGrath PJ, Unruh AM. Measurement and assessment of paediatric pain. In: Wall PD, Melzack R (Eds). *Textbook of Pain,* 4th ed. Edinburgh: Churchill Livingstone, 1999, pp 371–384.

McGrath PJ, Humphreys P, Keene D, et al. The efficacy and efficiency of a self-administered treatment for adolescent migraine. *Pain* 1992; 49:321–324.

Melzack R. The McGill Pain Questionnaire: major properties and scoring methods. *Pain* 1975; 1:277–299.

Melzack R, Katz J. Pain measurement in persons in pain. In: Melzack R, Wall PD (Eds). *Textbook of Pain,* 4th ed. Edinburgh: Churchill Livingstone, 1999, pp 409–426.

Mendelson G. Chronic pain and compensation issues. In: Wall PD, Melzack R (Eds). *Textbook of Pain,* 3rd ed. Edinburgh: Churchill Livingstone, 1994, pp 1387–1400.

Menon G, Yorkston EA. The use of memory and contextual cues in the formation of behavioral frequency judgements. In: Stone AA, Turkkan JS, Bachrach CA, et al. (Eds). *The Science of Self-Report: Implications for Research and Practice.* Mahwah, NJ: Lawrence Erlbaum, 1999, pp 63–79.

Morley S, Williams AC de C. Conducting and evaluating treatment outcome studies. In: Turk DC, Gatchel R (Eds). *Psychological Approaches to Pain Management: A Practitioner's Handbook,* 2nd ed. New York: Guilford Press, 2002, pp 52–68.

Peters ML, Sorbi MJ, Kruise DA, et al. Electronic diary assessment of pain, disability and psychological adaptation in patients differing in duration of pain. *Pain* 2000; 84:181–192.

Pincus T, Burton AK, Vogel S, Field AP. A systematic review of psychological factors as predictors of chronicity/disability in prospective cohorts of low back pain. *Spine* 2002; 27:E109–E120.

Price DD. *Psychological Mechanisms of Pain and Analgesia,* Progress in Pain Research and Management, Vol. 15. Seattle: IASP Press, 1999.

Prkachin KM, Hughes E, Schultz I, Joy P, Hunt D. Real-time assessment of pain behavior during clinical assessment of low back pain patients. *Pain* 2002; 95:23–30.

Reyes-Gibby CC, Aday L, Cleeland C. Impact of pain on self-rated health in the community-dwelling older adults. *Pain* 2002; 95:75–82.

Roland M, Morris R. A study of the natural history of back pain. Part I. Development of a reliable and sensitive measure of disability in low-back pain. *Spine* 1983; 8:141–144.

Romano JM, Turner HA, Friedman LS, et al. Sequential analysis of chronic pain behaviors and spouse responses. *J Consult Clin Psychol* 1992; 60:777–782.

Rosenthal R. Parametric measures of effect size. In: Cooper H, Hedges LV (Eds). *The Handbook of Research Synthesis.* New York: Russell Sage Foundation, 1994, pp 231–244.

Rudy TE, Lieber SJ, Boston JR, Gourley LM, Baysal E. Psychosocial predictors of physical performance in disabled individuals with chronic pain. *Clin J Pain* 2003; 19:18–30.

Ruta DA, Abdalla MI, Garratt AM, Coutts A, Russell IT. SF 36 health survey questionnaire: I. Reliability in two patient based studies. *Qual Health Care* 1994; 3:180–185.

Sackett DL, Haynes RB, Guyatt GH, Tugwell P. *Clinical Epidemiology: A Basic Science for Clinical Medicine.* Boston: Little, Brown and Co., 1991.

Sharp TJ, Nicholas MK. Assessing the significant others of chronic pain patients: the psychometric properties of significant other questionnaires. *Pain* 2000; 88:135–144.

Simmonds MJ, Olson SL, Jones S, et al. Psychometric characteristics and clinical usefulness of physical performance tests in patients with low back pain. *Spine* 1998; 23:2412–2421.

Skevington SM. Investigating the relationship between pain and discomfort and quality of life, using the WHOQOL. *Pain* 1998; 76:395–406.

Skevington SM, Carse MS, Williams AC de C. Validation of the WHOQOL-100: pain management improves quality of life for chronic pain patients. *Clin J Pain* 2001; 17:264–275.

Stone AA, Shiffman S, Schwartz JE, Broderick JE, Hufford MR. Patient compliance with paper and electronic diaries. *Control Clin Trials* 2003; 24:182–199.

Tait RC, Pollard CA, Margolis RB, Duckro PN, Krause SJ. The Pain Disability Index: psychometric and validity data. *Arch Phys Med Rehabil* 1987; 68:438–441.

Tait RC, Chibnall JT, Krause S. The Pain Disability Index: psychometric properties. *Pain* 1990; 40:171–182.

Turk DC, Melzack R (Eds). *Handbook of Pain Assessment,* 2nd ed. New York: Guilford Press, 2001a.

Turk DC, Melzack R. The measurement of pain and the assessment of people experiencing pain. In: Turk DC, Melzack R (Eds). *Handbook of Pain Assessment,* 2nd ed. New York: Guilford Press, 2001b, pp 3–11.

Turk DC, Okifuji A. Clinical assessment of the person with chronic pain. In: Jensen TS, Wilson PR, Rice ASC (Eds). *Clinical Pain Management: Chronic Pain.* London: Arnold, 2003, pp 89–100.

Vlaeyen JWS. Fear in musculoskeletal pain. In: Dostrovsky JO, Carr DB, Koltzenburg M (Eds). *Proceedings of the 10th World Congress on Pain,* Progress in Pain Research and Management, Vol. 24. Seattle: IASP Press, 2003, pp 631–650.

Vlaeyen JWS, Linton SJ. Fear-avoidance and its consequences in chronic musculoskeletal pain: a state of the art. *Pain* 2000; 85:317–332.

Von Korff M. Epidemiological and survey methods: assessment of chronic pain. In: Turk DC, Melzack R (Eds). *Handbook of Pain Assessment,* 2nd ed. New York: Guilford Press, 2001, pp 603–618.

Von Korff M, Ormel J, Keefe FJ, Dworkin SF. Grading the severity of chronic pain. *Pain* 1992; 50:133–149.

Wagner A, Sukiennik A, Kulich R, et al. Outcomes assessment in chronic pain treatment: the need to supplement the SF-36. *Abstracts: 8th World Congress on Pain.* Seattle: IASP Press, 1996, p 308.

Ware JE, Snow KK, Kosinski M, Gandek B. *SF-36 Health Survey: Manual and Interpretation Guide.* Boston: Health Institute, New England Medical Center, 1993.

Watson PJ. Non-physiological determinants of physical performance in musculoskeletal pain. In: Max M (Ed). *Pain 1999—An Updated Review.* Seattle: IASP Press, 1999, pp 153–157.

WHOQOL Group. The World Health Organization Quality of Life Assessment (WHOQOL): position paper from the World Health Organization. *Soc Sci Med* 1995; 41:1403–1409.

WHOQOL Group. Development of the World Health Organization WHOQOL-BREF quality of life assessment. *Psychol Med* 1998; 28:551–558.

Williams AC de C. Measures of function and psychology. In: Melzack R, Wall PD (Eds). *Textbook of Pain,* 4th ed. Edinburgh: Churchill Livingstone, 1999, pp 427–444.

Williams AC de C. Facial expression of pain: an evolutionary account. *Behav Brain Sci* 2003a; in press.

Williams AC de C. Selecting and applying pain measures. In: Breivik H, Campbell W, Eccleston C (Eds). *Clinical Pain Management: Practical Applications and Procedures.* London: Arnold, 2003b, pp 3–14.

Williams AC de C, Davies HTO, Chadury Y. Simple pain rating scales hide complex idiosyncratic meanings. *Pain* 2000; 85:457–463.

Correspondence to: Amanda C. de C. Williams, PhD, INPUT Pain Management Unit, Guy's and St. Thomas' Hospital, Lambeth Palace Road, London SE1 7EH, United Kingdom. Email: amanda.williams@kcl.ac.uk.

Psychosocial Aspects of Pain: A Handbook for Health Care Providers, Progress in Pain Research and Management, Vol. 27, edited by Robert H. Dworkin and William S. Breitbart, IASP Press, Seattle, © 2004.

6

The Role of Psychological Testing and Diagnosis in Patients with Pain

Robert N. Jamison

Pain Management Center, Brigham and Women's Hospital, and Departments of Anesthesia and Psychiatry, Harvard Medical School, Boston, Massachusetts, USA

This chapter presents an overview of psychological factors that influence chronic pain, emphasizing commonly used assessment techniques. The usefulness of psychometric measures of chronic pain patients is discussed, and areas considered critical to the psychological assessment are reviewed, including the semi-structured interview, behavioral analysis, neuropsychological testing, and measures of pain intensity, mood, activity interference, coping, quality of life, adverse effects, and substance abuse. Psychiatric diagnoses associated with pain syndromes are also presented. Finally, innovations in psychological assessment techniques are discussed.

In the United States, recent guidelines by the Joint Commission on Accreditation of Healthcare Organizations (JCAHO) suggest that pain should be assessed regularly as a "fifth vital sign" (along with blood pressure, temperature, heart rate, and respiration). Thus, recognition of the significance of pain has gained increasing attention in health care. President Clinton signed into law a bill declaring 2001–2010 as the Decade of Pain Control. Also, recent trends within health maintenance organizations have encouraged primary care physicians to take greater responsibility in monitoring and treating patients with intractable pain. These changes have stressed the importance of assessment of persons with chronic pain.

Several important factors must be considered in the psychological testing of persons with pain. First, the sensation of pain is a multifactorial personal experience that cannot be measured objectively. Because pain is a subjective state, its measurement can only rely on what the patient says and does in response to the pain. We also know that a number of psychosocial factors contribute to pain. These include attitudes, beliefs, cultural norms, moods, focus of attention, motivation, and personality traits. For example, persons who are anxious or depressed tend to report more intense pain than those who are experiencing minimal emotional distress (Jamison 1996). Conversely, persons with pain who have adequate psychological functioning exhibit a greater tendency to ignore their pain, to use coping self-statements, and to remain active in order to divert their attention from their pain (Jensen and Karoly 1991). Because pain is a complex, subjective experience, multiple measures of pain and psychosocial function are needed to reliably assess patients with persistent pain.

Second, it is generally unwarranted to assume that psychological factors are the cause of pain. Some still hold to the Cartesian notion that pain is a physiological response to tissue damage (see Main and Spanswick 2000). If physical findings are insufficient to account for a report of chronic pain, such pain is interpreted to be a largely psychological phenomenon. We know, however, that profound reactive changes in quality of life are associated with intractable chronic pain. Significant interference with memory, sleep, employment, social functioning, and daily activities is common. Chronic pain patients frequently report depression, anxiety, irritability, sexual dysfunction, and decreased energy. Family roles are altered, and worries about financial limitations and future consequences of a restricted lifestyle are prevalent. Chronic pain patients often present with a history of multiple medical tests with minimal physical findings, and clinicians are tempted to conclude, often wrongly, that psychological factors are the major precipitating cause for pain.

Finally, attempts to reliably distinguish between organic and psychogenic pain have been largely unsuccessful. Most pain specialists recognize that chronic pain is an interactive biopsychosocial phenomenon with biomedical, psychological, social, and behavioral influences. However, some clinicians still place the greatest emphasis on the biomedical component of pain and perceive this information as separate from psychological factors. They also mistakenly believe that the results of standardized psychometric measures will reflect whether a patient's chronic pain is related to a psychogenic pain problem. Unfortunately, a psychological evaluation cannot be relied upon to identify psychogenic pain.

PSYCHOLOGICAL ASSESSMENT OF CHRONIC PAIN

The International Association for the Study of Pain defines pain as "an unpleasant sensory and emotional experience associated with actual or potential tissue damage, or described in terms of such damage" (Merskey and

Bogduk 1994). This definition recognizes that pain is an emotional as well as a sensory phenomenon. Pain is the most common reason to see a physician, and epidemiological studies have independently documented that chronic noncancer pain is an international problem of immense proportions (Turk and Melzack 2001).

The initial assessment of a chronic pain patient entails assembling separate pieces of information and abstracting from them a prognosis and the best course of treatment. Important components that must be evaluated in this process include pain intensity, functional capacity, mood and personality, coping and pain beliefs, and medication usage. In addition, a behavioral analysis should be conducted, and information should be obtained on psychosocial history, adverse effects of treatment, and health care utilization. The following sections will highlight ways to assess each of these areas and will discuss strengths and weaknesses of the assessment process.

USEFULNESS OF PSYCHOMETRIC MEASURES

Standardized psychometric testing methods are frequently used to evaluate the psychological functioning of chronic pain patients. Unfortunately, most traditional testing tools were designed to evaluate psychopathology in persons with significant mental dysfunction. Although most chronic pain patients state that they are depressed and anxious, many of them have no history of long-standing psychiatric problems. Rather, their symptoms reflect their current condition.

One commonly encountered scenario involves an injury at a job that requires heavy lifting and bending. A worker experiences a sudden pain while lifting a particularly heavy object. During a few months of rest and recovery, the injured person may believe that the "muscle strain" will heal itself. After months or years of being evaluated by physicians and other health care professionals and after unsuccessful treatments and attempts to return to work, the patient begins to show signs of considerable emotional distress, including depression, anxiety, and anger. Often there are feelings of helplessness, low self-esteem, and isolation. Although chronic pain patients may exhibit certain personality traits that might contribute to their inability to cope with a chronic disabling condition, these traits do not always suggest significant psychopathology. Traditional assessment techniques, particularly projective tests, are not effective for assessing chronic pain patients. Rather, measures that more reliably evaluate the degree of reactive emotional distress are called for.

Ideally, only psychologists and other mental health personnel trained in issues related to chronic pain should administer, score, and interpret psychometric tests used in assessing chronic pain patients. A consideration of the components of the pain experience (see Table I) is crucial in determining the efficacy and course of treatment.

SEMI-STRUCTURED INTERVIEW

The most popular means of evaluating the psychological state of the patient is a semi-structured interview (Bradley and McKendree-Smith 2001), the results of which may frequently be given significant weight in a decision

Table I
Assessment categories and frequently used psychometric measures

1. Psychosocial History
    Comprehensive pain questionnaire
    CAGE questionnaire
    Michigan Alcoholism Screening Test (MAST)
    Self-Administered Alcoholism Screening Test (SAAST)
    Structured Clinical Interview for DSM-IV (SCID)

2. Pain Intensity
    Numerical rating scales (NRS)
    Visual analogue scales (VAS)
    Verbal rating scales (VRS)
    Pain drawings

3. Mood and Personality
    Minnesota Multiphasic Personality Inventory (MMPI)
    Symptom Checklist 90 (SCL-90)
    Millon Behavior Health Inventory (MBHI)
    Illness Behavior Questionnaire (IBQ)
    Beck Depression Inventory (BDI)
    Center for Epidemiologic Studies Depression Scale (CES-D)

4. Functional Capacity
    Sickness Impact Profile (SIP)
    Short-Form Health Survey (SF-36)
    Multidimensional Pain Inventory (MPI)
    Pain Disability Index (PDI)

5. Pain Beliefs and Coping
    Coping Strategies Questionnaire (CSQ)
    Pain Management Inventory (PMI)
    Pain Self-Efficacy Questionnaire (PSEQ)
    Survey of Pain Attitudes (SOPA)
    Inventory of Negative Thoughts in Response to Pain (INTRP)

6. Medication Monitoring and Adverse Effects
    Medication record
    Monitoring devices
    Side-effect checklist

regarding treatment. Self-report questionnaires can be used as adjuncts to the interview. Before meeting with the patient, the interviewer should review all referral information, including discharge summaries, testing results, previous physicians' notes, and medical history reports. Each of the following categories should be assessed during the interview: (1) pain intensity and description, (2) aggravating factors, (3) sleep and daily activity level, (4) relevant medical history, (5) social history, (6) past and current treatments, (7) education and employment history, (8) disability and compensation status, (9) history of drug or alcohol abuse, (10) history of psychiatric disturbance and past emotional trauma, (11) current emotional status and perceived support, and (12) motivation to take an active role in treatment. These areas have been identified as important in assessing candidacy for medical interventions for pain (Block 1996). Moreover, research has identified perceived support as an important variable in predicting positive treatment outcome and compliance with treatment (Jamison and Virts 1990; Turner and Romano 2001).

Preliminary demographic and medical history information can be obtained through the completion of a comprehensive questionnaire (Karoly and Jensen 1987; Main and Spanswick 2000). Additional information can be clarified at the time of the interview. It is important to consider and acknowledge factors such as the patient's gender, race, cultural background, and beliefs, all of which can greatly influence a person's perception of pain and coping mechanisms. Structured interview measures for the assessment of psychosocial aspects of pain include the Psychosocial Pain Inventory (PSPI; Getto et al. 1983). Instruments designed to assess alcoholism and drug abuse are described in the section "Substance Abuse Assessment" below. Interviews used to establish a psychiatric diagnosis include the Diagnostic Interview Schedule (DIS; Helzer and Robins 1988) and the Structured Clinical Interview for DSM-IV (SCID; Williams et al. 1992). Whenever possible, the patient's family members and/or significant other should also be interviewed.

BEHAVIORAL ANALYSIS

A thorough behavioral analysis is important in the successful rehabilitation of each chronic pain patient (Keefe et al. 2001). Fordyce (1976), one of the early proponents of behavioral assessment, put forward the learning theory of chronic pain, which highlights the important distinction between what pain patients say and what they do. Instead of relying solely on subjective measures of chronic pain, investigators should also evaluate objective, observable manifestations of how the patient responds to pain. A significant component of the learning theory of chronic pain is the distinction between "well" behaviors and "pain" behaviors. Further, it is essential to identify factors that perpetuate pain behaviors (Keefe and Block 1982; Egan 1989).

The first step in behavioral analysis is to identify overt behaviors in pain patients (Keefe et al. 2001), including posturing, limping, over-reliance on pain medication, and use of cervical collars, back braces, canes, and so on. All of these observable behaviors tend to perpetuate a disability identity. Other components of a behavioral analysis include self-monitored observations and use of electronic diaries (Follick et al. 1987; Jamison et al. 2001).

NEUROPSYCHOLOGICAL TESTING

As part of the psychological assessment, the clinician must determine a pain patient's neuropsychological status, especially in cases of physical trauma (such as head injury) or decreased cognitive functioning. Such an assessment may detect potential organic pathology that may limit the usefulness of cognitive interventions. A number of neuropsychological assessment tools exist for such evaluations (Wedding et al. 1986; Lezak 1995).

It may be necessary to measure cognitive function in pain patients in order to determine their ability to drive or operate other equipment while on pain medication. Short-term use of opioid medication in persons who have never taken opioids can adversely affect psychomotor performance (Kerr et al. 1991; Zacny et al. 1997; Chapman et al. 2002). Forrest and colleagues (1977) reported that subjects had a slowed reaction on the Finger Tapping Test and the Digit Symbol Substitution Test after receiving intramuscular morphine. As a result, many physicians recommend that individuals restrict their driving and use of motorized equipment while taking opioids for pain.

On the other hand, some studies and anecdotal evidence suggest that impairment in cognition after administration of opioids may be less severe in individuals with chronic pain than in individuals without pain (Lorenz et al. 1997; Zacny et al. 1997; Haythornthwaite et al. 1998). Many patients with chronic pain who have been taking opioids for an extended period indicate that opioids have no adverse effect on driving (Budd et al 1989; Stoduto et al. 1993). A recent study of 144 patients with low back pain assessed the psychomotor effects of chronic opioid use with the use of two neuropsychological tests—the Digit Symbol Substitution Test and the Trail Making Test (Jamison et al. 2003). All subjects completed the tests before being prescribed opioids for pain and repeated the tests at 90- and 180-day intervals after being prescribed long- and short-acting opioids. Test scores significantly improved from baseline while subjects were taking opioids, which suggests that the long-term use of opioids for pain does not significantly impair cognitive ability or psychomotor function. While cognitive impairment is not universal, physicians are compelled to recommend that individuals limit activities that may place them at risk of injury when taking opioids for pain, especially within the first 2 weeks of starting opioid therapy. Neuropsychological testing could help in documenting the presence or absence of cognitive deficits related to medication use.

ASSESSMENT TOOLS

PAIN INTENSITY MEASURES

Because one of the obvious primary goals of treatment for chronic pain is to decrease the intensity of the pain, it is important to monitor pain intensity both for a period before and throughout the course of treatment. There are various ways to measure pain intensity, including numerical pain ratings, the visual analogue scale (VAS), verbal rating scales, pain drawings, and a combination of standardized questionnaires. Pain intensity rating methods have evolved from designs originally developed by Budzynski et al. (1973) and Melzack (1975). Several studies have shown that self-monitored pain intensity ratings are both reliable and valid (Follick et al. 1984; Jensen et al. 1996; Jensen and Karoly 2001). The daily monitoring of multiple measures of pain intensity over a 1–2-week period before the start of therapy has a number of benefits. First, more information is obtained than can be gained from a single index of perceived pain intensity. More specifically, averaging multiple measures of pain intensity over time increases the reliability and validity of the assessment and is preferable to a single rating of pain intensity (Jensen and McFarland 1993; Jensen and Karoly 2001). Second, average pain intensity ratings can serve as a baseline to help establish whether continued treatment is needed after an appropriate trial period. Baseline measures are essential to making judgments about the overall impact of treatment for pain.

Numerical pain ratings often involve the patient's rating of his or her pain on a scale of 0–10 or 0–100. Ideally, the external validity of the measure is improved by descriptive anchors that help the patient understand the meaning of each numerical value. Another popular means of measuring pain intensity is the VAS (Fig. 1), which uses a straight line (often 10 cm long) with extreme limits of pain at either end (Karoly and Jansen 1987). The pain patient is instructed to place a mark at the point on the line that best indicates present pain severity. Scores are obtained by measuring the distance from the end labeled "no pain" to the mark provided by the patient. Evidence exists for the validity of the VAS (Jensen and Karoly 2001), but it is

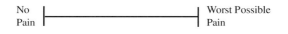

Fig. 1. Visual analogue scale.

time-consuming to score and can be difficult to use with older people (Jensen et al. 1986; see also D. Williams, this volume). These concerns have been addressed by the use of electronic VAS diaries, which are as reliable as paper measures (Jamison et al. 2002).

There are several verbal rating scales (Karoly and Jensen 1987; Jensen and Karoly 2001), which consist of phrases (as few as 4 or as many as 15, often ranked in order of severity from "no pain" to "excruciating pain") chosen by the patients to describe the intensity of their pain (Table II). Other descriptors can be used to describe the quality of pain (e.g., piercing, stabbing, shooting, burning, throbbing) (Table III; Jamison et al. 1987).

Among the self-report measures, numerical rating scales are most popular among professionals. However, there is no evidence to suggest that visual analogue or verbal rating scales are any less sensitive to treatment effects. All these types of measures have been shown to be acceptable in the quantification of clinical pain (Karoly and Jensen 1987; Jensen and Karoly 2001). For further discussion of the assessment of pain intensity, see A.C. de C. Williams (this volume).

Table II
Examples of verbal rating scales of pain intensity

1. No Pain	1. None	1. No Pain	1. Not noticeable	1. None
2. Mild	2. Mild	2. Mild	2. Just noticeable	2. Extremely weak
3. Moderate	3. Moderate	3. Discomforting	3. Very weak	3. Just noticeable
4. Severe	4. Severe	4. Distressing	4. Weak	4. Very weak
	5. Very severe	5. Horrible	5. Mild	5. Weak
		6. Excruciating	6. Moderate	6. Mild
			7. Strong	7. Moderate
			8. Intense	8. Uncomfortable
			9. Very strong	9. Strong
			10. Severe	10. Intense
			11. Very intense	11. Very strong
			12. Excruciating	12. Very intense
				13. Extremely intense
				14. Intolerable
				15. Excruciating

Table III
List of verbal pain descriptors

1. Piercing
2. Stabbing
3. Shooting
4. Burning
5. Throbbing
6. Cramping
7. Aching
8. Stinging
9. Squeezing
10. Numbing
11. Itching
12. Tingling
13. None

MOOD AND PERSONALITY

Psychopathology and extreme emotionality are considered contraindications for certain therapies (Savage 1993; Block 1996; Main and Spanswick 2000). Mental health professionals continue to debate the best way to measure psychopathology and emotional distress in chronic pain patients. Most measures are helpful in ruling out severe psychiatric disturbance, but unfortunately no measure can boast validity in predicting treatment outcome. The measures most commonly used to evaluate personality and emotional distress include the Minnesota Multiphasic Personality Inventory (MMPI-2; Bradley et al. 1978; Prokop et al. 1980; Leavitt 1985; Hathaway et al. 1989), the Symptom Checklist 90 (SCL-90-R; Derogatis 1977, 1983), the Millon Behavior Health Inventory (MBHI; Millon et al. 1979), the Illness Behavior Questionnaire (IBQ; Pilowsky and Spence 1975), and the Beck Depression Inventory (BDI; Beck et al. 1961).

The MMPI is the instrument most commonly used in assessing chronic pain patients (Hathaway et al. 1989). This measure consists of 567 true-false items and yields a distinct profile for each pain patient. Studies have shown that these profiles can predict return-to-work in males as well as response to surgical treatment (McCreary 1985). Although this test is widely used to measure psychopathology, the profiles obtained can be misinterpreted because of the physical symptoms frequently reported by these patients (Moore et al. 1988). Patients may also dislike the test's emphasis on psychopathology.

The SCL-90 is a 90-item checklist with a five-point scale that offers a global index score as well as nine subscale scores as a general assessment of emotional distress. It is a relatively brief measure that offers easy inspection of individual items that may pertain specifically to persons with chronic pain. However, its disadvantages include the high correlation between subscales and the absence of validity scales to detect subtle inconsistencies in responses (Jamison et al. 1988).

The MBHI, another popular measure for assessing mood and personality, includes 150 true-false items and offers 20 subscales that measure (1) styles of relating to providers, (2) psychosocial stressors, and (3) response to illness. The advantage of the MBHI is that the scales are not subject to misinterpretation due to physical symptoms. Unlike other measures, the MBHI emphasizes medical rather than emotional concerns.

The IBQ is commonly used to assess emotionality and illness behavior in chronic pain patients. This questionnaire includes 62 true-false items and yields seven subscales measuring symptoms and abnormal illness behavior. Patients whose organic pathology does not account for their pain tend to have higher IBQ scores. The IBQ is also correlated with anxiety measures.

The BDI assesses depressive symptoms in chronic pain patients. This 21-item self-report questionnaire measures the severity of depression and is commonly used to evaluate the outcome of treatment. It is easy to administer and score, though one limitation is the potential for misinterpretation of an elevated depression score as a result of the frequent endorsement of somatic items (e.g., fatigue, sleep disturbances, and loss of sexual interest) by chronic pain patients. The Center for Epidemiologic Studies Depression Scale (CES-D) is an additional tool for assessment of depressive symptoms in pain patients (Radloff 1977).

FUNCTIONAL CAPACITY AND ACTIVITY INTERFERENCE MEASURES

Some clinicians consider pain reduction meaningless unless accompanied by a noticeable change in function. Thus, some reliable measurement of functional capacity should be used before the onset of therapy. Research has shown that physical impairment is not very predictive of disability, and that beliefs about injury predict physical performance better than pain ratings (Turk et al. 1998). Measures that can be used to assess activity level and function include the Sickness Impact Profile (SIP; Bergner et al. 1981), the Short-Form Health Survey (SF-36; Ware and Sherbourne 1992), the West Haven-Yale Multidimensional Pain Inventory (WHYMPI, now referred to as MPI; Kerns et al. 1985), and the Pain Disability Index (PDI; Pollard 1984).

The SIP is a 136-item checklist with 12 subscales measuring levels of physical and psychosocial functioning. Each item is weighted, and the scales are correlated with other functional capacity measures. Shorter versions of the SIP (e.g., the Roland and Morris Disability Questionnaire; Roland and Morris 1983) are also suitable for the assessment of function in chronic pain patients.

The SF-36, which was initially developed from the Medical Outcomes Study to survey health status, includes eight scales that measure (1) limitations in physical activities due to health problems, (2) limitations in social activities due to physical and emotional problems, (3) limitations in usual role activities due to physical health problems, (4) bodily pain, (5) general mental health, (6) limitations in usual role activities due to emotional problems, (7) vitality (energy and fatigue), and (8) general health perceptions. The SF-36 is favored over the SIP because it is a shorter test with excellent reliability and validity. The SIP is preferred if the population being evaluated includes patients with extreme physical limitations.

The MPI is a 56-item measure made up of seven-point rating scales. The subscales assess activity interference, perceived support, pain severity, negative mood, and perceived control. The advantage of this self-report instrument is that it was created specifically for chronic pain patients and can be useful in classifying those patients into three types: dysfunctional, interpersonally distressed, and adaptive copers (Turk and Rudy 1988). Strong evidence supports the presence of these three types of chronic pain patients (Jamison et al. 1994).

Other functional measures include the Oswestry Disability Questionnaire (Leclaire et al. 1997), Chronic Illness Problem Inventory (Kames et al. 1984), the Waddell Disability Instrument (Waddell and Main 1984), the Functional Rating Scale (Evans and Kagan 1986), and the Back Pain Function Scale (Stratford and Binkley 2000). See A.C. de C. Williams (this volume) for additional discussion of the specific functional capacity scales.

PAIN BELIEFS AND COPING

Pain perception, beliefs about pain, and coping mechanisms are important in predicting the outcome of treatment. Unrealistic or negative thoughts about an ongoing pain problem may contribute to increased pain and emotional distress, decreased functioning, and greater reliance on medication. Certain chronic pain patients are prone to maladaptive beliefs about their condition that may not be compatible with the physical nature of their pain (DeGood and Shutty 1992; Waddell 1998). Patients with adequate psychological functioning exhibit a greater tendency to ignore their pain, use coping self-statements, and remain active in order to divert their attention from their pain (Jensen and Karoly 1991).

Since efficacy expectations have been shown to influence the efforts patients will make to manage their pain, measures of self-efficacy or perceived control are useful in assessing a patient's attitude (Jamison 1996). A number of self-report measures assess coping and pain attitudes. The most popular tests used to measure maladaptive beliefs include the Coping Strategies Questionnaire (CSQ; Rosenstiel and Keefe 1983), the Pain Management Inventory (PMI; Brown et al. 1989), the Pain Self-Efficacy Questionnaire (PSEQ; Lorig et al. 1989), the Survey of Pain Attitudes (SOPA; Jensen et al. 1987), and the Inventory of Negative Thoughts in Response to Pain (INTRP; Gil et al. 1990). Other instruments include the Pain Beliefs and Perceptions Inventory (PBPI; Williams et al. 1994), and the Chronic Pain Self-efficacy Scale (CPSS; Anderson et al. 1995). Patients who have a high score on the Catastrophizing Scale of the CSQ, who endorse passive coping on the PMI, who demonstrate low self-efficacy regarding their ability to manage their pain on the PSEQ, who describe themselves as disabled by their pain on the SOPA, and who report frequent negative thoughts about their pain on the INTRP are at greatest risk for poor treatment outcome. It is suspected that patients who have unrealistic beliefs and expectations about their condition are also poor candidates for pain treatment.

QUALITY OF LIFE ASSESSMENT

Pain and discomfort can make a significant impact on perceptions of general health-related quality of life (QOL; Skevington 1993). Those who are pain-free have significantly better QOL than those in pain. A longer duration of pain symptoms is associated with poorer QOL, and pain associated with increased emotional distress can be particularly detrimental. Assessment instruments should include a variety of social, psychological, and physical features in order to assess properly the QOL of persons with chronic pain.

A number of questionnaires, some of which have been adapted for computer use, have been developed to assess QOL from the patient's standpoint. Among the most widely cited are the General Health Questionnaire (GHQ; Bowling 1997), the Nottingham Health Profile (NHP; Coons et al. 2000), the Sickness Impact Profile (SIP; Bergner et al. 1981) and the SF-36 Health Survey (Ware and Sherbourne 1992).

Questionnaires of this type have been used widely to compare the quality of life of patients in chronic pain with that of healthy controls. The findings are clear and consistent in revealing the multi-factored impact of chronic pain on a person's perceived quality of life. In fact, the health-related quality of life of patients in chronic pain is among the lowest reported for any medical condition (Becker et al. 1997; Hill et al. 1999). In particular, low scores have been found for patients with pain due to chronic spinal disorders (Claiborne et al. 1999), multiple sclerosis (Vickrey et al. 1995), and headache (Wang and Fuh 2001). Elderly patients with osteoarthritis also have impaired QOL compared with peers without chronic illness, especially in the parameters of physical status, vitality, social functioning, and general health (Briggs et al. 1999). Relative to patients with diagnoses of chronic obstructive pulmonary disease, rheumatoid arthritis, atrial fibrillation, and advanced cancer, patients with fibromyalgia have been found to have lower scores on the Quality of Well-Being Scale (Kaplan et al. 2000). For more discussion of quality of life assessment, see A.C. de C. Williams (this volume).

MONITORING MEDICATION AND ADVERSE EFFECTS

Compliance is an important component in decisions about whether to continue, discontinue, or modify treatment for chronic pain. Clinicians ask patients to comply with their treatment protocol but are rarely prepared with a way to monitor compliance, particularly for medication usage. A patient's retrospective report of use of medication, although of value, is subject to inaccuracies (Jamison et al. 1989). Recall can be enhanced if the patient continuously monitors usage. In addition, both compliance and accuracy in reporting are improved if a family member assists with the monitoring. Medication records kept by patients often include the name of the medication, the date and time when it is taken, and the dosage (Steedman et al. 1992).

Adverse effects should be monitored regularly during treatment for chronic pain. The monitoring of side effects related to medication use in clinical trials can be as important as the monitoring of pain intensity. Adverse effects are often specific to a given medication. Opioid therapy, for instance, may contribute to constipation, tiredness, nausea, dizziness, itching, urinary retention, and breathing problems. Medications also influence mood and cognitive abilities (Bruera et al. 1989; Kerr et al. 1991; Banning et al. 1992). Periodic monitoring of adverse effects by means of a symptom checklist can provide relatively objective criteria useful in the assessment of treatment (Fig. 2). Each symptom can be rated on a scale from 0 (absent) to 10 (most severe). Although patients frequently report adverse reactions to medication during the initial stage of treatment, many of these reactions diminish over time (Jamison et al. 1998).

Portable monitors using customized software have made the collection and storage of serial data about health behaviors both convenient and

Do you have any of the following symptoms?
If so, rate them on intensity from 1 (minimal)
to 10 (most severe):

_____ Constipation   _____ Confusion
_____ Dizziness   _____ Nausea
_____ Drowsiness   _____ Nightmares
_____ Dry mouth   _____ Sneezing
_____ Headache   _____ Sweating
_____ Itching   _____ Visual problems
_____ Memory lapse   _____ Weakness

Fig. 2. Side-effect checklist.

affordable. Electronic diaries allow two-way communication between patients and providers and are an efficient means of evaluating and tracking medication use and associated symptoms (Jamison et al. 2001).

SUBSTANCE ABUSE ASSESSMENT

Structured interview measures have been published for the assessment of alcoholism and drug abuse. Whenever possible, the patient's family members and/or significant other should also be interviewed. The Structured Clinical Interview for DSM-IV (SCID; Williams et al. 1992) is a semi-structured diagnostic interview that assigns current and lifetime diagnoses based on DSM-IV criteria. For each positive identification of a symptom, the SCID uses a question sequence to determine whether the symptom meets severity criteria for diagnosis. Other substance abuse measures include the CAGE questionnaire, a four-item test with questions on Cutting down, Annoyance at criticism, Guilty feelings, and use of Eye-openers (Mayfield et al. 1974); the Michigan Alcoholism Screening Test (MAST; Selzer 1971), and the Self-Administered Alcoholism Screening Test (SAAST; Swenson and Morse 1975). Structured substance interviews for chronic pain patients have been proposed (Compton et al. 1998), although the validity and reliability of such measures are limited. For more discussion of substance abuse assessment, see Passik and Kirsh (this volume).

DSM-IV DIAGNOSES

In the fourth edition of the *Diagnostic and Statistical Manual of Mental Disorders* (DSM-IV) published in 1994, the American Psychiatric Association revised the classification of pain disorders. The diagnostic categories of earlier versions, *psychogenic pain disorder* (DSM-III) and *somatoform pain disorder* (DSM-III-R), were criticized for being only rarely applicable to patients with pain. In these versions, these diagnoses required a "preoccupation with pain, and pain which is grossly in excess of what would be expected from the physical findings." No attention was given to patients with acute pain or with psychological distress associated with "real" pain (i.e., pain with an objectively identifiable source). The other mental health diagnoses—conversion disorder, hypochondriasis, or somatization disorder—did little to resolve these problems.

Thus a new category, "pain disorder," was created for the DSM-IV. No longer were the terms *psychogenic* and *somatoform* combined with *pain disorder*. The following criteria must be met for a diagnosis of pain disorder: (1) There is pain in one or more anatomical site. (2) The pain causes clinically significant distress or impairment. (3) Psychological factors are judged to play an important role. (4) The symptom(s) are not intentionally produced. (5) The pain is not better accounted for by another psychiatric disorder.

Two mental health diagnoses for pain are given in the DSM-IV. "Pain disorder associated with psychological factors" (307.80) is the category used when psychological factors are judged to play the major role and medical conditions little or no role in the onset and maintenance of the pain. "Pain disorder associated with both psychological factors and general medical condition" (307.89) is used when both psychological factors and a general medical condition are judged to play important roles. For both codes, the duration of pain—less than 6 months (acute) or greater than 6 months (chronic)—must be specified.

These changes were welcomed by clinicians who worked predominantly with persons in pain. Other mental health diagnoses, such as somatization disorder, conversion disorder, hypochondriasis, body dysmorphic disorder, and factitious disorder, are still included in DSM-IV.

FOLLOW-UP AND EVALUATION

An important component of any intervention or group-based pain program is its ability to measure its own effectiveness. Several recommendations for effective program evaluation have been put forward by the Commission on the Accreditation of Rehabilitation Facilities (2000). A system should be in place for obtaining follow-up information from patients on the consumption of medications, use of health care services, return to gainful employment, functional activities, ability to manage pain, and subjective pain intensity. Provisions should also be made for periodic contact after discharge. A data-based system should be developed from which information on patients who have completed a program can be obtained on a regular basis. This type of system not only helps to determine how a program meets the needs of individual patients but also offers substantive information on overall efficacy. Program evaluation should encompass goals and objectives that are achievable and outcomes that are measurable. A program evaluation report should include primary objectives, measures, time of measurement, source of information, and expectations, as well as outcomes. Finally, program evaluation helps identify which services are most effective in the treatment of chronic pain patients.

Points to consider when implementing a program evaluation system include (1) a suitable patient sample from which follow-up data are collected, (2) standardized dependent measures, (3) valid and reliable psychometric instruments, (4) observational methods and self-report questionnaires, (5) experimental design with unbiased analyses, and (6) assessment of individual differences in outcome.

HEALTH CARE UTILIZATION

Insurance carriers and third-party payers are particularly interested in documenting health care utilization related to treatment for chronic noncancer pain. The Commission on the Accreditation of Rehabilitation Facilities (2000) has published standards for health care utilization by patients who have completed a pain program. The information gathered may include the number of health care professionals seen over the past month, the number of hospitalizations and surgeries, and whether or not the patient is employed or involved in a vocational rehabilitation program. This information is particularly useful in documenting whether reliance on other medical services decreases after a patient starts a new treatment or completes a pain program. Follow-up information is vital in establishing evidence for treatment efficacy. Some clinicians rely on return-to-work statistics to measure efficacy of treatment. They argue that without a change in function, the benefits of potentially harmful therapies do not justify the risks and possible adverse effects (Schofferman 1993).

FUTURE STUDIES

There has been a rapid change in the way health care services are offered in the United States. More and more decisions about treatment are made by employees of insurance carriers on the basis of financial resources rather than by heath care professionals on the basis of need. Brief, reliable measures are necessary to establish the need for care and to monitor outcome. An increasing need for accountability and efficacy has encouraged the implementation of cost-saving measures and program evaluation. Preference is given to programs that are tailored to the individual rather than to programs in which all group participants receive every treatment.

In light of the attention given to these changes, the economic efficiency of treatment for chronic noncancer pain is worthy of discussion. While evidence exists for the cost-effectiveness of therapy for chronic pain (Chapman et al. 2000), such treatment may not meet the criterion of increased benefit with very little cost. Prior classification of patients may help in identifying those individuals who will benefit most from pain therapy. No reported studies have satisfactorily addressed this issue, and outcome data are needed. Documentation of increased function and decreased health care utilization among certain patients as a result of pain therapy would support the continuation of pain management programs.

Electronic diaries have much promise for future psychological assessment of pain patients. They allow for improved communication between patients and providers and may be an efficient means of evaluating and tracking important clinical information. With the advent of desktop, laptop, and palmtop computers and the ability to capture time-stamped data and store it for uploading to the Web or to a larger computer, more clinicians are exploring options of capturing data throughout the day. Studies have shown that "natural" data are less prone to fabrication and may be a truer indicator of patient responses in the environment. Patients demonstrate remarkably high compliance with electronic diary monitoring (Jamison et al. 2001). Ever-evolving technological methods of tracking can address the need for improved evaluation and treatment of persons with chronic pain (Velikova et al. 1999; Tiplady et al. 2000).

REFERENCES

American Psychiatric Association. *Diagnostic and Statistical Manual of Mental Disorders.* Washington, DC: American Psychiatric Association, 1994.

Anderson KO, Dowds BN, Pelletz RE. Development and initial validation of a scale to measure self-efficacy beliefs in patients with chronic pain. *Pain* 1995; 63:77–84.

Banning A, Sjogren P, Kaiser F, Sjgren P. Reaction time in cancer patients receiving peripherally acting analgesics along or in combination with opioids. *Acta Anaesthesiol Scand* 1992; 36:480–482.

Beck AT, Ward CH, Mendelson M, Mock J, Erbaugh J. An inventory for measuring depression. *Arch Gen Psychiatry* 1961; 4:561–571.

Becker NA, Bondegaard TA, Olsen AK, et al. Pain epidemiology and health related quality of life in chronic non-malignant pain patients referred to a Danish multidisciplinary pain center. *Pain* 1997; 73:393–400.

Bergner M, Bobbitt RA, Carter WB, Gilson BS. The Sickness Impact Profile: development and final revision of a health status measure. *Med Care* 1981; 19:787–805.

Block AR. *Presurgical Psychological Screening in Chronic Pain Syndromes.* Mahwah, NJ: Lawrence Erlbaum Associates, 1996.

Bowling A. *Measuring Health: A Review of Quality of Life Measurement Scales.* Philadelphia: Open University Press, 1997.

Bradley LA, McKendree-Smith NL. Assessment of psychological status using interview and self-report instruments. In: Turk DC, Melzack R (Eds). *Handbook of Pain Assessment,* 2nd ed. New York: Guilford Press, 2001, pp 292–319.

Bradley LA, Prokop CK, Margolis R, Gentry WD. Multivariate analyses of the MMPI profiles of low back pain patients. *J Behav Med* 1978; 1:253–272.

Briggs A, Scott E, Steele K. Impact of osteoarthritis and analgesic treatment on quality of life of an elderly population. *Ann Pharmacother* 1999; 33:1154–1159.

Brown GK, Nicassio PM, Wallston KA. Pain coping strategies and depression in rheumatoid arthritis. *J Consult Clin Psychol* 1989; 57:652–657.

Bruera E, Macmillan K, Hanson JA, MacDonald RN. The cognitive effects of the administration of narcotic analgesics in patients with cancer pain. *Pain* 1989; 39:13–16.

Budd RD, Muto JJ, Wong JK. Drugs of abuse found in fatally injured drivers in Los Angeles County. *Drug Alcohol Depend* 1989; 23:153–158.

Budzynski T, Stoyva J, Adler LS, Mullaney DJ. EMG biofeedback and tension headache: a controlled study. *Psychosom Med* 1973; 35:484–496.

Chapman SL, Jamison RN, Sanders SH, Lyman DR, Lynch NT. Perceived treatment helpfulness and cost in chronic pain rehabilitation. *Clin J Pain* 2000; 16:169–177.

Chapman SL, Byas-Smith MG, Reed BA. Effects of intermediate- and long-term use of opioids on cognition in patients with chronic pain. *Clin J Pain* 2002; 18:S83–S90.

Claiborne N, Krause TM, Heilman AE, Leung P. Measuring quality of life in back patients: comparison of Health Status Questionnaire 2.0 and Quality of Life Inventory. *Soc Work Health Care* 1999; 28:77–94.

Commission on the Accreditation of Rehabilitation Facilities. *Standards Manual for Organizations Serving People with Disabilities.* Tucson, AZ: Commission on the Accreditation of Rehabilitation Facilities, 2000.

Compton P, Darakjian J, Miotto K. Screening for addiction in patients with chronic pain and "problematic" substance use: evaluation of a pilot assessment tool. *J Pain Symptom Manage* 1998; 16:355–363.

Coons SJ, Rao S, Keininger DL, Hays RD. A comparison review of generic quality-of-life instruments. *Pharmacoeconomics* 2000; 17:13–35.

DeGood DE, Shutty MS. Assessment of pain beliefs, coping, and self-efficacy. In: Turk DC, Melzack R (Eds). *Handbook of Pain Assessment.* New York: Guilford Press, 1992, pp 214–234.

Derogatis LR. *The SCL-90-R: Administration, Scoring and Procedures Manual,* Vol. I. Baltimore: Clinical Psychometric Research, 1977.

Derogatis LR. *The SCL-90-R Manual II: Administration, Scoring and Procedures.* Towson, MD: Clinical Psychometric Research, 1983.

Egan KJ. Behavioral analysis: the use of behavioral concepts to promote change of chronic pain patients. In: Loeser JD, Egan KJ (Eds). *Managing the Chronic Pain Patient: Theory and Practice at the University of Washington Multidisciplinary Pain Center.* New York: Raven Press, 1989, pp 81–93.

Evans JH, Kagan A II. The development of a functional rating scale to measure the treatment outcome of chronic spinal patients. *Spine* 1986; 11:277–281.

Ewings JA. Detecting alcoholism: the CAGE questionnaire. *JAMA* 1984; 252:1905–1907.

Follick MJ, Ahern DK, Laser-Wolston N. Evaluation of a daily activity diary for chronic pain patients. *Pain* 1984; 19:373–382.

Follick MJ, Ahern DK, Aberger EW. Behavioral treatment of chronic pain. In: Blumenthal JA, McKee DC (Eds). *Applications in Behavioral Medicine and Health Psychology: A Clinician's Source Book.* Sarasota, FL: Professional Resource Exchange, 1987, pp 237–270.

Fordyce WE. *Behavioral Methods for Chronic Pain and Illness.* St. Louis: C.V. Mosby, 1976.

Forrest WHJ, Brown BW Jr, Brown CR, et al. Dextroamphetamine with morphine for the treatment of postoperative pain. *N Engl J Med* 1977; 296:712–715.

Getto CJ, Heaton RK, Lehman RA. PSPI: A standardized approach to the evaluation of psychosocial factors in chronic pain. In: Bonica JJ, Lindblom U, Iggo A (Eds). *Proceedings of the Third World Congress on Pain,* Advances in Pain Research and Therapy, Vol. 5. New York: Raven Press, 1983, pp 885–889.

Gil K, Williams DA, Keefe F, Beckham JC. The relationship of negative thoughts to pain and psychological distress. *Behav Ther* 1990; 21:349–362.

Hathaway SR, McKinley JC, Butcher JN, et al. *Minnesota Multiphasic Personality Inventory-2: Manual for Administration.* Minneapolis: University of Minnesota Press, 1989.

Haythornthwaite JA, Menefee LA, Quatrano-Piacentini AL, Pappagallo M. Outcome of chronic opioid therapy for non-cancer pain. *J Pain Symptom Manage* 1998; 15:185–194.

Helzer JE, Robins LN. The Diagnostic Interview Schedule: its development, evaluations, and use. *Soc Psychiatry Psychiatr Epidemiol* 1988; 23:6–16.

Hill CL, Parson J, Taylor A, Leach G. Health related quality of life in a population sample with arthritis. *J Rheumatol* 1999; 26:2029–2035.

Jamison RN. *Mastering Chronic Pain: A Professional's Guide to Behavioral Treatment.* Sarasota, FL: Professional Resource Press, 1996.

Jamison RN, Virts KL. The influence of family support on chronic pain. *Behav Res Ther* 1990; 28:283–287.

Jamison RN, Vasterling JJ, Parris WC. Use of sensory descriptors in assessing chronic pain patients. *J Psychosom Res* 1987; 31:647–652.

Jamison RN, Rock DL, Parris WC. Empirically derived Symptom Checklist 90 subgroups of chronic pain patients: a cluster analysis. *J Behav Med* 1988; 11:147–158.

Jamison RN, Sbrocco T, Parris WC. The influence of physical and psychosocial factors on accuracy of memory for pain in chronic pain patients. *Pain* 1989; 37:289–294.

Jamison RN, Rudy TE, Penzien DB, Mosley TH. Cognitive-behavioral classifications of chronic pain: replication and extension of empirically derived patient profiles. *Pain* 1994; 57:277–292.

Jamison RN, Raymond SA, Slawsby EA, Nedeljkovic SS, Katz NP. Opioid therapy for chronic noncancer back pain. A randomized prospective study. *Spine* 1998; 23:2591–2600.

Jamison RN, Raymond SA, Levine JG, et al. Electronic diaries for monitoring chronic pain: 1-year validation study. *Pain* 2001; 91:277–285.

Jamison RN, Gracely RH, Raymond SA, et al. Comparison study of electronic vs. paper VAS ratings: a randomized, crossover trial using health volunteers. *Pain* 2002; 99:341–347.

Jamison RN, Schein JR, Vallow S, et al. Neuropsychological effects of long-term opioid use in chronic pain patients. *J Pain Symptom Manage* 2003; 26:913–921.

Jensen MP, Karoly P. Control beliefs, coping efforts, and adjustment to chronic pain. *J Consult Clin Psychol* 1991; 59:431–438.

Jensen MP, Karoly P. Self-report scales and procedures for assessing pain in adults. In: Turk DC, Melzack R (Eds). *Handbook of Pain Assessment.* New York: Guilford Press, 2001, pp 15–34.

Jensen MP, McFarland CA. Increasing the reliability and validity of pain intensity measurement in chronic pain patients. *Pain* 1993; 55:195–204.

Jensen MP, Karoly P, Braver S. The measurement of clinical pain intensity: a comparison of six methods. *Pain* 1986; 27:117–126.

Jensen MP, Karoly P, Huger R. The development and preliminary validation of an instrument to assess patients' attitudes toward pain. *J Psychosom Res* 1987; 31:393–400.

Jensen MP, Turner LR, Turner JA. The use of multiple-item scales for pain intensity measurement in chronic pain patients. *Pain* 1996; 67:35–40.

Kames LD, Naliboff BD, Heinrich RL, Schag CC. The chronic illness problem inventory: problem-oriented psychosocial assessment of patients with chronic illness. *Int J Psychiatry Med* 1984; 14:65–75.

Kaplan RM, Schmidt SM, Cronan TA. Quality of well being in patients with fibromyalgia. *J Rheumatol* 2000; 27:785–789.

Karoly P, Jensen MP. *Multimethod Assessment of Chronic Pain*. New York: Pergamon Press, 1987.

Keefe FS, Block AR. Development of an observation method for assessing pain behavior in chronic low back pain patients. *Behav Ther* 1982; 13:363–375.

Keefe FJ, Williams DA, Smith SJ. Assessment of pain behaviors. In: Turk DC, Melzack R (Eds). *Handbook of Pain Assessment.* New York: Guilford Press, 2001, pp 170–187.

Kerns RD, Turk DC, Rudy TE. The West Haven-Yale Multidimensional Pain Inventory (WHYMPI). *Pain* 1985; 23:345–356.

Kerr B, Hill H, Coda B, et al. Concentration-related effects of morphine on cognition and motor control in human subjects. *Neuropsychopharmacology* 1991; 5:157–166.

Leavitt F. The value of the MMPI conversion 'V' in the assessment of psychogenic pain. *J Psychosom Res* 1985; 29:125–131.

Leclaire R, Blier F, Fortin L, Proulx R. A cross-sectional study comparing the Oswestry and Roland-Morris Functional Disability scales in two populations of patients with low back pain of different levels of severity. *Spine* 1997; 22:68–71.

Lezak M. *Neuropsychological Assessment*, 3rd ed. New York: Oxford University Press, 1995.

Lorenz J, Beck H, Bromm B. Cognitive performance, mood and experimental pain before and during morphine-induced analgesia in patients with chronic non-malignant pain. *Pain* 1997; 73:369–375.

Lorig K, Chastain RL, Ung E, Shoor S, Holman HR. Development and evaluation of a scale to measure perceived self-efficacy in people with arthritis. *Arthritis Rheum* 1989; 32:37–44.

Main CJ, Spanswick CC. *Pain Management: An Interdisciplinary Approach.* Edinburgh: Churchill Livingstone, 2000.

Mayfield D, McLeod G, Hall P. The CAGE questionnaire: validation of a new alcoholism screening instrument. *Am J Psychiatry* 1974; 131:1121–1123.

McCreary C. Empirically derived MMPI profile clusters and characteristics of low back pain patients. *J Consult Clin Psychol* 1985; 53:558–560.

Melzack R. The McGill Pain Questionnaire: major properties and scoring methods. *Pain* 1975; 1:277–299.

Merskey H, Bogduk N (Eds). *Classification of Chronic Pain: Descriptions of Chronic Pain Syndromes and Definitions of Pain Terms,* 2nd ed. Seattle: IASP Press, 1994.

Millon T, Green CJ, Meagher Jr RB. The MBHI: a new inventory for the psychodiagnostician in medical settings. *Prof Psychol* 1979; 10:529–539.

Moore JE, McFall ME, Kivlahan DR, Capestany F. Risk of misinterpretation of MMPI schizophrenia scale elevations in chronic pain patients. *Pain* 1988; 32:207–213.

Pilowsky I, Spence ND. Patterns of illness behaviour in patients with intractable pain. *J Psychosom Res* 1975; 19:279–287.

Pollard CA. Preliminary validity study of the Pain Disability Index. *Percept Mot Skills* 1984; 59:974.

Prokop CK, Bradley LA, Margolis R, Gentry WD. Multivariate analysis of the MMPI profiles of patients with multiple pain complaints. *J Pers Assess* 1980; 44:246–252.

Radloff LS. The CES-D Scale: A self-report depression scale for research in the general population. *Appl Psychol Meas* 1977; 1:385–401.

Roland M, Morris R. A study of the natural history of back pain. Part I: Development of a reliable and sensitive measure of disability in low-back pain. *Spine* 1983; 8:141–144.

Rosenstiel AK, Keefe FJ. The use of coping strategies in chronic low back pain patients: relationship to patient characteristics and current adjustment. *Pain* 1983; 17:33–44.

Savage SR. Addiction in the treatment of pain: significance, recognition, and management. *J Pain Symptom Manage* 1993; 8:265–278.

Schofferman J. Long-term use of opioid analgesics for the treatment of chronic pain of nonmalignant origin. *J Pain Symptom Manage* 1993; 8:279–288.

Selzer ML. The Michigan Alcoholism Screening Test: the quest for a new diagnostic instrument. *Am J Psychiatry* 1971; 127:1653–1658.

Skevington SM. Investigating the relationship between pain and discomfort and quality of life, using the WHOQOL. *Pain* 1993; 76:395–406.

Steedman SM, Middaugh SJ, Kee WG. Chronic pain medications: equivalence levels and method of quantifying usage. *Clin J Pain* 1992; 8:204–214.

Stoduto G, Vingilis E, Kapur BM, et al. Alcohol and drug use among motor vehicle collision victims admitted to a regional trauma unit: demographic, injury, and crash characteristics. *Accid Anal Prev* 1993; 25:411–420.

Stratford PW, Binkley JM. A comparison Study of the Back Pain Functional Scale and the Roland Morris Questionnaire. *J Rheumatol* 2000; 27:1928–1936.

Swenson WM, Morse RM. The use of a self-administered alcoholism screen test (SAAST) in a medical center. *Mayo Clin Proc* 1975; 50:204–208.

Tiplady B, Jamieson AH, Cromptom GK. Use of pen-based diaries in an international clinical trial of asthma. *Drug Inform J* 2000; 34:129–136.

Turk DC, Melzack R. *Handbook of Pain Assessment,* 2nd ed. New York: Guilford Press, 2001.

Turk DC, Rudy TE. Toward an empirically derived taxonomy of chronic pain patients: integration of psychological assessment data. *J Consult Clin Psychol* 1988; 56:233–238.

Turk DC, Okifuji A, Sinclair JD, Starz TW. Differential responses by psychosocial subgroups of fibromyalgia syndrome patients to an interdisciplinary treatment. *Arthritis Care Res* 1998; 11:397–404.

Turner JA, Romano JM. Psychological and psychosocial evaluations. In: Loeser JD (Ed). *Bonica's Management of Pain.* Philadelphia: Lippincott Williams & Wilkins, 2001, pp 329–341.

Velikova G, Wright EP, Smith AB, et al. Automated collection of quality-of-life data: a comparison of paper and computer touch-screen questionnaires. *J Clin Oncol* 1999; 17:988–1007.

Vickrey BG, Hays RD, Harooni R, Myers LW. A health-related quality of life measure for multiple sclerosis. *Qual Life Res* 1995; 4:187–206.

Waddell G. *The Back Pain Revolution.* Edinburgh: Churchill Livingstone, 1998.

Waddell G, Main CJ. Assessment of severity in low-back disorders. *Spine* 1984; 9:204–208.

Wang S, Fuh J. Quality of life differs among headache diagnoses: analysis of SF-36 survey in 901 headache patients. *Pain* 2001; 89:285–292.

Ware JE, Sherbourne CD. The MOS 36-item Short Form Health Survey (SF-36). *Med Care* 1992; 30:473–483.

Wedding D, Horton AM Jr, Webster J. *The Neuropsychology Handbook.* New York: Springer, 1986.

Williams DA, Robinson ME, Geisser ME. Pain beliefs: assessment and utility. *Pain* 1994; 59:71–78.

Williams JB, Gibbon M, First MB, et al. The Structured Clinical Interview for DSM-III-R (SCID). II. Multisite test-retest reliability. *Arch Gen Psychiatry* 1992; 49:630–636.

Zacny JP, Conley K, Marks S. Comparing the subjective, psychomotor and physiological effects of intravenous nalbuphine and morphine in healthy volunteers. *J Pharmacol Exp Ther* 1997; 280:1159–1169.

Correspondence to: Robert N. Jamison, PhD, Pain Management Center, Brigham and Women's Hospital, 75 Francis Street, Boston, MA 02115, USA. Email: jamison@zeus.bwh.harvard.edu.

Psychosocial Aspects of Pain: A Handbook for Health Care Providers, Progress in Pain Research and Management, Vol. 27, edited by Robert H. Dworkin and William S. Breitbart, IASP Press, Seattle, © 2004.

7

Mood and Anxiety Disorders in Chronic Pain

Rollin M. Gallagher[a,b,c] and Sunil Verma[c]

[a]*Pain Medicine Service, Veterans Hospital of Philadelphia;* [b]*Departments of Psychiatry and Anesthesiology, University of Pennsylvania; and* [c]*Department of Psychiatry, Drexel University College of Medicine, Philadelphia, Pennsylvania, USA*

It is estimated that more than 50 million Americans suffer from chronic pain (U.S. Department of Health and Human Services 2001). Chronic pain is the most frequent symptom for which patients seek medical care and is associated with substantial economic and psychosocial costs. Many persons, including surgical patients, the elderly, and those suffering from cancer and chronic noncancer pain, receive inadequate treatment for their pain. Because persistent pain has an emotional component and is frequently accompanied by depression or anxiety, patients will benefit from a comprehensive assessment and from a multidisciplinary approach to treatment (Gallagher 1999; Staats 2002). Psychological factors play a significant role not only in chronic pain, but also in the suffering associated with acute pain, particularly in the transition to chronic problems. In a seminal paper in *Pain Medicine,* Rome and Rome (2000) have described the neuroscientific and clinical evidence for a close relationship between pain and mood states.

Fishbain (1999), in reviewing psychiatric problems in patients with pain disorders, proposed five major categories of comorbidity based upon the *Diagnostic and Statistical Manual of Mental Disorders* (DSM-IV; American Psychological Association 1994): (i) Axis I (major psychiatric disorders) comorbidities, e.g., depression and panic disorder; (ii) comorbidity of Axis I and Axis II (personality disorders), e.g., depression and antisocial personality disorder; (iii) Axis I psychoactive substance abuse disorder and other psychiatric disorders, e.g., alcohol dependence and depression; (iv) comorbidities within psychoactive substance abuse disorders, e.g., cocaine and alcohol dependence; and (v) comorbidity of Axis I disorders with a medical condition on Axis III, e.g., depression and coronary artery disease.

The psychiatric comorbidities that occur between chronic pain and Axis I disorders are perhaps most exhaustively studied and documented. Of the Axis I disorders, depression is the most common comorbid condition (Fishbain et al. 1997), with some authors reporting a prevalence rate approaching 100% (Romano and Turner 1985). The other common psychiatric comorbidities include substance abuse-related disorders, somatoform disorders, anxiety disorders, and a miscellaneous group comprising psychotic disorders, schizophrenia, delusional disorders, and bipolar affective disorders. This chapter will focus on management of depression and anxiety disorders associated with chronic pain.

PAIN AND DEPRESSION

Many studies and reviews have documented the high degree of comorbidity of depression with chronic pain in general as well as with specific pain diseases and disorders (Lindsey and Wycoff 1981; Krishnan et al 1985; Romano and Turner 1985; Magni et al. 1990; Gallagher et al. 1991; Wilson et al. 2002). Evidence suggests that the incidence of depression among persons with chronic pain is higher than for other chronic medical illnesses (Banks and Kerns 1996). Conversely, pain is one of the most common presenting symptoms of depression in medical practice, with the prevalence of depression increasing as the number of sites of pain in the body increases (Kroenke and Price 1993), and pain symptoms are reduced when depression is treated (Detke et al. 2002). Depression often follows chronic pain (Atkinson et al. 1991; Banks and Kerns 1996), even in patients without apparent risk factors for depression such as a personal or family history of depressive illness (Dohrenwend et al. 1999). Data from a family study of women with temporomandibular pain and dysfunction syndrome, which included community controls matched for socioeconomic status and first-degree relatives of both patients and controls, suggest the risk model for depression following chronic pain depicted in Fig. 1 (Dohrenwend et al. 1999).

Despite general acceptance of the high comorbidity of pain and depression, variability in the reported rates of depression in pain samples is considerable, ranging from 20% to 80%. Studies obtain variable rates because of methodological differences, such as using heterogeneous samples or discrete samples defined by regional anatomy (e.g., headache, facial pain, back pain), by disease (e.g., diabetic neuropathy, osteoarthritis, cancer) or by psychosocial factors (e.g., workers' compensation, disability, age) or employing different

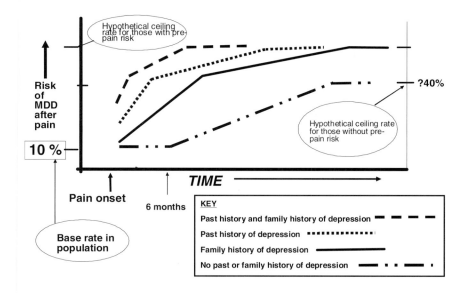

Fig. 1. Hypothetical risk model for major depressive disorder (MDD) in persons who develop chronic pain.

procedures for identifying cases of depression (Banks and Kerns 1996; Gallagher et al. 1991; Romano and Turner 1985). Methods of assessing depressive symptoms include psychometric instruments, often without adequate reliability and validity. Retrospective questionnaires used to establish the presence and timing of depressive and pain episodes are notoriously unreliable (Raphael and Marbach 1997). However, rates may also vary due to small differences in instruments. For example, studies using the DSM-III may underestimate the prevalence of depression because the DSM-III diagnosis of major depressive disorder (MDD) requires "depressed mood for 2 weeks" as a necessary criterion, whereas in DSM-III-R and DSM-IV, "loss of interest or pleasure" can substitute for "depressed mood." Thus, when DSM-III criteria are used, genuine cases of MDD may be missed by doctors who fail to ask about anhedonia and dismiss the possibility of depression when the patient disclaims depressed mood. Denial of depression is thought to be caused by the fear of appearing "weak" (not being able to stand up to the pain), or by unwillingness to be labeled with a "psychogenic" diagnosis and its consequences, such as loss of insurance coverage or workers' compensation benefits (Gallagher and Verma 1999). Many studies do not systematically assess the effects of confounding factors, such as medical illness or medication, on MDD case status. For example, pain and the medications used to treat it can cause several symptoms that are used to establish the

diagnosis of major depression, including sleep disturbance, change in appetite and weight, poor concentration, and fatigue. These factors also can
account for several of the items used in the Beck Depression Inventory, the
most commonly used scale for screening for depressive illness and for assessing the severity of depression. Semistructured instruments based upon
more recent classification schemas, such as the Structured Clinical Interview
for DSM-III-R (SCID) (Williams et al. 1994) also have problems when used
in studies of clinical pain populations, even when used by qualified clinicians. These instruments do not systematically account for confounding of
either individual diagnostic criteria or the diagnoses themselves by the effects of medication and by other medical problems (Gallagher et al. 1991,
1995a). Also, certain illnesses, such as fibromyalgia, have high rates of depressive symptoms with or without comorbid depression and are thought by
some to be somatic manifestations of mood disorder (Hudson et al. 1985).
One approach to diagnosing depression clinically in the face of the confounding effects of medical illness or drugs is to substitute emotional symptoms
(e.g., crying spells, guilty feelings) for physical symptoms (e.g., sleep disturbance, fatigue) to establish a threshold for case status of five out of nine
possible symptoms (Endicott 1984). This procedure is illustrated in Table I,
which lists the DSM-IV criteria along with appropriate substitute symptoms.

Additional problems in classifying psychiatric disorder in pain populations are inattention to diagnostic stability over time, or temporal validation,
and lack of inter-rater reliability. Most studies rely on a single measure of
depression by one interview or questionnaire and lack independent ratings
as well as repeated measures over time. It is quite common with mood
disorders to observe variances over time, for example from depressed to
normal or hypomanic moods or other variations. Many patients present differently from one point of assessment to another, as illustrated by a comparison of two depression prevalence studies in similar samples of disabled
persons with low back pain entering rehabilitation, the first conducted by
Polatin et al. (1993) in Texas and the second by Gallagher et al. (1995a) in
New York. Similar current prevalence rates of 45% and 44% were found,
respectively, using the same structured research interview, the SCID. However, when the New York study added patients diagnosed with MDD by the
clinical gold standard, detailed clinical assessment and treatment outcome
from daily contact for 6–12 weeks during rehabilitation, it found a final rate
of MDD of 72%, suggesting that cross-sectional diagnostic interviews such
as the SCID may overlook cases of MDD in chronic pain patients, and that
after the onset of chronic pain, clinicians as well as researchers should
repeatedly re-evaluate for hidden depression or for the emergence of a first
or recurrent depressive episode.

Table I
Diagnostic criteria for major depression

Questions to Elicit Symptom Criteria	Possible Substitute Symptom
A) Criteria of Major Depression (90–95% Sensitivity)	
Have you had a depressed mood or sadness most days for 2 or more weeks?	None
Do you lack enjoyment or interest in doing things most days for 2 or more weeks?	None
B) Other Symptoms of Depression	
Have you had, for 2 or more weeks, nearly every day, the following:	
Feelings of worthlessness or excessive guilt?	
Recurrent thoughts of death or of not wanting to live; thoughts or plans or an actual attempt to hurt yourself?	Unrealistic pessimism
Difficulty concentrating for 2 or more weeks?	
Fatigue or loss of energy?	Crying spells
Agitation and restlessness or profound slowing down for 2 or more weeks?	
Difficulty sleeping or excessive sleeping?	Lack of motivation in work, relationships, hobbies
Change in appetite or significant weight loss or gain without trying?	Irritability
Additional questions:	
Have you lost interest in sex?	
Are you more irritable at home or work?	

Note: At least one symptom from (A) is required to diagnose major depression; symptom cannot be accounted for by bereavement (within 2 months), substance use or medication, or general medical condition. Either three or four symptoms from (B), added to the one or two from (A), are needed to make a diagnosis of major depression (for a total of at least five symptoms).

MECHANISMS OF THE PAIN-DEPRESSION RELATIONSHIP

The mechanism for the established relationship of pain and depression is not yet clear. That depression is more likely to co-occur with chronic pain than with serious chronic illness without pain, such as cardiac or neurological disorders (Katon and Sullivan 1990), suggests that something more than just the effects of chronicity, perhaps an undiscovered biological mechanism, may account for this association. For example, seasonal fluctuations in chronic myofascial facial pain may be caused, in part, by seasonal fluctuations of mood (Gallagher et al. 1995b). Do nonspecific consequences of the pain, such as disability, loss of social support, and loss of mastery, cause demoralization, learned helplessness (Seligman 1975), and then depression?

Are individuals with chronic pain predisposed to depression because of a family tendency to develop it?

Fishbain et al. (1997), in a systematic review of pain and depression, found a statistical relationship between the presence of chronic pain and depression. Depression appeared to be more common among chronic pain patients than in healthy control patients without pain. The reviewed studies supported the relationship between severity of depression and the intensity of perceived pain as well as the relationship between pain and suicide. Regarding the question of whether depression preceded or followed the development of chronic pain, no unequivocal answer was forthcoming. However, there was more evidence for the "consequence hypothesis" (depression following chronic pain) than for the "antecedent hypothesis" (depression preceding pain). Some evidence supported the "scar hypothesis" (a history of depression causing vulnerability to pain disorders), and this was more likely in patients with a diagnosis of major depression than in patients with any other DSM diagnosis. However, it must be emphasized that the reviewed studies were heterogeneous in terms of the pain population group and the criteria used for diagnosing depression.

Family studies of depression and pain have shed light on the causal direction of the comorbidity model. Recent reviewers cite mounting evidence that patients with chronic nonmalignant pain disorders have elevated personal and family histories of clinical depression (Magni 1987; Banks and Kerns 1996; Kinney et al. 1996; Fishbain et al. 1997). France et al. (1986) showed that in a sample of patients with low back pain referred to a well-known tertiary care center, the relatives of patients with depression had higher rates of affective disorder as compared with relatives of patients without depression. This finding suggests that individuals with positive family histories of depression are more susceptible to developing depression once they develop chronic pain. The recent study by Dohrenwend et al. (1999), which employed a more sophisticated family study design, showed that the stress of living with pain may be causative of depression (see Fig. 1). This study's methodological advantages included a homogeneous chronic pain sample (women with myofascial facial pain), derived with standardized criteria (history and physical examination), and a same-sex control group (from the same community and with similar educational and socioeconomic status). The investigators conducted a direct psychiatric interview of at-risk cases, controls, and family members using the SCID to establish depression diagnosis, and added a semi-structured interview to evaluate confounding of depression diagnosis by physical factors (Gallagher et al. 1991, 1995a). They also included an independent comprehensive health interview and a review of medical records to help determine the timing of onset of pain and depression. As a group, women with depression beginning after the onset of pain did not have different family histories of mood disorder than women who had pain without depression or controls without pain or depression. The findings support the hypothesis that in most cases, the stress of living with chronic pain, not premorbid personal or familial depression, causes depression. However, in this pain sample, and we suspect in other samples, individuals with a personal or family history of depression, or both, developed depression sooner after pain onset than did those without such histories, suggesting the scar hypothesis or family vulnerability hypothesis.

When present, depression seems to play an important role in the experience of chronic pain. Patients with depression report higher levels of pain, tend to be less active, report greater disability and greater interference due to pain, and display more pain behaviors (Keefe et al. 1986; Haythornthwaite et al. 1991; Krause et al. 1994). A systematic review of prospective cohort studies in low back pain by Picus and colleagues (2002) showed that distress, depressed mood, and somatization are implicated in the transition from acute to chronic low back pain.

A number of studies also suggest that depression and depressive symptoms can augment the functional impairment related to pain and that depression persists in community populations despite access to excellent health care. In a prospective study of 228 well-insured older adults in a retirement community, Mossey and colleagues (2000) conducted sequential evaluations, every 6 months over 24 months, of pain, depression, physical impairment, and health care utilization. They found that pain and depressive symptoms were commonly comorbid, with increasing symptoms of depression associated with increasing pain-related impairment, that this comorbidity was usually sustained longitudinally (Mossey and Gallagher 2001), and that even mild depressive symptoms increased health care utilization over 2 years in older adults with pain (Gallagher and Mossey 2002).

Statistics on the relationship between specific common physical symptoms and depression in primary care patients further illustrate the pervasiveness of pain and depression comorbidity. Kroenke and Price (1993) found that the presence of any physical symptom increased the likelihood of a diagnosis of a mood or anxiety disorder in a sample of primary care patients by as much as threefold. Furthermore, 34% of patients with joint or limb pain, 38% of patients with back pain, 40% of patients with headache, 46% of patients with chest pain, and 43% of patients with abdominal pain also had a mood disorder.

A review of recent research suggests neurobiological mechanisms underlying the pain-depression relationship. Pain modulation and mood regulation are both influenced by the neurotransmitters norepinephrine and serotonin. Disturbances in these systems, and activation of the N-methyl-D-aspartate (NMDA)-receptor system in both chronic pain and depression, may underlie the close association of these conditions that we see clinically (Rome and Rome 2000; Blier and Abbott 2001; Verma and Gallagher 2002).

PSYCHIATRIC MANAGEMENT OF DEPRESSION IN PATIENTS WITH CHRONIC PAIN

The successful management of depression begins with a thorough initial assessment to establish the diagnosis and investigate potential biopsychosocial risks and strengths. Physicians initiating treatment have at their disposal a rapidly growing pharmacopeia, several psychotherapeutic techniques, electroconvulsive therapy, and other interventions. The specific components of psychiatric management that must be addressed for all patients are described in this section.

SCREENING FOR DEPRESSION

All patients with pain disorders should be screened for depression using simple diagnostic instruments such as the Beck Depression Inventory (Beck 1976) or by imbedding screening questions into the review of systems, which has the advantage of reducing systematic response bias (Gallagher and Verma 1999). Although all patients with chronic pain should be evaluated periodically for depression, particular attention should be paid to patients who have multiple sites of pain (Engel et al. 1996). If screening is positive, a more thorough diagnostic evaluation is needed to establish a more definitive diagnosis of a mood disorder, to formulate the relationship of depression to pain and its treatment, and to evaluate the presence of other comorbid psychiatric or medical conditions. Chronic pain can be considered a chronic disease associated with considerable risk for the onset of complicating or recurrent depressive illness. Hence, because initial evaluation may have a significant false-negative rate (Gallagher et al. 1995a), even when depression is not detected at first, clinicians should periodically screen for depression during treatment, particularly when there is a change in pain symptoms, impairment, or disability.

ESTABLISHING A DIAGNOSIS OF DEPRESSION

The diagnostic process should include a history of present illness and current symptoms; a past psychiatric history, including a history of depression or mania; a depression treatment history, including response to previous treatments; a general medical history and history of substance abuse; a family history of psychiatric illness; a personal history, which should include psychological development, coping skills, and response to previous life events; a mental status examination; and selective physical and laboratory examinations as indicated (Nurcombe and Gallagher 1986). So closely are pain and mood linked in the case of a person with chronic pain that a thorough assessment of the pain and its impact on mood and other aspects of quality of life must be integrated into the assessment for depression. This assessment should establish whether the patient has one or more of several possible mood disorder diagnoses: major depression, minor depression, dysthymia, bipolar illness, substance-induced mood disturbance, or mood disorder secondary to a medical condition (American Psychiatric Association 1994).

EVALUATING THE SAFETY OF THE PATIENT

Chronic pain can be a fatal disease because of its association with suicide (Fishbain 1996) and with violence (Bruns and DiSorbio 2000). A careful assessment of a patient's suicidal risk will have a direct bearing on whether he or she would be best treated in an inpatient or outpatient setting. Evidence is relatively strong that pain patients are at a greater risk for suicide than are nonpain patients (Fishbain 1996). The assessment of suicide risk should include presence of suicidal ideation, intent, plans made by the patient, and the availability and lethality of methods being contemplated. All suicidal patients should be evaluated by a professional with the proper training to assess suicidal risk and to arrange appropriate management. Pain clinicians should be aware that depression increases the risk of having anger attacks (Fava et al. 1991), that samples of persons with chronic pain who are in treatment have higher rates of violent ideation than do samples of community controls, and that depression increases this risk (Bruns and Disorbio 2000). Other factors associated with chronic pain that increase the risk of violence include job dissatisfaction, unemployment, workers' compensation, work rehabilitation programs, litigation, and a diagnosis of malingering (Fishbain et al. 2000b). Those of us involved with chronic pain patients are highly aware of the antagonistic relationships that pervade the triad of workers' compensation insurer, employer, and injured worker, and thus potentially threaten the very well-being of a patient's family. The physician should be aware of these risks and should always ask patients at evaluation, or during the course of treatment when there is a setback, if they are bothered by anger outbursts or angry thoughts, and whether they can control these thoughts.

ESTABLISHING AND MAINTAINING A THERAPEUTIC ALLIANCE

An effective working relationship starts with educating patients about their condition, the goals of treatment, and the rationale for different treatment choices, and defining the clinician's expectations of the patient's responsibilities for record-keeping, adherence, and follow-up. The trust in this relationship becomes critically important when dealing with matters of safety—drug toxicity, suicide, and violence. Creating a trusting and positive working relationship with the patient, and if possible with the family or significant others, is important to ensure safe and effective treatment, particularly in this era of rational polypharmacy. Successfully titrating medications to their analgesic and antidepressant potential requires that the clinician and patient communicate effectively about potential side effects, toxicity, drug interactions, and therapeutic targets.

EDUCATING THE PATIENT AND HIS OR HER FAMILY ABOUT DEPRESSION

Education concerning depression, pain, and the relationship between pain and depression should be provided to all patients and to the appropriate family members when indicated as well. Patients and families can be directed to an educational Web site, such as www.painconnection.org of the National Pain Foundation, to learn more about pain, including comorbid depression. Uninformed family members can sabotage the best of treatment plans by discouraging patients from taking psychotropic medication because of their fear of presumed side effects or addiction. Furthermore, in chronic pain patients, marital dissatisfaction and negative spousal responses to pain are related to depressive symptoms, suggesting that screening for marital problems may be important for treatment outcome in persons with chronic pain (Cano et al. 2000). In our clinical practice, we have found it useful to have time-limited pain management education groups for around 7–10 sessions in which we discuss various aspects of pain, mood, stress, anxiety, relationships, activities, and other pain-related issues, including the rational use of medications in these conditions (Gallagher 1999). Spouses may also benefit from these groups (Langelier and Gallagher 1989). Longitudinal open-ended support groups are also an important part of our clinical practice.

ENHANCING TREATMENT ADHERENCE

Successful treatment of depression requires close adherence to treatment plans for long or indefinite durations to assure full remission and to prevent relapse or recurrence (Kupfer 1991). However, particularly in the early stages of treatment, patients with pain and depression may be poorly motivated and unduly pessimistic about their chance of recovery. Asking patients to fill out pain diaries, scheduling frequent clinic visits or follow-up calls by staff, and enthusiastically educating patients and significant others about the mechanisms and importance of medication treatment may improve treatment adherence. In addition, side effects of medications must be carefully explained, because they may be an important reason for noncompliance.

PHARMACOLOGICAL MANAGEMENT OF DEPRESSION

With the introduction of escitalopram, 22 compounds have been approved by the U.S. Food and Drug Administration (FDA) as antidepressants, with two additional drugs (clomipramine and fluvoxamine) now being marketed outside the United States as antidepressants and having been approved by the FDA for obsessive-compulsive disorder (Richelson 2001). Reboxetine and duloxetine may be the next antidepressants approved for marketing in the United States. A classification and doses of the antidepressants are presented in Table II.

The plethora of medications for depression presents the practitioner with many choices. How must a clinician decide which drug is best for his or her patient? Are these drugs different in their efficacy? Are some antidepressants more efficacious when depression and pain are comorbid? The mechanism by which antidepressant medications achieve their therapeutic benefit is incompletely understood. No single drug has proved more effective than any other for the relief of depressive symptoms (Mulrow et al. 2000), although some recent evidence suggests that dual-action antidepressants with both noradrenergic and serotonergic re-uptake inhibition may have increased efficacy in achieving depression remission (Thase 2003). More than 80% of depressed patients have a response to at least one medication, although individual antidepressants are effective in only 50–60% of patients. Factors that may be considered in selecting a particular antidepressant include a previous response to that medication, a family history of a response to the same medication, and anticipated side effects (Depression Guideline Panel 1993). Anxiety and insomnia do not necessarily predict a better response to more sedating medications (Beasley et al. 1991; Tollefson et al. 1994; Simon et al. 1998). Although selective serotonin reuptake inhibitors (SSRIs) cost

Table II
Starting and usual doses of antidepressants (dose similar for anxiety
and depression titrate depending on clinical response)

Medication	Starting Dose (mg/day)	Usual Dose (mg/day)
Tertiary Amine Tricyclics		
Amitriptyline	25–50	100–300
Clomipramine*	25	100–300
Doxepin	25–50	100–300
Imipramine	25–50	100–300
Trimipramine	25–50	100–300
Secondary Amine Tricyclics		
Desipramine	25–50	100–300
Nortriptyline	25	50–200
Protriptyline	10	15–60
Tetracyclics		
Amoxapine	50	100–400
Maprotiline	50	100–225
Selective Serotonin Reuptake Inhibitors		
Citalopram	20	20–60
Escitalopram	10	10–20
Fluoxetine	20	20–60
Fluvoxamine*	50	50–300
Paroxetine	20	20–60
Sertraline	50	50–200
Dopamine-Norepinephrine Reuptake Inhibitors		
Bupropion	100 b.i.d.	150 t.i.d.
Bupropion (sustained release)	150 q.a.m.	150 b.i.d.
Bupropion (extended release)	150 q.a.m.	300 mg q.a.m.
Serotonin-Norepinephrine Reuptake Inhibitors		
Venlafaxine	37.5 bid	375
Venlafaxine (extended release)	37.5	225
Serotonin Modulators		
Nefazodone	50	150–300
Trazodone	50	75–300
Norepinephrine-Serotonin Modulator		
Mirtazapine	15	15–45
Monoamine Oxidase Inhibitors		
Irreversible, nonselective		
Phenelzine	15	15–90
Tranylcypromine	10	30–60
Reversible		
Moclobemide†	150	300–600
Selective Norepinephrine Reuptake Inhibitor		
Reboxetine‡		

* Approved for treatment of obsessive-compulsive disorder only.
† Not available in the United States. ‡ FDA approval anticipated.

more than tricyclic antidepressants (TCAs), the total costs of treatment with these two drug classes are usually similar because of the increased number of visits associated with switching to the more expensive SSRIs in some patients who begin with tricyclic agents but cannot tolerate their side effects or toxicity (Simon et al. 1999). The side-effect burden of antidepressant doses of TCAs increases with age, increasing the chances of an untoward reaction. Newer antidepressants are generally less toxic than TCAs in cases of overdose but do not reduce the overall risk of suicide (Jick et al. 1995).

How does one choose the best antidepressant for the patient with comorbid pain and depression? The issues of efficacy, remission rates, dosing, adherence, and cost are all important factors that must be considered together (Verma and Gallagher 2002). For example, if a physician prescribes an expensive antidepressant to a patient who cannot afford it, the patient is likely to discontinue it, leading to relapse and a recurrence of depression. Instead, looking at remission rates and cost together will help the clinician determine the best value for cost-sensitive patients. Dosing simplicity is also important in promoting adherence.

Due to the good efficacy rates and dosing simplicity, many patients with pain and depression receive SSRIs as initial treatment. As soon as antidepressants are started, it is important to follow the patient closely for a response. Patients, family, and physicians must not be impatient. If after a couple of weeks the patient is not responding to the recommended dose, the dose may be increased.

It is also important to confirm that the patient is in fact taking the medication (Mojtabai and Olfson 2003); clinicians should not assume that a patient is taking the drug as prescribed. Many patients have preset notions about the dangers and social implications of receiving antidepressants, and to avoid problems of noncompliance, the clinician should query patients about their attitudes toward taking medication for depression. Educating patients and their families (if possible and appropriate) about the benefits of the drug and the risk of relapse will help promote adherence. Furthermore, perpetuating factors such as stress, pain, and substance abuse must be addressed for successful outcomes.

If patients do not achieve remission with SSRIs, another category of antidepressants with a mixed mechanism of action should be tried. Thase and colleagues (2001) conducted a meta-analysis of eight randomized, double-blind trials to compare remission rates for depression during treatment with SSRIs versus venlafaxine, which acts as a dual reuptake inhibitor at high doses. Forty-five percent of patients achieved remission on venlafaxine compared to 35% of those taking SSRIs ($P < 0.001$); only 25% of patients who were randomized to receive placebo achieved remission (Thase 2003).

Animal and human studies suggest that antidepressants with dual nore-pinephrine and serotonin reuptake inhibition activity, such as venlafaxine and duloxetine, also provide superior pain relief compared with antidepressants that selectively act on either neurotransmitter alone (Max 1994; Fishbain et al. 2000a). In theory, these medications have the potential to help ameliorate symptoms of neuropathic pain and depression at the same time through their dual action.

These newer antidepressants with dual norepinephrine and serotonin reuptake inhibition, but with minimal activity at other receptor sites, are termed selective serotonin-norepinephrine reuptake inhibitors (SNRIs). They may prove to be advantageous clinically because of their combination of qualities including higher rates of depression remission, fewer side effects, fewer drug interactions, and in the case of duloxetine, the convenience of single dosing. Because of their effectiveness in neuropathic pain, their higher rates of depression remission, and their tolerability as compared with TCAs, many experienced clinicians consider SNRIs to be the drugs of first choice for patients with pain and depression, particularly when pain is neuropathic.

If antidepressants are equally efficacious as far as treating depression is concerned, are there any analgesic properties of antidepressants that can be utilized in treating patients with comorbid pain and depression? As suggested above, antidepressants have been used to treat various chronic non-neuropathic (nociceptive/inflammatory) and neuropathic pain conditions. In animal studies, using inflammatory and nerve injury models of persistent pain, which are of more relevance to human chronic pain conditions, antidepressants have demonstrated consistent analgesic properties (Sawynok et al. 2001). Analgesic effects are observed both when antidepressants are administered in the cerebral ventricles (Speigel et al. 1983; Sierralta et al. 1995; Schreiber et al. 1998) and when they are given spinally (Hwang and Wilcox 1987; Iwashita and Shimizu 1992; Eisenach and Gebhart 1995). More recent evidence indicates that peripheral administration of antidepressants produces analgesia (Sawynok et al. 1999a,b; Scott et al. 1999). The therapeutic effects of antidepressants in chronic pain conditions can be understood on the basis of the common neurotransmitters, norepinephrine and serotonin, that are implicated both in depression and pain. Antidepressants may be clinically effective in chronic pain through one or more of several mechanisms (Gallagher and Verma 1999). (1) Many antidepressant medications are thought to have direct analgesic effects by modulating pain perception through activity on noradrenergic and serotonergic neurophysiological systems that descend from the midbrain to the dorsal horn (Max 1994). Consistent with the mechanism of certain anticonvulsants, inhibition of sodium channel activity in the neuronal membrane may also contribute to the analgesic properties of antidepressants in neuropathic pain. (2) Comorbid depressive illnesses may worsen pain perception, interfere with coping, and contribute additional morbidity (France 1987; Gallagher and Verma 1999). Antidepressants could ameliorate pain through either of two purported mechanisms: first, by treating the "masked depression" in which pain is thought to be a symptom of the depression (Blumer and Heilbron 1982); and second, by treating manifest depression caused by the pain (Banks and Kerns 1996; Dohrenwend et al. 1999), which enables the patient to better tolerate the pain (Aronoff and Evans 1982). Panic disorder also specifically responds to antidepressants. (3) Antidepressants can reduce pain-related symptoms, including sleep disturbances and appetite disturbances, that can contribute significantly to chronic pain-related distress, psychological morbidity, and physical disability (Botney and Fields 1983; Gallagher and Woznicki 1993; Gallagher and Verma 2000).

TRICYCLIC AND TETRACYCLIC ANTIDEPRESSANTS

Data from 41 controlled trials indicate that tricyclic antidepressants are effective analgesics (Lynch 2001). Amitriptyline is the most thoroughly studied agent, although desipramine, imipramine, clomipramine, nortriptyline, and doxepin have also been well studied. Thirteen controlled trials have examined the analgesic effects of tricyclics in neuropathic pain. Consistent evidence shows that the tricyclics act as analgesics in diabetic neuropathy (Kvinesdale et al. 1984; Max et al. 1987, 1991; Sindrup et al. 1989; Joss 1999), postherpetic neuralgia (Watson et al. 1998), central pain syndromes (Panerai et al. 1990), poststroke pain (Leijon and Boivie 1989), and chronic headache (Tomkins et al. 2001). In addition, tricyclics may be effective not only in chronic pain syndromes but also as pre-emptive analgesics (Bowsher 1997) and in postoperative pain, where they can potentiate the effect of opioids (Levine et al. 1986).

As compared to the tricyclics, evidence is limited on the efficacy of the tetracyclics maprotiline (Lindsay and Olsen 1985) and amoxapine (Pfeiffer 1982) in treatment of pain disorders. Maprotiline appears to be more effective than paroxetine (Atkinson et al. 1999), but not superior to tricyclics (Eberhard et al. 1988; Watson et al. 1992; Vrethem et al. 1997).

Given that all tricyclic and tetracyclic antidepressants are equally effective in treating depression, and that most tricyclics and SNRIs are efficacious in pain disorders, the choice of a particular antidepressant is often influenced by its side-effect profile. Two factors that should always be kept in mind when prescribing tricyclics are *the potential for a lethal outcome in an overdose* and the *possibility of inducing a manic episode* in patients with and without history of mania. Common side effects of TCAs are described below.

Anticholinergic effects. These effects are common, though patients may develop tolerance for these effects with continued treatment. The anticholinergic effects include dry mouth, constipation, blurred vision, and urinary retention. Amitriptyline, imipramine, trimipramine, and doxepin are the most anticholinergic drugs; amoxapine, maprotiline, and nortriptyline are less anticholinergic; and desipramine is the least anticholinergic.

Sedation. This is a common side effect of tricyclics, although it may be welcomed in patients with sleep disturbances. Amitriptyline, doxepin, and trimipramine are the most sedating, while desipramine and protriptyline are the least sedating.

Autonomic effects. These effects are due to α_1- adrenergic blockade and result in orthostatic hypotension. Amitriptyline, doxepin, clomipramine, amoxapine, and nortriptyline, in that order, may be more likely to cause this side effect.

Cardiac effects. In therapeutic doses, tricyclics and tetracyclics may cause tachycardia, prolonged QT intervals, and depressed ST segments on EKGs. Thus their use is contraindicated in patients with prolonged conduction times. In patients with cardiac histories, these drugs should be initiated at low doses, with gradual dose increase and monitoring of cardiac functions.

SELECTIVE SEROTONIN REUPTAKE INHIBITORS

Fluoxetine was the first drug of this class to be introduced in the United States in 1988. Since then the SSRIs (fluoxetine, fluvoxamine, sertraline, paroxetine, and citalopram) have become the most frequently prescribed antidepressants owing to their favorable side-effect profile. However, their analgesic effects have not been as pronounced as those of drugs in the TCA class.

Ten studies have evaluated the efficacy of SSRIs in the treatment of chronic headache. Three of these studies found that SSRIs were no better than placebos, two studies reported them to be marginally better than placebos, and the others showed that although they resulted in some improvement, they were not better than the comparison drug (Jung et al. 1997). Three controlled trials have examined SSRIs in the treatment of painful diabetic neuropathy. The largest study, with 46 subjects (Max et al. 1992), found no difference between fluoxetine and placebo, and the other studies found both citalopram and paroxetine to be better than placebo (Sindrup et al. 1990, 1992). In studies that have examined both SSRIs and TCAs, the analgesia obtained with tricyclics was superior in every case (Lynch 2001). In an attempt to estimate the efficacy of different treatments, Sindrup and

Jensen (2000) identified all placebo-controlled drug trials involving treatment of pain in polyneuropathy. They calculated the number of patients they needed to treat (NNT) to obtain one patient with more than 50% pain relief. The NNT was 2.6 for tricyclics, 6.7 for SSRIs, 2.5 for anticonvulsant sodium channel blockers, 4.1 for the anticonvulsant calcium channel blocker gabapentin, and 3.4 for the mixed opioid and monoaminergic drug tramadol. The reviews of antidepressant analgesia suggest that antidepressants with both serotonin and norepinephrine reuptake inhibition show the greatest analgesic effect (Onghena and Van Houdenhove 1992; Fishbain et al. 2000a) and indicate that norepinephrine reuptake inhibition may be crucial for pain relief in diabetic and postherpetic neuralgia (Semenchuk and Davis 2000).

Although questions remain about the analgesic effects of SSRIs, there is no questioning their efficacy as antidepressants. SSRIs account for about 50% of all antidepressant prescriptions in the United States. Although they are not superior to the other antidepressants, they have a favorable side-effect profile as compared to tricyclics and monoamine oxidase (MAO) inhibitors as well as safety in overdoses, which often makes them the drug of first choice in the treatment of depression.

The major differences among the available SSRIs lie primarily in their pharmacokinetic profiles, specifically their half-lives. Fluoxetine has the longest half-life of 2–3 days; its active metabolite has a half-life of 7–9 days. The half-lives of other SSRIs are much shorter, about 20 hours. All SSRIs are metabolized in the liver by the cytochrome P450 (CYP) isoenzyme and therefore clinicians should be careful about drug interactions. Citalopram and escitalopram are least affected by CYP isoenzymes.

The most common side effects of SSRIs include agitation, anxiety, sleep disturbance, tremor, sexual dysfunction, and headache. Citalopram may have a lesser rate of sexual side effects than other SSRIs. Rarely, SSRIs have been associated with extrapyramidal symptoms, arthralgias, lymphadenopathy, inappropriate antidiuretic syndrome, agranulocytosis, and hypoglycemia. SSRIs can interact with MAO inhibitors to cause the central serotonin syndrome manifested by abdominal pain, diarrhea, sweating, fever, tachycardia, elevated mood, hypertension, altered mental state, delirium, myoclonus, increased motor activity, irritability, and hostility (Ener et al. 2003). For this reason, SSRIs should be prescribed with caution in patients taking tramadol for pain or triptans for migraine. Severe manifestation of this syndrome can include hyperemia, cardiovascular shock, and death. SSRIs are essentially devoid of the type 1A anti-arrhythmic effect of tricyclics, nor do they have any α-adrenergic antagonistic effect, and so they rarely are associated with orthostatic hypotension.

DOPAMINE-NOREPINEPHRINE REUPTAKE INHIBITORS

Bupropion was first synthesized in 1966, soon after TCAs entered widespread use, and emerged as an antidepressant without any anticholinergic or cardiac effects. However, increased incidence of drug-induced seizures in bulimic nondepressed subjects in one study delayed its marketing. Subsequent studies of depressed patients did not replicate this finding, and the drug was reintroduced in 1989. Evidence for the efficacy of bupropion in pain disorders comes from an open-labeled study (Semenchuk and Davis 2000) that reported significant reductions in pain levels at the end of 8 weeks, and from a double-blind, placebo-controlled crossover study (Semenchuk et al. 2001) that showed that bupropion in doses of 150–300 mg was effective and well tolerated for the treatment of neuropathic pain. Bupropion, because of its norepinephrine reuptake blockade, has the potential for being an analgesic antidepressant, although this possibility remains to be studied conclusively. As an antidepressant it as effective as other antidepressants with a unique side-effect profile, notably little psychosexual dysfunction. The adverse effects of bupropion are due to its potentiating effects on the dopaminergic system, namely, delusions and hallucinations and the risk of seizures, which affect about 5% of individuals taking doses of 450–600 mg a day.

SEROTONIN-NOREPINEPHRINE REUPTAKE INHIBITORS

Venlafaxine is an effective antidepressant that blocks the reuptake of norepinephrine and serotonin like the TCAs without the undesirable side effects associated with tricyclics. Its properties include a faster-than-usual onset of action and demonstrated efficacy in seriously depressed patients (e.g., patients with melancholic features). The norepinephrine reuptake-inhibiting properties of venlafaxine, particularly at the higher dosing schedules, along with its structural similarity to tramadol, an analgesic with both opioid agonist and monoaminergic activity (Markowitz and Patrick 1998), makes it a promising antidepressant that may benefit patients with chronic pain. In healthy volunteers, venlafaxine increased the pain tolerance threshold to electrical sural nerve stimulation and the threshold at which pain increases (pain summation). The impact of venlafaxine on pain summation in this experimental pain model of repetitive stimulation indicates a potential analgesic effect in clinical neuropathic pain (Enggaard et al. 2001). Several case reports suggest venlafaxine's efficacy in pain disorders (Songer and Schulte 1996; Davis and Smith 1999; Pernia et al. 2000; Tasmuth et al. 2002), but controlled studies are lacking. Venlafaxine is generally well tolerated. Its side effects include nausea (37%), somnolence (23%), dry mouth

(22%), and dizziness (22%). The most potentially worrisome adverse effect associated with venlafaxine is an increase in blood pressure, particularly in patients taking more than 300 mg a day.

Detke and colleagues (2002) recently conducted a multicenter, double-blind, placebo-controlled trial of duloxetine hydrochloride, a new dual reuptake inhibitor of serotonin and norepinephrine, in patients with major depression. Duloxetine proved significantly more effective than placebo ($P < 0.001$) in reducing depression and painful physical symptoms when compared with placebo. Preliminary studies indicate efficacy in diabetic neuropathy as well.

SEROTONIN MODULATORS

Trazodone and nefazodone are antidepressants that are structurally related to each other, but are unrelated to the TCAs, MAO inhibitors, and SSRIs. Trazodone is distinctive in its sedating properties and is used to treat insomnia in both pain and depression. Nefazodone is relatively free of this effect and is generally well tolerated and effective as an antidepressant; there are no human reports or randomized trials examining its analgesic effects. There are four placebo-controlled trials examining trazodone as an analgesic, and in general they support an analgesic effect (Lynch 2001). Nefazodone has a half-life of 2–4 hours and must be given in twice-daily doses. Its notable adverse reactions include liver failure, a drop in blood pressure, and in particular, interactions with the benzodiazepines triazolam and alprazolam, with the third-generation antihistamines terfenadine and astemizole, and with cisapride due to its inhibition of cytochrome P450 (CYP 3A4).

NOREPINEPHRINE-SEROTONIN MODULATOR

Mirtazapine is an antidepressant with a novel mechanism of action. By acting as an antagonist of the central presynaptic α_2-adrenergic receptors, it potentiates central noradrenergic and serotonergic transmission. It is an effective antidepressant, yet it lacks the anticholinergic effects of the TCAs and the anxiogenic effects associated with some SSRIs. Mirtazapine, because of its broad neurotransmitter profile, has the potential to be an analgesic antidepressant, but as far as we are aware, only a single case report has documented its efficacy in any pain disorder (Brannon and Stone 1999). The adverse effects associated with mirtazapine include somnolence, which is comparable to amitriptyline and may be welcome in patients with sleep disturbances, increased appetite with weight gain, increased serum cholesterol, and rarely agranulocytosis and neutropenia (affecting 0.3% of patients taking mirtazapine).

MONOAMINE OXIDASE INHIBITORS

Monoamine oxidase inhibitors act by increasing biogenic amine levels by inhibiting their degradation. The indication for MAO inhibitors is similar to those of TCAs. MAO inhibitors may be particularly effective for use in panic disorder with agoraphobia, post-traumatic stress disorder, eating disorders, social phobia, and atypical depression characterized by hypersomnia, hyperphagia, anxiety, and the absence of vegetative symptoms. There is one controlled trial in the literature involving 40 patients with atypical facial pain and depression, in which 45 mg of phenelzine led to a significant improvement in both pain and depression (Lascelles 1966). Animal studies support the analgesic effects of MAO inhibitors (Schreiber et al. 1998), but they have not been replicated in pain patients. The side effects of these agents and their potential for precipitating a toxic central serotonin syndrome when combined with other medications and certain foods limit their use to only treatment-resistant depression. Tyramine-induced hypertensive crisis in patients taking MAO inhibitors can be life threatening. Other side effects include orthostatic hypertension, weight gain, edema, sexual dysfunction, and insomnia.

ANTICONVULSANTS

Anticonvulsant drugs have an established role in the treatment of chronic neuropathic pain, especially when patients complain of shooting sensations. Anticonvulsant drugs have been used in pain management since the 1960s, very soon after they were first introduced in medicine, when they revolutionized the medical management of epilepsy. The clinical impression, supported by double-blind, placebo-controlled studies, is that they are useful for neuropathic pain, especially when the pain is lancinating or burning (Backonja 2000). The precise mechanisms of action of anticonvulsant drugs remain uncertain. The two standard explanations are enhanced γ-aminobutyric acid (GABA) inhibition or a stabilizing effect on neuronal cell membranes through sodium or calcium channel-blocking activity. A third possibility is action via NMDA-receptor sites. The newer anticonvulsants are now most often used in chronic pain conditions, including gabapentin, topiramate, and lamotrigine, all which have demonstrated efficacy in one or more neuropathic pain conditions (Backonja et al. 1998; Rowbotham et al. 1998, 2000; Sindrup and Jensen 1999; Eisenberg et al. 2001). Older anticonvulsants, such as phenytoin, clonazepam, and valproic acid, have not shown efficacy in clinical studies and because of their problematic toxicity, are generally not used, with the exception of carbamazepine, which has proved effective in trigeminal neuralgia.

Many of the anticonvulsants also have mood-stabilizing properties, but no controlled studies support the utility of mood-stabilizing agents as primary or augmentation therapy in depression (Christina 2000). Case reports, however, indicate marked improvement after, for example, the addition of carbamazepine to clomipramine and valproic acid to fluoxetine or fluvoxamine (Corrigan 1992; De la Fuente et al. 1992).

The anticonvulsants lamotrigine and gabapentin may have antimanic and antidepressant activity. Gabapentin seems to be safe and well tolerated; lamotrigine requires careful dosing and close monitoring because of potentially severe skin rash. Lamotrigine has been described as potentially useful in the treatment of various phases of refractory bipolar disorder (Calabrese et al. 1999a). Although presently it is an investigational drug for bipolar disorder, a growing number of clinicians appear to be adding it to the treatment regimens of bipolar patients with complex, treatment-resistant forms of illness. A double-blind study also showed lamotrigine at a dose of 50 or 200 mg/day to be superior to placebo for depression in patients with bipolar disorder (Calabrese et al. 1999b). In a placebo-controlled study (Eisenberg et al. 2001), lamotrigine was found to be effective and safe in relieving pain associated with diabetic neuropathy. Gabapentin has received recent attention as possible monotherapy or add-on treatment for bipolar illness by virtue of several factors, including its GABA-enhancing properties, favorable side-effect profile, possible anxiolytic effects, and virtual absence of drug interactions.

PSYCHOTHERAPY AND BEHAVIOR THERAPY FOR MOOD AND ANXIETY DISORDERS IN CHRONIC PAIN

Although psychopharmacological treatments of psychiatric comorbidities associated with chronic pain are helpful, they are almost never successful by themselves. This is because chronic pain not only has an anatomic and neurological substrate but also involves the conditioning of the neurophysiological system, both by pain itself and by its psychosocial contextual experience. The treatment of chronic pain is multidimensional, and psychotherapeutic interventions form one of the cornerstones of managing not only the psychiatric comorbidities but also pain itself (Gallagher 1999). The psychotherapeutic techniques that have been used in treating chronic pain patients,

which may exert some of their beneficial effects by regulating mood and
anxiety, have included methods focusing on pain education and supportive
psychotherapy, in which patients' existing coping strategies are strengthened. Important interventions, discussed in more detail below, include
cognitive-behavioral therapy, behavior therapy, interpersonal therapy, and
dynamic psychotherapy. Other useful types of therapy include family therapy
and couples therapy, which address the fact that chronic pain is such a
disruptive problem that it is likely to affect the entire family; and group
therapies, which can be either educational, psychotherapeutic, or both.

These psychosocial interventions are useful in managing depression and
anxiety associated with pain. Although these strategies are discussed in the
literature as distinct entities, such categorization is useful for heuristic purposes only. In clinical practice, psychotherapists use a combination of approaches that are individually tailored to meet the patient's circumstances.
The major forms of individual psychosocial interventions are described below.

Cognitive-behavioral therapy. This form of psychotherapy maintains
that irrational beliefs and distorted attitudes toward the self, the environment, and the future perpetuate depression. The goal of cognitive-behavioral
therapy is to reduce depressive symptoms by challenging these beliefs and
attitudes (Beck 1976). Besides focusing on patients' maladaptive cognitions,
the therapist can introduce behavioral techniques such as relaxation therapy
and assertiveness training, as described by Waters et al. (this volume). Cognitive-behavioral therapy can help patients with chronic pain recognize that
their emotional responses to pain are greatly influenced by their thoughts,
and that they can exercise some control over the disruption produced by an
unavoidable life event or chronic illness. Several investigators (Dworkin et
al. 1994; Keefe and Caldwell 1997) have suggested the value of providing
cognitive-behavioral interventions early in the course of a chronic pain condition so as to increase patients' confidence that they can manage many of
their own symptoms and reduce health care utilization.

Behavior therapy. This form of psychotherapy, based on behavior theory
and social learning theory, uses contingency management or operant conditioning, not to treat pain per se, but to help patients modify their pain-related
behavior. These methods can also be used to rehabilitate pain patients by
increasing their functional performance in daily life.

Interpersonal psychotherapy. Interpersonal psychotherapy was developed by Klerman and colleagues (1984) for treatment of depression. Focusing on social deficits and other interpersonal factors that may affect the
development of depression, this approach operates on the assumption that
because symptoms occur in a social context, addressing problems in the

patient's interpersonal life may help to alleviate symptoms. Interpersonal therapy for depression focuses on one of four interpersonal problem areas: (1) grief (a reaction to the death of a loved one), (2) role transition (giving up an old social role and adjusting to and embracing a new one), (3) role dispute (difficulty in a relationship arising from incompatible expectations), and (4) role deficits (a paucity of interpersonal relationships). These principles can be applied to patients with chronic pain who, because of their symptoms and disability, are constantly in a state of role transition, certainly exacerbated by comorbid depression or anxiety.

Psychodynamic psychotherapy. This approach includes a number of psychotherapeutic interventions that share a basis in psychodynamic theories regarding the etiological nature of psychological vulnerabilities. This form of psychotherapy is most often of long duration with goals beyond that of immediate symptom relief (Marmor and Woods 1980; Nurcombe and Gallagher 1986).

PSYCHIATRIC MANAGEMENT OF ANXIETY DISORDERS IN PATIENTS WITH CHRONIC PAIN

The anxiety disorders make up one of the most common groups of psychiatric disorders. Anxiety disorders are the most common form of mental illness in the United States, with one-fourth of the population endorsing current or past symptoms of an anxiety disorder compared with only one-fifth who report a lifetime history of a mood disorder (Brawman-Intzer 2001). Severe acute pain activates stress-related noradrenergic systems in the brain and is often accompanied by cognitive-emotional reactions such as fear and anxiety, which to some degree are contextually determined. For example, pain in childbirth often does not evoke fear or anxiety, whereas pain in traumatic injury, with uncertain outcome, often does. The association of pain, anxiety, and depression may have a common neurochemical substrate in the serotonergic systems (Blier and Abbott 2001). In an interesting study, Di Piero and colleagues (2001) studied cerebral blood flow by single photon emission computed tomography (SPECT), following induction of pain by the cold pressor test in healthy volunteers, with and without diazepam. Activation of the temporal regions during the test was interpreted as part of the affective-emotional component of pain response. After taking diazepam, subjects seemed to tolerate the pain better, and on SPECT this improvement was associated with lack of temporal lobe activation of sensory-discriminative pain-related brain regions (the contralateral hand region in the sensory motor cortex, premotor cortex, and thalamus, and the left anterior cingulate gyrus). This finding suggests that diazepam, which is useful in managing anxiety disorders, interferes with affective-emotional components of pain perception and modifies the temporal lobe activation pattern.

As mentioned earlier, anxiety disorders, along with depression and substance abuse, constitute the most common comorbid conditions in patients with chronic pain disorders. Anxiety symptoms may be prominent in patients with chronic pain for several reasons. Patients with pain conditions commonly experience anxiety because of the stress of living with pain. The stress of severe trauma, perhaps incurred in battle or in a motor vehicle accident, may lead to post-traumatic stress disorder or a driving phobia, which can be comorbid with injury-related pain. The presence of comorbid obsessive-compulsive disorder with chronic pain can make both conditions worse if the patient has to undertake compulsive motoric acts such as cleaning rituals, which can exacerbate pain conditions such as brachial plexopathy, to control the anxiety associated with the obsession (Kuch et al. 1996).

The DSM-IV lists the following anxiety disorders: panic disorder with or without agoraphobia, agoraphobia without history of panic disorder, specific and social phobias, obsessive-compulsive disorders, post-traumatic stress disorder, acute stress disorder, generalized anxiety disorder, anxiety disorders due to a general medical condition, substance-induced anxiety disorders, and anxiety disorders that are not otherwise classified. It is easy to see how these disorders can complicate a pain disorder and vice versa. The neurotransmitters implicated in panic disorders and phobic disorders—norepinephrine, serotonin, and GABA—are also implicated in pain modulation. It is also not hard to imagine the challenges posed by a chronic pain patient whose pain management and pacing of activities are thwarted by obsessive-compulsive disorder or post-traumatic stress disorder. The real and imagined consequences of disability can further complicate a pain disorder with comorbid generalized anxiety. The diagnostic criteria for common anxiety disorders are listed in Table III. In this section we will review some of the pharmacological and psychotherapeutic options available in managing anxiety disorders.

PHARMACOTHERAPY OF ANXIETY DISORDERS

The management of anxiety disorders requires a thorough assessment that should include a detailed history. As with other major psychiatric syndromes, other medical conditions that can present with symptoms of anxiety must be excluded on the basis of a physical examination and appropriate

Table III
Diagnostic criteria for anxiety disorders

Panic Disorder without Agoraphobia

A. 1) Discrete panic attacks during which at least four of the following symptoms developed abruptly and reached a peak within 10 minutes:

Sensation of shortness of breath or smothering

Feeling dizzy, unsteady, light-headed, or faint

Palpitations, pounding heart, or accelerated heart rate

Trembling or shaking

Sweating

Feeling of choking

Nausea or abdominal distress

Depersonalization or derealization

Numbness or tingling sensations (paresthesias)

Chills or hot flashes

Chest pain or discomfort

Fear of dying

Fear of losing control or going crazy

2) At least one of the attacks has been followed by a month or more of the following:

a) Persistent concerns about having another attack;

b) Worry about the implications of the attack or its consequences;

c) A significant change in behavior related to the attacks

B. Absence of agoraphobia

C. Not due to direct physiological effects of a substance or general medical condition

D. Not accounted for by another disorder such as social phobia, specific phobia, obsessive compulsive disorder, post-traumatic stress disorder, or separation anxiety disorder

Panic Disorder with Agoraphobia

Fear of being in places or situations from which escape might be difficult or embarrassing or in which help might not be available in the event of a panic attack; as a result, restricted activity.

Generalized Anxiety Disorder

A. Excessive anxiety and worry occurring more days than not for at least 6 months

B. Difficulty in controlling the worry

C. Associated with at least 3 of the following symptoms (some symptoms present most days for the past 6 months):

Difficulty concentrating or one's mind going blank

Muscle tension

Irritability

Sleep disturbance

Restlessness or feeling keyed up and on edge

Being easily fatigued

Table III
Continued

D. Not caused by another Axis I psychiatric disorder

E. Causing significant distress or impairment in social, occupational, and other important areas of functioning

F. Not due to the direct physiological effect of a substance or general medical condition, or occurring exclusively during mood disorder, psychotic disorder, or pervasive developmental disorder

Obsessive-Compulsive Disorder

A. Obsessions or compulsions

Obsessions:

Recurrent and persistent thoughts, impulses, or images that are intrusive and inappropriate and cause distress

Not simply excessive worries about real-life problems

The person attempts to ignore or suppress these

The person recognizes that the obsessions are the product of his/her mind

Compulsions:

Repetitive behaviors that a person feels driven to perform in response to an obsession

The behavior is aimed at preventing or reducing distress or preventing some dreaded event or situation, but is not realistic

B. At some point the person recognizes that obsessions or compulsions are excessive or unreasonable

C. Obsessions and compulsions cause marked distress, are time-consuming, or significantly interfere with the person's normal routine, occupational functioning, or usual social activities or relationships

D. Not restricted to association with another Axis I disorder

E. Not due to the direct physiological effects of a substance or general medical condition

Anxiety Disorder Due to a General Medical Condition

A. Prominent anxiety, panic attacks, or obsessions or compulsions

B. The direct physiological consequence of a general medical condition

C. Not better accounted for by another mental condition

D. Not occurring exclusively during delirium

E. Causes clinically significant distress or impairment in social, occupational, or other important areas of functioning

Substance-Induced Anxiety Disorder

A. Prominent anxiety, panic attacks, or obsessions or compulsions

B. Evidence for either: (1) symptoms developed during or within 1 month of substance intoxication or withdrawal; or (2) medication is directly related to the disturbance

C. Not accounted for by another anxiety disorder

Table III
Continued

Acute Stress Disorder

    A. Exposure to a traumatic event where the person experienced, witnessed, or was confronted by an event with actual or threatened death or serious injury or a threat to physical integrity, and also experienced intense fear, helplessness, or horror

    B. During or after the event, three or more of the following: a sense of numbing, detachment or absence of emotional responsiveness; a reduction in awareness of surroundings (in a daze); derealization; depersonalization; dissociative amnesia

    C. Event is persistently re-experienced in images, thoughts, dreams, illusions, flashbacks, or a sense of reliving event; or distress on exposure to reminders of event

    D. Marked avoidance of stimuli that arouse recollection of the trauma

    E. Marked anxiety or increased arousal

    F. Causes clinically significant distress or impairment in social, occupational, or other important areas of functioning

    G. Lasts for a minimum of 2 days and a maximum of 4 weeks, and occurs within 4 weeks of event

    H. Not due to the direct physiological effects of a substance or general medical condition

Specific Phobia

    A. Marked and persistent fear that is unreasonable, cued by the presence or anticipation of a specific object or situation

    B. Exposure to the phobic stimulus almost invariably provokes an immediate anxiety response

    C. The person recognizes that the fear is excessive or unreasonable

    D. The phobic situation is avoided or endured with intense anxiety or distress

    E. Significantly interferes with person's normal routine, occupational functioning, or social activities and relationships, or there is marked distress about having the phobia

    F. In an individual under 18, duration of at least 6 months

    G. Not accounted for by another disorder

Social Phobia

    A. Marked and persistent fear of one or more social or performance situations in which the person is exposed to unfamiliar people or by possible scrutiny by others

    B. Exposure to specific stimulus almost invariably provokes anxiety

    C. The person recognizes that the fear is excessive or unreasonable

    D. The feared situations are avoided or endured with intense anxiety or distress

    E. Significantly interferes with the person's normal routine (social activities, relationships) or causes marked distress about having the fear

    F. If under 18, duration of more than 6 months

    G. Not due to physiological effects of a substance or general medical condition

    H. The fear is not due an associated general medical or mental condition

Source: Adapted from the American Psychiatric Association (1994).

laboratory testing including imaging studies. Some of the medical conditions that can present with symptoms of anxiety include neurological disorders (cerebral neoplasm, cerebral vascular accident), systemic conditions (hypoxia, hypoglycemia, cardiac arrhythmias, and anemia), endocrine disturbances (thyroid, pituitary, and parathyroid), and deficiency states (B12 deficiency, pellagra). In addition it is also important to rule out anxiety secondary to drugs, toxins, and psychoactive substance abuse. The pharmacotherapy of each anxiety disorder will be briefly discussed below, with medication doses outlined in Table IV.

PANIC DISORDERS

Panic attacks occur in a variety of psychiatric disorders and, when recurrent or associated with significant apprehension and behavioral change, are the central manifestations of panic disorder. Because panic attacks by definition are abrupt and intense, with symptoms referable to several bodily systems, they very often present in the emergency room. The pharmacological treatment of panic disorder includes the use of high-potency benzodiazepines, TCAs, SSRIs, and MAO inhibitors. In general, experience has shown the superiority of the SSRIs and clomipramine over benzodiazepines, other TCAs, and MAO inhibitors in the treatment of panic disorder. A few reports have suggested the role of nefazodone, venlafaxine, and buspirone in panic disorder. Beta-adrenergic antagonists have not been found to be useful in the treatment of panic disorder.

One approach in managing patients with panic disorder is to start with an SSRI. If rapid control of anxiety symptoms is needed, a short-acting benzodiazepine should be used until the effects of the SSRI are felt, keeping in mind the abuse potential and other potential negative effects of prolonged use of benzodiazepines.

PHOBIC DISORDERS

Social phobia is persistent and disproportionate fear in a performance or a social setting. It may include intense anticipatory anxiety. Often, it is associated with hypersensitivity to criticism and low self-esteem, at times including the indirect criticism of others, as in test-taking. It may be generalized to involve multiple, slightly similar situations, or be specific for a particular event. It is quite often a lifelong problem that usually is handled by avoidance, which limits patients' life opportunities.

Only relatively recently has social anxiety disorder been taken seriously enough to justify active efforts in its diagnosis and treatment. New data

Table IV
Medications for anxiety disorders

Anxiety Disorder and Medication	Starting Dose (mg/day)	Usual Dose (mg/day)
Panic Disorder		
Alprazolam	0.25–0.5 t.i.d.	Max. 4
Lorazepam	0.5–2 q.6–8 h	Max. 10
Clonazepam	0.25–0.5 t.i.d.	Max. 4
Paroxetine	10	20–60
Sertraline	50	50–200
Fluvoxamine	50	50–300
Imipramine	25–50	100–300
Clomipramine	25	100–300
Desipramine	25–50	100–300
Phenelzine	15	15–90
Social Phobia		
Phenelzine	15	15–90
Tranylcypromine	10	30–60
Venlafaxine	37.5	225
Sertraline	50	50–200
Paroxetine	20	20–60
Buspirone	7.5 b.i.d.	Max. 60
Obsessive-Compulsive Disorder		
Fluvoxamine	50	50–300
Paroxetine	20	20–60
Fluoxetine	20	20–60
Clomipramine	25	100–300
Post-traumatic Stress Disorder		
Amitriptyline	25–50	100–300
Imipramine	25–50	100–300
Sertraline	50	50–200
Paroxetine	20	20–60
Generalized Anxiety Disorder		
Clonazepam	0.25–0.5 t.i.d.	Max. 4
Sertraline	50	50–200
Citalopram	20	20–60
Paroxetine	20	20–60
Buspirone	7.5 b.i.d.	Max. 60
Acute Situational Anxiety		
Alprazolam	0.25–0.5 t.i.d.	Max. 4
Lorazepam	0.5–2 q.6–8 h	Max. 10

indicate that the condition responds well to medication treatment and may benefit from specific behavioral treatments. SSRIs and high-potency benzo-diazepines currently are the treatments of choice. MAO inhibitors also are effective but now are used rarely because of their relative toxicity and food restrictions. Tricyclic antidepressants and β-blockers are not reliably better than placebo in generalized social phobia. Although they often are used in clinical practice, there is little scientific evidence to support their continued used in this subtype of phobia. Some anticonvulsants, notably gabapentin and perhaps divalproex sodium, appear to be useful in some cases and are reasonable options for patients who fail to benefit from the more conventional medications.

Paroxetine, fluvoxamine, and sertraline have been investigated in double-blind, placebo-controlled studies and found to be effective in social phobia. Only paroxetine, however, which has undergone sufficiently rigorous studies, has been approved to date by the FDA for this indication. Fluoxetine has been the subject of four open-label case series reports suggesting efficacy. Extended-release venlafaxine currently is under study in several large international trials in adult and adolescent social anxiety disorder, but these trials have not yet been completed. Citalopram has not yet been tested in social anxiety disorder.

OBSESSIVE-COMPULSIVE DISORDER

On a worldwide basis, it is estimated that 2% of the general population suffers from obsessive-compulsive disorder (Sasson et al. 1997). An obsession is a recurrent and an intrusive thought, feeling, idea, or sensation, while a compulsion is a conscious, standardized, recurring pattern of behavior. Persons with this disorder recognize that their reaction to these thoughts and acts are irrational and disproportionate.

Recognition and the beginning of appropriate treatment of this disease are very often much delayed. Like generalized anxiety disorder, this is a closet disorder, and there is often a great delay from the onset of the illness to the time of treatment. The generally accepted hypothesis about its mechanism is that it involves abnormal serotonergic function regulation. It is interesting to note that although both serotonergic and nonserotonergic antidepressants are effective in treating depression, only the serotonergic drugs are effective in treating obsessive-compulsive disorder. Fluoxetine, fluvoxamine, sertraline, and paroxetine have all been approved for the treatment of obsessive-compulsive disorder. Higher doses may be necessary, such as 80 mg/day of fluoxetine. Of the TCAs, clomipramine is the most selective for serotonin reuptake, and was the first FDA-approved drug for obsessive-compulsive disorder. Its limitation is its side-effect profile, which it shares with other TCAs. As with SSRIs in many psychiatric disorders, the best outcome in this disorder is seen in patients utilizing a combination of pharmacotherapy and behavior therapy.

POST-TRAUMATIC STRESS DISORDER

The DSM-IV criteria for post-traumatic stress disorder can be summarized as a traumatic experience, or exposure to a traumatic event that is then re-experienced persistently, resulting in avoidance of stimuli associated with the event and persistent symptoms of increased arousal. In the context of pain the comorbidity of this disorder has implications in terms of requiring an individualized rehabilitation protocol (Bryant et al. 1999).

Successful treatment requires that physicians give patients adequate time for disclosing their stories. Brief treatment does not mean rushed treatment. Education involves explaining to survivors and their families about the nature of post-traumatic stress and encouraging them to speak about their traumatic experience with family or friends to the extent that they wish to do so, yet not in a pressured way.

Pharmacotherapy of post-traumatic stress disorder includes a number of antidepressants. Amitriptyline, imipramine, and phenelzine have all proven beneficial (Davidson et al. 1990; Kosten et al. 1991). Among the SSRIs, fluoxetine and sertraline have been best studied in this disorder (van der Kolk et al. 1994; Connor et al. 1999b; Brady et al. 2000; Davidson et al. 2001). SSRIs modulate affects, memories, and impulses, conferring protection against their overwhelming intensity on the one hand and loosening excessive inhibitions on the other, and they often act rapidly.

Reports, which so far have been mostly uncontrolled and based on small samples, have suggested benefit for paroxetine (Marshall et al. 1998), citalopram hydrochloride (Seedat et al. 2000), fluvoxamine (Davidson et al. 1998), nefazodone hydrochloride (Hidalgo et al. 1999), trazodone hydrochloride (Canive et al. 1998), bupropion hydrochloride (Canive et al. 1998), and mirtazapine (Connor et al. 1999a). Non-SSRI drugs are now considered second-line or augmenting treatments, and trazodone has been suggested for managing insomnia in this disorder.

GENERALIZED ANXIETY DISORDER

Generalized anxiety disorder is a condition characterized by excessive worrying that is difficult to control and is associated with somatic symptoms such as muscle tension, irritability, difficulty sleeping, and restlessness.

The current FDA-approved agents for the treatment of anxiety include the benzodiazepines and buspirone (Kirkwood and Hayes 1997). Although well-controlled data are lacking, long-term benzodiazepine use for the treatment of anxiety may be associated with risks of tolerance, abuse, and dependence. Although buspirone is effective in the treatment of generalized anxiety disorder and avoids the disadvantages associated with benzodiazepines, it has a slower onset of action—typically 1–3 weeks. Antidepressants such as the tricyclics, SSRIs, trazodone, and nefazodone have been evaluated in generalized anxiety disorder (Kahn et al. 1986; Hoehn-Saric et al. 1988; Rickels et al. 1993; Hedges et al. 1996; Rocca et al. 1997), but data are extremely limited and, in some cases, are complicated by the inclusion of patients with major depression. Among the newer antidepressants, only venlafaxine extended-release formula has been shown to possess unequivocal efficacy in this disorder. The anxiolytic efficacy of this formula has been demonstrated in two clinical studies in a defined population of patients with generalized anxiety disorder without associated major depression (Davidson et al. 1999; Rickels et al. 2000).

PSYCHOTHERAPY FOR ANXIETY DISORDERS

The principles of psychotherapy for patients with anxiety disorders are similar to those with depression but with greater emphasis on behavioral methods. Chapters in this volume by Waters et al. and Andrasik provide detailed information about the use of these techniques in pain. The principles of treatment for anxiety and pain are similar in that the practitioner focuses on helping the patient learn specific cognitive and behavioral coping skills to prevent, abort, or ameliorate symptoms—in this case, anxiety. In panic disorder, cognitive therapy challenges the patient's false beliefs and information about panic attacks and is used in conjunction with breathing exercises, applied relaxation, and in vivo exposure and response prevention. In obsessive-compulsive disorder, behavior therapy may as effective as pharmacotherapy, with some suggestion that the beneficial effects are longer lasting. The principle behavioral approaches in this disorder are exposure and response prevention. Desensitization, thought stopping, flooding, and aversive conditioning have also been used. Psychodynamic psychotherapy may be useful in patients with post-traumatic stress disorder. In some cases the reconstruction of the traumatic event may be therapeutic. Other interventions for this disorder include cognitive therapy, behavior therapy, and hypnosis.

CONCLUSION

Pain activates emotions, and in certain situations, emotions activate pain. They are inextricably intertwined in the phenomenology of chronic pain diseases and disorders. Emotions and pain share common neuroanatomical and neurophysiological substrates. Managing unhealthy emotional responses to pain and its consequences is part and parcel of the pain physician's daily work. To treat pain without managing emotions, or to manage emotions without treating pain, is usually a futile exercise, dooming the patient to chronic suffering and the clinician to chronic frustration. Thus, to effectively manage most patients with chronic pain, clinicians must learn how to identify, diagnose, and treat common comorbidities such as uncomplicated depression. Because of the high prevalence of comorbid depression and anxiety, easy access to mental health professionals with experience in treating pain and comorbidities is critical to success in managing chronic pain in clinical practice. The physician must assure the patient that such referrals are common and expected in pain treatment and that they are critical to successful treatment. In the case of comorbidities, the physician should communicate that he or she will follow up the patient's emotional symptoms and psychosocial functioning with as much interest in outcomes as he or she has in the patient's pain symptoms. In the case of pain without existing depression or anxiety, the physician should educate the patient about the frequency of this comorbidity and explain that the patient should report immediately the onset of depressive or anxious symptoms. Because clinicians may choose from many pharmaceutical and psychotherapeutic strategies that are strongly supported by research, they should prescribe with the confidence that they can achieve a response, and with the realistic goal of achieving depression remission and effective control of many anxiety symptoms and disorders as well as pain.

REFERENCES

American Psychiatric Association. *Diagnostic and Statistical Manual of Mental Disorders,* 4th ed. Washington, DC: American Psychiatric Association Press, 1994.

Aronoff GM, Evans WO. Doxepin as an adjunct in the treatment of chronic pain. *J Clin Psychiatry* 1982; 43(8/Sec 2):42–45.

Atkinson JH, Slater MA, Patterson TL, Grant I, Garfin SR. Prevalence, onset, and risk of psychiatric disorders in men with chronic low back pain: a controlled study. *Pain* 1991; 45:111–121.

Atkinson JH, Slater MA, Wahlgren DR, et al. Effects of noradrenergic and serotonergic antidepressants on chronic low back pain intensity. *Pain* 1999; 83(2):137–145.

Backonja MM. Anticonvulsants (antineuropathics) for neuropathic pain syndromes. *Clin J Pain* 2000; 16:S67–S72.

Backonja M, Beydoun A, Edwards KR, et al. Gabapentin for the symptomatic treatment of painful neuropathy in patients with diabetes mellitus: a randomized controlled trial. *JAMA* 1998; 280:1831–1836.

Banks SM, Kerns RD. Explaining high rates of depression in chronic pain: a diathesis-stress framework. *Psychol Bull* 1996; 119:95–110.

Beasley CM Jr, Dornseif BE, Pultz JA, Bosomworth JC, Sayler ME. Fluoxetine versus trazodone: efficacy and activating-sedating effects. *J Clin Psychiatry* 1991; 52:294–299.

Beck AT. *Cognitive Therapy and the Emotional Disorders.* New York: International Universities Press, 1976.

Blier P, Abbott FV. Putative mechanisms of action of antidepressant drugs in affective and anxiety disorders and pain. *J Psychiatry Neurosci* 2001; 26(1):37–43.

Blumer D, Heilbron M. Chronic pain as a variant of depressive disease—the pain-prone disorder. *J Nerv Ment Dis* 1982; 170(7):381–406.

Botney M, Fields HL. Amitriptyline potentiates morphine analgesia by direct action on the central nervous system. *Ann Neurol* 1983; 13(2):160–164.

Bowsher D. The effects of pre-emptive treatment of post herpetic neuralgia with amitriptyline: a randomized double blind, placebo-controlled trial. *J Pain Symptom Manage* 1997; 13:327–331.

Brady KT, Pearlstein T, Asnis GM, et al. Efficacy and safety of sertraline treatment of posttraumatic stress disorder: a randomized controlled trial. *JAMA* 2000; 283:1837–1844.

Brannon GE, Stone KD. The use of mirtazapine in a patient with chronic pain. *J Pain Symptom Manage* 1999; 18(5):382–385.

Brawman-Intzer O. Generalized anxiety disorder. *Psychiatr Clin North Am* 2001; 24(1):11–12.

Bruns D, Disorbio M. Hostility and violent ideation: physical rehabilitation patient and a community samples. *Pain Med* 2000; 1:131–139.

Bryant RA, Marossezekey JE, Crooks J, Baguley IJ, Gurka JA. Interaction of posttraumatic stress disorder and chronic pain following traumatic brain injury. *J Head Trauma Rehabil* 1999; 14(6):588–594.

Calabrese JR, Bowden CL, McElroy SL, et al. Spectrum of activity of lamotrigine in treatment: refractory bipolar disorder. *Am J Psychiatry* 1999a; 156:1019–1023.

Calabrese JR, Bowden CL, Sachs GS, et al. A double-blind placebo-controlled study of lamotrigine monotherapy in outpatients with bipolar I depression. *J Clin Psychiatry* 1999b; 60:79–88.

Canive JM, Clark RD, Calaris LA, Quails C, Tuason VB. Bupropion treatment in veterans with posttraumatic stress disorder: an open study. *J Clin Psychopharmacol* 1998; 18:379–383.

Cano A, Weisberg J, Gallagher RM. Marital satisfaction and pain severity mediate the association between negative spouse behaviors and depressive symptoms in a chronic pain sample. *Pain Med* 2000; (1):35–43.

Christina MD. Antidepressant augmentation and combinations. *Psychiatr Clin N Am* 2000; 23(4):743–755.

Connor KM, Davidson JRT, Weisler AH, Ahearn EP. A pilot study of mirtazapine in posttraumatic stress disorder. *Int Clin Psychopharmacol* 1999a; 14:29–31.

Connor KM, Sutherland SM, Tupler LA, et al. Fluoxetine in post-traumatic stress disorder: randomized double-blind study. *Br J Psychiatry* 1999b; 175:17–22.

Corrigan FM. Sodium valproate augmentation of fluoxetine or fluvoxamine effects. *Biol Psychiatry* 1992; 31:1178–1179.

Davidson JRT, Kudler HS, Smith RD, et al. Treatment of posttraumatic stress disorder with amitriptyline and placebo. *Arch Gen Psychiatry* 1990; 47:259–266.

Davidson JRT, Weisler RH, Malik ML, Tupler LA. Fluvoxamine in civilians with posttraumatic stress disorder. *J Clin Psychopharmacol* 1998; 18:93–95.

Davidson JR, DuPont RL, Hedges D, Haskins JT. Efficacy, safety, and tolerability of venlafaxine extended release and buspirone in outpatients with generalized anxiety disorder. *J Clin Psychiatry* 1999; 60:528–535.

Davidson JRT, Rothbaum BO, van der Kolk BA, Sikes CR, Farfel GM. Multicenter, double-blind comparisons of sertraline and placebo in the treatment of posttraumatic stress disorder. *Arch Gen Psychiatry* 2001; 58:485–492.

Davis JL, Smith RL. Painful peripheral diabetic neuropathy treated with venlafaxine HCl extended release capsules. *Diabetes Care* 1999; 22(11):1909–1910.

De la Fuente JM, Mendlewicz J. Carbamazepine addition in tricyclic antidepressant-resistant unipolar depression. *Biol Psychiatry* 1992; 32:369–374.

Depression Guideline Panel. *Depression in Primary Care,* Clinical Practice Guideline No. 5. Rockville, MD: Agency for Health Care Policy and Research, 1993.

Detke MJ, Lu Y, Goldstein DJ, Hayes JR, Demitrack MA. Duloxetine, 60 mg once daily, for major depressive disorder: a randomized double-blind placebo-controlled trial. *J Clin Psychiatry* 2002; 63(4):308–315.

Di Piero V, Feracutti S, Sabatini U, et al. Diazepam effects on the cerebral responses to tonic pain: a SPET study. *Psychopharmacology* 2001; 158(3):252–258.

Dohrenwend B, Marbach J, Raphael K, Gallagher RM. Why is depression co-morbid with chronic facial pain? A family study test of alternative hypotheses. *Pain* 1999; 83:183–192.

Dworkin SF, Turner JA, Wilson L, et al. Brief group cognitive-behavioral intervention for temporomandibular disorders. *Pain* 1994; 59(2):175–187.

Eberhard G, von Knorring L, Nilsson HL, et al. A double-blind randomized study of clomipramine versus maprotiline in patients with idiopathic pain syndromes. *Neuropsychobiology* 1988; 19(1):25–34.

Eisenach JC, Gebhart GF. Intrathecal amitriptyline acts as a N-methyl-D-aspartate receptor antagonist in the presence of inflammatory hyperalgesia in rats. *Anesthesiology* 1995; 83:1046–1054.

Eisenberg E, Lurie Y, Braker C, Doud S, Ishay A. Lamotrigine reduces painful diabetic neuropathy: a randomized, controlled study. *Neurology* 2001; 57(3):505–509.

Endicott J. Measurement of depression in patients with cancer. *Cancer* 1984; 53(Suppl 10):2243–2249.

Ener RA, Meglathery SB, Van Decker WA, Gallagher RM. Serotonin syndrome and other serotonergic disorders. *Pain Med* 2003; 4(1):63–74.

Engel CC, von Korff M, Katon WJ. Back pain in primary care: predictors of high health-care costs. *Pain* 1996; 65(2–3):197–204.

Enggaard TP, Klitgaard NA, Gram LF, et al. Specific effect of venlafaxine on single and repetitive experimental painful stimuli in humans. *Clin Pharmacol Ther* 2001; 69(4):245–251.

Fava M, Anderson K, Rosenbaum JF. Anger attacks: possible variants of panic and major depressive disorders. *Am J Psychiatry* 1990; 147(7):867–870.

Fishbain DA. Current research on chronic pain and suicide. *Am J Public Health* 1996; 86(9):1320–1321.

Fishbain DA. Approaches to treatment decisions for psychiatric comorbidity in the management of the chronic pain patient. *Med Clin North Am* 1999; 83:737–760.

Fishbain DA, Cutler RB, Rosomoff HL, et al. Chronic pain associated depression: antecedent or consequence of chronic pain? A review. *Clin J Pain* 1997; 13:116–137.

Fishbain DA, Cutler R, Rosomoff HL, Rosomoff RS. Evidence-based data from animal and human experimental studies on pain relief with antidepressants: a structured review. *Pain Med* 2000a; 1(4):310–316.

Fishbain DA, Cutler R, Rosomoff HL, Rosomoff RS. Risk for violent behavior in patients with chronic pain: evaluation and management in the pain facility setting. *Pain Med* 2000b; 1:14–155.

France RD. The future of antidepressants; treatment of pain. *Psychopathology* 1987; 20(Suppl 1):99–113.

France RD, Krishnan KRR, Trainor M. Chronic pain and depression, III: Family history study of depression and alcoholism in chronic low back pain patients. *Pain* 1986; 24:185–190.

Gallagher RM. Integrating medical and behavioral treatment in chronic pain management. *Med Clin N Am* 1999; 83(5):823–849.

Gallagher RM, Mossey J. Inadequate pain care for elders: the need for a primary care-pain medicine community collaboration. *Pain Med* 2002; 3:180.

Gallagher RM, Verma S. Managing pain and co-morbid depression: a public health challenge. *Semin Clin Neuropsychiatry* 1999; 4(3):203–220.

Gallagher RM, Verma S. Treatment and rehabilitation of chronic orthopedic pain syndromes. In: Stoudemire A, Fogel B, Greenblatt D (Eds). *Psychiatric Care of the Medical Patient.* New York: Oxford University Press, 2000.

Gallagher RM, Woznicki M. Low back pain rehabilitation. In: Stoudemire A, Fogel BS (Eds). *Medical Psychiatric Practice,* Vol. 2. Washington, DC: American Psychiatric Association Press, 1993.

Gallagher RM, Marbach J, Raphael K, Dohrenwend B, Cloitre M. Is there co-morbidity between temporomandibular pain dysfunction syndrome and depression? A pilot study. *Clin J Pain* 1991; 7:219–225.

Gallagher RM, Moore P, Chernoff I. The reliability of depression diagnosis in chronic low back pain: a pilot study. *Gen Hosp Psychiatry* 1995a; 17:399–413.

Gallagher RM, Marbach J, Raphael K, Handte J, Dohrenwend B. Seasonal variation in chronic TMPDS pain and mood intensity. *Pain* 1995b; 61(1):113–120.

Haythornthwaite JA, Seiber WJ, Kerns RD. Depression and the chronic pain experience. *Pain* 1991; 46:177–184.

Hedges DW, Reimherr FW, Strong RE, Halls CH, Rust C. An open trial of nefazodone in adult patients with generalized anxiety disorder. *Psychopharmacol Bull* 1996; 32:671–676.

Hidalgo RB, Hertzberg MA, Mellman TA, et al. Nefazodone in post-traumatic stress disorder: results from six open-label trials. *Int Clin Psychopharmacol* 1999; 14:61–68.

Hoehn-Saric R, McLeod DR, Zimmerli WD. Differential effects of alprazolam and imipramine in generalized anxiety disorder: somatic versus psychic symptoms. *J Clin Psychiatry* 1988; 49:293–301.

Hudson JI, Hudson MS, Piner LF, Goldenberg DL, Pope HG. Fibromyalgia and major affective disorder: a controlled phenomenology and family history study. *Am J Psychiatry* 1985; 142(4):441–446.

Hwang AS, Wilcox GL. Analgesic properties of intrathecally administered heterocyclics. *Pain* 1987, 28:343–355.

Iwashita T, Shimizu T. Imipramine inhibits intrathecal substance P-induced behaviour and blocks spinal cord substance P receptors in mice. *Brain Res* 1992; 581:59–66.

Jick SS, Dean AD, Jick H. Antidepressants and suicide. *BMJ* 1995; 310:215–218.

Joss JD. Tricyclic antidepressant use in diabetic neuropathy. *Ann Pharmacother* 1999; 33(9):996–1000.

Jung AC, Staiger T, Sullivan M. The efficacy of selective serotonin reuptake inhibitors for the management of chronic pain. *J Gen Intern Med* 1997; 12(6):384–389.

Kahn RJ, McNair DM, Lipman RS, et al. Imipramine and chlordiazepoxide in depressive and anxiety disorders, II: efficacy in anxious outpatients. *Arch Gen Psychiatry* 1986; 43:79–85.

Katon W, Sullivan MD. Depression and chronic medical illness. *J Clin Psychiatry* 1990; 51(Suppl 6):3–11.

Keefe FJ, Caldwell DS. Cognitive behavioral control of arthritis pain. *Adv Rheumatol* 1997; 81:277–290.

Keefe FJ, Wilkins RH, Cook WA Jr, et al. Depression, pain and pain behavior. *J Consult Clin Psychol* 1986; 54:665–669.

Kinney RK, Gatchel RJ, Ellis E, Holt C. Major psychological disorders in chronic TMD patients: implications for successful management. *Psych Bull* 1996; 119:95–110.

Kirkwood CK, Hayes PE. Anxiety disorders. In: DiPiro JT, Talbert RL, Yee GC, et al. (Eds). *Pharmacotherapy,* 3rd ed. Stamford, Conn: Appleton & Lange, 1997, pp 1443–1462.

Klerman GL, Weissman MM, Rounsaville BJ, et al. *Interpersonal Psychotherapy for Depression.* New York: Basic Books, 1984.

Kosten TR, Frank JB, Dan E, McDougle CJ, Giller EL Jr. Pharmacotherapy for posttraumatic stress disorder using phenelzine or imipramine. *J Nerv Ment Dis* 1991; 179:366–370.

Krause SJ, Weiner RL, Tait RC. Depression and pain behavior in patients with chronic pain. *Clin J Pain* 1994; 10:122–127.

Krishnan KRR, France RD, Pelton S, et al. Chronic pain and depression I: classification of depression in chronic pain patients. *Pain* 1985; 22:279–287.

Kroenke K, Price RK. Symptoms in the community: prevalence, classification, and psychiatric comorbidity. *Arch Intern Med* 1993; 153:2474–2480.

Kuch K, Cox BJ, Evans RJ. Posttraumatic stress disorder and motor vehicle accidents: a multidisciplinary overview. *Can J Psychiatry* 1996; 41:429–434.

Kupfer DJ. Long-term treatment of depression. *J Clin Psychiatry* 1991; 52(Suppl):28–34.

Kvinesdale B, Molin J, Forland A, Gram LF. Imipramine in treatment of painful diabetic neuropathy. *JAMA* 1984; 251:1727–1730.

Langelier R, Gallagher RM. Group therapy for chronic pain patients and their spouses: the effects on marital satisfaction, locus of control, and pain perception. *Clin J Pain* 1989; 5(3):227–231.

Lascelles RG. Atypical facial pain and depression. *Br J Psychiatry* 1966; 112:651–659.

Leijon G, Boivie J. Central post-stroke pain: controlled trial of amitriptyline and carbamazepine. *Pain* 1989; 36:27–36.

Levine JD, Gordon NC, Smith R, et al. Desipramine enhances opiate postoperative analgesia. *Pain* 1986; 27:45–49.

Lindsay PG, Olsen RB. Maprotiline in pain-depression. *J Clin Psychiatry* 1985; 46(6):226–228.

Lindsey P, Wycoff M. The depression pain syndrome and response to antidepressants. *Psychosomatics* 1981; 22:511–517.

Lynch ME. Antidepressants as analgesics: a review of randomized controlled trials. *J Psychiatry Neurosci* 2001; 26(1):30–36.

Magni G. On the relationship between chronic pain and depression when there is no organic lesion. *Pain* 1987; 31:1–21.

Magni G, Caldieron C, Rigatti-Luchini S, Merskey H. Chronic musculoskeletal pain and depressive symptoms in the general population: an analysis of the 1st National Health and Nutrition Examination survey. *Pain* 1990; 43:299–307.

Markowitz JS, Patrick KS. Venlafaxine-tramadol similarities. *Med Hypotheses* 1998; 51(2):167–168.

Marmor J, Woods SM. *The Interface between the Psychodynamic and Behavioral Therapies.* New York: Plenum, 1980.

Marshall RD, Schneier FR, Fallon BA, et al. An open trial of paroxetine in patients with non-combat-related, chronic posttraumatic stress disorder. *J Clin Psychopharmacol* 1998; 18:10–18.

Max M. Antidepressants as analgesics. In: Fields H, Liebeskind JC (Eds). *Pharmacological Approaches to the Treatment of Chronic Pain: New Concepts and Critical Issues,* Progress in Pain Research and Management, Vol. 1. Seattle: IASP Press, 1994, pp 229–246.

Max MB, Cunane M, Scahfer SC, et al. Amitriptyline relieves diabetic neuropathy pain in patients with normal or depressed mood. *Neurology* 1987; 37:589–596.

Max MB, Kishore-Kumar R, Schaffer SC, et al. Efficacy of desipramine in painful diabetic neuropathy: a placebo-controlled tria l. *Pain* 1991; 45:3–9.

Max MB, Lynch SA, Muir J, et al. Effects of desipramine amitriptyline and fluoxetine on pain in diabetic neuropathy. *N Engl J Med* 1992; 326:1250–1256.

Mojtabai R, Olfson M. Medication costs, adherence, and health outcomes among Medicare beneficiaries. *Health Aff (Millwood)* 2003; 22(4):220–229.

Mossey JM, Gallagher RM. Longitudinal evaluation of the effects of pain and depression on the physical functioning of continuing care retirement community residents: implications for the treatment of pain in older individuals. *Pain Med* 2001; 2:246–247.

Mossey J, Gallagher RM, Tirumalasetti F. The effects of pain and depression on physical functioning in elderly residents of a continuing care retirement community. *Pain Med* 2000; 1:340–350.

Mulrow CD, Williams JW Jr, Chiquette E, et al. Efficacy of newer medications for treating depression in primary care patients. *Am J Med* 2000; 108:54–64.

Nurcombe B, Gallagher RM. *The Clinical Process in Psychiatry: Diagnosis and Management Planning.* Cambridge: Cambridge University Press, 1986.

Onghena P, Van Houdenhove B. Antidepressant-induced analgesia in chronic non-malignant pain: a meta-analysis of 39 placebo controlled studies. *Pain* 1992; 49:205–209.

Panerai AE, Monza G, Movilla P, et al. A randomized, within patient, crossover, placebo-controlled trial on the efficacy and tolerability of tricyclics antidepressants chlorimipramine and nortriptyline in central pain. *Acta Neurol Scand* 1990; 82:34–38.

Pernia A, Mico JA, Calderon E, Torres LM. Venlafaxine for the treatment of neuropathic pain. *J Pain Symptom Manage* 2000; 19(6):408–410.

Pfeiffer RF. Drugs for pain in the elderly. *Geriatrics* 1982; 37(2):67–69.

Picus T, Burton AK, Vogel S, Field AP. A systematic review of psychological factors as predictors of chronicity / disability in prospective cohorts of low back pain. *Spine* 2002; 27(5):E109–120.

Polatin PB, Kinney RK, Gatchel RJ, Lillo E, Mayer T. Psychiatric illness and chronic low back pain. *Spine* 1993; 18(1):66–71.

Raphael K, Marbach J. When did your pain start? Reliability of self-reported age of onset of facial pain. *Clin J Pain* 1997; 13:352–359.

Richelson E. Pharmacology of antidepressants. *Mayo Clin Proc* 2001; 76(5):511–527.

Rickels K, Downing R, Schweizer E, Hassman H. Antidepressants for the treatment of generalized anxiety disorder: a placebo-controlled comparison of imipramine, trazodone, and diazepam. *Arch Gen Psychiatry* 1993; 50:884–895.

Rickels K, Pollack MH, Sheehan DV, Haskins JT. Efficacy of extended-release venlafaxine in nondepressed outpatients with generalized anxiety disorder. *Am J Psychiatry* 2000; 157(6):968–974.

Rowbotham M, Harden N, Stacey B, et al. The Gabapentin Postherpetic Neuralgia Study Group. Gabapentin for the treatment of postherpetic neuralgia: a randomized controlled trial. *JAMA* 1998; 280:1837–1842.

Rowbotham MC, Petersen KL, Davies PS, et al. Recent developments in the treatment of neuropathic pain. *Proceedings of the 9th World Congress on Pain,* Progress in Pain Research and Management, Vol. 16. Seattle: IASP Press, 2000, pp 833–855.

Rocca P, Fonzo V, Scotta M, Zanalda E, Ravissa L. Paroxetine efficacy in the treatment of generalized anxiety disorder. *Acta Psychiatr Scand* 1997; 95:444–450.

Romano JM, Turner JA. Chronic pain and depression: does the evidence support the relationship. *Psychol Bull* 1985, 97:18–34.

Rome H, Rome J. Limbically augmented pain syndrome. *Pain Med* 2000; 1(1).

Sasson Y, Zohar J, Chopra M, et al. Epidemiology of obsessive-compulsive disorder: a world view. *J Clin Psychiatry* 1997; 58(Suppl 12):7–10.

Sawynok J, Esser MJ, Reid AR. Peripheral antinociceptive actions of desipramine and fluoxetine in an inflammatory and neuropathic pain test in the rat. *Pain* 1999a; 82(2):149–158.

Sawynok J, Reid AR, Esser MJ. Peripheral antinociceptive action of amitriptyline in the rat formalin test: involvement of adenosine. *Pain* 1999b; 80(1–2):45–55.

Sawynok J, Esser MJ, Reid AR. Antidepressants as analgesics: an overview of central and peripheral mechanisms of action. *J Psychiatry Neurosci* 2001; 26(1):21–29.

Schreiber S, Getslev V, Weizman A, Pick CG. The antinociceptive effect of moclobemide in mice is mediated by noradrenergic pathways. *Neurosci Lett* 1998; 253(3):183–186.

Scott MA, Letrent KJ, Hager KL, Burch JL. Use of transdermal amitriptyline gel in a patient with chronic pain and depression. *Pharmacotherapy* 1999; 19(2):236–2369.

Seedat S, Stein DJ, Emsley RA. Open trial of citalopram in adults with post-traumatic stress disorder. *Int J Neuropsychopharmacol* 2000; 3:135–140.

Seligman MEP. *Helplessness: On Depression, Development, and Death.* San Francisco: W.H. Freeman, 1975.

Semenchuk MR, Davis B. Efficacy of sustained-release bupropion in neuropathic pain: an open-label study. *Clin J Pain* 2000; 16(1):6–11.

Semenchuk MR, Sherman S, Davis B. Double-blind, randomized trial of bupropion SR for the treatment of neuropathic pain. *Neurology* 2001; 57(9):1583–1588.

Sierralta F, Pinardi G, Miranda HF. Effects of p-chlorophenylalanine and alpha-methyltyrosine on the antinociceptive effect of antidepressant drugs. *Pharmacol Toxicol* 1995; 77:276–280.

Simon GE, Heiligenstein JH, Grothaus L, Katon W, Revicki D. Should anxiety and insomnia influence antidepressant selection? A randomized comparison of fluoxetine and imipramine. *J Clin Psychiatry* 1998; 59:49–55.

Simon GE, Heiligenstein J, Revicki D, et al. Long-term outcomes of initial antidepressant drug choice in a "real world" randomized trial. *Arch Fam Med* 1999; 8:319–325.

Sindrup SH, Jensen TS. Efficacy of pharmacological treatments of neuropathic pain: an update and effect related to mechanism of drug action. *Pain* 1999; 83(3):389–400.

Sindrup SH, Jensen TS. Pharmacologic treatment of pain in polyneuropathy. *Neurology* 2000; 55(7):915–920.

Sindrup SH, Ejlertsen B, Forland A, et al. Imipramine in the treatment of diabetic neuropathy; relief of subjective symptoms without change in peripheral and autonomic nerve function. *Eur J Clin Pharmacol* 1989; 37:151–153.

Sindrup SH, Gram LF, Brosen K, et al. The selective serotonin reuptake inhibitor paroxetine is effective in the treatment of diabetic neuropathy symptoms. *Pain* 1990; 43:135–144.

Sindrup SH, BjerreU, Dejgaard A, et al. The selective serotonin reuptake inhibitor citalopram relieves the symptoms of diabetic neuropathy symptoms. *Clin Pharmacol Ther* 1992; 52:547–552.

Slater MA, Wahlgren DR, Williams RA, et al. Effects of noradrenergic and serotonergic antidepressants on chronic low back pain intensity. *Pain* 1999; 83(2):137–145.

Songer DA, Schulte H. Venlafaxine for the treatment of chronic pain. *Am J Psychiatry* 1996; 153(5):737.

Speigel K, Kalb R, Pasternak GW. Analgesic activity of tricyclic antidepressants. *Ann Neurol* 1983; 13:462–465.

Staats PS. Pain management and beyond: evolving concepts and treatments involving cyclooxygenase inhibition. *J Pain Symptom Manage* 2002; 24(Suppl 1):S4–9.

Tasmuth T, Hartel B, Kalso E. Venlafaxine in neuropathic pain following treatment of breast cancer. *Eur J Pain* 2002; 6(1):17–24.

Thase ME. Effectiveness of antidepressants: comparative remission rates. *J Clin Psychiatry* 2003; 64(Suppl 2):3–7.

Tollefson GD, Holman SL, Sayler ME, Potvin JH. Fluoxetine, placebo, and tricyclic antidepressants in major depression with and without anxious features. *J Clin Psychiatry* 1994; 55:50–59.

Tomkins GE, Jackson JL, O'Malley PG, Balden E, Santoro JE. Treatment of chronic headache with antidepressants: a meta-analysis. *Am J Med* 2001; 111(1):54–63.

U.S. Department of Health and Human Services. *Prescription Drugs: Abuse and Addiction.* NIH Publication Number 01-4881. Rockville, MD: U.S. Department of Health and Human Services, National Institutes of Health, 2001.

Van der Kolk BA, Dreyfuss D, Michaels M. Fluoxetine in posttraumatic stress disorder. *J Clin Psychiatry* 1994; 55:517–522.

Verma S, Gallagher RM. The psychopharmacologic treatment of depression and anxiety in the context of chronic pain. *Curr Pain Headache Rep* 2002; 6:30–39.

Vrethem M, Boivie J, Arnqvist H, et al. A comparison of amitriptyline and maprotiline in the treatment of painful polyneuropathy in diabetics and nondiabetics. *Clin J Pain* 1997; 13(4):313–323.

Watson CP, Chipman M, Reed K, Evans RJ, Birkett N. Amitriptyline versus maprotiline in postherpetic neuralgia: a randomized, double-blind, crossover trial. *Pain* 1992; 48(1):29–36.

Watson CP, Vernich L, Chipman M, Reed K. Nortriptyline versus amitriptyline in postherpetic neuralgia: a randomized trial. *Neurology* 1998; 51(4):1166–1167.

Wilson KG, Eriksson MY, D'Eon JL, Mikail SF, Emery PC. Major depression and insomnia in chronic pain. *Clin J Pain* 2002; 18:77–83.

Williams JBW, Gibbon M, First M, et al. The structured clinical interview for DSM-III-R (SCID): II. Multisite test-retest reliability. *Arch Gen Psychiatry* 1994; 49:630–636.

Correspondence to: Rollin M. Gallagher, MD, MPH, 1129 Rock Creek Road, Gladwyne, PA 19035, USA. Email: rmg3@comcast.net.

Psychosocial Aspects of Pain: A Handbook for Health Care Providers, Progress in Pain Research and Management, Vol. 27, edited by Robert H. Dworkin and William S. Breitbart, IASP Press, Seattle, © 2004.

8

Somatoform Disorders and Pain Complaints

Vicenzio Holder-Perkins[a] and Thomas Wise[b,c]

[a]Inpatient Psychiatric Services and Department of Psychiatry and Behavioral Sciences, The George Washington University, Washington, DC, USA; [b]Department of Psychiatry and Behavioral Sciences, Johns Hopkins University School of Medicine, Baltimore, Maryland, USA; [c]Department of Psychiatry, Inova Fairfax Hospital, Falls Church, Virginia, USA

Pain is frequently a "ticket of admission" to seek medical care. Pain is best defined as "an unpleasant sensory and emotional experience associated with actual or potential tissue damage or described in terms of such damage" (Merskey and Bogduk 1994). This definition highlights two essential aspects of this inherently subjective experience. First, pain is unpleasant; those who enjoy it are labeled masochistic. Second, pain may be associated with a clearly defined disease. Pain is subjective and is reported in both quality and intensity by the patient. Objective signs that indicate painful states include guarding of a painful limb, abdominal rigidity, or withdrawal from painful stimuli. In addition, individuals in acute or chronic pain may express their distress in a variety of ways such as facial grimacing or verbal expressions of pain.

When objective causes for unexplained pain are not found, health care providers may tend to discount the problem or may suspect a psychological cause. The patient, however, often requires validation of such a problem and may continue a search for a satisfactory explanation, usually within the somatic realm. At the same time, the health care provider seeks to discover the causes of medically unexplained complaints of pain or physical discomfort, and may use many tests and studies that are not necessary. This course of action derives from the clinical educational experience wherein health care providers learn to distinguish between signs and symptoms. Signs are more or less definitive and obvious, and are independent of the patient's impressions. Symptoms are subjective and usually are not objectively verifiable.

Clinicians are taught that a sign should validate the subjective report of a physical complaint. When symptoms occur without objective evidence or are determined to be in excess of any detectable biological findings, patients may be labeled "hypochondriacal worriers," "somatizers," or "malingerers." Nevertheless, such somatic complaints and euphemistic or pejorative labels may indicate the presence of a psychiatric disorder.

Many pain complaints are not explained by a medical etiology. In the Epidemiologic Catchment Area Study, Kroenke and Price (1993) documented that the lifetime prevalence of pain was 25% for chest pain, 24% for abdominal pain, 25% for headache, and 32% for back pain. To be noted in the survey, such complaints had to be considered problematic to the individual. More than 80% of the time, pain symptoms had prompted respondents to see a health care provider, take medication, or reduce normal activities. Thus, pain complaints without any clear medical etiology are particularly common. Such situations may suggest a psychiatric disorder such as the somatoform disorders (Table I). Frequently pain is among the chief complaints of these disorders. In a review of relevant studies, Dworkin and Caligor (1988) noted prevalence rates ranging from 16% to 53% for somatoform disorders among chronic pain populations. Both Katon et al. (1985) and Reich et al. (1983) reported that nearly one-third of their chronic pain samples merited a diagnosis of what is now referred to in the fourth volume of the *Diagnostic and Statistical Manual of Mental Disorders* (DSM-IV; American Psychiatric Association 1994) as "pain disorder with psychological features." In a prospective study, Owen-Salters et al. (1996) assessed 100% of their chronic back pain patients as having a somatoform pain disorder.

Psychiatric disorders where pain may be reported include the somatoform disorders and a condition known as factitious disorder or malingering, where pain or discomfort is feigned. Patients with a somatoform disorder are likely to switch from clinician to clinician and from one medical setting to another in search of an etiology for their unexplained medical complaint, hoping for its ultimate relief, which does not seem to come. Compared with patients who are not somatically preoccupied, they have a greater number of outpatient visits, more frequent hospitalizations, and higher overall health care expenditures (Barsky et al. 1991; Bass and Murphy 1991; Fink 1992; Craig et al. 1993). Kellner (1991) estimated that 10–20% of the U.S. medical budget is spent on patients who somatize or have hypochondriacal concerns. These patients are likely to seek relief in nonpsychiatric settings, where they can be elusive because many health care providers are trained only in the identification and treatment of physical illness. Malingerers have similar patterns of health care utilization, but they fake symptoms in order to gain

Table I
Somatoform disorders

Somatization Disorder
Many physical complaints occurring over a period of several years before age 30 and
resulting in treatment being sought
All of the following physical complaints occurring at any time during the disturbance:
1) history of pain related to at least four sites or functions
2) two gastrointestinal symptoms
3) one sexual function and
4) one pseudoneurological symptom

Undifferentiated Somatoform Disorder
One or more physical complaints with a duration of a least 6 months

Conversion Disorder
One or more symptoms or deficits affecting voluntary motor or sensory function that
suggest a neurological or other general medical condition associated with
psychological factors

Pain Disorder
Pain in one or more anatomical sites is the predominant focus of the clinical
presentation; psychological factors are judged to have an important role

Hypochondriasis
Preoccupation with fear of having a serious disease based on misinterpretation of
symptoms for at least 6 months; the patient is not reassured by a negative medical
evaluation

Body Dysmorphic Disorder
An excessive preoccupation with an imagined deficit in appearance

Somatoform Disorder Not Otherwise Specified
Somatoform symptoms that do not meet criteria for other somatoform disorders,
including unexplained complaints of less than 6 months' duration

Source: Adapted from American Psychiatric Association (1994).

something of obvious value or avoid something obviously painful. Pain expression in a medical clinical setting should be conceptualized not only as a manifestation of an organic disease but as a possible correlate to psychopathology, a marker of functional impairment, or a link to the patient's assessment of his or her health status. How patients with hypochondriasis and somatization perceive their health is paramount because this perception is most likely related to their distress, disability, and high utilization of health care services. Noyes et al. (1993) found that patients with hypochondriasis rated themselves worse than control subjects on measures of functioning including physical, psychological, work, social, and sexual aspects and overall health, and also reported more disabilities than did patients with panic disorder on the Functional Status Questionnaire (Barsky et al. 1994).

This chapter is designed to help clinicians identify patients with somatoform disorders and to provide ways in which to effectively provide care. It is important to demonstrate a caring interest that will help the patient move from the "maddening" search for a "cure" to an ability to cope with the symptoms. The following discussion will review the somatoform disorders that include hypochondriasis, somatization disorder, conversion disorder, and pain disorder. Neurasthenia, a diagnosis in the International Classification of Disease iterations (World Health Organization 1992), will also be discussed. But first it will be useful to distinguish various terms that are often used interchangeably but have different meanings.

CATEGORIES AND PROCESSES

The terms *hypochondriasis* and *somatization* are often used interchangeably, but they differ. *Hypochondriasis* denotes a categorical psychiatric disorder involving a preoccupation with fears of having, or the idea that one has, a serious disease based on the patient's misinterpretation of bodily symptoms despite appropriate medical evaluation and reassurance. *Somatization,* on the other hand, is a common phenomenon that has different meanings in different cultures. In some cultures it does not signify a psychiatric disorder but is a culturally coded expression of distress, a metaphor for experience, or a medium of social positioning, and as such may not constitute a medical or psychiatric problem (Kirmayer and Young 1998). In Nigeria, for example, "brain fag" is a syndrome involving sensations of heaviness or heat in the head associated with the efforts of studying. This problem has been noted among students who are the first to be formally educated and in the process have been psychologically and physically separated from their families and communities of origin. Somatization is thus best understood as a somatic idiom of psychosocial distress (Lipowski 1987). It occurs in a variety of psychiatric disorders such as anxiety, depression, and various somatoform disorders including hypochondriasis. The comorbidity between hypochondriasis and somatization is high (Kellner 1991), and the relationship between the two is not well understood. However, it is useful to conceptualize hypochondriasis as a discrete categorical designation rather than as a dimension of somatizing. Another way of identifying the difference is defining hypochondriasis in terms of cognitive and emotional symptoms, whereas the definition of somatization emphasizes somatic symptoms (see Table I).

Hysteria and *hysterical* are also terms with different meanings that are often confused. The development of hysteria in many ways mirrors the history of psychiatry. Hysteria as a categorical disorder has been in use since the times of Hippocrates; it is characterized by recurrent, multiple somatic complaints, often described dramatically, that do not fit the pattern of any known clinical disorders. Its current operational definition is discussed below. *Hysterical* as an adjective denotes a dramatic emotional style, and this epithet may often stigmatize a patient and can be used to rationalize ceasing to investigate an organic cause for a patient's complaint.

Jean Marie Charcot (1890) popularized the category of hysteria by demonstrating the dramatic pseudoseizures of his female patients in his clinical rounds at the Saltpietre Hospital in Paris. Modern medical historians have questioned whether some of the patients he described were consciously simulating the disorders rather than having a "true" unconscious disorder. Sigmund Freud, who observed Charcot on his clinical rounds, further developed the concept and emphasized the role of conversion (a process) into hysteria (a disorder) (Breuer and Freud 1936). Thus the terms *conversion* and *hysteria* are widely found in psychoanalytic literature, often used interchangeably. Freud proposed the term *conversion* to denote the repression of a painful idea, which according to Freud weakened its affect by diverting its energy into somatic channels. *Conversion* for some has been a synonym for *hysteria,* leading to difficulties in demarcating somatization from similar phenomena. This confusion probably stems from the fact that hysteria was Freud's central concern during the early years of psychoanalysis, ultimately resulting in the identification of conversion symptoms with hysteria. Many psychoanalysts consider hysteria a simulation of illness designed to work out unconscious conflicts. In the absence of specific diagnostic criteria and systematic studies, the use of the terms *hysteria* and *conversion* was inconsistent during the early years of psychoanalysis. A conversion phenomenon is now used to describe symptoms within the neurological system that have no clear focal or physiological basis. *Hysteria* is a term best abandoned by clinicians other than mental health professionals because it stigmatizes the patient. Concurrently, the clinician may become frustrated and see the "hysterical" patient as difficult to help.

THE SOMATOFORM DISORDERS

Somatoform disorders are present in at least 10–15% of primary care patients (Kellner 1985; Kirmayer and Robbins 1991; Spitzer et al. 1994). The somatoform disorders share the common feature of physical symptoms that suggest a medical disorder but are not fully explained by organic pathology or by the direct effects of a drug or another psychiatric disorder, such as rapid heart rate and panic disorder. Given the role of physical symptoms as the unifying feature of somatoform disorders, it is not surprising that pain is commonly found among the various disorders. The somatoform disorders described in the DSM-IV include somatization disorder, undifferentiated somatization disorder, conversion disorder, pain disorder, hypochondriasis, body dysmorphic disorder, and somatoform disorder not otherwise specified (Table I). Except for body dysmorphic disorder, characterized by a preoccupation with an imagined or exaggerated defect in physical appearance, all the other entities frequently have pain as part of the presenting complaint. Pain expression among those identified with these disorders is challenging and difficult to treat. This difficulty might be attributed to the fact that the etiology of pain is judged to be psychogenic. Moreover, potential physiological parameters are devalued, and the patient and clinician become entangled in an adversarial relationship notable for disagreement and distrust. Many of the negative outcomes for chronic pain treatment can be attributed to this failure of therapeutic rapport (Roth 2000). Noyes et al. (1999) observed that patients with hypochondriasis rated their health problems as having been less thoroughly evaluated, less completely explained, and less adequately treated, and also rated their response to treatment as having been less satisfactory, viewed the physician as having been less interested or concerned, and reported less overall satisfaction with their health care than did control subjects who were attending an internal medicine clinic.

HYPOCHONDRIASIS

Hypochondriasis is among the most common somatoform disorders found in primary care settings (Bridges and Goldberg 1991). The DSM-IV defines hypochondriasis as a disorder in which ruminative fears of a serious illness are based on misinterpretation of subjective bodily symptoms. To meet the criteria for hypochondriasis, the preoccupation with such fears must persist despite appropriate medical evaluation and reassurance for at least 6 months and cause social, occupational, or other limitations in functioning.

Epidemiological studies estimate the prevalence of hypochondriasis at 0.4–14% in primary care settings and at 3–13% in the community, depending on the population surveyed and the methods used (Bearber and Rodney 1984; Kellner 1985, Barsky et al. 1990). Gerdes et al. (1996) found that the identification of hypochondriasis by physicians does occur without formal diagnostic labeling, despite their awareness of their patients' fears of disease and bodily preoccupations.

Most hypochondriacal complaints concern the head and neck, abdomen, and chest (Kenyon 1976). Nearly all complaints center on the experience of pain. Most importantly for clinicians, the hypochondriacal patient is concerned with the meaning of the pain rather than the sensation itself. For example, the hypochondriac who complains about headaches is more concerned with the "tumor" that is "causing" the headache than with the headache pain itself.

Persons with hypochondriasis are likely to be found among patients in primary care settings. Because hypochondriasis is defined in terms of psychological symptoms, the somatic presentation by such patients may be confusing for clinicians trained to identify physical illness. Hypochondriacal patients feel chronically ill and endure significant role impairment. In most nonpsychiatric settings, there is usually a shortened time frame in which to gather data. Nevertheless, obtaining an accurate history is paramount.

At the first session with the somatically preoccupied patient, the physician should undertake a careful evaluation to understand the evolution of the patient's illness and health-related experiences. The way symptoms are disclosed to physicians is shaped by the social context within which they are experienced and to whom they are disclosed. An illness is organized through an evolving interaction between physician and patient (Balint 1957).

Information obtained from the history will help clinicians recognize patients with unreasonable fear of illness. The somatically preoccupied patient may present with a history of a great number of outpatient visits (Barsky et al. 1991), frequent hospitalizations (Craig et al. 1993), and repetitive subspecialty referrals (Blackwell and De Morgan 1996). A medical record release may result in a "thick" record revealing multiple medications, a large number of diagnoses, and many diagnostic studies. This record is a concrete manifestation of the somatically preoccupied patient's high utilization of health care. Despite these findings, such patients find their extensive care ineffective and unsatisfactory.

A past medical history of the following symptoms or syndromes has been associated with somatic preoccupation: chronic fatigue syndrome; fibromyalgia; irritable bowel syndrome; atypical chest pain; hyperventilation; pelvic, abdominal, and low back pain; headache; and nonulcer dyspepsia (Katon 1991; Blackwell 1992; Walker et al. 1995). A history of multiple drug allergies and extreme sensitivity to medication side effects also may indicate somatic preoccupation. The clinician should search for diagnosable psychiatric disorders, particularly anxiety and depression (Leibbrand et al. 1999). The hypochondriac with pain preoccupations might be anxious. The existence of both comorbid disorders often impairs the management of pain and the patient's functional status. Anxiety can change pain threshold and tolerance and increase pain ratings. Anxiety in the hypochondriac might also demonstrate apprehensive self-scrutiny and a sense of physical jeopardy, which could make symptoms more worrisome (Barsky 1996). Early recognition and treatment of anxiety will address the goals most commonly identified for the pain patient, namely pain control and improved functional status. A family history of anxiety and depressive disorder might be another clue from the patient's history to indicate an excessive fear of illness (Noyes et al. 1997). The patient's social history might also identify risk factors for somatic preoccupation including being a single parent, social isolation, unemployment, urban living, and substance abuse (Bhui and Hotopf 1997). Additional associations include childhood exposure to models of illness behavior such as having a parent with chronic illness or pain and exposure to physical or sexual abuse (Stuart and Noyes 1999).

SOMATIZATION DISORDER

Pain complaints are necessary components of the diagnostic criteria for somatization disorder, which refers to multiple recurrent physical symptoms and complaints in multiple organ systems that cannot be objectively validated through physical examinations or diagnostic studies or cannot be fully explained based on known medical conditions or on the direct effect of a substance. These "unexplained" physical complaints must begin before 30 years of age and assume a chronic and fluctuating course. In addition the physical symptoms and complaints are usually of sufficient severity to impair social, occupational, or other important areas of functioning. In order to make the diagnosis, according to DSM-IV the following criteria must also be met, with the presence of several symptoms in four major categories: (1) Four pain symptoms related to at least four different sites (head, abdomen, back, joints, extremities, chest, or rectum) or functions (menstruation, sexual intercourse, or urination). (2) Two gastrointestinal symptoms other than pain (nausea, bloating, vomiting other than during pregnancy, diarrhea, or intolerance of several different foods). (3) One sexual symptom other than pain, such as sexual indifference, erectile or ejaculatory dysfunction, irregular menses, excessive menstrual bleeding, or vomiting throughout pregnancy. (4) One pseudoneurological symptom or deficit suggesting a neurological condition not limited to pain, such as paralysis or numbness, impaired coordination or loss of balance, difficulty swallowing, loss of voice, visual or auditory deficits, seizures, loss of consciousness, amnesia, or hallucinations.

Patients' presentation of these symptoms is classically described as being colorful, with much flair for the dramatic. Kaminsky and Slavney (1976) describe the characteristics of somatizing patients not in terms of the number or severity of their medically unexplained symptoms, but in terms of their dramatic and persistent complaints about them. However, some patients express their physical complaints with no emotional concerns; this sign can be designated *la belle indifference.*

Information obtained from the history will assist in the recognition of patients with somatization disorder. They may present with a history similar to that of the hypochondriac, with a great number of outpatient visits, frequent hospitalizations, and repetitive subspecialty referrals. It is imperative that the health care provider not skim the past medical history and miss the diagnosis. Unlike hypochondriacs, patients with somatization disorder often lead chaotic lives, and their histories often reveal impulsive or manipulative behaviors and even suicide attempts or gestures. Difficulties with interpersonal relations often emerge during the interview. These patients demonstrate less introspection, are more likely to deny psychological causes of somatic symptoms than to deny psychosocial presenters of distress, and are more likely to discount common somatic symptoms by endorsing normal conditions or environmental circumstances than are patients without somatization disorder (Keeley et al. 2000).

The patient's psychiatric and family history also might provide clues. Anxiety and depression are often associated with somatization disorder (Chiles et al. 1983; Polatin et al. 1991). Chronic anxiety can change pain threshold and tolerance and increase pain ratings. Depressive symptomatology in chronic pain patients has been associated with role impairment and loss of function. The pain syndrome observed in patients with somatization disorder is usually chronic in nature. It appears that comorbidly depressed chronic pain patients may be more sensitive to acute pain stimuli. Katon et al. (1985), working with a sample of 37 chronic pain patients, observed that almost two-thirds of their sample had a first-degree relative with chronic pain. Implicit from this study is the social learning theory of modeling of illness behavior. Children exposed to their parents' maladaptive illness behavior adopt the responses to pain and illness that they observe. Simply stated, children exposed to parents who deal with pain and illness in a maladaptive manner are likely to exhibit similar behaviors. Bass and Murphy (1991) noted that over half of their adult patients with somatization disorder had been exposed to physical disability in one or both parents. A family history of childhood exposure to models of illness behavior such as a parent with chronic illness and the presence of a personality disorder in one or both of the parents will be important diagnostic information. Katon et al. (1985) also documented a strong association between a past history of alcohol abuse and the future development of chronic pain. The data on alcohol abuse demonstrated a high past rate of alcohol abuse (35.1%) and dependence (16.2%). Most of the alcohol problems had preceded the onset of chronic pain by several years. It is probable that the chronic pain reported in this sample may be an expression of these patients' chronic psychiatric illness. An example would be the patient with depression who focuses on the somatic component of the depressive syndrome, such as headache, and denies the affective component. The authors concluded that many of the patients' current depressive episodes were secondary to chronic pain.

CONVERSION DISORDER

The formal diagnosis of conversion disorder does not mention pain. Sensory changes are "pseudoneurological" in the DSM-IV text; loss of sensory modalities, including pain, is more common. The pain observed as a sensory dysfunction in conversion disorder tends to be localized to the abdominal cavity or the genital area, or may have the pattern of a fatal illness. If pain is a symptom of conversion disorder, other symptoms must be present. Pain disorder would be the proper diagnosis if pain is the only complaint and the other criteria for that disorder are met.

Conversion phenomena occur in somatization disorder, which often has pain complaints inherent in its diagnosis. It is essential for the clinician to recognize conversion as a categorical disorder. It now denotes a syndrome where the predominant symptom is loss of voluntary muscle or sensory function that is not explained by an organic disease state, and it is not an element of somatization disorder. Ziegler and Imboden (1962) noted that pain is a modern presentation of the traditional conversion disorders. The DSM-IV does not reflect this impression and classifies pain disorder separately from conversion phenomena.

Conversion phenomena include defects with no medical explanation that affect the voluntary motor or sensory functions. A conversion phenomenon is now thought to be most appropriate for symptoms within the neurological system that have no clear focal or physiological basis. Symptoms or signs that seem to have no obvious neurological basis do not rule out organic disease, however. One study found that nearly 70% of patients diagnosed with conversion disorder had evidence of a preceding or coexisting neurological disorder (Barsky 1989). Patients with multiple sclerosis, myasthenia gravis, and central nervous system tumors have often been previously mislabeled as having "conversion symptoms."

Conversion reaction may occur more often in rural settings, where patients may be naive about medical and psychological issues. The disorder is observed more commonly in lower socioeconomic groups, in those with little education or little knowledge of medical concepts, and in military personnel exposed to combat situations. In some cultures, conversion symptoms may be viewed as acceptable and credible ways to express distress. In addition to reviewing demographic data of patients with suspected conversion phenomena, the clinician should, as with other clinical situations, obtain a medical history. The most common medical finding is a history of head trauma. Bowman (1993) found that 66% of patients reported a history of head injuries and that 55% had experienced loss of consciousness. In the social history one might recognize experiences of physical or sexual abuse. A detailed psychosocial history is essential in the process of making the diagnosis because the clinician may find a connection between the symptom and any psychological conflict or stressor.

The onset of conversion disorder is usually acute, with variable progression of symptoms. It often occurs in connection with a psychological stressor. In most instances, the duration of the symptoms and associated pain is brief, with remission usually occurring within 2 weeks if the stressor is addressed or removed, although the condition sometimes has a remitting and relapsing course.

PAIN DISORDER

Pain disorder was outlined in the DSM-IV as a syndrome where pain is the predominant focus of the clinical picture and causes impairment in social, occupational, or other areas of functioning. An essential feature of pain disorder is that psychological factors are judged to play a significant role in the onset, severity, exacerbation, or maintenance of pain. The pain is not better accounted for by another disorder (mood disorder, anxiety, or psychosis). Acute pain is most often associated with anxiety regarding the cognitive derivative of fear of what the pain might represent, such as a life-threatening disorder. In acute painful states, anxiety may make the pain far worse. As the pain becomes more protracted and enters a chronic stage, depression often is a result and increases the discomfort. Another criterion needed to establish the diagnosis of pain disorder is that it is not intentionally produced or feigned as in malingering (described below).

The subtypes of pain disorder include those associated with psychological factors, with a general medical condition, or with combined medical and psychological factors. Sullivan (2000) has cogently argued against this diagnosis. He notes that partitioning organic from psychogenic causes of pain is particularly difficult and inherently unsound because severe pain syndromes, clearly caused by organic factors, obviously have a psychological reaction. Furthermore, there have been few reliability and validity studies of the DSM-IV pain disorders. Nevertheless, although pain disorder is within the somatoform disorder section, it is difficult to truly partition it from other disorders. Individuals with somatization disorder have a variety of pain complaints.

Adjustment disorder with anxiety or depression may better capture the reality of those with clear-cut organic pain. Finally, this diagnosis may minimize the true suffering the patient experiences and limit the empathy of the physician (Sullivan 2000).

The clinical conundrum of the pain disorder category in the DSM-IV is nowhere better demonstrated than in the clinical category of low back pain. Approximately 80% of individuals will, at some point in their life, complain of low back pain (Deyo et al. 1991). There is dramatic disability within the entity and wide variation in treatment response. Medical and psychological approaches to low back pain have been reported, both separately and in combination. Such patients often have comorbid depressive disorders that may best be diagnosed as adjustment disorders. Noncardiac chest pain also reflects the complexities of pain and of attributing such a complaint to psychiatric categories. Mayou et al. (1997) have reported upon the chronic nature of pain in such patients, who feel generally dissatisfied with their medical care. Both panic disorder and somatization disorder may be associated with such chest pain. Nonspecific disorders in the gastrointestinal tract, such as "nutcracker" esophagus on motility study, and musculoskeletal abnormalities also may co-occur with such disorders. Management involves active treatment of comorbid depression or anxiety, reassurance that the pain is not indicative of coronary disease, and relaxation exercises. It is also effective to address the cognitive-behavioral element of catastrophic thinking that may arise from automatic thoughts when the pain is experienced (Salkovskis 1992).

OTHER DIAGNOSES SUGGESTIVE OF PHYSICAL DISORDER

Malingering is a forensic topic, but it is a focus of clinical attention because persons who consciously feign symptoms or exaggerate them for secondary gain seek treatment in clinical settings. Malingering, unlike hypochondriasis and somatization, is not an expression of factors as various as personality characteristics, learned patterns of behaviors, coping styles, and psychiatric disorders. It is not a psychosomatic expression, and thus not a psychiatric disorder. In malingering, attaining the sick role is the immediate goal of simulations that are consciously intended. Back and neck pain are disabilities often reported by a malingerer. One may suspect feigned pain when the onset of symptom coincides with a large financial gain, when the patient does not cooperate with the diagnostic workup or prescribed treatment, and when objective medical tests do not confirm the patient's complaints. In a prospective study ($n = 350$ subjects), Waddell et al. (1980) were able to distinguish between physical and behavioral causes of back pain complaints. They identified eight signs that are consistently reliable and reproducible for identifying nonstructural problems in patients with back pain. A finding of three or more positive signs increases the predictive value of the Waddell signs.

Direct confrontation with the observed clinical findings not suggestive of an organic etiology is punitive at best. The clinician must cultivate a constant awareness that what appears initially to be a nonorganic cause might later turn out to be the contrary, and should reexamine the patient at scheduled visits, focusing on the reportedly painful areas, and perform a more complete examination if the findings change significantly over time.

Neurasthenia is a syndrome that is not included in DSM iterations but appears in the ICD-10 (World Health Organization 1992). It is subsumed in the DSM-IV as "undifferentiated somatoform disorder." The predominant symptom in neurasthenia is fatigue after either mental or physical effort. It is also accompanied, however, by pain, often muscular in nature, as well as by "tension headaches." Neurasthenia is not used as a formal diagnosis to any great extent in the United States or Western Europe, but it has been used commonly in Asia. It has a high degree of comorbidity, especially with depression, and could be considered a character style, as well as a discrete syndrome. Whether neurasthenia is another term for functional somatic syndromes such as fibromyalgia or chronic fatigue remains to be better defined (Hickie 2002).

CONCLUSION

Pain is a common complaint within the somatoform disorders. These disorders are usually encountered in primary care settings. When patients with somatoform disorders are referred to a psychiatrist, the patients often feel that their primary care physician does not fully appreciate their suffering. Conjoint treatment must be emphasized to avoid fears of abandonment. It is the task of the psychiatrist to fully understand the nature of the pain complaint with respect to its onset, characteristics, aggravating factors, and any comorbidity, either medical or psychiatric. A careful and complete history will allow a better diagnosis and help forge a treatment alliance. Each category within the somatoform disorders has its specific features, which will challenge both patient and physician alike.

REFERENCES

American Psychiatric Association. *Diagnostic and Statistical Manual of Mental Disorders,* 4th ed. Washington, DC: American Psychiatric Association, 1994.

Balint M. *The Doctor, His Patient and the Illness.* New York: International Universities Press, 1957.

Barsky AJ. Hypochondriasis: medical management and psychiatric treatment. *Psychosomatics* 1996; 37:48–56.

Barsky AJ, Wyshak G. Hypochondriasis and related health attitudes. *Psychosomatics* 1989; 30:412–420.

Barsky AJ, Wyshak G, Klerman GL, Latham KS. The prevalence of hypochondriasis in medical outpatients. *Soc Psychiatry Psychiatr Epidemiol* 1990; 25:89–94.

Barsky AJ, Wyshak G, Latham KS, Klerman GL. Hypochondriacal patients, their physicians, and their medical care. *J Gen Intern Med* 1991; 6:413–419.

Barsky AJ, Barnett MC, Cleary PD. Hypochondriasis and panic disorder: boundary and overlap. *Arch Gen Psychiatry* 1994; 51:918-925.

Bass C, Murphy M. Somatisation disorder in a British teaching hospital. *Br J Clin Pract* 1991; 45:237–244.

Bearber RJ, Rodney WM. Underdiagnosis of hypochondriasis in family practice. *Psychosomatics* 1984; 25:39–46.

Bhui K, Hotopf M. Somatization disorder. *Br J Hosp Med* 1997; 58:145–149.

Blackwell B. Sick-role susceptibility. *Psychother Psychosom* 1992; 58:79–90.

Blackwell B, De Morgan NP. The primary care of patients who have bodily concerns. *Arch Fam Med* 1996; 5:457–463.

Breuer J, Freud S. *Studies in Hysteria,* Nervous and Mental Disease Monographs. Brill AA (Trans). New York, 1936.

Bridges K, Goldberg D, Evans B, Sharpe T. Determinants of somatization in primary care. *Psychol Med* 1991; 21:473–483.

Charcot JM. *Ouevres Completes de JM Charcot,* Tome IX. Paris: Lecrosnier et Babe, 1890.

Chiles JA, Ward NG, Becker J. Depressive illness and medical practice. In: Carr JE, Dengerink HA (Eds). *Behavioral Science in the Practice of Medicine.* New York: Elsevier Biomedical, 1983, p 347.

Craig TK, Boardman, AP, Mills K, et al. The South London Somatization Study. I: Longitudinal course and the influence of early life experiences. *Br J Psychiatry* 1993; 163:579–588.

Deyo RA. The early diagnostic evaluation of patients with low back pain. *J Gen Intern Med* 1986; 1:328–338.

Deyo RA, Cherkin D, Conrad D, Volinn E. Cost, controversy, crisis: low back pain and the health of the public. *Annu Rev Public Health* 1991; 12:141–156.

Dworkin RH, Caligor E. Psychiatric diagnosis and chronic pain: DSM-III-R and beyond. *J Pain Symptom Manage* 1988; 3:87–98.

Fink P. The use of hospitalizations by somatizing patients. *Psychol Med* 1992; 22:173–180.

Gerdes TT, Noyes R Jr, Kathol RG, et al. Physician recognition of hypochondriacal patients. *Gen Hosp Psychiatry* 1996; 18:106–112.

Hickie I. Neurasthenia: prevalence, disability and health care characteristics in the Australian community. *Br J Psychiatry* 2002; 181:56–61.

Kaminsky MJ, Slavney PR. Methodology and personality in Briquet's syndrome: a reappraisal. *Am J Psychiatry* 1976; 133:85–88.

Katon WJ. The development of a randomized trial of consultation—liaison psychiatry trial in distressed high utilizers of primary care. *Psychiatry Med* 1991; 9:577–591.

Katon W, Egan K, Miller D. Chronic pain: lifetime psychiatric diagnoses and family history. *Am J Psychiatry* 1985; 142:1156–1160.

Keeley R, Smith M, Miller J. Somatoform symptoms and treatment nonadherence in depressed family medicine outpatients. *Arch Fam Med* 2000; 9:46–54.

Kellner R. Functional somatic symptoms and hypochondriasis: a survey of empirical studies. *Arch Gen Psychiatry* 1985; 42:821–833.

Kellner R. *Psychosomatic Syndromes and Somatic Symptoms.* Washington, DC: American Psychiatric Press, 1991, pp 189–225.

Kenyon FE. Hypochondriacal states. *Br J Psychiatry* 1976; 129:1–14.

Kirmayer LJ, Robbins JM. Three forms of somatization in primary care: prevalence, co-occurrence and sociodemographic characteristics. *J Nerv Ment Dis* 1991; 179:647–655.

Kirmayer LJ, Young A. Culture and somatization: clinical, epidemiological, and ethnographic perspectives. *Psychosom Med* 1998; 60:420–430.

Kroenke K, Price RK. Symptoms in the community prevalence, classification, and psychiatric comorbidity. *Arch Intern Med* 1993; 153:2474–2480.

Leibbrand R, Hiller W, Fichter M. Effect of comorbid anxiety, depressive, and personality disorders on treatment outcome of somatoform disorders. *Compr Psychiatry* 1999; 40(3):203–209.

Lipowski ZJ. Somatization: the experience and communication of psychological distress as somatic symptoms. *Psychother Psychosom* 1987; 47:160–167.

Mayou RA, Bryant BM, Sanders D, et al. A controlled trial of cognitive behavioural therapy for non-cardiac chest pain. *Psychol Med* 1997; 27:1021–1031

Merskey H, Bogduk N. *Classification of Chronic Pain: Description of Chronic Pain Syndromes and Definition of Pain Terms,* 2nd ed. Seattle: IASP Press, 1994.

Noyes R, Kathol RG, Fisher MM, et al. The validity of DSM-III-R hypochondriasis. *Arch Gen Psychiatry* 1993; 50:961–970.

Noyes R, Holt CS, Happel RL, et al. A family study of hypochondriasis. *J Nerv Ment Dis* 1997; 185:223–232.

Noyes R, Langbehn DR, Happel RL, et al. Health attitude survey: a scale for assessing somatizing patients. *Psychosomatics* 1999; 40:470–478.

Owen-Salters E, Gatchel RJ, Polatin PB, et al. Changes in psychopathology following functional restoration of chronic low back pain: a prospective study. *J Occup Rehab* 1996; 6:215–223.

Polatin PB, Kinney RK, Gatchel RJ. Premorbid psychopathology in somatoform pain syndrome. In: *Abstracts of the American Psychiatric Association 144th Annual Meeting,* p 181.

Reich I, Rosenblatt RM, Turpin J. DSM-III: a new nomenclature for classifying patients with chronic pain. *Pain* 1983; 16:201–206.

Roth RS. Psychogenic models of chronic pain: a selective review and critique. In: Massie MJ (Ed). *Pain: What Psychiatrists Need to Know,* Review of Psychiatry, Vol. 19. Washington, DC: American Psychiatric Press, 2000, pp 89–131.

Salkovskis PM. Psychological treatment of noncardiac chest pain: the cognitive approach. *Am J Med* 1992; 92(5A):114S–121S.

Spitzer RL, Williams JBW, Kroenke K, et al. Utility of a new procedure for diagnosing mental disorders in primary care: the PRIME-MD 1000 study. *JAMA* 1994; 272:1749–1756.

Stuart S, Noyes Jr R. Attachment and interpersonal communication in somatization. *Psychosomatics* 1999; 40:34–43.

Sullivan MD. DSM-IV Pain disorder: a case against the diagnosis. *Int Rev Psychiatry* 2000; 12:91–98.

Waddell G, McCulloch JA, Kummel E, et al. Nonorganic physical signs in low back pain. *Spine* 1980; 5(2):117–125.

Walker EA, Gelfand AN, Gelfand MD, et al. Psychiatric diagnoses, sexual and physical victimization, and disability in patients with irritable bowel syndrome or inflammatory bowel disease. *Psychol Med* 1995; 25:1259–1267.

World Health Organization. *The ICD-10 Classification of Mental and Behavioural Disorders: Clinical Descriptions and Diagnostic Guidelines.* Geneva: World Health Organization, 1992.

Ziegler FJ, Imboden JB. Contemporary conversion reactions to a conceptual model. *Arch Gen Psychiatry* 1962; 6:279.

Correspondence to: Thomas Wise, MD, Department of Psychiatry, Inova Fairfax Hospital, 3300 Gallows Road, Falls Church, VA 22042, USA. Email: thomas.wise@inova.com.

Psychosocial Aspects of Pain: A Handbook for Health Care Providers, Progress in Pain Research and Management, Vol. 27, edited by Robert H. Dworkin and William S. Breitbart, IASP Press, Seattle, © 2004.

9

Screening Pain Patients for Invasive Procedures: A Review of the Evidence and Recommendations for Clinical Practice

Robert J. Gatchel, Ann Matt Maddrey, and Richard C. Robinson

Department of Psychiatry, The University of Texas Southwestern Medical Center at Dallas, Dallas, Texas, USA

Pain is a complex and debilitating medical condition that affects over 50 million people in the United States alone. As pain moves from an acute problem to a chronic condition, the scope of its impact widens, to the detriment of more and more areas of psychological and social functioning. In addition to the cost in human suffering, pain-related treatment costs and lost productivity are staggering (Gatchel and Turk 1996). Pain accounts for approximately 80% of all physician visits (Gatchel and Turk 1996), and an estimated 176,000 patients in the United States seek more intensive treatment at pain clinics each year (Marketdata 1995). Conservative estimates of the cost of chronic pain for Americans in terms of health care and lost productivity exceed U.S.$70 billion annually (Gatchel and Turk 1996). In fact, Frymoyer and Durett (1997) estimated that over $125 billion was spent in the United States on medical charges and hospitalization costs related to chronic pain. The complexity of pain and the absence of any one simple method to treat it necessitates examination into which treatments will have the highest likelihood of success for any given patient.

INVASIVE PROCEDURES

SURGICAL PROCEDURES

Much of what we know about acute and chronic pain is derived from years of investigation into back pain. Chronic low back pain is the most common form of chronic pain, and it affects 70% of Americans at some point during their lives. Fortunately, the vast majority of individuals who develop back pain recover without the need for major invasive procedures. However, an estimated 300,000 to 400,000 pain sufferers in the United States will undergo some form of spine surgery each year (Gatchel 2001).

Several surgical procedures are commonly used to treat back pain, but these procedures typically are used only after more conservative approaches have been attempted. A *laminectomy/diskectomy,* or simply a *laminectomy,* involves the removal of a section of bone from the patient's lamina. Disk tissue is then removed that is pressing on the patient's nerve root. A similar procedure, *microdiskectomy,* uses small incisions and intraoperative magnification to accomplish results similar to that of a laminectomy. A *facet rhizotomy* ablates the nerve that innervates the facet joints. A *foraminotomy* entails relieving pressure on an exiting nerve root by increasing the opening of a narrowed foramen. Finally, a *spinal fusion* essentially entails eliminating motion of a painful spinal segment; it can be accomplished through several techniques. In addition to the surgical procedures listed above, *intradiskal electrothermal therapy* (IDET) and disk replacement are newer procedures that have received a great deal of attention in the last few years (Block et al. 2003).

Spinal surgery is a necessary and beneficial procedure for many back pain sufferers. However, success rates vary according to the procedure and problem (Mayer et al. 1998). Success is typically measured in reduction of pain and improvement in functional ability. For a laminectomy/diskectomy, the success rate is 80–90% (Deyo et al. 1992), but for a spinal fusion it is only 70–80% (Turner et al. 1992). Atlas and colleagues (1996) conducted a 4-year follow-up in patients with lumbar spinal stenosis and found that those treated surgically had significantly less back and leg pain and had greater satisfaction than did those treated nonsurgically. In addition, Malter and colleagues (1998) found that quality of life for patients with herniated lumbar disks who had a diskectomy was significantly better than that of patients who were treated conservatively. This study found that the cost-effectiveness of a diskectomy was significantly greater than that of such procedures as a coronary artery bypass graft for single artery disease and medical therapy for moderate hypertension.

Unfortunately, a significant proportion of individuals who have undergone previous surgery may be classified as suffering from "failed back surgery syndrome." This syndrome may be diagnosed in individuals with back pain who have undergone at least one previous surgery with an unsatisfactory outcome (Block et al. 2003). Oaklander and North (2001) suggest that the most common cause of this syndrome is operating on patients who have many psychological risk factors or who have less than clear pathological indications. However, other reasons for the syndrome include issues related to the procedure, recurrent spinal problems, and scar tissue. Unfortunately, even when patients are appropriately selected and a technically sound surgery is performed, certain patients may remain in significant pain and be functionally impaired despite no discernible physical reason (Block et al. 2003). Surgeries to correct failed back surgery syndrome typically are successful only 60% of the time (Deyo et al. 1992).

IMPLANTABLE MODALITIES

Laminectomies, spinal fusions, and other surgical procedures are not the only invasive procedures used to treat pain. Implantable modalities have received increasing attention as a means for decreasing pain and suffering. Implantable devices, which are usually reserved for patients who have tried other nonsurgical and surgical techniques, typically provide either *neurostimulation* or *neuraxial drug administration*. With neurostimulation, electrodes placed on appropriate nerves are used to decrease pain by stimulating pain pathways; the patient is able to control the stimulation within certain parameters (Prager and Jacobs 2001). Depending on the type of stimulation unit, patients with neuropathic pain may achieve successful treatment with neurostimulation between 30% and 70% of the time (North et al. 1993).

Neuraxial drug administration allows opioids to be administered directly to opioid receptors. Intraspinal infusion of opioids decreases pain while minimizing the dose, thus reducing potential side effects. Implantable drug delivery systems come in many forms and are tailored to the needs of the patient based on diagnosis and individual situations (Prager and Jacobs 2001). Many chronic pain patients who have failed other treatments may be eager to try an implantable pump, despite variables that might interfere with their successful recovery or before conservative measures have been fully explored.

PSYCHOSOCIAL SCREENING

THE BIOPSYCHOSOCIAL PERSPECTIVE

With advances in technology, it may become easy for individuals to forget the complex nature of pain. Clinicians from all specialties know that certain patients believe that their pain can simply be "fixed," or that a procedure they saw on a news show will be the one that finally "cures" their pain. However, pain must be understood from a biopsychosocial perspective that takes into account the medical diagnosis and other relevant biological variables as well as psychosocial issues. Indeed, this biopsychosocial perspective is now accepted as the most heuristic approach to the understanding, assessment, and treatment of pain. It views physical disorders such as pain as a result of a complex and dynamic interaction among physiological, psychological, and social factors that perpetuate and may worsen the clinical presentation. Each individual experiences pain uniquely. A range of socioeconomic factors can interact with physical pathology to modulate a patient's report of symptoms and subsequent disability. The development of this biopsychosocial approach has grown rapidly during the past decade, and a great deal of scientific knowledge has emerged in this short period of time concerning the best care of individuals with complex pain problems, as well as pain prevention and coping strategies. Some recent comprehensive articles have reviewed the biopsychosocial perspective of pain (e.g., Turk and Monarch 2002).

PSYCHOSOCIAL ASSESSMENT FOR SURGICAL PROCEDURES

As noted by Epker and Block (2001), results of spinal surgery rely not only on medical factors but on the patient's environment, incentives or disincentives to recovery, and emotional functioning. Block and colleagues (2003) delineated several reasons for preoperative assessment: (1) Improve overall treatment outcome by excluding patients with a strong potential to experience a poor outcome; (2) provide a strong, empirically validated rationale for avoiding invasive procedures in cases where the surgeon feels uncomfortable about operating; (3) reduce average treatment duration and cost by helping avoid ineffective procedures; (4) improve outcome in patients undergoing surgery by identifying and, when necessary, treating emotional and behavioral problems; (5) identify patients who are likely to develop medication abuse or compliance problems; and (6) reduce the number of problem patients in a surgeon's practice. Although much of what will be presented in this section relates to surgical procedures, much can also be applied to implantable devices.

MMPI and personality. "Personality" refers to a set of beliefs, feelings, and behaviors that remain stable over time. The Minnesota Multiphasic Personality Inventory (MMPI) and its revised edition, the MMPI-2, have long been used to examine the way personality and emotional factors affect treatment outcomes. The MMPI-2 is a 567-item, true-false test that asks individuals about thoughts, beliefs, likes, and dislikes. The original MMPI was developed in the 1940s, and what made the instrument so unique was that the items were selected by comparing patients with a certain diagnosis, such as hysteria or hypochondriasis, to individuals who were believed to be free of psychopathology (McKinley and Hathaway 1940). The final MMPI consisted of three validity scales and 10 standard scales that represented eight clinical diagnoses, as well as two other nonclinical scales. A patient's MMPI profile is developed by calculating a *t*-score on each of the individual scales. Using a *t*-score allows clinicians to determine how far an individual deviates from the normative sample group (see Fig. 1). A score that is two standard deviations above the mean is considered clinically significant for the MMPI, and a score one and a half standard deviations above the mean is considered clinically significant for the MMPI-2. Much of the research with the original MMPI applies to the MMPI-2, published in 1989. However, the MMPI-2 was developed to update the wording of some of the test items and, most importantly, to develop a more representative normative sample than the MMPI. The MMPI-2 normative sample closely matches the gender, age, and socioeconomic characteristics of the United States based on 1980 census data (Friedman et al. 2001).

The first three clinical scales (hypochondriasis, depression, and hysteria) intuitively appear the most relevant for chronic pain patients and, in fact, have repeatedly been investigated with this population. McKinley and Hathaway (1940) defined Scale 1 (hypochondriasis) as an abnormal concern with one's health. Persons with elevations on Scale 1 tend to be whining and demanding (Butcher and Williams 1993).

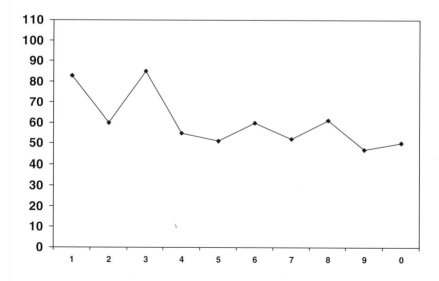

Fig. 1. Example of a "conversion V" profile on an MMPI, with the vertical axis representing *t* scores. Scale 1 (hypochondriasis) and scale 3 (hysteria) are two standard deviations above the mean.

The clinical group for Scale 2 (depression) consisted mostly of bipolar patients during a depressive episode (Butcher and Williams 1993). While many individuals with elevations on Scale 2 are depressed, an individual can have an elevated score on Scale 2 without meeting the criteria for a major depressive disorder. Rather, Scale 2 may be thought of as an indication of the degree to which individuals are satisfied with themselves, their life, or their current situation. Individuals with an elevated Scale 2 score tend to be unhappy, pessimistic, self-deprecating, and sluggish. In addition, they may have many of the neurovegetative symptoms consistent with a depressive disorder, including fatigue and mental dullness (Butcher and Williams 1993).

Scale 3 (hysteria) was developed to aid in the detection and diagnosis of conversion hysteria. People with an elevated score on this scale tend to react to stress with physical symptoms and have limited insight into their feelings and motivations, although they may lack anxiety and depression (Butcher and Williams 1993). Further, these individuals may be immature, childish, and egocentric, often requiring excessive attention and affection from others (Butcher and Williams 1993). Elevations on Scale 3 may reflect a difficulty acknowledging or accepting aggressive or hostile aspects of oneself. Therefore, hostility may be expressed through indirect or passive means, or else acted out with little insight into one's behavior. While these individuals may demonstrate good interpersonal skills, the quality of their relationships is likely to be superficial (Butcher and Williams 1993). These three scales are likely to be elevated in almost every chronic pain patient. It is when these elevations exceed what is expected for a patient, given his or her unique circumstances, that potential problems are indicated.

The MMPI has been studied to help predict who will respond well to treatment and who will have difficulty. The types of treatment studied have ranged from spinal fusions to comprehensive pain treatment or functional restoration programs. Initially, these studies focused attention on scale elevations as a predictor. For example, Wilfling et al. (1973) studied 26 male subjects from a population of veterans who had received lumbar intervertebral fusions for relief from low back pain. Subjects were assigned to three groups, either a "good" group, a "poor" group, or a "fair" group, based on the success or failure of the fusion in restoring the patient to normal functioning. The orthopedist based the decision on employment, pain, motor signs, and the patient's self-report. As expected, the "good" group produced a relatively normal MMPI profile. However, the "poor" group had clinically significant elevations on Scales 1 (hypochondriasis) and 2 (depression), with a near-clinically significant elevation on Scale 3 (hysteria). The "fair" group had clinically significant elevations on Scales 1 and 3, with a near-clinically significant elevation on Scale 2. The "poor" and "fair" groups also showed lower scores on the Ego Strength Scale (Wilfling et al. 1973), a subscale of the MMPI that, when elevated, reflects an ability to cope with daily stressors and difficult life situations (Graham 1993).

Whereas Wilfling et al. (1973) examined MMPI profiles after treatment, Wiltse and Rocchio (1975) examined the MMPI profiles of low back pain patients prior to chemonucleolysis (the use of a proteolytic agent to dissolve the nucleus pulposus of a herniated intervertebral disk). In addition to the MMPI, the researchers used surgeon ratings, patient biographical data, and scores from the Cornell Medical Index and the Quick Test. The patients' outcomes were rated 1 year after the chemonucleolysis based on organic and symptomatic aspects of success. Scales 1 (hypochondriasis) and 3 (hysteria) of the MMPI were found to be the best predictors of treatment outcome. In addition, reviewing data from 274 patients who had been hospitalized for persistent back pain symptoms, these researchers concluded that scores on Scales 1 and 3 tended to increase as the number of back operations increased (Wiltse and Rocchio 1975). The list of subsequent studies that have found the first three scales relevant to surgical outcomes is relatively large (e.g., Blumetti and Modesti 1976; Gentry et al. 1977; Long 1981; Herron and Pheasant 1982).

Scale 3 (hysteria) has been described as a character scale and, as such, is believed to measure a relatively stable trait (Trimboli and Kilgore 1983). While little can be reliably and conclusively drawn from this fact, it raises the notion that a person's characteristic ways of handling negative emotions and general psychological distress are important. Individuals with an elevated score on Scale 3 have limited insight into their psychological functioning and often react to stress with physical symptoms. Further, they rely heavily on other people and have difficulty directly expressing negative emotions. Rather, their negative feelings may occur as passive-aggressive or indirect behavior. For instance, a chronic low back pain patient with an elevated score on Scale 3 may deny any dissatisfaction with a spouse who has continually been critical of the patient's absence from work. Rather than voicing anger at the spouse's less than supportive stance, the patient may stop performing some of the minor household chores he or she previously performed, complaining of a decrease in physical functioning.

Scale 2 (depression) is also relevant to the examination of potential surgical candidates. Epker and Block (2001) have summarized the research on the depression scale by highlighting the fact that depressed individuals are more likely to focus on and expect negative results, have a lower threshold for pain, and are likely to report reduced functioning. The Beck Depression Inventory has also been used to demonstrate the relationship between surgical outcome and depression (Kjelby-Wendt et al. 1999).

Elevations on Scale 4 (psychopathic deviate) have also been associated with poor outcomes for invasive procedures (Epker and Block 2001). Individuals who have elevated scores on this scale are rebellious, tend to have difficulty with authority figures, and are also likely to be angry and resentful. A pain patient with an elevated Scale 4 score often blames others for his or her current situation and is quite angry about it. Complicating matters is the fact that pain patients often have reasons to be upset with employers or with the workers' compensation system. However, when anger interferes with a patient's ability to improve, or if the rebelliousness results in non-compliance with treatment recommendations, it is no wonder that these patients may be at increased risk for poor outcomes with invasive procedures. A common clinical observation is that if a patient begins to feel better then his or her employer is "off the hook" and the patient's months or years of suffering and anger have been for nothing.

Lastly, Scale 7 (psychasthenia) is also related to poor outcomes (Epker and Block 2001). Individuals with high scores on this scale tend to be ruminative and obsessive in nature, and may experience tension and anxiety. Fear and worry over re-injury present major obstacles to these patients' ability to recover from their medical problems.

Medical history. Several factors that can be obtained from a patient's history may improve the physician's ability to make an appropriate decision about surgery. Patients with a history of a mental health disturbance tend to respond poorly to surgery (Manniche et al. 1994). Polatin and colleagues (1993) found that, of 200 chronic low back pain patients, 77% met lifetime diagnostic criteria for psychiatric disturbances. The most common diagnoses were depression, substance abuse, and anxiety disorders. In addition, 51% of the patients met criteria for a personality disorder. Gatchel et al. (1994) examined 152 chronic low back pain patients before they began an intensive 3-week interdisciplinary treatment program, and found that 90% of these patients met criteria for a lifetime diagnosis of a disorder on Axis I of the DSM, the most prevalent diagnoses being major depression and substance abuse. In fact, evidence indicates that a history of alcohol or pain medication abuse or dependence may place an individual at risk for a poor surgical outcome (Spengler et al. 1980). Finally, a history of sexual or physical abuse increases one's chance for a poor surgical outcome as well (Schofferman et al. 1992).

Coping. Coping strategies are methods used to manage life's stresses and problems. The Coping Strategies Questionnaire (CSQ) is a widely studied instrument that has been used to determine coping strategies in patients with chronic pain. The CSQ is psychometrically sound and comprises several cognitive and behavioral scales. Coping strategies assessed by the CSQ include making coping self-statements, ignoring pain sensations, praying or hoping, catastrophizing, and increasing one's activity level; the instrument also assesses patients' perceived ability to control pain (Rosenstiel and Keefe 1983). Gross (1986) administered the CSQ to 50 patients who were scheduled to receive a laminectomy. Patients who felt that they had some sense of control and felt they could do something about their pain had better surgical outcomes (Gross 1986). Mahomed and colleagues (2002) used the SF-36 and the Western Ontario-McMaster University Osteoarthritis Index to explore the relationship among patients' expectations, functional outcomes, and satisfaction in total joint arthroplasty. These investigators studied 102 patients receiving total hip arthroplasty and 89 patients receiving total knee arthroplasty. They reported that expectation of pain relief prior to surgery predicted better physical functioning and greater decrease in pain 6 months after surgery.

The role of catastrophizing in the prediction of chronic pain and disability has gained increased attention in recent years. Catastrophizing involves thinking negatively, and in an exaggerated fashion, about events and stimuli. This term can be applied to how individuals perceive their pain or to their ability to cope with their pain (Sullivan et al. 1998). In one of the first studies to address this variable, Butler et al. (1989) evaluated cognitive strategies and postoperative pain in a sample of general surgical patients, and found that increased catastrophizing was associated with higher levels of postoperative pain intensity. Main and Waddell (1991) found a strong relationship between catastrophizing and depressive symptoms in a sample of low back pain patients. Furthermore, of the cognitive variables investigated by the authors, catastrophizing was determined to have the "greatest potential for understanding current low back symptoms" (Main and Waddell 1991). Jacobsen and Butler (1996) also examined the role of catastrophizing in 59 women who had undergone surgery for breast cancer, and found that increased catastrophizing was associated with more intense pain and greater use of analgesic medications. In addition, age emerged as an important predictor of both catastrophizing and postoperative pain, with younger patients being more likely to catastrophize and to report greater levels of pain.

Family. Evidence gathered over the years suggests that families can inadvertently have a negative impact on a patient's pain-related behavior. Specifically, when spouses or family members are overly solicitous toward a pain patient, they may be reinforcing pain behaviors. Eventually, spouses may even serve as a cue for pain behavior to be exhibited (Block et al. 1983). In addition, pain serves as a stressor not only for the patient, but often for the entire family. Decreased functioning and financial strain, which are often associated with chronic pain, can produce an environment in which patients and their family feel misunderstood and perhaps resentful of one another. Often, resentment may be directed toward health care professionals, which can reduce the patient's trust of his or her health care providers and ultimately impair treatment compliance.

Occupational and legal issues. The impact of occupational and legal issues must be taken into account during screening for invasive procedures. Schade and colleagues (1999) examined a host of variables predicting 2-year outcomes of lumbar diskectomy for 46 patients. In this study, several psychological aspects of work had strong associations with outcome. High levels of job satisfaction, a low level of occupational mental stress, and "job-related resignation" (acceptance that one must work even though the job is not desirable) were significant positive predictors of return to work. These same factors, to varying degrees, also predicted pain relief and overall outcome. The results of Schade et al.'s study and of other research (Vingard et al. 2000) suggest that individuals who perceive their work environments as being aversive, especially if their jobs involve heavy physical demands, may be particularly at risk for poor outcome after spine surgery.

In study after study, patients whose injuries have placed them within the workers' compensation system have tended to have poorer results from spine surgery. For example, Klekamp et al. (1998) examined 82 patients who underwent lumbar diskectomy and found that 81% of nonworkers' compensation patients achieved a good result, compared with only 29% of workers' compensation patients. Workers' compensation status is thus a significant risk factor for poor spinal surgery results. This effect may be mediated by the multitude of physical and emotional problems faced by patients with job-related injuries.

In further evidence that litigants have poorer surgical response, Finneson and Cooper (1979) found that both a history of lawsuits and secondary gain from disability predicted inferior diskectomy results. Taylor and colleagues (2000) found that whereas about two-thirds of spinal fusion patients reported improvement in functional ability and quality of life a year after surgery, several litigation-associated variables (including consultation with an attorney) contributed significantly to less favorable results. Similar reductions in surgical outcome have emerged in a number of other studies (Davis 1994; Manniche et al. 1994).

Environmental and historical factors. Epker and Block (2001) reviewed a host of medical and lifestyle factors that also may affect response to a surgical intervention. These factors include the duration of pain, previous surgery, the destructiveness of the surgery, and multiple medical problems. In addition, smoking (Manniche et al. 1994) and obesity appear to be risk factors for spinal surgery. Lastly, the observance of "nonorganic" signs (i.e., signs that should not be present given the pain complaint) is associated with poor surgical outcome (Greenough and Fraser 1989).

PSYCHOSOCIAL ASSESSMENT FOR IMPLANTABLE DEVICES

The psychosocial variables listed to this point have focused on screening for invasive surgeries. Although more research is needed, the selection of appropriate candidates for implantable modalities should take into consideration the factors that have already been discussed. However, unlike most surgical procedures, implantable devices can be tested in an individual patient in a brief clinical trial before the hardware is permanently implanted.

Prager and Jacobs (2001) reviewed the procedure for determining appropriate candidates for a trial of neuraxial medication or neurostimulation. According to the authors, two questions are fundamental with regard to a neuraxial medication trial: "(1) Is the patient's pain responsive to the therapy? and (2) Can the patient tolerate the planned modality?" Similar questions are posed for a neurostimulation trial. The authors suggested that the surgeon should outline the expectations and goals of therapy and clear up any misconceptions before proceeding with implantation. Further, the authors recommended that implantation be considered only when the trial yields at least 50% reduction in pain.

Although research is scarce on screening for implantable devices, Neben and colleagues (1996) published clinically sound guidelines for screening candidates for implantation of a spinal cord stimulator. The following criteria should be used to exclude patients from consideration: (1) active psychosis; (2) active suicidality; (3) active homicidality; (4) untreated or poorly treated major mood disorders such as major depression; (5) an unusually high level of somatization or other somatoform disorders; (6) substance abuse disorders; (7) unresolved workers' compensation or litigation cases; (8) lack of appropriate social support; and (9) cognitive defects that compromise adequate reasoning and memory. Obviously, the above potential exclusion criteria may be quite limiting for patients who otherwise might be candidates for implantable devices. Neben and associates (1996) also reviewed a host of other psychosocial parameters that need to be considered. More recently, Doleys (2002) provided a comprehensive overview of the vital importance of pretrial psychological evaluations and preparation of chronic pain patients who are being considered for implantable devices.

APPROACHES TO ASSESSMENT

DISTRESS AND RISK ASSESSMENT METHOD

Recent years have seen attempts to create brief paper-and-pencil screening tools to more systematically identify spine surgery candidates who are likely to benefit from referral for more comprehensive assessment. The most well-developed and most extensively researched of these tools is the Distress and Risk Assessment Method (DRAM; Main et al. 1992). The DRAM combines two previously developed brief instruments: a modified version of the Zung Depression Inventory (Zung 1965) and the Modified Somatic Perception Questionnaire (MSPQ; Main 1983). The DRAM involves 45 items and requires about 10 minutes to complete. It has been applied to the screening of chronic pain surgery candidates and has shown good predictive validity in some studies. For example, Trief et al. (2000) administered the DRAM to 102 subjects, most of whom underwent lumbar fusion. Regression analyses showed that the DRAM (combined with duration of pain) predicted daily functioning and the ability to sustain work and leisure activities, as well as improvement in back and leg pain. Distressed groups showed less improvement than the normal groups on all these measures, and the results of an "at-risk" group fell between the two.

SCORECARD METHODS

Several investigators have recommended the use of a "scorecard" approach. In one study of 280 patients receiving lumbar surgery, several psychosocial and medical factors were assigned a score (Finneson and Cooper 1979). The authors reported that patients with better scorecard numbers had an increased likelihood of obtaining desired surgical outcomes. Manniche and colleagues (1994) confirmed the value of Finneson and Cooper's scorecard approach.

In a similar study, Spengler and colleagues (1980) examined variables to help predict who would have a successful lumbar diskectomy. The predictive variables used included sciatic root tension, radiographic variables, and psychosocial factors from the MMPI. The MMPI factors were among the strongest predictors of success or failure, and the scorecard correctly classified 40% of patients. Block and colleagues (1983) studied 204 patients who underwent laminectomies/diskectomies. Variables examined included MMPI elevations on the depression (2), hysteria (3), psychopathic deviate (4), psychasthenia (7), and schizophrenia (8) scales, as well as poor coping, spousal reinforcement, workers' compensation, a history of psychological treatment, and heavy job requirements. The researchers correctly classified 83% of the patients by utilizing a multiple regression equation.

THE STEPWISE APPROACH

Recently, Gatchel (2001) recommended a "stepwise approach" in the biopsychosocial assessment of patients. Clinicians must not make the assumption that a single instrument or technique can serve as the best overall assessment method. For many patients, several assessment steps will be necessary. Rather than asking what method should be used, a better question is: "What sequence of testing or risk assessment should I consider in order to develop the best understanding of potential biopsychosocial problems that might be encountered with this patient?"

Fig. 2 presents a flow chart for a stepwise biopsychosocial process of screening patients who may be candidates for pain management intervention. Let us consider the patient who has symptoms of a potential herniated disk. If there is good evidence of a herniated disk, then surgery should be seriously considered. If there are signs that call for immediate intervention, then surgery should be conducted immediately. However, if no such emergency signs are present, than a prescreening evaluation could be administered

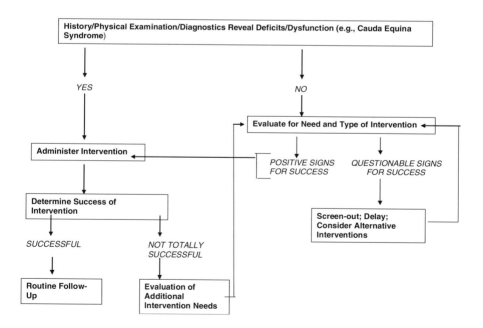

Fig. 2. Stepwise biopsychosocial screening.

in order to determine the surgery's relative chances of success. Positive signs for success would be an indication for surgery, whereas any questionable signs would call for a delay in surgery and possibly the consideration of alternative interventions such as functional restoration. After a period of more conservative care or other presurgical preparation, the physician can reevaluate the potential risk for surgical intervention. The final treatment outcomes should always be subsequently evaluated to determine the success of the intervention, both for surgical and nonsurgical interventions. Mayer et al. (2000) presented a systematic method for evaluating treatment outcomes, taking into account self-report, functional variables, and socioeconomic outcomes. In the event that this evaluation indicates that additional intervention is required, the patient will need to be "recycled" back up to the "Evaluate for Need and Type of Intervention" step in the Fig. 2 flow chart (Gatchel 2001).

This biopsychosocial screening process could be adapted for any type of intervention strategy, such as long-term opioid management. The important feature of this flow chart is that it provides health care professionals with a standard protocol to use in the management of all chronic pain patients. The consistent use of such a protocol could lead to a more unified approach to the assessment of risk factors and subsequent pain management in patients across various clinical facilities. This consistency would help facilitate a more structured standard of care in the evaluation and treatment of patients with chronic pain. Indeed, some national organizations are starting to heed this advice. For example, the North American Spine Society has developed clinical guidelines for multidisciplinary spine care specialists to improve quality and efficiency of care through efficient evaluation and treatment of patients suffering from herniated disk, spondylolisthesis, lytic spondylolisthesis, degenerative spondylolisthesis, and unremitting low back pain. In years to come, it would be encouraging to see other medical specialties develop similar guidelines (Gatchel 2001).

CONCLUSION

More research is clearly needed in the area of screening for invasive procedures, and the application of sophisticated statistical techniques, such as path analysis, will aid in our ability to develop empirically sound protocols for assessment. However, every patient presents with a unique set of circumstances, and the importance of clinical judgment should not be overlooked. There will always be cases where the outcome of a surgical procedure is successful in a patient who would not be predicted to do well.

Unfortunately, the opposite will remain true. With careful examination of the psychosocial and medical variables described in this chapter, clinicians have an opportunity to more appropriately select candidates for invasive procedures in order to increase their chances for successful treatment.

ACKNOWLEDGMENTS

R.J. Gatchel was supported by grants from the National Institutes of Health (MH46452, MH01107, and DE10703).

REFERENCES

Atlas S, Deyo R, Keller R, et al. The Maine lumbar spine study, part II. One year outcomes of surgical and nonsurgical management of sciatica. *Spine* 1996; 21(15):1777–1786.

Block AR, Kremer EF, Gaylor M. Behavioral treatment of chronic pain: the spouse as a discriminative cue for pain behavior. *Pain* 1983; 9:243–252.

Block A, Gatchel RJ, Deardorff WW, Guyer RD. *The Psychology of Spine Surgery.* Washington, DC: American Psychological Association, 2003.

Blumetti AE, Modesti LM. Psychological predictors of success or failure of surgical intervention for intractable back pain. In: Bonica JJ, Albe-Fessard D (Eds). *Proceedings of the Second World Congress on Pain,* Advances in Pain Research and Therapy, Vol. 3. New York: Raven Press, 1976, pp 220–248.

Butcher JN, Williams CL. *Essentials of MMPI-2 and MMPI-A Interpretation.* Minneapolis: University of Minnesota Press, 1993.

Butler RW, Damarin FL, Beaulieu C, Schwebel AI, Thorn BE. Assessing cognitive coping strategies for acute pain. *Psychol Assess* 1989; 1:41–45.

Davis RA. A long-term outcome analysis of 984 surgically treated herniated lumbar discs. *J Neurosurgery* 1994; 80:415–421.

Deyo RA, Cherkin DC, Loeser JD, Bigos SJ, Ciol MA. Morbidity and mortality in association with operations on the lumbar spine: the influence of age, diagnosis, and procedure. *J Bone Joint Surg* 1992; 74(4):536–543.

Doleys DM. Preparing patients for implantable technologies. In: Turk DC, Gatchel RJ (Eds). *Psychological Approaches to Pain Management.* New York: Guilford Press, 2002, pp 334–348.

Epker J, Block A. Presurgical psychological screening in back pain patients: a review. *Clin J Pain* 2001; 17:200–205.

Finneson BE, Cooper VR. A lumbar disc surgery predictive score card: a retrospective evaluation. *Spine* 1979; 4:141–144.

Friedman AF, Lewak R, Nichols DS, Webb JT. *Psychological Assessment with the MMPI-2.* Mahwah, NJ: Lawrence Erlbaum, 2001, p 688.

Frymoyer JW, Durett CL. The economics of spinal disorders. In: Frymoyer JW (Ed). *The Adult Spine,* 2nd ed. Philadelphia: Lippincott-Raven, 1997.

Gatchel RJ. A biopsychosocial overview of pretreatment screening of patients with pain. *Clin J Pain* 2001; 17:192–199.

Gatchel RJ, Turk DC (Eds). *Psychological Approaches to Pain Management: A Practitioner's Handbook.* New York: Guilford Press, 1996.

Gatchel RJ, Polatin PB, Mayer TG, Garcy PD. Psychopathology and the rehabilitation of patients with chronic low back pain disability. *Arch Phys Med Rehabil* 1994; 75(6):666–670.

Gentry WD, Newman MC, Goldner JL, Von Baeyer C. Relation between graduated spinal block technique and MMPI for diagnosis and prognosis of chronic low back pain. *Spine* 1977; 2:210–213.

Graham JR. *MMPI-2. Assessing Personality and Psychopathology,* 2nd ed. New York: Oxford University Press, 1993.

Greenough CG, Fraser RD. The effects of compensation on recovery from low-back injury. *Spine* 1989; 14:947–955.

Gross AR. The effect of coping strategies on the relief of pain following surgical intervention for lower back pain. *Psychosom Med* 1986; 48:228–239.

Herron LD, Pheasant HC. Changes in MMPI profiles after low back surgery. *Spine* 1982; 7:591–597.

Jacobsen PB, Butler RW. Relation of cognitive coping and catastrophizing to acute pain and analgesic use following breast cancer surgery. *J Behav Med* 1996; 19:17–23.

Kjelby-Wendt G, Styf JR, Carlsson SG. The predictive value of psychometric analysis in patients treated by extirpation of lumbar intervertebral disc herniation. *J Spinal Disord* 1999; 12:375–379.

Klekamp J, McCarty E, Spengler D. Results of elective lumbar discectomy for patients involved in the workers' compensation system. *J Spinal Disord* 1998; 11:277–282.

Long C. The relationship between surgical outcome and MMPI profiles in chronic pain patients. *J Clin Psychol* 1981; 37:744–749.

Mahomed NN, Liang MH, Cook EF, et al. The importance of patient expectations in predicting functional outcomes after total joint arthroplasty. *J Rheumatol* 2002; 29(6):1279–1279.

Main CJ. The Modified Somatic Perception Questionnaire (MSPQ). *J Psychosom Res* 1983; 27:503–514.

Main CJ, Waddell G. A comparison of cognitive measures in low back pain: statistical structure and clinical validity at initial assessment. *Pain* 1991; 56:287–298.

Main CJ, Wood PLR, Hollis S, Spanswick CC, Waddell G. The Distress and Risk Assessment Method: a simple patient classification to identify distress and evaluate the risk of poor outcome. *Spine* 1992; 17:42–52.

Malter AD, McNeney B, Loeser JD, Deyo RA. 5-year reoperation rates after different types of lumbar spine surgery. *Spine* 1998; 23(7):814–820.

Manniche C, Asmussen KH, Venterberg H, et al. Analysis of preoperative prognostic factors in first-time surgery for lumbar disc herniation, including Finneson's and Spengler's score systems. *Dan Med Bull* 1994; 41:110–115.

Marketdata. *Chronic Pain Management Programs: A Market Analysis.* Valley Stream, NY: Marketdata Enterprises, 1995.

Mayer T, McMahon MJ, Gatchel RJ, et al. Socioeconomic outcomes of combined spine surgery and functional restoration in workers' compensation spinal disorders with matched controls. *Spine* 1998; 23(5):598–606.

Mayer TG, Prescott M, Gatchel RJ. Objective outcomes evaluation: methods and evidence. In: Mayer TG, Gatchel RG, Polatin PB (Eds). *Occupational Musculoskeletal Disorders: Function, Outcomes, and Evidence.* Philadelphia: Lippincott-Williams and Wilkins, 2000.

McKinley JC, Hathaway SR. A multiphasic personality schedule (Minnesota): II. A differential study of hypochondriasis. *J Psychol* 1940; 10:255–268.

Neben DV, Kennington M, Novy DM, et al. Psychological selection criteria for implantable spinal cord stimulators. *Pain Forum* 1996; 5:93–103.

North RB, Kidd DH, Zahurak M, James CS, Long DM. Spinal cord stimulation for chronic, intractable pain: experience over two decades. *Neurosurgery* 1993; 32:384–395.

Oaklander AL, North RB. Failed back surgery syndrome. In: Loeser J, Butler SH, Chapman CR, Turk DC (Eds). *Bonica's Management of Pain,* 3rd ed. Philadelphia: Lippincott, Williams, and Wilkins, 2001, pp 1540–1549.

Polatin PB, Kinney RK, Gatchel RJ, Lillo E, Mayer TG. Psychiatric illness and chronic low-back pain. The mind and the spine—which goes first? *Spine* 1993; 18(1):66–71.

Prager J, Jacobs M. Evaluation of patients for implantable pain modalities: medical and behavioral assessment. *Clin J Pain* 2001; 17:206–214.

Rosenstiel A, Keefe F. The use of coping strategies in low back pain patients: relationship to patient characteristics and current adjustment. *Pain* 1983; 17:33–40.

Schade V, Semmer N, Main CJ, Hora J, Boos N. The impact of clinical, morphological, psychosocial and work-related factors on the outcome of lumbar discectomy. *Pain* 1999; 80:239–249.

Schofferman J, Anderson D, Hines R, Smith G, White A. Childhood psychological trauma correlates with unsuccessful lumbar spine surgery. *Spine* 1992; 17(S6):138–144.

Spengler DM, Freeman CW, Westbrook R, Miller JW. Low-back pain following multiple lumbar spine procedures: failure of initial selection? *Spine* 1980; 5:536–560.

Sullivan MJ, Stanish W, Waite H, Sullivan M, Tripp DA. Catastrophizing, pain and disability in patients with soft-tissue injury. *Pain* 1998; 77:253–260.

Trief PM, Grant W, Fredrickson B. A prospective study of psychological predictors of lumbar surgery outcome. *Spine* 2000; 25:2616–2621.

Trimboli F, Kilgore RB. A psychodynamic approach to MMPI interpretation. *J Pers Assess* 1983; 47:614–626.

Turk DC, Monarch ES. Biopsychosocial perspective on chronic pain. In: Turk DC, Gatchel RJ (Eds). *Psychological Approaches to Pain Management.* New York: Guilford Press, 2002, pp 3–29.

Turner J, Ersek M, Herron L, et al. Patient outcomes after lumbar spinal fusions. *JAMA* 1992; 268:907–911.

Vingard E, Alfredsson L, Hagberg M, et al. To what extent do current and past physical and psychological occupational factors explain care-seeking for low back pain in a working population? *Spine* 2000; 25:493–500.

Wilfling FJ, Klonoff H, Kokan P. Psychological, demographic and orthopaedic factors associated with prediction of outcome of spinal fusion. *Clin Orthop* 1973; 90:153–160.

Wiltse LL, Rocchio PD. Preoperative psychological tests as predictors of success of chemonucleolysis in the treatment of the low back syndrome. *J Bone Joint Surgery* 1975; 57(A):478–483.

Zung W. A self-rating depression scale. *Arch Gen Psychiatry* 1965; 12:63–70.

Correspondence to: Robert J. Gatchel, PhD, Department of Psychiatry, The University of Texas Southwestern Medical Center at Dallas, 5323 Harry Hines Boulevard, Dallas, TX 75390-9044, USA. Email: robert.gatchel@utsouthwestern.edu.

Part III

Treating Pain Patients

Psychosocial Aspects of Pain: A Handbook for Health Care Providers, Progress in Pain Research and Management, Vol. 27, edited by Robert H. Dworkin and William S. Breitbart, IASP Press, Seattle, © 2004.

10

What Are the Goals of Pain Treatment?

Mark D. Sullivan

Department of Psychiatry and Behavioral Sciences, School of Medicine, University of Washington, Seattle, Washington, USA

GOALS OF HEALTH CARE AND GOALS OF PAIN CARE

Health care has multiple goals. Their importance shifts from patient to patient and during the care of a single patient. Goals listed for health care typically include the following: (1) restoration of health, (2) relief of physical and psychological symptoms (e.g., pain and suffering), (3) restoration or maintenance of function, (4) saving or prolonging of life, (5) advising the patient of his or her prognosis, and (6) avoiding harm to the patient (Jonsen et al. 2002). While simultaneous achievement of these goals may represent the clinical ideal, these goals often compete with each other. Indeed, most common ethical dilemmas in modern clinical medicine stem from competition among these goals.

In *Clinical Ethics,* Jonsen and colleagues (2002) describe three different types of diseases encountered in clinical practice and the differing goals of intervention for each. They name each type of disease by an acronym: ACURE, CARE, and COPE. The first is ACURE, which stands for acute, critical, unexpected, responsive, and easily diagnosed and treated. One example of this kind of situation is a college student presenting to an emergency room with a high fever, headache, stiff neck, and cough. The student is diagnosed with meningitis and pneumonia and treated. Such ACURE situations offer physicians the chance to meet most of the above goals of the medical encounter without conflict. Because a cure is available and usually is desired by patient and physician, there is often little debate about clinical goals in these situations. Ethical conflicts can still arise if the patient's decision-making capacity becomes impaired or if the patient has other medical problems that provide competing goals.

The care of acute pain generally follows the ACURE model. Aggressive analgesia can almost always achieve adequate pain control in acute illness. There are always complexities to diagnosis and treatment, but these respond to the rational application of pathophysiological and pharmacological principles. Sometimes analgesia needs to be delayed to promote diagnosis, such as in acute abdominal pain, but rarely is there an enduring conflict between disease treatment and pain treatment. The time-limited nature of acute pain offers little opportunity for conflict between pain relief and functional restoration in these patients. Deliberate undertreatment of acute pain due to fears of iatrogenic addiction has been widely discredited (Greer et al. 2001). Innovations such as patient-controlled analgesia have recently improved pain relief and patient satisfaction in the treatment of acute pain (Gagliese et al. 2000).

The second type of disease, designated by the acronym CARE, is critical, active, recalcitrant, and eventual. An example of this type of disease is a 34-year-old man with a 15-year history of multiple sclerosis with episodic but progressive physical impairment. CARE illnesses are either acute or chronic, but they are incurable, progressive, and usually fatal. CARE illnesses can arise as the acute exacerbation of a chronic illness or at the end stage of a chronic, progressive disease. These are not the purely acute illnesses of ACURE, nor the purely chronic illnesses of COPE. Because cure is not possible with CARE illnesses, other clinical goals move to the forefront. These include prolongation of life, relief of pain and suffering, preservation of function, and enhancement of control and dignity for the patient. These goals can come into conflict, especially as the patient nears the end of life. Decisions to withhold or withdraw life-sustaining care in these situations require the physician to balance competing clinical goals. The central challenge in CARE illnesses is when and how to accommodate the death of the patient.

The treatment of chronic cancer pain generally follows the CARE model, and clinical decisions in terminal cases are invariably shaped by the fact that the disease is ultimately fatal. When the cancer is curable, however, pain control takes on the shape of the COPE illnesses described below. The costs and benefits of cancer pain control are framed by the time-limited and often fatal nature of the illness (Neumann 2001). Some balancing of symptom relief and functional preservation is necessary so that the patient may have adequate pain control while continuing to live a satisfying life. What constitutes adequate pain control must be decided in collaboration with the patient, who chooses how to balance pain control with diminishment of physical and cognitive function. As death approaches, pain control must also be balanced against any potential shortening of life. However, the challenge of balancing pain control with life's other interests over the long term is generally absent from cancer pain management.

The third type of disease is designated by the acronym COPE: chronic, outpatient, palliative, and efficacious. COPE is the basic model for outpatient chronic disease management. It thus comprises the bulk of family medicine or internal medicine practice. An example of this type of disease is a 42-year-old woman with a 17-year history of type 1 diabetes mellitus. She is actively engaged in her insulin, diet, and exercise regimen. However, she has developed early retinopathy and some painful neuropathy in her feet. The defining feature of COPE illnesses is their chronic character: cure is not possible, and death is not in sight. The patient has lived with the disease, its symptoms, and associated impairments for some time. Hospitalizations can be necessary for acute exacerbations, but the vast majority of care is delivered in the outpatient setting. Patients have more control and discretion in these COPE illnesses than they do in the more acute ACURE and CARE illnesses, which are often managed in the hospital. COPE illnesses are a central part of patients' lives and must be managed in accord with their values. The doctor-patient relationship is more developed in these COPE illnesses and offers a means for negotiation. COPE illnesses offer many options for prioritizing the goals of clinical care. Many opportunities may arise for conflict among goals and also among persons assigning differing priorities to these goals.

The care of chronic nonmalignant pain generally follows the COPE model. Cure is very rarely possible. Conflict between clinical goals and negotiations among persons with competing sets of priorities dominate patient care. Deciding on the goals of chronic nonmalignant pain care offers the greatest ethical and clinical challenges of the three types. It will be my focus for the remainder of this chapter.

WHOSE GOALS FOR PAIN TREATMENT?

Because chronic pain has such pervasive effects on the lives of those who suffer with it, multiple parties have an interest in the priorities of its care. Patient, family, care provider, employer, insurer, and society itself are stakeholders in chronic pain care. Patients might give the highest priority to reducing pain intensity. Families might prefer to limit sedation and confusion. Care providers might prefer to keep patients away from hospitalizations and emergency rooms. Employers might want the patient back at work, but only if he or she is fully functional. Insurers might want the least expensive care. Society might prefer to spend more on care and less on disability benefits. Each party feels entitled to its particular set of priorities. At present no method has been agreed upon by all parties for adjudicating between these priorities. It is not surprising that pain is among the most common reasons for patients and other stakeholders to go to court (Rich 2002).

CONCEPTUAL DIMENSIONS OF THE
PATIENT-CENTERED APPROACH

It is the patient who directly suffers with chronic pain, so it makes sense for the patient to dictate the goals of chronic pain care. Indeed, over the last 30 years an extensive body of medical literature has emerged advocating a "patient-centered" approach to medical care. Writing in the *Journal of the American Medical Association,* Laine and Davidoff (1996) called for patient-centered care that is "closely congruent with, and responsive to, patients' wants, needs and preferences." Informed consent has become the standard way in which patients' preferences and their capacity for having preferences are honored in medicine. But calls for patient-centered medicine take us beyond bioethical calls to respect patient autonomy. Proponents of this new paradigm not only want the patient to be able to make the best choice from the various medical care options, but seek to reshape those options so that they are conceived from the patient's perspective.

Mead and Bower (2000) recently identified five conceptual dimensions to patient-centeredness that are relevant to chronic pain care. These are: (1) a biopsychosocial perspective, (2) the concept of patient-as-person, (3) sharing power and responsibility, (4) establishing a therapeutic alliance, and (5) the concept of doctor-as-person. The biopsychosocial perspective means directing clinical attention beyond disease and strictly biomedical concerns "to become involved in the full range of difficulties that patients bring to their doctors." This broader scope is especially important in chronic pain care, where it is common to find no disease that can explain the magnitude of the patient's pain. Reassuring a patient with chronic pain who does not have identifiable pathology that "there is nothing medically wrong" can exacerbate his or her suffering.

Attending to the patient as a person means acknowledging that in order to understand illness and alleviate suffering, medicine must first understand the personal meaning of the illness for the patient. Rather than thinking of a patient as a diabetic, for example, the clinician might view her as a 35-year-old single mother struggling with homelessness, diabetes, and painful feet. Chronic pain has time to insinuate itself into all aspects of a patient's life. Its meaning can become as unique as the patient's biography itself. The biopsychosocial perspective emphasizes that it is not adequate to identify the disease behind the pain. The patient-as-person principle emphasizes that a provider must ask about more than pain intensity to discover what meaning the pain has for that person.

Sharing of power and responsibility is part of a modern egalitarian doctor-patient relationship. It is a necessary part of chronic disease care, which is provided largely by the patient at home. If patients are not active participants in the care of their chronic disease, outcomes will be poor, with deteriorating adherence to self-management, medication, and monitoring regimens. Because cure usually cannot be achieved in chronic pain, collaboration in choosing and achieving clinical goals is essential. Although sharing power and responsibility is essential, it is fraught with difficulty. Conflicts about the priorities assigned to symptom relief versus functional improvement create some of this difficulty. Disagreements about the appropriateness of various treatments, such as surgery or opioids, to achieve these goals may compound the problem. In the case of chronic opioids, patient contracts have been devised "to improve care through dissemination of information, facilitate a mutually agreed-upon course, or enhance compliance" (Fishman et al. 1999). However, the most common elements of these contracts are terms of treatment, behaviors from which patients are prohibited, and reasons for termination of care. Thus these contracts may exist primarily to clarify responsibilities rather than share power. We will return to the special difficulties in applying a patient-centered model to long-term opioids for chronic pain below.

The therapeutic alliance is an important component of patient-centered care. Given that chronic disease care is without a self-evident endpoint such as cure, negotiation is necessary to define therapeutic goals. If patient and physician cannot agree upon these goals and form an alliance to achieve them, care will not be successful. However, many aspects of chronic pain care can hamper the achievement of a solid therapeutic alliance. The difficulty in defining a clear medical diagnosis can make the purpose of the alliance unclear at the outset. The adversarial medicolegal atmosphere within which much chronic pain care takes place is another prime reason why the patient does not feel that the physician is an ally. Another reason for difficulty is the potential harm of many pain treatments such as neuroablative procedures and dependence-inducing medications. Physicians who refuse to administer these treatments feel they are protecting patients, but patients may feel that they are being denied the only treatments that might help.

The pain doctor is a person. Anyone who has cared for many patients with chronic pain will tell you how personal the work is. These patients are in a personal predicament and the physician must engage with that predicament in order to help. But engaging means getting wrapped up not only in patients' pain, but in their anger, their sadness, and their desperation. It is not surprising that pain physicians feel "burned out" or become angry or depressed. These feelings cannot be prevented, but can be managed in a way that does not damage the physician or the patient. Psychiatrists and psychologists have long been trained to recognize and handle these "countertransference" feelings. There is some indication that other physicians are recognizing the importance of physicians' emotions as well (Novack et al. 1997).

OUTCOMES OF PATIENT-CENTERED CARE

Patient-centered medicine is usually advocated for moral reasons as a more humane medicine. Some also advocate it as a more effective medicine. Some recent studies in cardiology (Fremont et al. 2001) and general practice (Little et al. 2001) have found improved clinical outcomes such as reduced symptom burden, improved self-rated health, and greater patient satisfaction with patient-centered care. Another study, which attended carefully to potential confounding factors, found no benefit for patient satisfaction or empowerment in general practice (Mead et al. 2002). These conflicting findings suggest that the crucial aspects of patient-centered care and how they are linked with clinical outcomes remain to be defined.

LIMITATIONS OF PATIENT-CENTERED CARE

Patient-centered care for chronic pain is difficult to implement in practice. For a number of reasons, it may need to be qualified by other considerations. First and foremost, physicians should not simply accept patient goals for treatment, but must educate and negotiate with patients. It is often not possible to accept the goals for care initially presented by the patient. It is common for patients arriving at our pain clinic to state that they want "no pain" or "to be like I was before the injury." These requests for cure cannot be met. It is necessary to engage in a process of negotiation about which goals are possible and what trade-offs are necessary given the current state of medicine. It is also essential to clarify the dangers inherent in aggressively pursuing a pain-free state through medications or surgery.

Even after patients have relinquished the goal of a pain-free state, it is often necessary to educate and negotiate them about the priority of pain relief among other clinical goals such as functional improvement and well-being. Patients often believe that pain relief is necessary before any of these other goals can be achieved. They can be taught that functional improvement generally occurs before pain relief in a pain rehabilitation program, and learn that regaining a feeling of control over one's life may precede rather than follow a reduction in pain intensity. Indeed, the role of pain intensity reduction in recovery from chronic pain is complex and poorly understood. Patients completing our 3-week structured pain program will, on average, have their pain change from 6. 5 to 5. 5 on an 11-point numerical rating scale. Individual patients will often report after treatment that "my pain is the same." Given that they have dramatically decreased their opioid intake and substantially increased their activity level during the program, it is unclear what this statement means. It may mean that patients did not get the reduction in pain intensity that they expected or hoped for, but it may also mean that they are now focusing on what is happening in their lives other than pain.

The proper goals of pain treatment are at issue in the currently active debate concerning the use of long-term opioids for chronic nonmalignant pain. Harden (2002) has described the two dominant theories of chronic pain treatment as palliative versus rehabilitative. The palliative theory prioritizes symptom relief, while the rehabilitative theory prioritizes functional restoration. He argues that these approaches imply strongly contrasting views on the values of long-term opioids. "If the doctor's primary goal is to palliate, chronic opioid therapy is an expedient way to achieve this goal. If the primary goal is to rehabilitate and restore the patient to optimal functioning, opioids may be contraindicated." It appears that rheumatologists and general practitioners are more likely to prescribe long-term opioids and endorse a palliative theory than are surgeons, neurologists, or physiatrists (Turk et al. 1994). Central to Harden's argument are the potential trade-offs between pain relief from opioids and functional improvement. The few randomized trials of chronic opioids suggest little functional improvement or return to work, but the long-term studies necessary to fully address these questions have not been conducted (Moulin et al. 1996).

Even estimating the amount of pain relief achieved with chronic opioid therapy can be clinically difficult due to the dependence-inducing properties of the medications (Jasinski 1997). The risks of iatrogenic addiction have received a great deal of attention in the pain literature, and appear to be low for most patients (Portenoy 1996). However, the issue of psychological dependence has been less well studied (Fordyce 1992). The average pain reduction achieved by chronic opioids is quite modest. In controlled studies the average pain reduction from long-term opioids is only 32% when weighted by sample size (Turk et al. 2002). Patients in clinical practice will often acknowledge that their pain is not well relieved, but maintain that the opioids are essential because they "take the edge off." The extreme reluctance of some patients to taper off opioids given these modest levels of pain relief suggest that the opioids may be primarily relieving *fear* of pain rather than pain itself (Keefe et al. 2001). This statement is not meant to minimize what the opioids are achieving. Many of these patients have been completely overwhelmed by pain and desperately want to avoid this happening again. Consistent with this fear is the fact that many patients overestimate how severe their pain will be when they are tapered off opioids. I have seen many patients who are surprised at how high a price they were paying in side effects for incomplete pain relief. All these issues raise the question of who is the best judge of the efficacy of chronic opioids: the patient while on opioids, the patient after tapering off opioids, the spouse, or the physician? I believe that negotiation toward consensus is necessary. To simply focus on patients' reports of pain intensity is a misapplication of patient-centered medicine.

WHICH GOALS FOR PAIN TREATMENT?

Given that providing pain relief almost always involves compromising some legitimate clinical goals to achieve others, can anything be said in general about these trade-offs? Has consensus been achieved about when these are appropriate, or do we need to rely on individual patient, family, or physician choice in each individual case? (Sullivan 2002).

PAIN RELIEF VERSUS QUANTITY OF LIFE:
THE "DOUBLE EFFECT"

Largely due to their capacity to induce respiratory depression during aggressive short-term use, opioids can potentially shorten life. This is a significant issue in the use of opioids in cancer pain and at the end of life in general. Consensus is broad in the current bioethical literature that aggressive use of opioids to relieve suffering at the end of life is permissible, even if it shortens life. The Catholic Church developed the doctrine of "double effect" in the Middle Ages to allow such unintended shortening of life. This doctrine remains controversial but is commonly cited in order to ethically distinguish between intentional and unintentional shortening of life. According to this doctrine, administering high-dose opioids to treat a terminally ill patient's pain may be acceptable even if the medication causes the patient's death. In contrast, the rule does not authorize physician-assisted suicide or voluntary euthanasia. Recent commentators have criticized the doctrine for its absolute prohibitions against intentionally causing death, its unrealistic characterization of physicians' intentions as being purely about relieving suffering rather than hastening death, and its failure to account for patients' wishes to hasten death (Quill et al. 1997).

ROLE OF PAIN IN QUALITY OF LIFE

In chronic nonmalignant pain care, the clinical dilemma involves *quality* of life rather than *quantity* of life. Quality of life, or the more narrowly defined health-related quality of life (HRQOL), is a concept designed to try to capture the overall value of medical care from the patient's perspective (Sullivan 2003). The role of pain in patients' HRQOL is complex. The World Health Organization, for example, uses a disability-adjusted life year concept to compare HRQOL across different countries (Murray and Lopez 1996). Such a metric assumes that the effects of pain (and other aversive symptoms) on HRQOL are wholly mediated by their effects on disability. But this assumption appears to underestimate the role of pain in HRQOL (Sullivan et al. 2000). Aversive symptoms are significant factors in quality of life in their own right. Pain relief has direct value to the patient, but it still must be balanced against other components of quality of life. Compromises in cognitive, emotional, or physical functional status need to be weighed by the patient against any reduction in pain. This weighing may be difficult because patients are often either inexperienced with the treatment or already compromised by its side effects.

This process of weighing pain relief against its cost is also complicated by the fact that this balance must be achieved over the long term, often the remainder of the patient's life. Patients overwhelmed by pain are typically unable to do this dispassionately and may seek heroic treatments with negative long-term consequences, such as ablative neurosurgical procedures. Problems with dispassionate weighing of long-term consequences may apply to more common surgical procedures as well. In one recent review of lumbar surgery for work-related injuries, 71% of those with a single procedure and 95% of those with multiple procedures had not returned to work 4 years after the operation due to persistent pain (Berger 2000). An aggressive therapy offering a small chance of relief can seem enticing to a desperate patient. Medications that provide pain relief may also obscure the patient's ability to discern his or her own cognitive or emotional impairment. Psychological dependence on medications may distort a patient's judgment of cost versus benefit for a given medication regime. Because the same person must undergo treatments and judge their efficacy, it is difficult for that person to be fully informed about a treatment's effects and yet be objective or impartial about efficacy. Even if we accept the patient as the authoritative judge of his or her quality of life, and therefore of pain treatment efficacy, when is the definitive judgment of efficacy made? Again, some synthesis of multiple perspectives is necessary to achieve the most valid judgment of efficacy.

With the multiplicity of relevant outcomes for pain treatment, it can be difficult to distinguish predictors of outcomes from preferences for outcomes. In one study of a pain management program, having the goal of returning to work was the best predictor of return-to-work outcome (Tan et al. 1997). Patients who are more committed to a self-management strategy for chronic pain do better in a program focused on teaching self-management skills (Kerns et al. 2000). A decrease in the belief that one is disabled predicts improvement in self-reported disability after multidisciplinary pain management (Jensen et al. 2001). Primary care providers typically address medical safety and medication issues, but do not adequately address patient concerns or functional limitations. On the other hand, patients randomized to a self-care program showed significantly greater reductions in fear-avoidance beliefs and back-related worry, but more modest reductions in pain intensity and activity interference (Moore et al. 2000). Although improved HRQOL is a universally valid goal for pain treatment, determining which of its components are most important will vary among patients with different pain problems and life goals.

QUALITY OF LIFE ASSESSMENT METHODS

Because there is no single definitive outcome measure for chronic pain treatment, choice of outcome can be as important as efficacy of treatment in deciding whether a treatment has been successful. One way to synthesize HRQOL into a single patient-generated value is through the determination of health-state utilities, wherein various strategies are used to determine what fraction of a healthy life year is equal to a year in one's current health state. Standard gamble, time trade-off, and rating scales are methods used to help patients generate these fractions or discount variables. In the standard gamble procedure, for example, patients are asked what risk of death they would be willing to face to obtain a complete cure for their condition. These discount variables describing quality of life can be combined with mortality measures describing effects on quality of life to generate summary measures of the value of a health intervention such as number of quality-adjusted life years (QALYs) gained from a particular intervention. However, it is difficult to obtain similar utility values from different assessment methods. In a study of 133 fibromyalgia patients and 148 patients with chronic nonspecific low back pain, the mean utility score for the health state at baseline was 0.43 with the rating scale and 0.78 for the standard gamble. The correlation between both methods was poor ($r = 0.21$). Domain-specific measures about pain and functional impairment were also administered. Multiple regression analyses demonstrated that 32% of the variance in rating scale values and only 13% of the variance in standard gamble utilities could be explained by domain-specific measures (Goossens et al. 1999). This result suggests that patients' overall valuation of their health state by these methods is only partially captured by the domain-specific measures (e.g., pain intensity and activity interference) that are commonly used as outcomes in pain management studies. Therefore, a consensus among patient, family, and providers about which treatments maximize patient HRQOL is most likely the best clinical guide.

COST-EFFECTIVENESS: BALANCING PAIN TREATMENT WITH OTHER SOCIAL GOALS

It was not long ago that mentioning cost in the process of making medical treatment decisions was considered to be in poor taste. But the days when medicine had an unqualified claim on the public purse are over. Society clearly cannot afford all that medicine has to offer; certainly not if it is to pursue other laudable objectives such as education, safety, and housing. Now medicine must demonstrate efficiency as well as efficacy for its treatments. The most common way of quantifying efficiency is in terms of cost-effectiveness. One popular metric applicable to a wide array of medical interventions is cost per QALY gained. In fact, medical interventions can be ranked in league tables according to how much it costs to gain a QALY through each intervention. Because chronic pain has little effect on mortality, the QALY may not be the most appropriate metric by which to compare treatments.

Turk (in press) has recently summarized data on the cost-effectiveness of the most common means of treating chronic pain, combining a wide variety of studies with heterogeneous patient populations and intervention strategies. None of the currently available treatments eliminate pain for the majority of patients receiving them. Pain rehabilitation programs provide comparable reduction in pain to long-term opioids, surgery, spinal cord stimulators, and intrathecal pumps. However, they provide better outcomes with respect to medication use, health care utilization, functional activities, return to work, and closure of disability claims. They also have fewer iatrogenic injuries and adverse events. Nevertheless, these are expensive programs that generally fail to provide more than 50% pain relief for more than 50% of the patients treated. It is also important to remember that only a small percentage of those with chronic pain are ever referred to a multidisciplinary pain center and of those referred, fewer than 25% successfully complete the program (Weir et al. 1992).

Sometimes a health intervention saves dollars that would otherwise be spent elsewhere in the health care system. This net reduction in direct medical costs is called a cost offset. There is some suggestion that multidisciplinary pain treatment may provide a cost offset. Flor and colleagues (1992) conducted a meta-analysis of these programs that suggested that patients completing the programs had one-third as many surgical interventions and hospitalizations as patients managed by other means. Simmons et al. (1988) found that those treated with a multidisciplinary program had 62% lower medical costs in the following year. It is important to remember that lowering health care costs is likely to be a low priority for patients themselves. Society, on the other hand, is very interested in lowering costs associated with pain. Direct health care costs are a small fraction of the overall costs of chronic pain. Frymoyer and Durett (1997) estimated the costs for back pain in the United States to be (in 1993 U.S. dollars) $33.6 billion for health care, $11–43 billion for disability compensation, $4.6 billion for lost productivity, and $5 billion for legal services. These dollar figures create a huge incentive for cost containment with respect to chronic pain. This situation prompts policy makers to sometimes talk as if reducing costs were the only goal for chronic pain care. The challenge is to lower costs for the sake of society while improving pain and functional limitations for the sake of patients.

The challenge now being taken up in primary care health systems is how to deliver effective pain care at a reasonable cost. The Northwest Region of Kaiser Permanente estimates that 15% of its 40,000 members seek care for a chronic pain condition in a given year. Intensive multidisciplinary or interventional strategies are not affordable for even the most distressed 2,000 patients with chronic pain. This system experimented with a series of six group visits directed by a multidisciplinary team (Donovan et al. 1999). Results were mixed, with 30% attrition and marginally significant reductions in pain and functional interference, but clear cost savings of about $1,100 per member per year. An earlier study in the same health maintenance organization was unable to show added benefit (on pain, mood, or disability) of a 16-hour, 8-week class teaching cognitive-behavioral techniques to patients with chronic pain compared to a minimal-treatment control group. However, patient satisfaction was significantly higher in those receiving the class (McCarberg and Wolf 1999). Given that chronic pain can very rarely be cured, fostering self-care appears to be in everyone's interest. However, it is tempting for health care organizations to minimize care and costs. It is up to patients and society to demand adequate care.

NEGOTIATING THE GOALS OF PAIN TREATMENT

Patients and others, naive concerning the complexities of chronic pain treatment, often think of success simply in terms of reduced pain intensity. But chronic pain is a more complex and pervasive problem than this. Incomplete achievement of outcomes and trade-offs among the various desired outcomes are the norm. There are multiple stakeholders in pain treatment that often have competing sets of priorities. Negotiating these priorities is itself one of the most important tasks for chronic pain care.

NEGOTIATING WITH PATIENTS

Naive patients with chronic pain often approach physicians with a set of priorities appropriate for acute pain (e.g., the ACURE illness model). These beliefs dictate that pain relief and rest will promote healing and functional restoration with time. Education about how a chronic illness model better fits chronic pain is an essential first step in successful care. This task is difficult because it involves taking away the patient's hope for a cure. The hope for cure can be replaced with a hope for less pain, better function, and an improved life. This switch can be difficult for many patients, and they may go "doctor shopping" rather than accept it. Primary care studies indicate that patients feel that physicians do not listen to what they are saying about their pain (Miller et al. 1994). It is likely that their frustration is a result of differing explanatory models and incentives surrounding care. Better training in listening and communication skills might help physicians better bridge this gap (Schers et al. 2001).

More experienced chronic pain patients can arrive at their physician's office already feeling embattled and defensive. They can feel as if physicians either do not believe or do not care about their pain. This adversarial position makes the establishment of a workable treatment alliance much more difficult. The communication task at this point is not simply education, but a form of power sharing. Many primary care encounters about chronic pain appear to be characterized by a competition for control of the conversation (Eggly and Tzelepis 2001). These conversations can be characterized by anger and other negative emotions with which physicians are uncomfortable and for which they are poorly equipped. All of us find it difficult to compromise when feeling angry and defensive. Yet it is often important for physicians to compromise in favor of patients' short-term needs for pain relief while urging patients that these needs must be balanced against long-term quality of life.

It is important to remember that it is suffering rather than pain that motivates patients to seek health care (Loeser 2000). Physicians need to be able to acknowledge, engage with, and manage this suffering if they are to establish a solid treatment alliance with patients whose lives are dominated by chronic pain. It is only within such an alliance that successful negotiation about the goals of chronic pain treatment can take place.

NEGOTIATING WITH HEALTH CARE SYSTEMS

Because chronic pain is associated with such a complex array of biological, psychological, and social factors, organized health care is unsure how much responsibility it must take for chronic pain. Parts of the system have tried to disavow chronic pain as malingering or purely mental. This view has not succeeded as official policy, but it persists in the minds of many physicians. However, even if the health care system cannot reject all of chronic pain as nonmedical, it cannot afford to take on the entire burden of chronic pain and associated suffering. Some line needs to be drawn between what suffering should be addressed through the medical system and what should be addressed in nonmedical ways. Over the past century, we have tried to draw this line with laboratory and imaging tests such as X-rays, computed tomography scans, and magnetic resonance imaging. But this demarcation effort has clearly failed, most obviously in the case of back pain (Deyo 2002).

Some other, as yet unformulated, method must be found for determining the responsibilities of professional health care for chronic pain and therefore the goals for chronic pain care within the health care system. This determination must be achieved by a process that is both scientific and political. It will be informed by new scientific information about the central nervous system biology of chronic pain. It will also be shaped by a political process that decides which kinds of suffering we can bring to the medical system and which kinds we must manage ourselves.

ACKNOWLEDGMENTS

Supported by a grant from the National Institute of Mental Health (K01-MH-01351).

REFERENCES

Berger E. Late postoperative results in 1000 work related lumbar spine conditions. *Surg Neurol* 2000; 54(2):101–106.

Deyo RA. Diagnostic evaluation of LBP: reaching a specific diagnosis is often impossible. *Arch Intern Med* 2002; 162(13):1444–1447.

Donovan MI, Evers K, Jacobs P, Mandleblatt S. When there is no benchmark: designing a primary care-based chronic pain management program from the scientific basis up. *J Pain Symptom Manage* 1999; 18(1):38–48.

Eggly S, Tzelepis A. Relational control in difficult physician-patient encounters: negotiating treatment for pain. *J Health Commun* 2001; 6(4):323–333.

Fishman SM, Bandman TB, Edwards A, Borsook D. The opioid contract in the management of chronic pain. *J Pain Symptom Manage* 1999; 18(1):27–37.

Flor H, Fydrich T, Turk DC. Efficacy of multidisciplinary pain centers: a meta-analytic review. *Pain* 1992; 49:221–230

Fordyce WE. Opioids, pain, and behavioral outcomes. *APS J* 1992; 1:282–284.

Fremont AM, Cleary PD, Hargraves JL, et al. Patient-centered processes of care and long-term outcomes of myocardial infarction. *J Gen Intern Med* 2001; 16(12):800–808.

Frymoyer J, Durett C. The economics of spinal disorders. In: Frymoyer J (Ed). *The Adult Spine*. Philadelphia: Lippincott Raven, 1997, pp 143–150.

Gagliese L, Jackson M, Ritvo P, Wowk A, Katz J. Age is not an impediment to effective use of patient-controlled analgesia by surgical patients. *Anesthesiology* 2000; 93(3):601–610.

Goossens ME, Vlaeyen JW, Rutten-van Molken MP, van der Linden SM. Patient utilities in chronic musculoskeletal pain: how useful is the standard gamble method? *Pain* 1999; 80(1–2):365–375.

Greer SM, Dalton JA, Carlson J, Youngblood R. Surgical patients' fear of addiction to pain medication: the effect of an educational program for clinicians. *Clin J Pain* 2001; 17(2):157–164.

Harden RN. Chronic opioid therapy: another reappraisal. *APS Bull* 2002; 12(1):8–12.

Jasinski DR. Tolerance and dependence to opiates. *Acta Anaesthesiol Scand* 1997; 41(1 Pt 2):184–186.

Jensen MP, Turner JA, Romano JM. Changes in beliefs, catastrophizing, and coping are associated with improvement in multidisciplinary pain treatment. *J Consult Clin Psychol* 2001; 69(4):655–662.

Jonsen A, Siegler M, Winslade W. *Clinical Ethics,* 5th ed. New York: McGraw Hill, 2002.

Keefe FJ, Lumley M, Anderson T, et al. Pain and emotion: new research directions. *J Clin Psychol* 2001; 57(4):587–607.

Kerns RD, Rosenberg R. Predicting responses to self–management treatments for chronic pain: application of the pain stages of change model. *Pain* 2000; 84(1):49–55.

Laine C, Davidoff F. Patient-centered medicine: a professional evolution. *JAMA* 1996; 10:275(2):152–156.

Little P, Everitt H, Williamson I, et al. Observational study of effect of patient centredness and positive approach on outcomes of general practice consultations. *BMJ* 2001; 323(7318):908–911.

Loeser JD. Pain and suffering. *Clin J Pain* 2000; 16(Suppl 2):S2–6.

McCarberg B, Wolf J. Chronic pain management in a health maintenance organization. *Clin J Pain* 1999; 15:50–57.

Mead N, Bower P. Patient-centeredness: a conceptual framework and review of the empirical literature. *Soc Sci Med* 2000; 51:1087–1110.

Mead N, Bower P, Hann M. The impact of general practitioners' patient-centredness on patients post-consultation satisfaction and enablement. *Soc Sci Med* 2002; 55(2):283–299.

Miller WL, Yanoshik MK, Crabtree BF, Reymond WK. Patients, family physicians, and pain: visions from interview narratives. *Fam Med* 1994; 26(3):179–184.

Moore JE, Von Korff M, Cherkin D, Saunders K, Lorig K. A randomized trial of a cognitive-behavioral program for enhancing back pain self-care in a primary care setting. *Pain* 2000; 88(2):145–153.

Moulin DE, Iezzi A, Amireh R, et al. Randomised trial of oral morphine for chronic non-cancer pain. *Lancet* 1996; 347(8995):143–147.

Murray CJL, Lopez AD. *The Global Burden of Disease*. Cambridge: Harvard University Press, 1996.

Neumann JL. Ethical issues confronting oncology nurses. *Nurs Clin North Am* 2001; 36(4):827–841.

Novack DH, Suchman AL, Clark W, et al. Calibrating the physician: personal awareness and effective patient care. Working Group on Promoting Physician Personal Awareness, American Academy on Physician and Patient. *JAMA* 1997; 278(6):502–509.

Portenoy RK. Opioid therapy for chronic nonmalignant pain: a review of the critical issues. *J Pain Symptom Manage* 1996; 11(4):203–217.

Quill TE, Dresser R, Brock DW. The rule of double effect—a critique of its role in end-of-life decision-making. *N Engl J Med* 1997; 337(24):1768–1771.

Rich BA. Moral conundrums in the courtroom: reflections on a decade in the culture of pain. *Camb Q Healthc Ethics* 2002; 11(2):180–190.

Schers H, Wensing M, Huijsmans Z, van Tulder M, Grol R. Implementation barriers for general practice guidelines on low back pain a qualitative study. *Spine* 2001; 26:E348–353.

Simmons JW, Avant WS Jr, Demski J, Parisher D. Determining successful pain clinic treatment through validation of cost effectiveness. *Spine* 1988; 13(3):342–344.

Sullivan MD. The illusion of patient choice in end-of-life care. *Am J Geriatr Psychiatry* 2002; 10:1–8.

Sullivan MD. The new subjective medicine: taking the patient's point of view on health and health care. *Soc Sci Med* 2003; 56:1595–1604.

Sullivan MD, Kempen GIJM, Van Sonderen E, Ormel J. Models of health-related quality of life in a population of community-dwelling Dutch elderly. *Qual Life Res* 2000; 9:801–810.

Tan V, Cheatle MD, Mackin S, Moberg PJ, Esterhai JL Jr. Goal setting as a predictor of return to work in a population of chronic musculoskeletal pain patients. *Int J Neurosci* 1997; 92(3-4):161–170.

Turk DC. Clinical effectiveness and cost effectiveness of treatments for chronic pain patients. *Clin J Pain*; in press.

Turk DC, Brody MC, Okifuji EA. Physicians' attitudes and practices regarding the long-term prescribing of opioids for non-cancer pain. *Pain* 1994; 59:201–208.

Turk DC, Loeser JD, Monarch ES. Chronic pain: purposes and costs of interdisciplinary pain programs. *Economics Neurosci* 2002; 4:64–69.

Weir R, Browne GB, Tunks E, Gafni A, Roberts J. A profile of users of specialty pain clinic services: predictors of use and cost estimates. *J Clin Epidemiol* 1992; 45(12):1399–1415.

Correspondence to: Mark D. Sullivan, MD, PhD, Department of Psychiatry and Behavioral Sciences, Box 356560, University of Washington School of Medicine, 1959 NE Pacific Street, Seattle, WA 98195-6560, USA. Tel: 206-685-3184; Fax: 206-221-5414; email: sullimar@u.washington.edu.

Psychosocial Aspects of Pain: A Handbook for Health Care Providers, Progress in Pain Research and Management, Vol. 27, edited by Robert H. Dworkin and William S. Breitbart, IASP Press, Seattle, © 2004.

11

Principles of Psychopharmacology in Pain Treatment

J. Hampton Atkinson, Jr., Jonathan M. Meyer, and Mark A. Slater

Psychiatry Services, VA San Diego Healthcare System, San Diego, California; and Department of Psychiatry, School of Medicine, University of California, San Diego, La Jolla, California, USA

The prevalence, morbidity, and treatment costs associated with chronic pain syndromes call for simple, safe, and effective therapy. Two classes of psychotropic medications—antidepressants and anticonvulsants/mood stabilizers—may help meet the needs of many pain patients, although it could be argued that these drugs historically have been overused or misused for pain treatment. Fortunately, data from the past decade of clinical trials and clinical psychopharmacology research provide better guidance for the use of psychotropics, permitting clinicians to realize much more of the potential of these agents for pain management.

The aim of this chapter is to convey an understanding of the indications, efficacy, and clinical pharmacology of selected antidepressants and mood stabilizers with demonstrated effectiveness in pain disorders, along with a rational approach to treatment. Among the important principles guiding treatment with psychotropics are understanding the functional classification (putative mechanism of action) of these drugs; considering these agents as part of a treatment program, rather than a sole or primary treatment; following evidence-based practices; using patient factors (e.g., side-effect profiles), illness factors (e.g., pain diagnosis and mechanisms), and drug-specific factors to guide therapy; and analyzing treatment outcomes. Included within this chapter is a focused review of the literature, based on recent meta-analyses of placebo-controlled clinical trials, which summarizes the efficacy data for antidepressants and anticonvulsants in treatment of the most prevalent chronic pain diagnoses. Comparisons of efficacy, side-effect profiles, and drug interactions will also be presented to assist in treatment selection, along with approaches to managing side effects, evaluating outcomes, and responding to treatment failure.

CLASSIFICATION OF PSYCHOTROPICS AS A GUIDE TO TREATMENT

Over 20 antidepressant agents are available and many more are on the horizon, but these newer agents are just now being tested in controlled trials for chronic pain. Nonetheless, an understanding of their mechanism of action is helpful in interpreting the developing literature because most antidepressants share one of a small number of therapeutic mechanisms. While antidepressants can be classified by criteria corresponding either to drug structure (e.g., tricyclic rings) or function (e.g., selective serotonin reuptake inhibitor), the function criterion is becoming the more useful approach because it relates to putative mechanism of action and can be used to conceptualize treatment strategies (Stahl 1998; Richelson 2001). Classification by function, by helping to predict side effects and tolerability, also may assist the clinician in matching the patient with the right drug. Classified according to function, the classic tricyclic antidepressants or TCAs (e.g., amitriptyline and imipramine) are termed nonselective serotonin-norepinephrine reuptake inhibitors because besides blocking presynaptic transport of these monoamines, they also have antimuscarinic-anticholinergic, α_1-adrenergic antagonist, and histamine-1 (H_1) antihistaminic properties. The primary metabolites of amitriptyline (nortriptyline) and imipramine (desipramine) block norepinephrine reuptake more selectively than do the parent compounds, and have somewhat less potent effects on muscarinic, α_1-adrenergic, and H_1 receptors. By contrast, the selective dual serotonin and norepinephrine reuptake inhibitors (SNRIs) (e.g., venlafaxine and duloxetine) block both serotonin and norepinephrine reuptake transporters, but do not markedly affect other neurotransmitter systems and therefore generally have a more favorable side-effect profile. The selective serotonin reuptake inhibitors (SSRIs) (e.g., fluoxetine, citalopram, sertraline, and paroxetine) primarily block the serotonin transporter. Selective norepinephrine reuptake inhibitors (NRIs) also are available (e.g., reboxetine and atomoxetine). Another group is the norepinephrine agonist/dopamine reuptake inhibitors (NDRIs), of which there is only one example (bupropion). The remaining major class is the serotonin type 2A (5-HT_{2A}) receptor antagonist/serotonin reuptake inhibitors (SARIs; e.g., mirtazapine, nefazodone, and trazodone) (for an overview, see Stahl 1998, Richelson 2001). Although this classification system is appealing and useful, the clinical pharmacology of these drugs is complex, and additional drug properties are beginning to be identified. It is becoming clear that antidepressant categories of function may be more dynamic than once thought. For example, venlafaxine is termed a dual serotonergic and noradrenergic agent, but at a low dose it is serotonin selective, whereas at higher doses (150–225 mg or more daily) it has effects on norepinephrine and serotonin reuptake. Drugs classified as SARIs may also block serotonin reuptake directly (e.g., nefazodone), or may increase norepinephrine and serotonin neurotransmission (e.g., mirtazapine) without effects on reuptake. Paroxetine is usually classified as an SSRI, but new data indicate that at very high doses it potently blocks the norepinephrine reuptake transporter (Gilmor et al. 2002), although the clinical significance of this finding is not clear. A better appreciation of the properties of these drugs, along with data on the efficacy of newer antidepressants as analgesics, may lead to important advances in therapy.

The analgesic mechanism of action of antidepressants is unknown. It has been pointed out that the standard explanation—that they act on norepinephrine and serotonin systems—is not thoroughly compelling (McQuay and Moore 1997). Some nonselective reuptake blockers also inhibit postsynaptic *N*-methyl-D-aspartate receptors, and may reduce neuronal hypersensitivity by this mechanism. Many classical antidepressants (e.g., TCAs) block sodium or calcium channels, or both, while some SSRIs appear to block calcium channels. Which of these properties, or other properties, are most crucial to analgesic efficacy is unknown.

Agents that have anticonvulsant and mood-stabilizing properties also have promise as analgesics. These agents include carbamazepine, gabapentin, lamotrigine, phenytoin, and valproate. In general neurological practice they are prescribed as anti-epileptics, but in psychiatric settings they are used as mood-stabilizing medications to treat the manic or depressive phases of bipolar disorder, and sometimes major depression. All of these anticonvulsants appear to have ion-channel-blocking effects with resulting neuronal membrane stabilization, and these effects seem to correlate with their analgesic properties. In general, calcium or sodium channel blockade may alter the release of neurotransmitters (e.g., serotonin, norepinephrine, and glutamate) and of excitatory amino acids thought to be important in pain modulation, although one must bear in mind that different types or subtypes of ion channels exist that are localized to specific tissues. For example, there are at least eight subtypes of voltage-gated sodium channels and five subtypes of calcium channels, of which the N-type and T-type channels appear to be localized to neurons that play a role in pain modulation. Gabapentin may exert its analgesic properties by binding to calcium channel subunits and modulating calcium currents in neurons, but carbamazepine, lamotrigine, valproate, and phenytoin mostly act at sodium channels. Of course, new drugs with more potent or selective ion-channel-blocking properties may lead to new therapies. Combination treatment with agents affecting two or more systems modulating pain, such as one drug affecting monoaminergic systems and another affecting ion channels, might result in improved outcomes, but as will be discussed below, evidence from clinical data must be used to guide decision-making.

PSYCHOTROPICS AS ADJUNCTIVE TREATMENT

Chronic pain patients must cope not only with pain itself, but also with its effects on vocational, family, and social life. Therefore, pain treatment must be evaluated in terms of analgesia as well as life quality and everyday functioning. Little research addresses these so-called "secondary outcomes." Some evidence suggests that psychotropic agents, by reducing pain, also improve life quality (Farrar et al. 2001). However, it unusual for these drugs to alleviate pain completely. And, even though they usually reduce pain intensity at least moderately, it is not clear that they reliably improve rates of return to work, decrease absenteeism, or enhance other aspects of everyday functioning. For these reasons, psychotropics are best considered adjunctive rather than definitive treatment.

Although it seems logical that once pain is reduced a patient should be able to resume normal activities, many patients will require behavioral interventions to return to functioning. Behavioral treatments described by Waters et al. and Andrasik et al. in this volume are often crucial to success; these include setting goals for physical reactivation, scheduling daily activities, self-monitoring progress, using problem-solving techniques to remove barriers to recovery, and learning relaxation techniques. Exploring work demands, work satisfaction, and vocational goals can enhance rehabilitation. Marital or family intervention may be needed to help the family assist in this process.

USE OF EVIDENCE-BASED MEDICINE

Clinical practices based on the best available information and recommendations derived from these data are often referred to as *evidence-based medicine* (Evidence Based Medicine Working Group 1992; Cook et al. 1995). Larger-scale randomized trials offer the strongest evidence (Level I) of treatment efficacy and thus are appropriate to apply to individual patients (Cook et al. 1995). A systematic review that uses statistical approaches to combine the results of previous randomized trials (a meta-analysis) can provide even greater assurance for making treatment decisions that will apply to diverse groups of patients (Cook et al. 1995), by minimizing chance effects and offsetting the unique characteristics of any individual study. A meta-analysis may be particularly helpful when, as in the chronic pain literature, the sample in individual randomized trials is often small and the estimate of the treatment effect is imprecise. Combining the results in a meta-analysis may provide a more precise estimate of the treatment effect. Until the past decade most of the level of evidence for treatment of chronic pain consisted of small-scale randomized trials with imprecise estimates of treatment effect (Level II) or various nonrandomized cohort studies (Levels III, IV) or case series (Level V). Chronic pain can be so resistant to treatment that positive expectancy for a "new" therapy may bias both clinicians and patients toward reporting improvement. Because the placebo effect, even in chronic pain, can be profound (Turner et al. 1994; see also Fields, this volume), the end result can be proliferation of useless therapy, unless evidence is based on controlled studies (Deyo 1983). The clinician should evaluate reports of drug efficacy using criteria thought to be essential for establishing the validity and generalizability of analgesic research. The criteria include: (a) representative, diagnostically homogeneous clinical samples described with sufficient demographic and clinical detail; (b) use of reliable methods to measure pain intensity; (c) an appropriate control or reference standard to compare with the experimental drugs; (d) random allocation; (e) blinded outcome assessment, with testing adequacy of the masking procedure; (f) documentation of concurrent interventions; (g) assessment of compliance or adherence; (h) adequate statistical power to detect an effect; (i) analysis by intent-to-treat; and (j) consideration of statistical and clinical significance of outcome (e.g., see Deyo 1983). Clinical trials cited in this review meet most of these requirements.

PAIN DIAGNOSIS AS A GUIDE TO DRUG SELECTION

Data from meta-analyses and individual controlled trials of antidepressants and anticonvulsants/mood stabilizers are available for the most prevalent pain syndromes (see Tables I and II). Results are presented by two methods: as standardized differences (effect sizes) and as numbers needed to treat (NNT). Effect sizes show the differences between the mean scores (e.g., pain intensity) for the treated and control groups, adjusted (standardized)

Table I
Meta-analyses of randomized trials of antidepressant analgesia
in chronic pain syndromes

Pain Syndrome	Treatment	Meta-analysis	No. of Studies	Pain Outcome	
				NNT*	Effect Size†
Diabetic neuropathy	Tricyclics SSRIs	Sindrup and Jensen 1999, 2000	9 3	1.4–2.4 6.7	>1.0
Postherpetic neuralgia	Tricyclics	Sindrup and Jensen 1999		2.3	>1.0
Peripheral nerve injury	Tricyclics	Sindrup and Jensen 1999		2.5	
Central pain	Tricyclics	Sindrup and Jensen 1999		2.5	
Chronic back pain	Tricyclics	Salerno et al. 2002	9	2.5	
Migraine/tension headaches	Tricyclics‡ SSRIs	Tomkins et al. 2001	19 7	2.5–4.3* 4	>0.6
Fibromyalgia	Tricyclics SSRIs	O'Malley et al. 2000	10 3	4*	0.5§
Functional/irritable bowel syndrome	Tricyclics	Jackson et al. 2000	9	3.2	0.9

* NNT = number needed to treat for >50% improvement. From cited meta-analyses.
† Effect size = improvement in pain intensity. Adapted from Max (1994).
‡ Includes other nonselective noradrenergic-serotonergic agents.
§ Combines results of all antidepressants.

for the variation in the scores. For the pain literature, effect sizes >1 indicate definitely responsive syndromes, and effect sizes of 0.5–0.6 suggest probable or possible efficacy (Max 1994). NNT is the number of patients one needs to treat with a particular drug to obtain one patient with a specified magnitude of pain relief beyond that expected from a placebo, calculated as NNT = 1/([goal achieved$_{active}$/total$_{active}$] – [goal achieved$_{placebo}$/total$_{placebo}$]). An alternative statement is NNT = 1/(percentage improved by active treatment) – (percentage improved by placebo). The usual definition of "improvement" is "at least 50% relief." Although this approach has its limitations, it allows evaluation of the relative analgesic efficacy of various drugs within and across diagnostic conditions (e.g., McQuay and Moore 1997; Sindrup and Jensen 1999).

Several generalizations follow from these tables. First, at least for initial treatment, it may be useful to select a specific class of antidepressants for a specific pain diagnosis, rather than taking the approach that all antidepressants are generally analgesic for any chronic pain state. The nonselective serotonin-norepinephrine reuptake inhibitors (i.e., TCAs) are clearly broadly efficacious, with evidence for efficacy compared to placebo in nine specific pain diagnoses. Depending upon the method used to ascertain relative efficacy, the most responsive syndromes may be neuropathic states, although migraine headache, irritable bowel syndrome, and chronic back pain also respond at least moderately. On the other hand, although there is some preliminary evidence of SSRI efficacy in migraine headache (Tomkins et al. 2001) and fibromyalgia (O'Malley et al. 2000) studies in diabetic neuropathy (Max et al. 1991) and chronic back pain (Atkinson et al. 1999) suggest that SSRIs are not more effective than placebo for these conditions. Specific classes of antidepressants thus may be effective in some pain syndromes, but not in others. Second, evidence is emerging for the efficacy of some, but not all, anticonvulsants/mood stabilizers (Table II). Most studies evaluating gabapentin and lamotrigine have found efficacy for neuropathic pain roughly comparable to that of the nonselective serotonin-norepinephrine reuptake inhibitors (e.g., amitriptyline, imipramine). Phenytoin, carbamazepine, and valproate (Kochar et al. 2002) may also be as effective in some neuropathies, but there is only one trial for each drug (see Sindrup and Jensen 2000). Much additional study is needed to determine whether anticonvulsants will be as broadly effective across several pain disorders as are the classical antidepressants. Third, the outlines of rational sequential treatment of some conditions are beginning to emerge, should response to the first agent selected be unsatisfactory. For example, in neuropathic pain there is efficacy for three classes of antidepressants (nonselective serotonin-norepinephrine reuptake inhibitors and one trial each of the SNRI venlafaxine and the NDRI bupropion) as well as for one or more agents from another drug category,

Table II
Selected summary of randomized trials demonstrating the efficacy of anticonvulsants/mood stabilizers as analgesics in chronic pain syndromes

Pain Syndrome	Treatment	Study	NNT*
Diabetic neuropathy	Carbamazepine	Rull et al. 1969	3.3
	Gabapentin	Backonja et al. 1998	4.1
	Lamotrigine	Eisenberg et al. 2001	4
	Phenytoin	Chadda and Mathur 1978	2.1
	Valproate	Kochar et al. 2002	4.0
HIV-associated neuropathy	Lamotrigine	Simpson et al. 2000	3.0
Postherpetic neuralgia	Gabapentin	Rowbotham et al. 1998	3.2
		Rice and Maton 2001	3.0
Central poststroke pain	Lamotrigine	Vestergaard et al. 2001	3.3

Source: Results summarized in part from Sindrup and Jensen (1999, 2000).
* Pain outcome; NNT = number needed to treat for 50% improvement.

the anticonvulsants/mood stabilizers (gabapentin and lamotrigine). In migraine headache there is evidence for efficacy of one class of antidepressants, the nonselective noradrenergic-serotonergic reuptake inhibitors, and at least some trials that are positive for SSRIs. The corollary generalization is that relatively few studies of SSRIs or other classes of antidepressants or anticonvulsants have been conducted, limiting our ability to make informed decisions about these drugs. Clearer approaches to matching diagnosis and drug treatment depend upon evaluating the efficacy of newer antidepressants (SNRIs, NDRIs, and NRIs) and anticonvulsants in diagnostically homogeneous samples.

It is also important to note that the efficacy of classical antidepressants across diverse neuropathic pain states (e.g., diabetes, herpes zoster, and trauma) leads some authorities to argue that underlying common mechanisms of pain pathophysiology may be more relevant than diagnostic etiology for drug selection (Woolf and Mannion 1999; Sindrup and Jensen 2000). In addition, patients diagnosed with a specific neuropathy may experience several types of pain, such as constant pain, paroxysmal pain, and touch-evoked pain. These sensations may be related to distinct pathophysiological mechanisms independent of etiology (e.g., ectopic firing of peripheral neurons or increased sensitivity to noxious or normal stimuli). Matching treatment to underlying mechanisms rather than diagnosis may result in better outcomes (Sindrup and Jensen 2000). Although it is not yet possible to base treatment selection on mechanisms, careful attention to both diagnoses and mechanisms may be increasingly important to therapeutic success.

For various painful conditions, the efficacy of psychotropics has not been well established, either because evidence is insufficient or because a preponderance of trials are negative. For example, nonselective noradrenergic-serotonergic antidepressants are effective for some neuropathies (e.g., diabetic neuropathy and postherpetic neuralgia), but results are negative for cisplatin-induced and HIV-related painful neuropathies. This failure has been attributed to differences in pain mechanism. Known responsive syndromes are all small-fiber disorders, whereas the antineoplastic drug cisplatin may cause a large-fiber neuropathy; moreover, HIV pain may be attributed to myelopathy. Additionally, evidence of efficacy is thin for some orofacial pain states, including temporomandibular disorder, atypical odontalgia (pain in the teeth), and oral dysesthesia (disturbed taste, dry mouth, and burning tongue). Evidence also is sparse for other conditions, including what may be termed chronic psychogenic pain disorder or somatoform pain disorder, depending on the diagnostic system used. The key feature of psychogenic or somatoform pain disorder is that psychological factors are thought to be important in the onset, severity, or maintenance of pain, but that the symptom is not intentionally produced or feigned. One extremely thorough meta-analysis of 11 randomized trials representing 832 patients concluded that psychogenic pain was responsive to antidepressants (Fishbain et al. 1998). Nevertheless, at least five of these trials, which included 565 subjects (68% of the total) studied tension headaches, which are known to respond to antidepressants. The reason these trials were included in the meta-analysis is that the original authors had diagnosed the patients as having "psychogenic" (tension) headache. Given what is now known about tension-migraine headache syndromes, this label of psychogenicity seems unjustified. As a result, it is unclear that psychogenic pain responds to antidepressants, given that the conclusion of the meta-analysis may have been heavily influenced by favorable outcomes for chronic headache syndromes. Additional research is needed to determine whether antidepressants show efficacy for all of these diagnoses or whether responsive diagnostic subgroups exist. There may be limits to the generalizability of antidepressant-associated analgesia.

ISSUES OF COMPARATIVE EFFICACY AND DOSING

NONSELECTIVE VERSUS SELECTIVE ANTIDEPRESSANTS

The initial rationale for using antidepressants as analgesics was based on the hypothesis that both norepinephrine and serotonin mediate pain control systems (Basbaum and Fields 1978; Max 1994). In accordance with this model one might generate two other hypotheses: first, that agents with balanced noradrenergic and serotonergic effects will outperform those blocking only one transporter; and second, that both noradrenergic and serotonergic agents will be effective. Most of the data addressing the first proposition come from samples of patients with diabetic and postherpetic neuropathies or headache syndromes. In these disorders the effects of amitriptyline, an agent with rather equivalent or balanced (Max 1994) effects on norepinephrine and serotonin reuptake, could not be distinguished statistically from those of desipramine (Max et al. 1992) or maprotiline (Watson et al. 1992), which potently block norepinephrine reuptake but have comparatively little effect on serotonin. Desipramine also has been shown to be equivalent to other balanced agents (imipramine and clomipramine) (e.g., Sindrup et al. 1990). Calculations using NNT provide another perspective. In painful neuropathy, agents with combined serotonin and norepinephrine reuptake inhibition (i.e., imipramine, amitriptyline) have an NNT of 2.7 (2.2–3.3), compared to an NNT of 2.5 for drugs with relatively more selective norepinephrine reuptake inhibition (e.g., desipramine, maprotiline) (see Sindrup and Jensen 1999, 2000). The noradrenergic-dopaminergic agent bupropion is roughly comparable (Semenchuk et al. 2001). Two points stand out from these data. First, it seems (at least for these neuropathy diagnoses) that there are no pronounced differences in efficacy within the class of nonselective (e.g., tricyclic) antidepressants: the parent compounds amitriptyline and imipramine are equivalent in efficacy, and the primary metabolites of these compounds (nortriptyline and desipramine) are equivalent to each other and as effective as the parent compound, even though they have more selective effects on monoamine transport. The main difference is in the side-effect profile. Second, it seems clear that noradrenergic action is crucial to efficacy (Max 1994).

The data on the role of serotonergic action is more complex. In two of four studies of neuropathy and one study in chronic back pain, selective noradrenergic drugs were effective whereas standard doses of SSRIs were ineffective. The SSRIs that proved ineffective were fluoxetine for diabetic neuropathy (Max et al. 1992), zimelidine for postherpetic neuralgia (Watson and Evans 1985), and paroxetine for back pain (Atkinson et al. 1998). Yet in two other studies, SSRIs (citalopram and high-dose paroxetine) were effective (Sindrup et al. 1990, 1992). Although it is possible that paroxetine analgesia was mediated by its known noradrenergic effects at doses greater than 30–40 mg daily, this possibility would not explain the efficacy of the most selective serotonin reuptake inhibitor, citalopram, which appears to have negligible noradrenergic action (Richelson 2001). A substantial number of studies support the efficacy of nonselective (tricyclic) agents in migraine and tension headache, fibromyalgia, and irritable bowel syndrome, but the efficacy of SSRIs such as fluoxetine, femoxetine, and fluvoxamine remains open to question because of a lack of data. Although the overall effect size for SSRIs is comparable to that of TCAs for headache (Tomkins et al. 2001) and fibromyalgia (O'Malley et al. 2000), there are only six studies in headache, three in fibromyalgia, and none in irritable bowel syndrome (Jackson et al. 2000). Drugs with selective serotonergic effects, while not as reliably effective as those with noradrenergic activity across the spectrum of chronic pain disorders (Max 1994), may have a role in specific syndromes. Larger trials studying these diagnoses are needed to clarify this issue.

ANTIDEPRESSANTS VERSUS ANTICONVULSANTS

The effect sizes and NNT calculations suggest that nonselective antidepressants and gabapentin, an anticonvulsant, have equivalent efficacy in specific neuropathic pain syndromes (e.g., see Tables I and II; also see Rowbotham et al. 1998). Results from meta-analyses are supported by one randomized, double-blind, crossover, head-to-head trial comparing 6 weeks of amitriptyline (25–75 mg daily) or gabapentin (900–1800 mg daily) in patients with painful diabetic peripheral neuropathy (Morello et al. 1999). The extensive literature on antidepressants suggests that they may be first-line agents for painful neuropathy (Sindrup and Jensen 2000), but data for gabapentin also are strong. Gabapentin is an alternative for those who fail to respond to antidepressant treatment or who have medical comorbidity (e.g., heart block) or are unable to tolerate the side effects of antidepressants. Data from other syndromes are too sparse to gauge the comparative efficacy of anticonvulsants.

ROLE OF SERUM CONCENTRATION-RESPONSE RELATIONSHIPS

A better understanding of the serum concentration-response relationships of psychotropic-related analgesia would clarify questions of comparative efficacy and improve treatment (Max 1994). For example, such data might identify therapeutic windows of efficacy to enhance precision of therapy, reduce toxicity, or suggest minimum thresholds that must be attained for effectiveness. Such data would also direct responses to treatment failure by noting whether dose modification is warranted if one dose does not provide relief. Yet few studies examine concentration-response relationships for antidepressants or anticonvulsants, and almost none have used a prospective design wherein subjects are randomly assigned to specific concentrations and followed for outcome. Thus the evidence is insufficient to determine the role of concentration-response relationships for any drug in any pain syndrome (Max 1994). As a result, one cannot assume that changing doses (concentrations) will convert a nonresponding patient into a responder, or will improve the analgesia already achieved by a responder. However, one study provides some potentially valuable guidance for use of antidepressants. Patients with diabetic neuropathy were assigned to ascending doses of imipramine, escalated at 1-week intervals (Sindrup et al. 1990) to achieve either maximum relief, or a target maximum concentration of around 120 ng/mL. The difficulty in interpreting such studies is that with forced dose escalation, analgesia may have occurred at a low concentration, but due to delayed onset of response it might be attributed to a higher concentration achieved later. Most responses occurred at concentrations of around 50 ng/mL (corresponding to a dosage of 50–75 mg daily). The optimal strategy for diabetic neuropathy may be to use a low dose to minimize side effects and improve adherence, to consider escalation to moderate concentrations only after 2–4 weeks on treatment, then to escalate to even higher doses (e.g., 150 mg or more) only in the absence of a response to a trial of moderate-dose therapy. In the absence of additional data, this approach may also be considered in other pain syndromes. Plasma concentrations may be used to check compliance, diminish toxicity, or detect unsuspected drug interactions. Obtaining a determination may be useful after steady state is achieved (5–7 days) if no benefit is evident after 4 weeks or if side effects are unusually severe.

As for anticonvulsants, although there are no formal concentration-response studies, studies of gabapentin suggest that daily doses of 1800–2400 mg provide equivalent relief for some neuropathic pain, as do doses of 3600 mg (e.g., Rowbotham et al. 1998; Rice and Maton 2001), although it is not clear that low-dose strategies (900 mg daily) are therapeutic. Because gabapentin is generally well tolerated, most studies have employed the higher dose schedule, and this may be a reasonable clinical approach. For lamotrigine, relatively low doses of 200 mg daily appear to be efficacious (Eisenberg 2001). It is not known whether higher doses (e.g., up to 600 mg) are associated with increased likelihood of efficacy, but toxicity is certainly increased.

APPROACH TO PARTIAL RESPONSE
OR TREATMENT FAILURE

The meta-analyses presented here suggest that 50–75% of patients treated for a condition known to be responsive to antidepressants and anticonvulsants will achieve at least a 50% reduction in pain intensity. Onset of therapeutic effects is usually within 2–4 weeks. This outcome leaves a considerable number of patients who may be partial responders (e.g., 25–49% decrease) or truly treatment resistant (Hirschfeld et al. 2002). (Distinguishing true from apparent treatment resistance is discussed below.) The theory underlying combining two or more drugs, or of switching from one class of drugs to another is straightforward. The concept behind combination therapy is that the action of the first drug is enhanced or the second drug delivers a new pharmacological effect. Combination treatment is generally reserved for those who experience at least a partial response to first-line therapy and for whom there is a risk of losing the partial response if that therapy is withdrawn. Switching is conceptually most appropriate for those who fail or are intolerant of first-line treatment (Hirschfeld et al. 2002). The physician might select another agent in the same class of drugs (e.g., within nonselective noradrenergic-serotonergic transport blockers) or another category of antidepressants (e.g., switching from nonselective agents to selective SSRIs or SNRIs) or another class of drugs (e.g., anticonvulsants). Although switching within the same drug class would not seem promising, data from studies of chronic pain (Watson et al. 1992) and other disorders treated with antidepressants (i.e., major depression) suggest that this strategy might be viable (see Hirschfeld et al. 2002). Unfortunately, we have few data to guide switching or combination therapies. Neuropathic pain syndromes respond to the nonselective serotonin-norepinephrine class of antidepressants, so partial response of one of these agents might be addressed by use of an anticonvulsant (i.e., gabapentin). Treatment failure with a nonselective serotonin-norepinephrine or norepinephrine reuptake inhibitor would suggest switching to an anticonvulsant. Another consideration would be use of a selective serotonin-norepinephrine reuptake inhibitor (SNRI, e.g., venlafaxine) or a selective noradrenergic-dopaminergic agent (NDRI, e.g., bupropion), given evidence of their efficacy (Semenchuk et al. 2001; Sindrup et al. 2003). A possible but less proven approach would be switching to the one "pure" SSRI (i.e., citalopram) with strong evidence for efficacy. Some evidence indicates that adding a second anticonvulsant (i.e., lamotrigine) to treat partial response to another anticonvulsant may be effective (Zakrzewska et al. 1997). For chronic headache syndromes and fibromyalgia, a partial response to a nonselective antidepressant might be followed by switching to an SSRI, given that some trials support their efficacy. Combining an SSRI with a nonselective antidepressant might be attempted on the grounds that it would "double boost" serotonergic action, but no data support this method, and any combination of nonselective reuptake inhibitors and SSRIs should be carefully reviewed for drug interactions, as noted below. In chronic back pain, partial response to or treatment failure with a nonselective antidepressant might warrant treatment with another drug of the same class or an SNRI (e.g., venlafaxine), because there is no evidence for efficacy of SSRIs and we lack published data of randomized trials with anticonvulsants for back pain. The same strategy might be employed for irritable bowel syndrome.

CONDUCTING AND ANALYZING TREATMENT TRIALS

Selecting appropriate therapy depends on patient-specific factors and drug-specific factors (Marangell et al. 2003). Analysis of possible reasons for less than fully successful outcomes, a process that will guide the next step in therapy, likewise involves both patient- and drug-specific elements.

Patient factors include consideration of pain diagnosis, comorbid medical or other disorders, and history of response and side effects with prior treatments. Moreover, pain patients who enter specialty clinics commonly are taking many agents for symptomatic treatment, including hypnotics for sleep, anxiolytics for distress, and primary analgesics. Simplifying the drug regimen by eliminating agents is often extremely useful. Two essential patient-physician factors are forming a therapeutic alliance and defining goals of treatment (Fait et al. 2001; Marangell et al. 2003).

The importance of a therapeutic alliance between patient and physician is perhaps the most critical yet overlooked ingredient to successful pharmacotherapy (Fait et al. 2001; Marangell et al. 2003). This alliance implies that the patient and physician interact and agree to a course of action, expecting a positive outcome. The process of prescribing involves exploring patient attitudes, both favorable and negative, toward drug treatment, and offering drug therapy as a choice. The physician's failure to inquire about biases against drugs, and to attempt to clarify issues and resolve concerns, may lead to patient nonadherence. Involving key family members in the process is often essential. The more the patient and family understand about the pain disorder and the reason a specific drug has been chosen, the more likely the patient is to be adherent and the family is to be supportive (Marangell et al. 2003). Much of this involves education about the special properties of psychotropics, with regard to the need for daily dosing, delayed development of therapeutic action, durability of analgesia, and desirability of pacing one's resumption of activities. This information will assist the patient in understanding that these agents must be taken daily, not just when pain is intense; that 2 weeks or more of treatment may be necessary for onset of noticeable therapeutic effects, so treatment should not be judged or abandoned prematurely; that benefits will not persist if the drug is stopped; and that there may be the temptation to resume full activity at the first sign of pain relief, so caution is needed in certain conditions such as back pain so as to avoid re-injury. Another component of education is the importance of treatment adherence. Tips to enhance compliance include incorporating pill-taking into one's daily routine, on a set schedule (e.g., keyed to bedtime, meals, or other activities). Pillboxes are very useful aides; posting of cues or reminders at key locations can help patients remember to take their pills. Side effects are a major source of nonadherence and dropout from treatment. Education about side effects, and availability of methods to eliminate or reduce them, may greatly improve adherence and outcomes.

Before beginning a trial of a psychopharmacological agent it is important for the patient and physician to agree on treatment goals. This step strengthens the therapeutic alliance and assists in treatment planning. For example, if part of the definition of success includes both pain relief and return to functioning, then behavioral or cognitive-behavioral therapy may at some point be crucial. As mentioned above, much of the literature defines successful outcome as a 50% or better reduction in pain intensity (e.g., Sindrup and Jensen 2000). Meaningful improvement in life quality is associated with a reduction in chronic pain intensity of 30% or more (Farrar et al. 2001).

The following section on drug-specific factors describes methods for using the major classes of agents in a treatment trial, including an overview of properties, side effects, consideration of specific drug interactions, and pretreatment evaluation. Because management of side effects is so important, the most common ones, and approaches to their management, are summarized in Table III.

ANTIDEPRESSANTS

NONSELECTIVE SEROTONIN-NOREPINEPHRINE REUPTAKE INHIBITORS

Properties and side effects. The focus will be on the classical, tricyclic, nonselective reuptake inhibitors because they have the broadest side-effect profile. Beyond blocking serotonin and norepinephrine reuptake presynaptically, these agents have strong -antimuscarinic (M_1) and anticholinergic, antihistaminic (H_1), and α_1-adrenergic antagonist properties, producing autonomic, cardiac, and central nervous system (CNS) side effects. Autonomic effects include dry mouth, blurred vision, constipation, ileus, and urinary retention. Cardiovascular effects include orthostatic hypotension, increased heart rate, and repolarization abnormalities on the electrocardiogram (Q-T interval prolongation and T-wave inversion or flattening). Atrial and ventricular arrhythmias, as well as conduction delay with bundle branch block, may occur. This effect results from prolongation of the H-V interval, the time from activation of the bundle of His to activation of the ventricular myocardium. These effects resemble the properties of type I cardiac antiarrhythmics, such as quinidine and procainamide (Risch et al. 1981). These antidepressants also can depress myocardial contractility. CNS effects can include agitated states in elderly patients related to decreased plasma protein binding of the drug and higher plasma concentration, and even delirium caused by central anticholinergic effects on the brain, again primarily in the elderly. Other common side effects are weight gain, and in men delayed ejaculation and impotence. In general, anticholinergic, cardiac, and CNS side effects are more common with tertiary amines (amitriptyline, imipramine) than with demethylated secondary amines (nortriptyline, desipramine, and others). Thus desipramine is the least anticholinergic and sedating of the tricyclic drugs. Patients with agitation or insomnia may benefit more from sedating drugs. All these agents will increase heart rate secondary to adrenergic and anticholinergic effects. Furthermore, imipramine

Table III
Major side effects of antidepressants and their management

Receptor	Side Effects*	Antidepressants	Possible Treatments†
Alpha-1 antagonism	Orthostatic hypotension	Classical TCAs; rarely SSRIs, venlafaxine, trazodone	9-α-fluorohydrocortisone 0.025–0.05 mg q.d., b.i.d.
Alpha-2 presynaptic agonism	Sexual dysfunction (erectile dysfunction, delayed ejaculation, anorgasmia, reduced libido)	Classical TCAs	Sexual dysfunction due to TCAs: bethanechol 10–20 mg, yohimbine 5.4–16.2 mg; impotence: sildenafil 50–100 mg
Histamine (H_1) antagonism	Sedation, weight gain, hypotension		Sedation: bedtime dosing, caffeine; weight gain: exercise, nutritional counseling, dose reductions, consider switching to venlafaxine
Muscarinic antagonism	Dry mouth, blurred vision, urinary retention, constipation	Classical TCAs; rarely SSRIs, venlafaxine, trazodone	Dry mouth: sugar-free candies or gum; constipation: exercise, fluid intake, stool softeners (docusate sodium 100–200 mg q.d.); all muscarinic effects may respond to bethanechol 10–50 mg q.d, q.i.d.
$5HT_2$, $5HT_3$ agonism	Anxiety; insomnia; erectile and ejaculatory dysfunction or delayed orgasm, hypotension, nausea	Classical TCAs, SSRIs, venlafaxine	Anxiety/jitters: wait for tolerance; short-term lorazepam 0.5 mg t.i.d.; insomnia: morning dosing; hypnotic agent (e.g., zolpidem 5–10 mg at bedtime); sexual dysfunction from SSRIs or trazodone: cyproheptadine 4–12 mg before sex, or bupropion augmentation; impotence: sildenafil 50–100 mg
Norepinephrine agonism	Hypertension, tachycardia tremors		Hypertension: dose reduction or antihypertensives; tachycardia tremors: dose reduction
Multiple/ unclear	Headache	SSRIs, venlafaxine, rarely TCAs	Due to SSRIs: amitriptyline 25–50 mg q.d.
	Paresthesia	TCAs, SSRIs	Dose reduction; pyridoxine 50–150 mg q.d.

* Persistent side effects, which usually do not attenuate over time, are hypotension and sexual side effects. Others are often manageable by slow dose escalation, or attenuate over time. † Treatments are adapted from McElroy et al. (1995).

suppresses ventricular arrhythmias (ectopy), so patients on quinidine may need a revised dosage of that agent. Because of these effects, this class of drugs is generally not used in patients with cardiac disease. If used, careful monitoring (e.g., serial EKGs) is indicated. Some evidence indicates that nortriptyline is less likely to depress H-V conduction and less likely to produce orthostatic hypotension than other drugs in this class (Bigger et al. 1978; Roose et al. 1987). If an agent in this class is used, nortriptyline may be preferred in patients with bradyarrhythmias, heart block, or prolonged Q-T interval. Safer alternatives might be an SNRI (e.g., venlafaxine).

Selected pharmacokinetic and pharmacodynamic interactions. The importance of understanding drug interactions has been impressed upon clinicians during the past decade with the highly publicized withdrawal from market of cisapride and the nonsedating antihistamines, terfenadine and astemizole. These medications are metabolized via the hepatic cytochrome P450 (CYP) isozyme 3A4, with multiple cases of fatal or potentially lethal tachyarrhythmias (e.g., torsades de pointes) reported when patients taking any of the above drugs were prescribed strong CYP 3A4 inhibitors, such as ketoconazole or erythromycin. Given the narrow therapeutic index for TCAs, serious side effects have also been reported when these drugs are co-administered with agents that inhibit their hepatic metabolism (Sawada and Ohtani 2001). While the list of medications and over-the-counter herbal preparations that inhibit various P450 enzymes is daunting, the recent publication of small handbooks devoted to cytochrome P450 drug interactions (Cozza and Armstrong 2001), reviews of drug interactions involving herbal remedies (Ioannides 2002), and the availability of pharmacopoeia programs for handheld computers obviate the need to commit to memory the P450 relationships for each medication. However, it is worthwhile knowing the basic metabolic pathways for the few TCAs that a clinician might commonly employ, because this knowledge will narrow the search for possible pharmacokinetic interactions with other medications and substances a patient may be taking.

Most TCAs undergo oxidative metabolism through more than one cytochrome P450 isozyme, but these agents utilize a limited number of pathways (Olesen and Linnet 1997; Rudorfer and Potter 1999). Table IV illustrates the common P450 isozymes involved in the metabolism of various TCAs, with the primary pathways for each TCA in italics. As one can see, CYP 2D6 is implicated in the hepatic metabolism of most TCAs, with CYP 1A2 and 2C19 also playing important roles.

Routine inquiry into use of other medications, particularly nonprescribed herbal remedies, is important to discern the potential for pharmacokinetic interactions with TCAs. It is also worthwhile to ask if the patient has a

Table IV
Cytochrome P450 isozymes involved in tricyclic antidepressant metabolism

1A2	2C9	2C19	2D6	3A4
Amitriptyline *Imipramine*	Amitriptyline	*Amitriptyline* *Imipramine*	*Amitriptyline* *Imipramine* *Desipramine* *Nortriptyline*	Amitriptyline Nortriptyline Desipramine

Note: Italic type = primary metabolic pathway(s).

history of sensitivity to TCAs or other drugs taken in usual doses, because this may indicate a genetic polymorphism in a particular CYP isozyme that markedly reduces activity. These polymorphisms can be found in 7–10% of Caucasian patients at CYP 2D6, and in 15–30% of Asians at CYP 2C19. Kinetic studies recommend a 50% reduction of the full therapeutic dose for such poor metabolizers to prevent unwanted side effects and toxicity (Kirchheiner et al. 2001).

Drugs that may interact with TCAs include: (1) Sympathomimetic amines. TCAs potentiate the pressor response of direct-acting amines such as phenylephrine (Boakes et al. 1973), with a possible hypertensive crisis characterized by hypothermia, sweating, severe headache, and cerebrovascular accident. (2) Neuroleptics. Because TCAs and neuroleptics compete for the same hepatic metabolic pathways, their anticholinergic and hypotensive properties may be additive or potentiated (Thornton and Pray 1975). (3) Propranolol. TCAs may potentiate propranolol-induced depression of myocardial contractility and hypotension from central vasomotor regulatory centers (Griffin and O'Arcy 1975). (4) Opioids. There is an additive increase in the anticholinergic effects of opioids.

Pretreatment evaluation. Patients over 50 years old or who have a history of cardiovascular disease (stroke, myocardial infarction, angina, congestive heart failure, syncope, or arrhythmias) should have an electrocardiogram (EKG) and standing and supine blood pressures if treatment with TCAs is considered. Careful assessment of the risk/benefit ratio and cardiology consultation is indicated in the presence of bradyarrhythmias, heart block, or very long Q-T intervals. Orthostatic blood pressure changes of over 10 mm Hg before drug treatment are associated with pronounced postural changes during treatment, and these patients should be carefully observed. A careful drug history should be obtained, not only to assess possible drug interactions, but also to determine past response and side effects. Additional laboratory investigation should include a complete blood count with differential and liver function tests.

Treatment technique for chronic pain. Patients without evidence of complicating medical or psychiatric disorders are generally started on a dose of nortriptyline or desipramine at 10–25 mg at night, with 10–25-mg increases every 5 days to a dose of 50–75 mg daily. Failure of an adequate trial (e.g., plasma concentrations of 50–100 ng/mL) for 2–4 weeks can be addressed by dose escalation (i.e., 150 mg or more daily) (Dworkin and Schmader 2003). The drug is usually given at bedtime to take advantage of any sedating effects, although doses initially may be divided if a single dose produces excessive side effects. Elderly patients or those with cardiovascular disease should receive a 10–25-mg test dose and have orthostatic blood pressure determinations taken 1 hour later.

Because these agents are often poorly tolerated, careful dose titration and close follow-up are essential to assure adherence and maintain the patient in a course of therapy. Otherwise, it is common for the discontinuation rate to approach 30%. If a trial at steady state proves ineffective, tapering rather than abrupt discontinuation is indicated to avoid anticholinergic rebound, which creates a withdrawal syndrome. Tapering by dose reduction of 25–50% every 5 days is generally sufficient.

SELECTIVE NORADRENERGIC-SEROTONERGIC AND NORADRENERGIC-DOPAMINERGIC AGENTS

The SNRIs and NDRIs may become an attractive alternative to TCAs, given their superior side-effect profile. One randomized trial each of venlafaxine (Sindrup et al. 2003) and bupropion (Semenchuk et al. 2001) in diabetic neuropathic pain shows efficacy comparable to standard treatment. Venlafaxine at low and high doses inhibits serotonin reuptake, while at high doses (>225 mg daily) it potently inhibits norepinephrine uptake. In contrast to the classical antidepressants, venlafaxine does not interact with adrenergic, muscarinic cholinergic, histaminergic, or serotonergic receptors, nor with fast sodium channels of cardiac cells. This profile makes venlafaxine more tolerable and much safer for the medically ill than the older nonselective drugs. At low doses, side effects are similar to those seen with an SSRI (see below); at high doses noradrenergic effects of hypertension, tremor, and diaphoresis are evident. Given that noradrenergic activity is important to analgesia at least in some syndromes, doses should be in the higher range. Venlafaxine's disadvantages are induction of hypertension at high doses (in up to 3% of cases), which requires checks of blood pressure during the first 2 months of treatment, and the need for twice-daily dosing (Horst and Preskorn 1998).

Bupropion inhibits dopamine reuptake and increases norepinephrine neurotransmission without affecting serotonin mechanism, or α_1-adrenergic, muscarinic cholinergic, or H_1 receptors. Its side-effect profile includes dry mouth, dizziness, constipation, and agitation. It has no effects on cardiac conduction. Seizures are associated with doses exceeding 450 mg daily; the combination of fluoxetine with bupropion increases the likelihood of seizures. One disadvantage of bupropion is the need for twice-daily dosing (Horst and Preskorn 1998).

SELECTIVE SEROTONIN REUPTAKE INHIBITORS

Properties and side effects. The SSRIs have little affinity for muscarinic cholinergic receptors, α_1-adrenergic receptors, H_1 receptors, or voltage-dependent ion channels in the myocardium (Goodnick and Goldstein 1998). The resultant lack of significant sedation, anticholinergic effects, orthostasis, and QRS widening make the SSRIs safer and more tolerable agents.

Nonetheless, SSRIs are not without side effects, with sexual dysfunction in both men and women and gastrointestinal upset being common complaints. Sexual dysfunction may present in both sexes as delayed orgasm or anorgasmia, and in men as erectile difficulty (Cheer and Goa 2001). The gastrointestinal complaints are related to the propensity of serotonin to increase motility. Hence, patients may complain of frequent or loose bowel movements, nausea, "sour stomach," or dyspepsia. Early in treatment, patients may also note the relatively stimulating quality of these agents, and complain of initial insomnia, nervousness, or headache, all of which tend to dissipate after the first 1–2 weeks. Unfortunately, gastrointestinal and sexual side effects may persist despite attempts at dose reduction, and often represent a reason for termination of SSRI therapy (Goodnick and Goldstein 1998).

A rare and sometimes fatal side effect known as the serotonin syndrome may occur when multiple serotonergic agonist medications are used concomitantly, particularly the combination of SSRI antidepressants and monoamine oxidase inhibitors used primarily for refractory major depression (Figgitt and McClellan 2000). The presenting symptoms include muscular rigidity, hyperthermia, and autonomic instability, often with fluctuating vital signs and alterations in level of consciousness, and should prompt immediate discontinuation of the suspecting agents and hospitalization. The triptan antimigraine medications are agonists at the serotonin 1D receptor, so patients on these medications (almotriptan, frovatriptan, naratriptan, rizatriptan, sumatriptan, and zolmitriptan) should be warned about the possible interaction with SSRIs, as milder forms of the serotonin syndrome have been described when triptans are taken together with SSRI antidepressants.

Lastly, hyponatremia has rarely been reported in patients on SSRIs, with elderly females being the group most at risk. The elderly are also sensitive to the anorectic effects of SSRIs and may experience significant weight loss.

This unwanted weight loss may become an issue in more frail elderly patients (Muijsers et al. 2002).

SSRI antidepressants possess identical mechanisms of action, and are thus differentiated based upon their pharmacokinetics and inhibitory effects at various CYP isozymes (Baumann 1996a,b; Richelson 1997; Sproule et al. 1997; Sawada and Ohtani 2001). As can be seen in Table V, all of these agents, with the exception of fluvoxamine, have sufficiently long half-lives to be dosed on a daily basis, while fluoxetine and its major active metabolite norfluoxetine have an exceptionally long half-life and may be given as infrequently as once or twice per week. Both paroxetine and fluoxetine are available in extended-release forms, which are rarely prescribed due to the significant additional expense without any obvious therapeutic benefit.

Pharmacokinetic and pharmacodynamic drug interactions relevant to pain. The potential for pharmacokinetic drug interactions varies across the class of SSRI antidepressants, with fluoxetine being the agent most likely to incur such interactions due to its strong affinity for multiple CYP isozymes, and its extraordinarily long half-life. Fluoxetine should not be co-prescribed with TCAs, phenytoin, methadone, or propranolol (drugs dependent on CYP 2D6 for clearance), because reduction in clearance may result in serious toxicity. Sertraline and citalopram and its s-enantiomer (escitalopram) are the SSRIs least likely to cause significant drug interactions, and sertraline exhibits modest antagonism of CYP 2D6 that is unlikely to be of clinical relevance for most patients (von Moltke et al. 1999, 2001; Parker and Brown 2000). Although many SSRIs are highly protein bound, their site affinity rests primarily on glycoproteins, and not on albumin or prealbumin, and therefore the SSRIs have not been associated with toxicity related to displacement of protein-bound drugs with narrow therapeutic indices.

Table V
Kinetic properties of selected SSRI antidepressants

Drug	Dosage	Half-Life	Cytochrome P450 Inhibition
Fluoxetine*	20–60 mg p.o., q.d.	15 d	2C9, 2C19, 2D6, 3A4 (modest)
Citalopram	40–80 mg p.o., q.d. or q.h.s.	33 h	2C19 (weak)
Escitalopram	10–20 mg p.o., q.d. or q.h.s.	30 h	2C19, 2D6 (weak)
Sertraline	50–150 mg p.o., q.d.	26 h	2D6 (modest)
Paroxetine	20–60 mg p.o., q.d. or q.h.s.	21 h	2D6
Fluvoxamine	50–100 mg p.o., b.i.d.	22 h	1A2, 2C19 3A4

* Includes its active metabolite norfluoxetine.

Pretreatment evaluation. As with other antidepressants, a prior history of mania should be considered a relative contraindication to SSRI use without careful psychiatric consultation, and such a history should be ruled out before initiating therapy. No other pretreatment evaluation is necessary for patients commencing SSRI therapy beyond an initial scrutiny of currently prescribed medications and over-the-counter preparations for possible interactions.

Treatment technique. To minimize the initial complaints of nervousness or headache, SSRI therapy is typically initiated at one-half of the average therapeutic dosage, and titrated up over the course of 1–2 weeks. Patients with a history of panic disorder are exquisitely sensitive to the initial anxiety-inducing effects of SSRIs and should be started at one-fourth of the typical starting dose to prevent exacerbation of this effect, and titrated more slowly. Except for fluoxetine, all of the SSRIs will reach steady-state serum levels within 1 week after dose increase.

Although discontinuation side effects are not as prevalent as with TCAs, there is a distinct but usually mild serotonin withdrawal syndrome characterized by restlessness, anxiety, dizziness or dysequilibrium, paresthesias, nausea, and tremor. These symptoms occur most often in patients withdrawn abruptly from the shorter half-life SSRIs, but have been reported with all agents except fluoxetine (Bull et al. 2002). The symptoms are reversed upon resumption of the prior medication, but can be avoided by gradually tapering the SSRI over 1–2 weeks. Occasionally patients will report that one SSRI is more tolerable than another, so many clinicians who wish to switch will simply cross-taper the two agents. All of the SSRIs, with one notable exception, will be cleared within 1 week after the last dose, and thus will have no further potential for drug interactions; however, patients stopping fluoxetine will have therapeutic serum levels of its active metabolite norfluoxetine for several weeks after discontinuation, thereby posing ongoing pharmacokinetic issues during that time frame.

ANTICONVULSANTS/MOOD STABILIZERS

PROPERTIES AND SIDE EFFECTS

Four anticonvulsants are widely used for the treatment of chronic pain disorders (gabapentin, lamotrigine, valproate, and carbamazepine). As noted previously, lamotrigine, valproate, and carbamazepine slow the recovery rate in voltage-dependent sodium channels. Gabapentin appears to modulate the calcium flux through Ca^{2+}-dependent channels, as may lamotrigine. Gabapentin and valproate may also indirectly enhance neurotransmission at inhibitory γ-aminobutyric acid (GABA) synapses through reduction of GABA breakdown or stimulating increased presynaptic release (Leppik 2002). Which of these pharmacodynamic effects is necessary for the antinociceptive properties of the anticonvulsants is not clear, so the choice of agent is guided exclusively by results of clinical trials.

Anticonvulsants also have some common side effects, particularly the CNS properties of sedation, dizziness, and ataxia, which become more prevalent at higher serum levels. Table VI outlines the typical dosages, serum levels where appropriate, and side effects for the commonly used anticonvulsants for chronic pain conditions. Among the rare but important idiosyncratic side effects to be aware of are hyperammonemia with valproate, particularly in patients with urea cycle enzyme deficiencies, and Stevens-Johnson syndrome (erythema multiforme) with lamotrigine. Hyperammonemia should be suspected when a patient on valproate presents with ataxia delirium, which may evolve as the drug is titrated upwards, but which also may be episodic (e.g. post-dose confusion that resolves after several hours). Obtaining a serum ammonia level during a suspected episode is diagnostic

Table VI
Properties of anticonvulsants commonly used for pain

Drug	Dosing (Serum Level)	Common Side Effects	Pharmacokinetic Interactions
Carbamazepine	400–800 mg p.o. b.i.d. (6–12 μg/mL)	Bone marrow: transient leukopenia 10%; rare purpura, thrombo-cytopenia; hyponatremia; neurological: dizziness, ataxia, sedation	Induces CYP 1A2, 2C19, 3A4; 75% protein bound
Lamotrigine	50–200 mg p.o. b.i.d.	CNS: sedation, ataxia, diplopia, headache; benign rash 11%; Stevens-Johnson <0.1% (risk increased by rapid titration or concurrent valproate)	None (see valproate)
Gabapentin	100–1200 mg p.o. t.i.d.	CNS: sedation, ataxia, dizziness	None
Valproate	500–1000 mg p.o. b.i.d. or 1000–2000 mg h.s. for extended-release form (50–100 μg/mL)	CNS: sedation, tremor, dizziness, ataxia; nausea (especially with valproate sodium); weight gain; elevated transaminases; thrombocytopenia; rare: hyperammonemia, pancreatitis	80–94% protein bound; inhibits metabolism of 10,11 epoxide metabolite of carbamazepine; increases lamotrigine levels 2–3-fold

(Jensen 2002). While Stevens-Johnson syndrome occurs in fewer than 1% of patients on lamotrigine, a rash of any type may be seen in 10%, so the clinician is obliged to consider discontinuing lamotrigine if a suspect rash develops to prevent evolution from a benign rash to the potentially life-threatening Stevens-Johnson syndrome. As noted below, slow dose titration and significant dose reduction with concomitant valproate therapy helps minimize the risk of Stevens-Johnson syndrome in patients starting lamotrigine (Jensen 2002).

DRUG INTERACTIONS RELEVANT TO PAIN

Unlike the SSRI antidepressants, which tend to inhibit CYP 450 activity, carbamazepine may interfere with the action of other medications through its ability to induce the activity of CYP 3A4, thereby decreasing the serum levels of agents that rely upon 3A4 for at least 50% of their metabolism (Spina et al. 1996). None of the other anticonvulsants used for pain have significant effects on CYP 450 enzymes, but they may displace highly protein-bound medications, thereby increasing the free fraction available. Gabapentin has no significant drug interactions at all because it is excreted renally, it neither induces nor inhibits P450 isozymes, and it has low protein binding.

PRETREATMENT EVALUATION

Manufacturers of many anticonvulsants have a list of recommended baseline laboratory evaluations to perform, which should be followed in most patients. Renal impairment (i.e., creatinine > 1.8 mg/dL) is a relative contraindication to gabapentin, although dosing guidelines are available to address its use in such patients. Lamotrigine does not necessitate any pretreatment evaluation. For carbamazepine, the following should be obtained prior to treatment and monitored periodically during therapy: complete blood count with platelets, serum sodium, and transaminases.

TREATMENT TECHNIQUE

Rapid dose titration tends to maximize the CNS side effects of these agents, especially sedation, and in the case of lamotrigine significantly increases the risk for developing Stevens-Johnson syndrome. Generally, most anticonvulsants can be titrated over 2–4 weeks to average clinical dosages, bearing in mind the wide dosage range for some compounds such as gabapentin (Leppik 2002). Lamotrigine, however, must be titrated over 1 month or more using the following schedule for patients who are not receiving concurrent valproate therapy: 50 mg/day for 2 weeks, then 100 mg/day for 2 weeks. If necessary, the dose can increase by 100 mg/day weekly to a maximum dose of 500 mg/day. In those receiving valproate, this titration is decreased fourfold to 25 mg every other day for 2 weeks, then 25 mg/day for 2 weeks. Increases of 25 mg/day weekly can occur after the initial 4-week titration to a maximum dosage of 150 mg/day (Leppik 2002). Although there are well-defined serum levels for employing many of these agents in epilepsy treatment, serum levels should be used mostly as guides to patient compliance and as an indication of the maximum tolerable serum level, because pain conditions may respond at dosages that are considered subtherapeutic for control of seizure disorders.

TREATMENT DISCONTINUATION

In patients without a history of seizure disorder, abrupt discontinuation of anticonvulsants carries a low risk for withdrawal seizures. Nevertheless, it is best to taper patients off of medication over 4–7 days whenever possible. Cross-tapering of anticonvulsant agents can occur with the following caveats: CYP 3A4 enzyme induction from carbamazepine will take approximately 2 weeks to resolve after discontinuation, so dosage adjustment may be necessary for new or ongoing drug therapy with medications metabolized via CYP 3A4 (Spina et al. 1996); the steady state half-life of valproate is 12–16 hours in adults, so one should allow a minimum of 5 days to elapse after the last dose of valproate before commencing lamotrigine to lessen the risk of pharmacokinetic drug interactions in patients switching to lamotrigine.

ANALYSIS OF TREATMENT RESULTS

In psychiatric literature, true treatment resistance can be defined as "inadequate response to two successive courses of monotherapy with pharmacologically different drugs given with adequate doses for a sufficient duration" (Hirschfeld et al. 2002). This is also a reasonable definition for chronic pain, but it is important to distinguish true nonresponse from apparent treatment failure or resistance. Leading sources of apparent treatment resistance are presented in Table VII. Minimizing and managing side effects is crucial to adherence and to retaining patients in treatment (McElroy et al. 1995). Many patients will not spontaneously report side effects, sometimes because of embarrassment in the case of sexual side effects, so standardized inquiry for side effects is advisable because it may uncover complaints that otherwise

Table VII
Leading sources of treatment failure

Intolerance of side effects
Nonadherence
Comorbid psychiatric disorder
Comorbid substance use disorder
Improper drug selection/dose
Inadequate treatment duration
Misdiagnosis

Source: Adapted from Hirschfeld et al. (2002).

would lead to silent dropout from treatment (Rosen and Marin 2003). Successful treatment of chronic pain is virtually impossible in the face of concurrent alcohol or drug abuse or dependence. Diagnosis usually depends on a high index of suspicion and careful history from patients and family members, although laboratory testing may be helpful (elevated γ-glutamyltransferase [GGT] and positive urine toxicology). Major depression, being associated with reports of increased pain intensity and poor daily functioning, may limit treatment efficacy. Major depression often responds to the drugs and dosages proven effective for selected chronic pain diagnoses, so even undiagnosed depression could be inadvertently but successfully treated, although 30% of major depressive disorders do not respond to the first antidepressant trial, and a greater proportion of cases are only partially responsive. Management of treatment-resistant depression requires expert psychiatric consultation (Hirschfeld et al. 2002). Panic disorder, another source of failure to return to function, is associated with at least one chronic pain state, namely migraine headache. Treatment efficacy for each of the psychotropics depends on establishing at least a modest serum concentration, while onset of response may take up to 2 weeks or more. It is crucial to determine whether patients took medications irregularly, on an "as-needed" basis, or for less than the minimum duration. Nevertheless, given a therapeutic alliance, careful attention to matching of diagnosis and patient-specific factors, and a systematic approach, one can expect satisfying results when psychotropics are used as adjuncts in the treatment of many chronic pain disorders.

ACKNOWLEDGMENT

Supported in part by the Department of Veterans Affairs.

REFERENCES

Atkinson JH, Slater MA, Williams RA, et al. A placebo-controlled randomized clinical trial of nortriptyline for chronic low back pain. *Pain* 1998; 76(3):287–296.

Atkinson JH, Slater MA, Wahlgren DR, et al. Effects of noradrenergic and serotonergic antidepressants on chronic low back pain intensity. *Pain* 1999; 83:137–145.

Backonja M, Beydoun A, Edwards KR, et al. Gabapentin for the symptomatic treatment of painful neuropathy in patients with diabetes mellitus: a randomized controlled trial. *JAMA* 1998; 280:1831–1836.

Basbaum AI, Fields HL. Endogenous pain control mechanisms: review and hypothesis. *Ann Neurol* 1978; 4:451–462.

Baumann P. Pharmacokinetic-pharmacodynamic relationship of the selective serotonin reuptake inhibitors. *Clin Pharmacokinet* 1996a; 31:444–469.

Baumann P. Pharmacology and pharmacokinetics of citalopram and other SSRIs. *Int Clin Psychopharmacol* 1996b; 11(Suppl 1):5–11.

Bigger JT, Kantor SJ, Glassman AH, Perel JM. Cardiovascular effects of tricyclic antidepressant drugs. In: Lipton MA, DeMascio A, Killam KF (Eds). *Psychopharmacology: A Generation of Progress.* New York: Raven Press, 1978.

Boakes AJ, Laurence DR, Teoh PC, et al. Interactions between sympathomimetic amines and antidepressant agents in man. *BMJ* 1973; 1:311–315.

Bull SA, Hunkeler EM, Lee JY, et al. Discontinuing or switching selective serotonin-reuptake inhibitors. *Ann Pharmacother* 2002; 36:578–584.

Chadda VS, Mathur MS. Double blind study of the effects of diphenylhydantoin sodium on diabetic neuropathy. *J Assoc Phys Ind* 1978; 26:403–406.

Cheer SM, Goa KL. Fluoxetine: a review of its therapeutic potential in the treatment of depression associated with physical illness. *Drugs* 2001; 61:81–110.

Cook DJ, Guyatt GH, Laupacis A, Sackett DL, Goldberg RJ. Clinical recommendations using levels of evidence for antithrombotic agents. *Chest* 1995; 108(Suppl 4):227S–230S.

Cozza KL, Armstrong SC. *Concise Guide to the Cytochrome P450 System: Drug Interaction Principles for Medical Practice.* Washington, DC: American Psychiatric Press, 2001.

Deyo RA. Conservative therapy for low back pain: distinguishing useful from useless therapy. *JAMA* 1983; 250:1057–1062.

Dworkin RH, Schmader KE. Treatment and prevention of postherpetic neuralgia. *Clin Infect Dis* 2003; 36:877–882.

Eisenberg E, Lurie Y, Braker C, Daoud D, Ishay A. Lamotrigine reduces painful diabetic neuropathy: a randomized, controlled study. *Neurology* 2001; 57:505–509

Evidence Based Medicine Working Group. Evidence-based medicine: a new approach to teaching the practice of medicine. *JAMA* 1992; 268:2420–2425.

Fait ML, Wise MG, Jachna JS, Lane RD, Gelenberg AJ. Psychopharmacology. In: Wise MG, Rundell JR (Eds). *Textbook of Consultation-Liaison Psychiatry.* Washington, DC: American Psychiatric Publishing, 2001, pp 939–987.

Farrar, JT, Young JP, LaMoreaux L, Werth JL, Poole RM. Clinical importance of changes in chronic pain intensity measured on an 11-point numerical pain rating scale. *Pain* 2001; 94:149–158.

Figgitt DP, McClellan KJ. Fluvoxamine: an updated review of its use in the management of adults with anxiety disorders. *Drugs* 2000; 60:925–954.

Fishbain DA, Cutler RB, Rosomoff HL, Rosomoff RS. Do antidepressants have an analgesic effect in psychogenic pain and somatoform pain disorder? A meta-analysis. *Psychosom Med* 1998; 60:503–509.

Gilmor ML, Owens MJ, Nemeroff CB. Inhibition of norepinephrine uptake in patients with major depression treated with paroxetine. *Am J Psychiatry* 2002; 159:1702–1710.

Goodnick PJ, Goldstein BJ. Selective serotonin reuptake inhibitors in affective disorders—I. Basic pharmacology. *J Psychopharmacol* 1998; 12:S5–20.

Griffin JP, O'Arcy PF (Eds). *A Manual of Adverse Drug Interactions.* Bristol: John Wright and Sons, 1975.

Hirschfeld RMA, Montgomery SA, Aguglia E, et al. Partial response and nonresponse to antidepressant therapy: current approaches and treatment options. *J Clin Psychiatry* 2002; 63:826–837.

Horst WD, Preskorn SH. Mechanisms of action and clinical characteristics of three atypical antidepressants: venlafaxine, nefazodone, bupropion. *J Affect Disord* 1998; 51:237–254.

Ioannides C. Pharmacokinetic interactions between herbal remedies and medicinal drugs. *Xenobiotica* 2002; 32:451–478.

Jackson JL, O'Malley PG, Tomkins G, et al. Treatment of functional gastrointestinal disorders with antidepressant medications: a meta-analysis. *Am J Med* 2000; 108:65–72.

Jensen TS. Anticonvulsants in neuropathic pain: rationale and clinical evidence. *Eur J Pain* 2002; 6(Suppl A):61–68.

Kirchheiner J, Brosen K, Dahl ML, et al. CYP2D6 and CYP2C19 genotype-based dose recommendations for antidepressants: a first step towards subpopulation-specific dosages [erratum appears in *Acta Psychiatr Scand* 2001 Dec;104(6):475]. *Acta Psychiatr Scand* 2001; 104:173–192.

Kochar DK, Jain N, Agarwal RP, et al. Sodium valproate in the management of painful neuropathy in type 2 diabetes: a randomized placebo controlled study. *Acta Neurol Scand* 2002; 106:248–252.

Leppik IE. *Contemporary Diagnosis and Management of the Patient with Epilepsy,* Handbooks in Health Care. Newtown, PA: Associates in Medical Marketing, 2002.

Marangell LB, Silver JM, Goff DC, Yudofsky SC. Psychopharmacology and electro-convulsive therapy. In: Hales R, Yudofsky SC (Eds). *Textbook of Clinical Psychiatry*, 4th ed. Washington, DC: American Psychiatric Publishing, 2003, pp 1041–1180.

Max MB. Antidepressants as analgesics. In: Fields HL, Liebeskind JC (Eds). *Pharmacological Approaches to the Treatment of Chronic Pain: New Concepts and Critical Issues,* Progress in Pain Research and Management, Vol. 1. Seattle: IASP Press, 1994, pp 229–246.

Max MB, Kishore-Kumar R, Schafer SC, et al. Efficacy of desipramine in painful diabetic neuropathy: a placebo-controlled trial. *Pain* 1991; 45:3–9.

Max MB, Lynch SA, Muir J, et al. Effects of desipramine, amitriptyline and fluoxetine on pain in diabetic neuropathy. *N Engl J Med* 1992; 326:1250–1256.

McElroy SL, Keck PE, Friedman LM. Minimizing and managing antidepressant side effects. *J Clin Psychiatry* 1995; 56(Suppl 2):49–55.

McQuay HJ, Moore RA. Antidepressants and chronic pain. *BMJ* 1997; 314:763–764.

Morello CM, Leckband SG, Stoner CP, Moorhouse DF, Sahagian GA. Randomized double-blind study comparing the efficacy of gabapentin with amitriptyline on diabetic peripheral neuropathy pain. *Arch Intern Med* 1999; 159:1931–1937.

Muijsers RB, Plosker GL, Noble S. Sertraline: a review of its use in the management of major depressive disorder in elderly patients. *Drugs Aging* 2002; 19:377–392.

Olesen OV, Linnet K. Metabolism of the tricyclic antidepressant amitriptyline by cDNA-expressed human cytochrome P450 enzymes. *Pharmacology* 1997; 55:235–243.

O'Malley PG, Balden E, Tomkins G, et al. Treatment of fibromyalgia with antidepressants: a meta-analysis. *J Gen Intern Med* 2000;15:659–666.

Parker NG, Brown CS. Citalopram in the treatment of depression. *Ann Pharmacother* 2000; 34:761–771.

Rice AS, Maton S. Gabapentin in postherpetic neuralgia: a randomised, double blind, placebo controlled study. *Pain* 2001; 94:215–224.

Richelson E. Pharmacokinetic drug interactions of new antidepressants: a review of the effects on the metabolism of other drugs. *Mayo Clin Proc* 1997; 72:835–847.

Richelson E. Pharmacology of antidepressants. *Mayo Clin Proc* 2001; 76:511–527.

Risch SC, Groom GP, Janowsky DS. Interfaces of psychopharmacology and cardiology, Part I and II. *J Clin Psychiatry* 1981; 42:23–34, 47–59.

Roose SP, Glassman AH, Giardina EG, et al. Tricyclic antidepressants in depressed patients with cardiac conduction disease. *Arch Gen Psychiatry* 1987; 44:273–275.

Rosen RC, Marin H. Prevalence of antidepressant-associated erectile dysfunction. *J Clin Psychiatry* 2003; 10:5–10.

Rowbotham M, Harden N, Stacey B, Bernstein P, Magnus-Miller L. Gabapentin for the treatment of postherpetic neuralgia: a randomized controlled trial. *JAMA* 1998; 280:1837–1842.

Rudorfer MV, Potter WZ. Metabolism of tricyclic antidepressants. *Cell Mol Neurobiol* 1999;19:373–409.

Rull JA, Quibrera R, Gonzalez-Millian H, Castaneda OL. Symptomatic treatment of peripheral diabetic neuropathy with carbamazepine (Tegretol®): double blind crossover trial. *Diabetologia* 1969; 5:215–218.

Salerno SM, Browning R, Jackson JL. The effect of antidepressant treatment on chronic back pain: a meta-analysis. *Arch Intern Med* 2002; 162:19–24.

Sawada Y, Ohtani H. Pharmacokinetics and drug interactions of antidepressive agents. *Nippon Rinsho* 2001; 59:1539–1545.

Semenchuk MR, Sherman S, Davis B. Double-blind, randomized trial of bupropion SR for the treatment of neuropathic pain. *Neurology* 2001; 57:1583–1588.

Simpson DM, Olney R, McArthur JC, et al. A placebo-controlled trial of lamotrigine for painful HIV-associated neuropathy. *Neurology* 2000; 54:2115–2119.

Sindrup SH, Jensen TS. Efficacy of pharmacologic treatments of neuropathic pain: an update and effect related mechanism of drug action. *Pain* 1999; 83:389–400.

Sindrup SH, Jensen TS. Pharmacologic treatment of pain in polyneuropathy. *Neurology* 2000; 55:915–920.

Sindrup SH, Gram LF, Broen K, Eshoj O, Mogensen DF. The selective serotonin reuptake inhibitor paroxetine is effective in the treatment of diabetic neuropathy symptoms. *Pain* 1990; 42:135–144.

Sindrup SH, Bjerre U, Dejgaard A, et al. The selective serotonin reuptake inhibitor citalopram relieves the symptoms of diabetic neuropathy. *Clin Pharmacol Ther* 1992; 52:547–552.

Sindrup SH, Bach FW, Madsen C, Gram LF, Jensen TS. Venlafaxine versus imipramine in painful polyneuropathy: a randomized, controlled trial. *Neurology* 2003; 60:1284–1289.

Spina E, Pisani F, Perucca E. Clinically significant pharmacokinetic drug interactions with carbamazepine: an update. *Clin Pharmacokinet* 1996; 31:198–214.

Sproule BA, Naranjo CA, Brenmer KE, Hassan PC. Selective serotonin reuptake inhibitors and CNS drug interactions: a critical review of the evidence. *Clin Pharmacokinet* 1997; 33:454–471.

Stahl SM. *Psychopharmacology of Antidepressants*. London: Martin Dunitz, 1998.

Thornton WE, Pray RJ. Combination drug therapy in psychopharmacology. *J Clin Pharmacol* 1975; 15:511–517.

Tomkins GE, Jackson JL, O'Malley PG, Balden E, Santoro JE. Treatment of chronic headache with antidepressants: a meta-analysis. *Am J Med* 2001; 111:54–63.

Turner JA, Deyo RA, Loeser JD, Von Korff M, Fordyce WE. The importance of placebo effects in pain treatment and research. *JAMA* 1994; 20:1609–1614.

Vestergaard K, Andersen G, Gottrup H, Kristensen BT, Jensen TS. Lamotrigine for central poststroke pain. *Neurology* 2001; 56:184–190.

von Moltke LL, Greenblatt DJ, Grassi JM, et al. Citalopram and desmethylcitalopram in vitro: human cytochromes mediating transformation, and cytochrome inhibitory effects. *Biol Psychiatry* 1999; 46:839–849.

von Moltke LL, Greenblatt DJ, Giancarlo GM, et al. Escitalopram (S-citalopram) and its metabolites in vitro: cytochromes mediating biotransformation, inhibitory effects, and comparison to R-citalopram. *Drug Metab Dispos* 2001; 29:1102–1109.

Watson CPN, Evans RJ. A comparative trial of amitriptyline and zimelidine in postherpetic neuralgia. *Pain* 1985; 23:387–394.

Watson CPN, Chipman M, Reed K, Dvans RJ, Birkett N. Amitriptyline versus maprotiline in postherpetic neuralgia: a randomized, double-blind, crossover trial. *Pain* 1992; 48:29–36.
Woolf CJ, Mannion FJ. Neuropathic pain: aetiology, symptoms, mechanisms, and management. *Lancet* 1999; 353:1959–1964.
Zakrzewska JM, Chaudhry Z, Nurmikko TJ, Patton DW, Mullens EL. Lamotrigine (lamictal) in refractory trigeminal neuralgia: results from a double-blind placebo controlled crossover trial. *Pain* 1997; 73:223–230.

Correspondence to: J. Hampton Atkinson, MD, Department of Psychiatry, School of Medicine, University of California, San Diego, 9500 Gilman Drive, La Jolla, CA 92039, USA.

Psychosocial Aspects of Pain: A Handbook for Health Care Providers, Progress in Pain Research and Management, Vol. 27, edited by Robert H. Dworkin and William S. Breitbart, IASP Press, Seattle, © 2004.

12

The Essence of Cognitive-Behavioral Pain Management

Sandra J. Waters, Lisa C. Campbell, Francis J. Keefe, and James W. Carson

Department of Psychiatry, Duke University Medical Center, Durham, North Carolina, USA

Over the past 25 years, cognitive-behavioral treatment has emerged as a viable and empirically validated approach to managing patients with persistent pain (Compas et al. 1998). Cognitive-behavioral treatment protocols are effective for disease-related pain conditions such as arthritis (Keefe et al. 2002), cancer (Syrjala et al. 1995), and sickle cell disease (Gil et al. 1989) as well as for nonmalignant chronic pain conditions such as low back pain (Morley et al. 1999), tension headache, and migraine headache (Compas et al. 1998).

Most protocols for cognitive-behavioral pain management have been developed, refined, and utilized by psychologists with expertise in pain management. Reports documenting the efficacy of cognitive-behavioral treatment have appeared in psychology and behavioral science journals. As a result, many health professionals working in pain management, such as physicians, nurses, occupational therapists, and physical therapists, are relatively unfamiliar with the principles and methods used in cognitive-behavioral therapy.

This chapter provides health professionals who are not versed in cognitive-behavioral therapy with a description of the basic elements of this treatment approach. The chapter is divided into three sections. In the first section, we describe behavioral therapy techniques that form the foundation of cognitive-behavioral treatment. We outline the basic steps involved in implementing each technique and present methods for troubleshooting common problems that may arise. In the second section, we provide a similar description of cognitive therapy techniques used in pain management. The third section discusses ways in which behavioral and cognitive therapy techniques can be integrated into clinical practice.

BEHAVIORAL THERAPY TECHNIQUES

Behavioral therapy techniques are based on learning principles derived from instrumental or operant conditioning (Keefe and Lefebvre 1999). Fordyce (1976) was the first to clearly articulate how these principles could be applied to the understanding and treatment of patients with persistent pain. He maintained that learning principles are especially relevant in understanding learned pain behavior patterns. Fordyce used the term *pain behavior* to refer to behaviors that serve to communicate to others the fact that pain is being experienced. Such behaviors might include verbal descriptions or complaints of pain, excessive bed rest, guarded movement, or pain-related facial expressions (Keefe and Lefebvre 1999). Pain behaviors frequently occur in the context of acute pain, where it can be quite adaptive in terms of reducing pain and eliciting help from others. However, for some patients, pain behaviors persist long after the normal healing time for an injury (Keefe and Lefebvre 1999). Behavioral therapists maintain that, in such cases, social learning processes can affect the maintenance of pain behaviors (Keefe and Lefebvre 1994). Avoidance of activity, for example, can be reinforced by an overly solicitous spouse or by being relieved of unwanted home or work responsibilities. Behavioral therapists argue that learning processes are particularly likely to play an important role in maintaining pain behaviors that are excessive or inappropriate given the extent of the underlying tissue pathology (Keefe and Lefebvre 1994).

Behavioral techniques for managing chronic pain have two major goals (Keefe et al. 1986). The first is to increase the frequency of *well behaviors*—adaptive behaviors that are incompatible with pain behavior. For sedentary patients one of the most important well behaviors is "uptime" (time spent out of the reclining position). Activity-pacing interventions can be helpful in increasing uptime (Gil et al. 1988). Given that many patients lead very restricted lifestyles, another key aim is to increase their involvement in valued and pleasurable activities through activity scheduling (Lewinsohn et al. 1990; Rohde et al. 2001). The second major goal of behavioral treatment is to decrease maladaptive pain behaviors. Behavioral techniques such as activity pacing, social reinforcement, and time-contingent medications are often used to reduce excessive bed rest, limit reliance on pain medication, and diminish inappropriate verbal pain behaviors such as excessive "pain talk" and motor pain behaviors such as exaggerated pain-avoidant posturing (Keefe 2000).

Although the behavioral therapy techniques described below were initially developed for patients with nonmalignant chronic pain whose pain behavior was exaggerated or inconsistent, over the past 15 years these techniques have found broader application (Gil et al. 1989; Keefe et al. 2002).

Behavioral methods are increasingly used as part of the treatment of patients with disease-related pain conditions such as cancer pain. Although the disease itself may place limits on the goals of behavioral therapy, techniques such as activity pacing and social reinforcement can improve function and help patients adjust to pain.

ACTIVITY PACING

A primary goal of behavioral therapy is to increase the activity of chronic pain patients who have developed an overly sedentary and restricted lifestyle (Gil et al. 1989). To accomplish this goal, therapists must teach patients how to increase their activity level by pacing their activities. Activity pacing involves dividing the day into activity and rest cycles (periods of limited activity followed by limited rest) and then, over time, gradually increasing the time spent engaging in activity and decreasing rest time. Activity pacing involves four steps.

Step 1: Establish a baseline level of activity. To establish a baseline measure of daily activity, the clinician should ask the patient to keep a daily diary record. In this daily record, the patient should note the amount of time spent hourly engaging in three categories of activity (sitting, standing or walking, and reclining). To provide a baseline estimate of activity, the clinician should graph the daily amount of uptime from 5 to 7 days of record keeping and examine patterns of activity level to calculate an average level of uptime.

Step 2: Establish a target level of uptime. Analysis of the baseline data should yield a specific target level of daily uptime (usually 10–15% less than the baseline). In addition, specific time goals for activity-rest cycles should be set. Each cycle is broken down into an activity period that is manageable for the patient (e.g., 30 minutes up and out of the reclining position) and a limited rest period (e.g., 15 minutes resting or reclining). The patient is instructed to pace daily activities using the activity-rest cycle.

Step 3: Repeat the activity-rest cycle. The patient should repeat the activity-rest cycle frequently throughout about 70% of the waking day. Over the course of treatment, the duration of the activity portion of the activity-rest cycle is increased while the amount of rest is decreased. Over a matter of weeks, a patient might build from an initial activity-rest cycle of 30 minutes up and 15 minutes down to 75 minutes up and 5 minutes down. To provide a visual record of progress, the clinician should keep a graph of the total daily uptime and review this graph in treatment sessions with the patient.

Step 4: Troubleshoot. Several common problems occur in implementing an activity-rest cycle (Gil et al. 1989; Waters et al. 2002). First, the patient may overestimate the baseline level of activity, perhaps because of inaccurate record keeping. As a result, the initial activity goals may be set too high. To avoid this problem, initial activity goals should be set 10–15% below the average for the baseline. Also, if initial activity goals appear too high, the clinician should reduce them to a lower level as soon as possible. Second, the patient may become engrossed in an activity and forget that is time to take a rest. The fact that activity can be so distracting is a positive sign that suggests that activity is self-reinforcing. However, the danger is that patients will lapse back into a pain cycle pattern by persisting with the activity until their pain becomes so severe that they have to stop. The best way to solve this problem is to encourage the patient to purchase a countdown timer so that he or she can program the duration of the activity period and receive a warning beep when the session comes to an end. Third, the patient may fall asleep during the rest period, particularly if it is taken in bed in a fully reclining position or if the patient is experiencing drowsiness as a medication side effect. To avoid this problem, the patient can rest in a busy area of the house and remain alert while resting. Careful adjustment of the patient's medication intake may also be required to address side effects.

PLEASANT ACTIVITY SCHEDULING

Many patients with persistent pain significantly reduce their involvement in once-pleasurable activities (Ross et al. 1988; Waters et al. 2002). As a result, their days are uneventful and provide few, if any, distractions from pain. A decrease in pleasant activities can bring increased depression and physical deconditioning. Pleasant activity scheduling provides a systematic method for gradually increasing the frequency and range of distracting activities.

Step 1: Brainstorm. During brainstorming, patients are encouraged to develop a broad list of activities they consider meaningful and pleasurable (Waters et al. 2002). Helpful brainstorming rules include: (a) anything goes—patients should list any activity they can think of, regardless of whether they currently engage in it, and clinicians should avoid making critical or evaluative comments about any activity; (b) the more the merrier—patients should try to identify at least 20 to 30 different pleasant activities; and (c) mix and match—patients should be encouraged to mix together different pleasant activities in imaginative and creative ways.

Step 2: Identify activity goals. In this step patients evaluate the list generated during brainstorming and identify specific activity goals that can be completed within the coming week. Typically, two to three goals are identified. The patient should be taught how to set goals that are specific, measurable, and achievable. Over time, the number and difficulty of activity goals are gradually increased as a means of helping patients reach their long-term objectives.

Step 3: Monitor and reinforce goal attainment. In this step, a simple graph is used to track the number of goals accomplished each week (Ross et al. 1988). Graphing and discussing the goals attained can be very beneficial and can serve to reward a patient's effort and progress. As goals are accomplished, patients are encouraged to use pleasant activities to reward themselves. For example, a patient who has increased his tolerance for walking might reward himself with a trip to his favorite art museum.

Step 4: Troubleshoot. The major impediment to implementing pleasant activity scheduling is that the patient selects activity goals that are too physically demanding. When the therapist suspects that a given goal is too difficult, he or she should actively encourage the patient to modify the goal to make it achievable. For example, a patient with limited sitting tolerance who sets a goal of going out to a restaurant for a 2-hour dinner with his wife might be encouraged to set a more realistic initial goal of a 30-minute coffee and dessert outing. Another problem is that patients who have been inactive for a long time or who are depressed often have difficulty identifying potentially pleasurable goals. One strategy we have found helpful in dealing with this problem is to look through newspaper listings of local events together and discuss activities that might be enjoyable. Such discussions often lead to a broader exploration of the patient's interests and can be helpful in identifying specific short- and long-term activity goals.

SOCIAL REINFORCEMENT

Behavioral therapists maintain that social reinforcement can have a major influence on pain behaviors and well behaviors (Fordyce 1976; Moore and Chaney 1985; Keefe et al. 1996). For example, a health care professional who shows interest in a patient's progress with an exercise program can increase the likelihood that the patient will persevere. Alternatively, an overly solicitous spouse or family member who criticizes the patient for trying to do household chores can increase the likelihood that the patient will spend more time reclining. Social reinforcement can be used as part of a behavioral therapy program to help patients achieve their goals (Keefe et al. 1996). It is important that those involved in the treatment team as well as those in the home environment receive systematic training in reinforcement techniques.

Step 1: Present rationale and training to increase well behaviors. An important step in behavioral treatment is teaching significant others to reinforce the well behaviors, including participation in pleasant activities, that are the key targets of treatment (Fordyce 1976). Significant others typically show a propensity to respond to pain behaviors and worry that increasing activity will increase the patient's pain. Training should focus on the long-term benefits, for both the patient and his or her significant other, of the patient's return to a more active lifestyle. Patients and their partners should identify specific well behaviors that are the targets for social reinforcement efforts (e.g., engaging in exercise, or going out of the house each day). They also should be encouraged to develop innovative strategies for delivering daily reinforcement (e.g., a hug, a squeeze of the hand, or a brief kiss). Intermittent reinforcers can also be built into the program: for example, a spouse might purchase exercise clothes for the patient who has followed through on his or her exercise program for several weeks.

Step 2. Present rationale and training to decrease pain behaviors. Discussions with the patient and significant others are typically needed to identify the specific maladaptive pain behaviors that are reinforced by the significant other (Fordyce 1976; Keefe and Lefebvre 1999). The short-term effects of reinforcing these behaviors (e.g., providing temporary pain relief for the patient or reducing distress for a solicitous spouse) are then contrasted with the long-term effects of reducing reinforcement (e.g., increasing the patient's tolerance for activity or reducing his or her dependency on the spouse). Role playing is often used to teach significant others how to reduce attention to and reinforcement of pain behaviors, while simultaneously increasing reinforcement for well behaviors.

Step 3: Troubleshoot. Giving and receiving positive reinforcement from a significant other can be more challenging than one would think. Before putting a social reinforcement program into effect it is important to discuss how the patient and others involved feel about this approach to behavior change. A number of issues typically arise. A spouse, for example, may view the systematic use of praise or encouragement as a form of bribery. It is often helpful to point out that the definition of bribery is to use something positive to induce someone to engage in a behavior that is illegal or immoral. Thus, the use of praise to help someone better adjust to pain does not constitute bribery. Social reinforcement can be likened to a crutch—a tool that is used temporarily to help someone to achieve a goal, but is put aside once that goal is achieved. Second, the patient may feel uncomfortable receiving verbal praise (e.g., "good job") from a partner. In such a case, it is often helpful to have the patient and partner work out other potentially effective ways of providing reinforcement (e.g., engaging the patient in a pleasant conversation, turning on a favorite music selection, or providing a hug). Finally, it is important that the schedule of social reinforcement be reduced over time. During the initial stages of a behavioral program, positive reinforcement should be immediate and consistent. However, once the patient has made progress and is following through with many elements of the program, social reinforcement should be provided on a more intermittent basis.

TIME-CONTINGENT MEDICATIONS

Time-contingent medication scheduling is a method of breaking the learned associations between increased pain and pain behavior and delivery of pain-relieving medications (Keefe and Lefebvre 1994).

Step 1: Provide a rationale. Patients with persistent pain may be skeptical of the benefits of time-contingent pain medications, and thus it is important to provide a credible rationale for this intervention. One rationale for using a time-contingent dosing schedule is that it maintains a steadier blood level of pain medications, thereby providing better pain relief with fewer side effects. A second rationale is that time-contingent medication scheduling enables patients to gradually reduce their pain medication intake. Finally, time-contingent medications break learned associations between pain behavior and pain medication intake, thereby disrupting the tendency for medication to reinforce high levels of pain and pain behavior.

Step 2: Estimate pretreatment pain medication intake. A baseline estimate of pain medication intake can be obtained by having the patient record times and amounts of medication taken. Typically, medication intake is recorded along with data on activity level so that comparisons between activity patterns and medication use can be readily made. Typically, a 5-7-day period is needed to establish a reliable baseline estimate of pain medication intake.

Step 3: Implement the time-contingent medication program. To implement the time-contingent medication program, average daily baseline pain medication intake is divided into equal amounts to be delivered at regular intervals (e.g., every 6 hours) over a 24-hour period. Time-contingent medications are usually administered in a pill form, although a liquid format ("pain cocktail") may be used in some cases (Fordyce 1976). The main advantage of the pain cocktail is that it masks the exact amount of medication so that daily reductions in dose levels can be made without the patient's awareness. Whether medications are delivered as a pill or in a cocktail, the amount of medication is often reduced over a period of days or weeks until the dosage has been reduced to a level that enables the patient to maintain a moderately active lifestyle while experiencing good pain control and minimizing side effects.

Step 4: Troubleshoot. Many health care professionals utilize formal contracts when implementing a pain medication program (Portenoy 1991; Fishman et al. 2002). These contracts clearly outline dosing and refill schedules as well as the responsibilities of the patient and physician. When used in the context of a behavioral therapy program, such contracts should address not only the pharmacological aspects but also the behavioral components of treatment. A formal contract is helpful in clearly outlining treatment goals and minimizing misunderstandings. Habit-forming medications always carry a potential for abuse, and health professionals must screen patients carefully before implementing any pain medication regimen. Patients having histories of problems with addiction present special challenges and need to be carefully monitored.

COGNITIVE TECHNIQUES

Cognitive therapy techniques are based on the notion that a person's cognitions can have a major impact on their mood, behavior, and physiology (Beck et al. 1979). Numerous studies have shown that patients who frequently have overly negative thoughts about themselves, others, and the future are much more likely to experience high levels of depression, low levels of activity, and increased tension (Sullivan et al. 2001). Cognitive techniques used in pain management are designed to help patients notice and modify the negative thought patterns that contribute to pain, emotional distress, and pain behavior.

The use of cognitive therapy techniques is indicated in a variety of circumstances, including (a) when evidence of tissue damage is clear and there is correspondingly less evidence that environmental factors (e.g., attention from loved ones during pain episodes) are maintaining a patient's condition; (b) when patients are distressed because of medical uncertainty about the cause of their pain, or about when and if their pain will be alleviated; (c) when there are indications that maladaptive thoughts and feelings, such as exaggerated perception of loss or danger, poor self-esteem, or persistent anger, are interfering with a patient's ability to effectively cope and adapt; and (d) when patients have relatively high levels of functioning and are receptive to learning new strategies for controlling and managing their pain.

Cognitive therapy techniques used in pain management focus on cognitive factors—thoughts, beliefs, and expectations—that contribute to overwhelming emotions such as depression, guilt, anxiety, and anger that compound the suffering component of the chronic pain experience (Turk 1997). Cognitive techniques have two goals in common: (1) building awareness of how negative thoughts affect mood, behavior, and pain; and (2) challenging or modifying these thoughts so as to promote improved pain coping. Cognitive therapy techniques frequently used in pain management include cognitive restructuring, problem solving, distraction, and relapse prevention.

COGNITIVE RESTRUCTURING

Cognitive restructuring is the process of altering one's perception of a situation or experience so as to reveal possible solutions that were not previously apparent (Burns 1980). Cognitive restructuring consists of four steps.

Step 1: Identify automatic thoughts. Automatic thoughts, often outside our conscious awareness, are closely linked to our moods. Automatic thoughts about pain tend to be negative and extreme: "I can't stand it anymore" or "It's never going to end" (Gil et al. 1990). Such thoughts are important because they are associated with negative mood states such as depression and anxiety that, in turn, are associated with increased pain. Automatic negative thoughts are most likely to occur when pain is severe or when patients are experiencing strong negative emotions (Gil et al. 1990). When automatic thoughts are brought into awareness they can be examined and modified.

The most common automatic thoughts tend to fall into categories of irrational thinking called cognitive distortions (Beck 1995). Organizing these thoughts into categories can help patients identify, evaluate, and alter them. Categories of cognitive distortions include: (1) All-or-nothing thinking: interpreting a situation only in extremely positive or negative terms (complete success or complete failure) without regard for the range of interpretations falling between the two extremes. (2) Overgeneralization: assigning global implications to a specific event. (3) Catastrophizing: focusing on the worst-case scenario. (4) "Should" statements: having inappropriate expectations of oneself based on personal standards or what one perceives others' expectations to be. (5) Disqualifying the positive: ignoring positive experiences and selectively attending to the negative.

Step 2: Identify the negative emotions that follow from negative thoughts. Increased awareness of automatic thoughts and cognitive distortions is often accompanied by a growing awareness of negative emotional states that follow from these thought patterns. However, for many patients, the thought-mood connection will need to be clearly demonstrated. A tool that is often used for this purpose is a thought record (Beck 1995). Simply put, a thought record is a way for patients to record their reactions to troubling events like pain flares in an organized and systematic manner. A typical thought record includes columns for writing down the event ("pain flare after going for a walk"), thoughts ("I'll never be able to walk; I am going to end up in a wheelchair"), mood ("depressed, anxious"), and behavior ("went to bed and took extra pain medication"). When patients review the thought record, they can see the thought-mood connection more clearly.

Patients with chronic pain often have trouble identifying their negative thoughts. A useful tool for identifying negative pain-related thoughts is a questionnaire instrument developed in our laboratory known as the Inventory of Negative Thoughts in Response to Pain (INTRP) (Gil et al. 1990). The INTRP consists of 21 items measuring negative thoughts commonly reported by patients with chronic pain. Respondents are asked to rate each item, indicating how often they have the thought when having a pain flare.

Table I
The Inventory of Negative Thoughts in Response to Pain

Negative Self-Statements
  I am useless
  Other people have to do everything for me
  I can no longer do anything
  I am worthless
  My pain is getting worse
  I am afraid to do anything
  My family has taken over all my responsibilities
  I am going to become an invalid
  I can't do anything for others
  I am a burden on my family
  I know if I do anything it will make my pain worse

Negative Social Cognitions
  No one cares about my pain
  Other people do not believe I have pain
  It is not fair that I have to live this way
  No one cares about me anymore
  No one wants to hear about my problems
  I cannot control this pain
  I can't stand depending on my family and friends any
    more

Self-Blame
  I must have done something to bring on this pain
  It is my own fault I hurt like this
  I've injured myself again

Source: Gil et al. (1990).

Table I provides a list of each of the items. Factor analysis of the INTRP has revealed three factors: negative self-statements, negative social cognitions, and self-blame. Patients scoring high on the negative self-statements and negative social cognitions scales of the INTRP report much more severe pain and psychological distress (Gil et al. 1990). Clinically, the INTRP can be used to help patients identify specific negative thoughts that they have during pain flares. These thoughts can then be monitored using the thought record described above.

Step 3: Challenge negative thoughts and develop coping thoughts. When patients in pain become aware of the thought-mood connection, they are often more open to the idea that they can reduce emotional distress by developing alternative, coping thoughts (Turk 1997). Coping thoughts are deliberate and accurate versions of reality that tend to incorporate more information than negative automatic thoughts ("It is true I had more pain walking today; I think I need to adjust my walking goal as my therapist suggested, and will try again tomorrow"). Patients are instructed to monitor their negative thoughts and, each time they occur, to replace them with alternative coping thoughts. The thought record is typically used to monitor the effect of applying coping thoughts.

Step 4: Troubleshoot. While some patients readily generate alternative thoughts and almost immediately notice a positive impact on their mood, other patients need more help to develop alternative thoughts. Beck (1995) found that an effective strategy for developing alternative thoughts is to actively challenge the negative thought by asking questions such as: "What is the evidence against this thought?" "Is this thought true 100% of the time?" "If I heard my best friend express this thought, what would I tell him/her?" "Am I overgeneralizing?" "Am I thinking in terms of 'all' or 'nothing'"?

Patients may have difficulty remembering coping thoughts when they are upset. In such cases, patients can be encouraged to write positive thoughts on index cards (Keefe and Lefebvre 1999). Patients can use these "coping cards" during problematic situations to deliberately disrupt thought patterns that may be working against them and replace them with thoughts that work for them.

Another common problem is that patients may not fully believe the alternative thoughts, particularly if their content was suggested by the therapist rather than self-generated. In so far as possible, clinicians should ensure that patients produce their own alternative thoughts and also check whether they are believable. The level of belief in coping thoughts often increases when patients apply them in a challenging situation and discover how applicable and effective they are.

PROBLEM SOLVING

Problem-solving techniques can help pain patients to reinterpret their pain experience in terms that make solutions more evident (Goldfried and Davidson 1976). While we all solve problems daily, few of us have experience with formal problem-solving approaches. A four-step approach to problem solving is as follows:

Step 1: Identify the problem. This step often involves breaking down a larger problem into smaller, more manageable problems that can be tackled one by one. Specificity is a key to this aspect of problem identification. The more specific the description, the more targeted the solutions can be.

Step 2: Analyze the impact of the problem. This step is an extension of step 1, and may help some patients to identify their problems. It involves taking stock of how a specific problem is affecting one's life, namely one's actions, thoughts and feelings, and body. For example, a patient may fear returning to work because working creates specific challenges in terms of: (1) activities—problems tolerating sitting at a desk or standing at a work bench and difficulties responding to coworkers' questions about the pain; (2) thoughts and feelings—dealing with thoughts of worthlessness, feeling guilty about not meeting work demands, and worrying about job security; and (3) body responses—dealing with fatigue and muscle tension. When patients identify the impact of a pain-related problem in such a fashion, it is often much easier to come up with solutions. Problems related to activities, for example, often respond to behavioral interventions such as activity pacing, while those in the realm of thoughts and feelings often respond to cognitive interventions such as cognitive restructuring.

Step 3: Generate a list of solutions that can be applied to the problem. Brainstorming can generate a wide range of solutions to any problem that is identified (Waters et al. 2002). It is important to promote mastery by reminding patients that they have been successful with problem solving in the past and that these experiences can be brought to bear in managing their pain. Patients trained in behavioral and cognitive pain management techniques can be encouraged to adapt those skills in novel ways so as to meet the challenges of the specific problem. It is important to generate a wide array of solutions. Some of these are likely to be more feasible than others, but in the spirit of brainstorming all solutions are placed on a list and judgments on their utility are withheld.

Step 4: Pick the most appropriate solution, implement it, and evaluate it. Each solution is critically analyzed to determine its likelihood of success. Creativity and flexibility are encouraged. An effective component of one solution can often be integrated with an effective component of another to generate the most appropriate plan. Once the best solution has been identified, patients are encouraged to implement the plan. A follow-up session serves to evaluate the effect of the patient's problem-solving plan, to make adjustments, and to encourage the patient to continue to implement the plan until the problem is resolved satisfactorily.

Step 5: Troubleshoot. Not uncommonly, patients approach problem solving in an unsystematic manner and consequently do not develop a greater sense of self-efficacy in solving problems. We therefore recommend that patients follow a formal step-by-step approach to problem solving in which they carefully attend to each of the steps outlined above and write down their responses on a problem-solving handout or notebook. The written records provide a concrete guide to a specific problem and a reminder of how successful the solution was. We have found that patients value these written records and refer back to them whenever they encounter similar problems.

DISTRACTION TECHNIQUES

Distraction techniques reduce patients' preoccupation with pain and other bodily symptoms by diverting their attention (McCaul and Malott 1984). Patients with chronic pain often use distraction methods in a haphazard fashion and can benefit from systematic guided training. Distraction techniques commonly used in cognitive-behavioral treatment protocols include imagery, progressive muscle relaxation, concentration on a focal point, and listening to music (Turk 1997). We discuss training in imagery as a way to illustrate how these techniques are used.

Imagery involves generating a detailed mental image of a pleasant scene involving all of the senses—sound, sight, touch, smell, and taste. This technique can be particularly helpful during pain flares and episodes of increased pain. Imagery is typically taught using the following steps:

Step 1: Begin with a progressive muscle relaxation exercise. One of the most effective ways to teach imagery is to pair it with training in progressive relaxation techniques. The essential elements of progressive relaxation training are reviewed in detail by Andrasik (this volume). Basically, the technique involves inducing relaxation through a guided exercise involving the systematic tensing and relaxing of the major muscle groups. During the exercise patients are encouraged to focus their attention on sensations that occur. During this early phase of training, it is important to talk patients through the exercise so as to demonstrate the steady, calming pace that is desired.

Step 2: Add visual imagery. After a patient has achieved a more relaxed state, the therapist describes a pleasant image such as walking by a mountain stream or reclining on a sunny ocean beach. Patients are asked to actively imagine the sensations that might occur in this scene. Using the image of walking by a mountain stream, they would be asked to focus on what they might see (running water, blue sky, green grass), hear (a burbling brook, birds chirping), feel (the warmth of the sun), and smell (the smell of pine trees in the air). Patients are reminded that they are in control of the scene and can linger on parts of it for as long as they like, or change it in any way that makes it more personal. Creativity is an important part of building an effective image and helps patients master this technique.

Step 3: Encourage home practice. Patients are typically given a tape recording of guided imagery exercises and are encouraged to listen to it twice daily at home. In addition, patients are also trained in a brief imagery exercise to enable them to generalize learned imagery skills to daily situations where pain may become a problem. This exercise involves first letting go of tension throughout the body for 20 seconds and then focusing on a pleasant image for 20 seconds. The brief imagery exercise can be repeated up to 20 times per day in a variety of situations. We give patients reminder cues such as adhesive dots to place in their homes to remind them to do a brief imagery exercise. The goal is to gradually build up to 20 brief imagery practice sessions per day. Once patients reach this level, they typically report that the use of imagery has become a habitual and much more natural part of their pain-coping regimen.

Step 4: Troubleshoot. Many patients enjoy imagery, while others have little affinity for this technique. A patient's affinity for imagery is often apparent soon after this technique is introduced. It is important to explore the patient's responses to the initial imagery exercises in order to assess personal preferences and tailor subsequent exercises accordingly. For example, the imagery scene can be scripted or self-generated, and can be used with or without relaxation training. Whatever their individual preferences, patients should be encouraged to use imagery only to the extent to which they find it beneficial.

RELAPSE PREVENTION

Relapse prevention focuses on long-term maintenance of the behavioral and cognitive coping skills reviewed above (Keefe and Van Horn 1993). It falls within the domain of cognitive techniques because it involves awareness and modification of cognitive factors that can disrupt continued practice of pain management skills. This strategy involves teaching patients to (1) identify high-risk situations that might lead to a lapse in coping efforts, (2) self-monitor coping efforts, (3) plan for how they will deal with lapses in coping and problems that may arise, (4) behaviorally rehearse coping strategies, and (5) troubleshoot (Marlatt and Gordon 1985; Keefe and Van Horn 1993). These steps are elaborated below.

Step 1: Identify high-risk situations. Patients are encouraged to make a list of high-risk problem situations or stressful events such as pain flares that have led to a lapse in the use of their coping skills. They also are encouraged to identify problems or stressors that they are likely to encounter in the future. Patients' responses to previous problem situations should be discussed in detail in order to identify both problematic and effective ways of coping with future events (Marlatt and Gordon 1985).

Step 2: Encourage self-monitoring of coping efforts. Self-monitoring involves keeping a record of the frequency of practice of learned coping skills as well as internal and external cues that are signs of distress. The therapist should work with the patient to develop a personalized self-monitoring format. This might take the form of a daily diary, a week-at-a glance recording sheet, or even a monthly calendar. The patient should record each of the coping skills used on a given day, such as activity pacing, cognitive restructuring, and imagery. In addition, the patient should note any internal or external cues that might serve as warning signs to indicate that coping efforts are not working well. The therapist should work with the patient to develop a list of such cues. Internal cues might include negative thoughts and emotions such as depression, anxiety, or frustration. External cues might include feedback from a spouse and other family members regarding social withdrawal, increased irritability, or other changes in social behavior.

Step 3: Develop a relapse prevention plan. A relapse prevention plan consists of a list of behavioral and cognitive techniques that can prevent problems from occurring or lessen the impact of unavoidable or unforeseen problems (Keefe and Van Horn 1993). Key elements of such a plan could include the use of: (1) cognitive restructuring to deal with typical negative thoughts that occur during a setback or relapse ("Nothing I am doing is working; I'll never be able to cope with this pain"), (2) activity pacing to interfere with the tendency to revert to excessive bed rest as a way of coping with pain, (3) increased practice with imagery and relaxation methods to reduce high levels of tension and anxiety that accompany setbacks, (4) a decision-making technique that contrasts the consequences of continuing coping efforts versus stopping them, and (5) seeking social support by informing family and friends that the relapse is occurring and obtaining instrumental and emotional support for coping efforts.

Step 4: Use behavioral rehearsal. This technique can enhance the patient's self-efficacy with regard to preventing and managing relapses. In behavioral rehearsal, the therapist role-plays how the patient might effectively respond to a problem situation. The patient then is asked to role-play how he or she might respond to the same situation. After receiving corrective feedback, the patient role-plays the situation once again. The process continues until the patient has mastered the skills needed to deal with the problem situation. Behavioral rehearsal can be quite effective, particularly because it provides concrete examples of how to apply cognitive and behavioral pain-coping skills to challenging situations.

Step 5: Troubleshoot. It is not unusual for patients to misunderstand the rationale for relapse prevention training. One erroneous assumption is that the clinician is teaching relapse prevention because he or she believes that failure to maintain skills is inevitable. If this assumption is not corrected, patients can become less confident in their ability to self-manage their pain in the long term. To prevent or counter this potential problem, it is important to stress that lapses in practicing pain management techniques are common and can be addressed through the development of a coping plan that addresses early recognition of reduced coping and emphasizes early intervention to minimize the impact of lapses on long-term self-management of pain.

Another challenge in relapse prevention training relates to the specificity of the coping plan. Some patients will benefit most from a problem-specific coping plan (an "if X, then Y" approach). Other patients may choose to develop a more general coping plan that can address a wide range of challenges or problems. Rather than dictate a particular approach to relapse prevention, it is best to accommodate individual preferences in finding a set of coping skills with which the patient feels comfortable.

INTEGRATING BEHAVIORAL AND COGNITIVE-BEHAVIORAL THERAPY TECHNIQUES INTO CLINICAL PRACTICE

Traditionally, the behavioral and cognitive-behavioral methods described above have been delivered in formal individual or group therapy sessions conducted by a counselor who is highly trained and experienced. Recognition is growing, however, of the benefits that can be obtained by integrating these techniques into clinical practice. In this section we provide some practical guidelines on how these therapy techniques can be integrated into primary care.

BEHAVIORAL THERAPY TECHNIQUES

Fordyce and colleagues (1986) were among the first to test the effects of behavioral techniques in treating pain in the primary care setting. These investigators compared the efficacy of behavioral pain management with that of routine pain management in the treatment of acute back pain. Workers who had recently experienced an episode of back pain following a work-related injury were randomly assigned to one of two groups. For patients in the routine medical care group, pain medications and return visits were scheduled on a p.r.n. basis, and patients determined their exercise and activity level on a daily basis. For patients in the behavioral pain management group, medications were given on a time schedule (e.g., every 6 hours), exercise was scheduled in a graded fashion (e.g., beginning with 10 repetitions per day and increasing by one repetition per day until reaching 20 repetitions), weekly activity quotas were determined, and a set schedule of return visits was implemented. Data analysis revealed that patients in these two conditions did not differ in outcome at 9 weeks, but at 1-year follow-up those who had received behavioral pain management were much more likely to have returned to work; this group also reported fewer pain-related limitations. These findings are interesting for several reasons. First, persons in both conditions received access to the same interventions, with the exception that in one group the interventions were delivered according to behavioral principles (i.e., on a time-contingent basis) rather than on a more typical p.r.n. basis. Second, primary care physicians delivered the behavioral intervention in the course of their routine treatment.

When should behavioral techniques be used? As noted earlier, these techniques are most appropriate for patients whose pain behavior is excessive or inappropriate given the evidence of underlying disease tissue damage. The patient with persistent lower back pain who has no physical findings on physical examination, but who has developed an overly sedentary and dependent lifestyle, is likely to be a good candidate for behavioral intervention. Other good candidates for treatment are patients whose pain behavior consistently increases when they are in the presence of a solicitous spouse or family member.

Behavioral therapy techniques, like most pain management approaches, are not as effective for patients who are involved in ongoing litigation, disability hearings, or compensation claims. In such cases, it is important to closely monitor patients' progress. Patients who experience difficulty following through with treatment assignments may require more intensive treatment or may benefit from delaying treatment until the outcome of their pending claim is settled. Also inappropriate for behavioral therapy are patients with significant psychopathology (e.g., psychosis or severe depression) or addiction problems (e.g., drug or alcohol addiction). Finally, patients with very long-standing, entrenched, or complicated pain problems are likely to require referral to a specialist for behavioral treatment. Psychologists specializing in behavioral treatment are available in many tertiary pain management programs. Referrals of behavioral and cognitive-behavioral therapists can also be obtained by contacting the Association for the Advancement of Behavioral Therapy (www.aabt.org).

When in the course of treatment should behavioral techniques be considered? Early intervention, before maladaptive pain behavior patterns develop, is likely to be optimal. Most acute pain problems resolve in a matter of days or weeks and thus are inappropriate for behavioral treatment. If pain is likely to persist (e.g., low back pain following a back injury) and there is evidence of excessive or inappropriate pain behavior, then it is likely that early intervention with behavioral techniques can be helpful.

How can behavioral therapy techniques be integrated into practice? Table II provides a list of guidelines for utilizing behavioral techniques in clinical practice. An overriding principle is that interventions should be delivered on a time-contingent, rather than a symptom-contingent, basis. As the study by Fordyce et al. (1986) suggests, the practitioner should avoid telling patients to "let pain be your guide" when scheduling doctor visits, pain medications, and activities. Although such an approach is often the norm in primary care practice, it provides many opportunities for learned associations to develop between severe pain and potentially reinforcing consequences. Whenever possible, return visits, pain medications, and activation efforts such as participating in exercise or returning to work should be scheduled on a time-contingent basis.

Another key principle guiding the use of behavioral therapy methods in clinical practice is that patients do not change independently of their social environment. Significant others—a spouse or other family members—need to be educated about the role they can play in pain management. Clinicians should explain to them the benefits of encouraging the patient to engage in

Table II
Guidelines for integrating behavioral therapy techniques in pain management programs

Schedule time-contingent visits	Avoid p.r.n. visits for patients
Prescribe time-contingent pain medications	Avoid p.r.n. pain medications
Socially reinforce well behaviors	Do not reinforce inappropriate pain behavior
Encourage family and significant others to reinforce progress	Do not ignore family and significant others in treatment plan
Encourage use of relaxation methods or refer the patient for formal training	Do not rely solely on medications for tension and anxiety reduction
Set clear and concrete goals for activities	Do not use pain as a guide for activity selection

well behaviors (e.g., by joining the patient in an exercise program) while reducing social reinforcement for pain behaviors (e.g., by refusing to take over activities the patient is capable of doing, such as tying her shoes or getting her medication). These behavioral changes can be difficult, so it is important to routinely involve significant others in treatment sessions and to reinforce the progress of both the patient and significant others.

Patients who are excessively fearful about becoming more active often request p.r.n. prescriptions for sedative or hypnotic agents. It is important to teach patients to avoid relying on these medications. Research shows that significant reductions in fear, anxiety, and pain occur when patients with chronic pain expose themselves to activities they have been avoiding (Vlaeyen et al. 2002). By pacing their activities, most patients experience success in increasing their activity level. Patients whose excessive fears cause them to avoid activities may benefit from systematic training in relaxation methods or from a referral for more intensive and formal behavioral therapy intervention.

COGNITIVE-BEHAVIORAL THERAPY TECHNIQUES

When should cognitive therapy techniques be used in primary care settings? As noted earlier, these techniques are most appropriate for patients whose behavioral and emotional responses to pain appear to be more strongly influenced by negative and distorted thoughts than by environmental factors. A patient with arthritis pain who ruminates on the thought that she may become wheelchair bound and thus feels discouraged and distressed is likely to benefit from cognitive therapy techniques. Cognitive therapy can help patients with severe psychopathology such as major depression or personality disorders; however, these patients should be seen by specialists who can conduct a formal course of cognitive therapy.

When in the course of treatment should cognitive techniques be considered? Cognitive therapy techniques, like behavioral therapy techniques, are most effective if applied early in the course of a persistent pain problem. If a patient develops a pattern of overly negative and unrealistic thinking that appears to be contributing to his problems in coping with persistent pain, then cognitive intervention is warranted.

How can cognitive therapy techniques be integrated into practice? Table III lists several practical methods for utilizing cognitive-behavioral techniques in clinical practice. A key strategy used to counter unrealistic thoughts is to provide patients with educational information about the cause and future trajectory of their pain. Patients need to be reassured that the health care provider accepts that they have a "real" pain problem and that the focus of treatment will be in managing this pain. It is important to avoid suggesting that the primary cause of their pain lies in their thought processes. Patients need to be given a rationale that explains how thoughts and feelings influence their pain. Along these lines, the clinician can provide a brief review of the gate control theory of pain (Melzack and Wall 1984), which describes how brain centers responsible for cognition and emotion can block pain signals coming from the site of an injury by sending nervous impulses to block pain at the level of the spinal cord. This theory helps patients understand the link between mind and body and often opens them to the possibility that cognitive therapy techniques can influence their pain.

The most challenging cognitive therapy technique to integrate into clinical practice is cognitive restructuring. To effectively alter thought patterns requires patience and repeated effort on the part of the both the patient and clinician. The cognitive model maintains that maladaptive and distorted thoughts are learned and that systematic training is needed to foster the learning of new and more adaptive ways of thinking (Turk 1997). Cognitive restructuring requires a formal and structured approach that relies on home practice with thought records. In reviewing these records during therapy sessions, it is important that the clinician adopt the role of a collaborative

Table III
Guidelines for integrating cognitive-behavioral techniques
in pain management programs

Educate patients about the powerful influence that thoughts can have on pain, emotions, and behavior	Avoid suggesting that patients' thoughts are the primary cause of their pain (e.g., "this is all in your head")
Introduce problem solving as an enhancement to abilities that patients already have	Avoid conveying the impression that patients are incompetent at solving their problems
Use a guided discovery approach to help patients systematically identify potential solutions to problems	Avoid directive recommendations or solutions
Encourage patients to consider progressive muscle relaxation as a time to focus on sensations of relaxation rather than those of pain	Avoid promoting progressive muscle relaxation as an effortful exercise that will eliminate pain
Let patients' personal preferences determine the make-up of imagery exercises	Avoid imposing an imagery approach on patients
Tailor each long-term maintenance plan around the skills at which the individual patient has been most successful and is most motivated to continue	Avoid automatically including all skills in each long-term maintenance plan
As part of maintenance plans, develop an individualized skill practice schedule for each patient	Avoid general recommendations to practice skills that are not anchored within a specific schedule and maintenance plan

teacher and guide, rather than an authority who dictates what the patient must think or do.

Problem solving, in contrast to cognitive restructuring, is relatively easy to adapt for use in primary care settings. Primary care clinicians often use informal problem-solving approaches in their work with patients. When using the more formal problem-solving steps outlined in this chapter, it is important to introduce this approach as a way to build upon patients' current problem-solving abilities. This approach serves to reinforce patients' current coping efforts and avoids sending the message that patients are unable to cope with or solve their own problems. The key is teaching patients to solve their own problems. The problem-solving steps provide a general framework that, with practice, the patient can use to deal with a wide variety of problematic issues.

Primary care clinicians vary in their own background in using imagery techniques. The clinician who is familiar with these techniques can integrate them into primary care settings either through brief in-session training or by making an audiotape for the patient. A key point is to be sure that the imagery is tailored to take into account the patient's personal preferences. A cardinal principle for imagery is that any associated relaxation and relief cannot be forced. Although patience and persistent practice are needed, these techniques must be approached with a nonstriving attitude, a willingness to engage in the exercises and let the results come on their own.

Relapse prevention training represents a special application of problem-solving methods to issues of maintenance and coping with setbacks and lapses. A special effort is needed to tailor each patient's relapse prevention plan to his or her own needs and problems. In particular, a realistic plan must be developed for ongoing practice with learned coping skills. Clinicians must avoid applying a cookie-cutter approach where the same recommendations are given to each patient. Incorporating coping skills training into a patient's treatment program could expand the pain clinician's repertoire and enhance treatment success.

REFERENCES

Beck AT, Rush AJ, Shaw BF, Emery G. *Cognitive Therapy of Depression*. New York: Guilford Press, 1979.

Beck JS. *Cognitive Therapy: Basics and Beyond*. New York: Guilford Press, 1995.

Burns DD. *Feeling Good: The New Mood Therapy*. New York: Signet, 1980.

Compas BE, Haaga DAF, Keefe FJ, Leitenberg H, Williams DA. A sampling of empirically supported psychological treatments from health psychology: smoking, chronic pain, cancer, and bulimia nervosa. *J Consult Clin Psychol* 1998; 66:89–112.

Fishman SM, Mahajan G, Jung, S-W, Wilsey BL. The trilateral opioid contract: bridging the pain clinic and the primary care physician through the opioid contract. *J Pain Symptom Manage* 2002; 24:335–344.

Fordyce WE. *Behavioural Methods for Chronic Pain and Illness.* St. Louis: C.V. Mosley, 1976.

Fordyce WE, Brockway JA, Bergman JA, Spengler D. Acute back pain: a control-group comparison of behavioral versus traditional methods. *J Behav Med* 1986; 9:127–140.

Gil KM, Ross SL, Keefe FJ. Behavioral treatment of chronic pain: four pain management protocols. In: France RD, Krishnan KR (Eds). *Chronic Pain.* New York: American Psychiatric Press, 1988, pp 376–413.

Gil KM, Abrams MR, Phillips G, Keefe FJ. Sickle cell disease pain: the relationship of coping strategies to adjustment. *J Consult Clin Psychol* 1989; 57:725–731.

Gil KM, Williams DA, Keefe FJ, Beckham JC. The relationship of negative thoughts to pain and psychological distress. *Behav Ther* 1990; 21:349–362.

Goldfried MR, Davidson GC. *Clinical Behavior Therapy.* New York: Holt, Rinehart and Winston, 1976.

Keefe FJ. Can cognitive-behavioral treatments succeed where medical treatments fail? In: Devor M, Rowbotham MC, Wiesenfeld-Hallin Z (Eds). *Proceedings of the 9th World Congress on Pain,* Progress in Pain Research and Management, Vol. 16. Seattle: IASP Press, 2000, pp 1069–1084.

Keefe FJ, Lefebvre J. Pain behavior concepts: controversies, current status, and future directions. In: Gebhart G, Hammond DL, Jensen TS (Eds). *Proceedings of the 7th World Congress on Pain,* Progress in Pain Research and Management, Vol. 2. Seattle: IASP Press, 1994, pp 127–147.

Keefe FJ, Lefebvre JC. Behaviour therapy. In: Melzack R, Wall P. *Textbook of Pain.* London: Churchill Livingstone, 1999, pp 1445–1462.

Keefe FJ, Van Horn Y. Cognitive-behavioral treatment of rheumatoid arthritis pain. *Arthritis Care Res* 1993; 6:213–222.

Keefe FJ, Crisson JE, Maltbie A, Bradley L, Gil KM. Illness behavior as a predictor of pain and overt behavior patterns in chronic low back pain patients. *J Psychosom Res* 1986; 30:543–551.

Keefe FJ, Caldwell DS, Baucom D, et al. Spouse-assisted coping skills training in the management of osteoarthritic knee pain. *Arthritis Care Res* 1996; 9:279–291.

Keefe FJ, Smith SJ, Buffington ALH, et al. Recent advances and future directions in the biopsychosocial assessment and treatment of arthritis. *J Consult Clin Psychol* 2002; 70:640–655.

Lewinsohn PM, Clarke GN, Hops H, Andrews JA. Cognitive-behavioral treatment for depressed adolescents. *Behav Ther* 1990; 21:385–401.

Marlatt GA, Gordon JR. *Relapse Prevention.* New York: Guilford Press, 1985.

McCaul KD, Malott JM. Distraction and coping with pain. *Psychol Bull* 1984; 95:516–533.

Melzack R, Wall P. *The Challenge of Pain.* New York: Penguin Press, 1984.

Moore JE, Chaney EF. Outpatient group treatment of chronic pain: effects of spouse involvement. *J Consult Clin Psychol* 1985; 53:326.

Morley S, Eccleston C, Williams A. Systematic review and meta-analysis of randomized controlled trials of cognitive behaviour therapy and behaviour therapy for chronic pain in adults, excluding headache. *Pain* 1999; 80:1–13.

Portenoy R. The effect of drug regulation on the management of cancer pain. *NY State J Med* 1991; 91:13S–18S.

Rohde P, Clarke GN, Lewinsohn PM, Seeley JR, Kaufman NK. Impact of comorbidity on a cognitive-behavioral group treatment for adolescent depression. *J Am Acad Child Adolesc Psychiatry* 2001; 40:795–802.

Ross SL, Gil KM, Keefe FJ. Learned responses to chronic pain: behavioral, cognitive and psychophysiological. In: France RD, Krishnan KR (Eds). *Chronic Pain.* New York: American Psychiatric Press, 1988, pp 228–243.

Sullivan MJ, Thorn B, Haythornthwaite JA, et al. Theoretical perspectives on the relation between catastrophizing and pain. *Clin J Pain* 2001; 17:52–64.

Syrjala KL, Donaldson GW, Davis MW, Kippes ME, Carr JE. Relaxation and imagery and cognitive-behavioral training reduce pain during cancer treatment: a controlled clinical trial. *Pain* 1995; 63:189–198.

Turk DC. Psychological aspects of pain. In: *Springhouse Guide: Expert Pain Management.* Springhouse, PA: Springhouse Corporation, 1997.

Vlaeyen JWS, de Jong J, Geilen M, Heuts PHTG, van Breukelen G. The treatment of fear of movement/(re)injury in chronic low back pain: further evidence on the effectiveness of exposure *in vivo*. *Clin J Pain* 2002; 18:251–261.

Waters SJ, McKee DC, Keefe FJ. Cognitive behavioral approaches to the treatment of pain. *Trends Evidence-Based Neuropsychiatry* 2002; 4:57–63.

Correspondence to: Francis J. Keefe, PhD, Box 3159, Duke University Medical Center, Durham, NC 27710, USA. Email: keefe003@mc.duke.edu.

Psychosocial Aspects of Pain: A Handbook for Health Care Providers, Progress in Pain Research and Management, Vol. 27, edited by Robert H. Dworkin and William S. Breitbart, IASP Press, Seattle, © 2004.

13

The Essence of Biofeedback, Relaxation, and Hypnosis

Frank Andrasik

Institute for Human and Machine Cognition, University of West Florida, Pensacola, Florida, USA

Pain is a complex experience that typically requires a multifaceted, multidisciplinary approach. Biofeedback, relaxation, and hypnosis are often components of treatment. Although this chapter focuses on these modalities separately, they are rarely applied in isolation. Often combined with one another and with allied psychological and medical interventions, they are some of the many options open to patients and therapists.

Biofeedback, relaxation, and hypnosis share common features. This chapter provides a detailed description of biofeedback. Sections discussing relaxation and hypnosis are less detailed because many of the comments made regarding biofeedback apply equally well to relaxation and hypnosis. These treatments rely less on physical procedures applied by others and place a correspondingly greater emphasis on patient involvement and personal responsibility. They expand the scope of treatment to include emotional, mental, behavioral, and social factors that affect pain, with the goal of enabling patients to cope more effectively with pain and associated symptoms. Patients who take an active role in their treatment can gain increased confidence in their abilities to prevent and manage pain, and thus may experience less pain-related disability (French et al. 2000).

THE ESSENCE OF BIOFEEDBACK

BIOFEEDBACK DEFINED

Biofeedback has been defined as "a process in which a person learns to reliably influence physiological responses of two kinds: either responses which are not ordinarily under voluntary control or responses which ordinarily are easily regulated but for which regulation has broken down due to trauma or disease" (Blanchard and Epstein 1978).

The process of biofeedback involves three operations: (1) detection and amplification of a biological response by using certain measurement devices (or transducers) and electronic amplifiers; (2) conversion of these bioelectrical signals to a form that the patient can easily understand and process; and (3) immediate feedback of the signal to the patient. Feedback is most often auditory or visual and is presented in either binary or continuous proportional fashion. Binary feedback uses a signal that comes on or goes off at a specified threshold value, whereas continuous feedback involves a decreasing tone or slower rate of clicking as physiological relaxation occurs. On occasion, a combination of both types of signal may be used. The practitioner must adequately prepare areas for sensor placement and place the measurement devices on the proper locations. Electrode sites may need to be cleaned and lightly abraded, and a conductive gel may be applied to facilitate conductance and reduce measurement artifact. More detailed discussion of the physiology, electrical theory, and basis of the primary responses used in biofeedback may be found in Peek (2003) and various chapters within Cacioppo et al. (2000) and Stern et al. (2001). Several theories have been put forth to explain the mechanism of biofeedback, ranging from operant learning to cognitive and expectancy models (Schwartz and Schwartz 2003).

Three different rationales have been offered for the use of biofeedback in pain management (Belar and Kibrick 1986; Flor 2001; Andrasik and Flor 2003). For simplicity, this chapter describes them as general, specific, and indirect approaches.

GENERAL APPROACH TO BIOFEEDBACK

The general approach, which employs biofeedback to lower overall arousal and promote a generalized state of relaxation, is based on two assumptions. The first is that a reduction in general arousal will lead to reduced central processing of peripheral sensory inputs. The second assumption derives from the observed association of anxiety with decreased pain tolerance and increased reports of pain. Achievement of a more relaxed state, it is argued, reduces anxiety and thus will enhance pain tolerance and decrease pain reports. A case can be made that most pain patients could benefit from relaxation and tension reduction, especially those whose pain is associated with increased muscle tension. This approach is probably the most common, and also requires the least technical proficiency.

Examples of biofeedback as a general aid to relaxation

Any response modality indicative of heightened arousal theoretically can serve as a target for promoting relaxation, although three responses are used most commonly—muscle tension (electromyographic or EMG), skin conductance (or sweat gland activity), and peripheral temperature. These modalities, termed the "workhorses" of the biofeedback general practitioner (Andrasik 2000), are easily collected, quantified, and interpreted. Other responses, such as heart rate, respiration, and blood volume, can be useful, but will not be addressed further in this chapter (see Flor 2001 for discussion).

EMG-assisted relaxation. The rationale for employing muscle tension (and skin conductance) feedback to facilitate relaxation is straightforward. The EMG signal is based on the small electrochemical changes that occur when a muscle contracts. These changes can be monitored by placing a series of electrodes along the muscle fibers to assess the muscle action potentials associated with the ion exchange across the membrane of the muscles. When EMG is used for generalized relaxation, large-diameter sensors are typically placed on the forehead to pick up muscle tension from adjacent areas, possibly down to the upper rib cage (Basmajian 1976). Once it was believed that reductions in forehead muscle tension would automatically generalize to most other untrained muscles, promoting a state of "cultivated low arousal." This response does not occur automatically, however (Surwit and Keefe 1978), so clinicians may need to train patients to reduce tension in several body sites in the course of general relaxation treatment (or else combine biofeedback with other approaches).

Factors affecting measurement include sensor type and size, sensor placement on the muscle, distance between sensors, adiposity, and bandpass or recording range.

Skin-conductance-assisted relaxation. Electrical activity of the skin, or sweating, has long been thought to be associated with arousal. In the late 1800s Romain Virouroux included measures of skin resistance when working with cases of hysterical anesthesias (Neumann and Blanton 1970; Peek 2003). In the early 1900s Carl Jung used electrodermal activity in word-association experiments, a technique that became popular as a way to "read the mind." Sensors are typically placed on body surface areas that are most densely populated with eccrine sweat glands (such as the palm of the hand or the fingers), which are innervated by the sympathetic branch of the autonomic nervous system and respond primarily to psychological stimulation (Boucsein 1992; Stern et al. 2001). Conductance measures (in micro-ohms or microsiemens) have a linear relationship to the number of sweat glands that are activated and are preferred to resistance measures in clinical application. The explanation to patients is straightforward: as arousal increases, so does skin conductance; focusing on decreasing skin conductance helps to lower arousal and to achieve a state of relaxation.

Skin-temperature-assisted relaxation. Why skin temperature feedback is useful for general relaxation is not readily apparent. The first clinical application resulted from a serendipitous finding by clinical researchers at the Menninger Clinic. During a laboratory evaluation, Sargent et al. (1972) observed that spontaneous termination of a migraine was accompanied by flushing in the hands and by a rapid and sizable rise in surface hand temperature. This finding inspired Sargent's team to test a new treatment procedure wherein patients received feedback for attempts to raise their hand temperatures as a way to regulate stress and reduce headache activity. Treatment was augmented by components of autogenic training (see subsequent section), leading to a procedure that was termed "autogenic feedback." Given that constriction of peripheral blood flow is modulated by the sympathetic branch of the nervous system, these researchers reasoned that decreases in sympathetic outflow cause increased vasodilation and blood flow and a resultant rise in peripheral temperature (due to the warmth of the blood). Thus, temperature feedback may best be considered another way to facilitate general relaxation. Other biofeedback approaches for migraine headache, including using EEG or measures of blood flow in various arteries, are based on the assumption of a more direct tie to the underlying pathophysiology. These approaches will not be discussed further because they are quite specialized and have not been the focus of extensive research.

SPECIFIC APPROACH

The specific approach seeks to directly modify the physiological dysfunction or response system assumed to underlie the pain condition. This approach has its origins in the pain-spasm-pain cycle first described by Bonica (1957). To apply this approach, therapists assess psychophysiological responses in the modalities assumed to be relevant to the condition under varied stimulus conditions. The following text will restrict comments to peripheral measures that have garnered the greatest attention by researchers and clinicians (see Flor 2001 for information concerning central measures of pain).

Flor (2001) has pointed out the functions, utility, and advantages of collecting psychophysiological data in the specific biofeedback approach to the treatment of chronic pain. Data from a psychophysiological assessment demonstrate the role of psychological factors in maladaptive physiological functioning and provide justification for the use of biofeedback therapy. The assessment process allows therapists to tailor treatments to individual patients, to document treatment efficacy, and to identify predictors of treatment response. The process also motivates patients; when they realize that their own thoughts, emotions, and actions influence bodily process, their feelings of helplessness decrease and they become more open to trying psychological approaches.

Psychophysiological assessment

This approach begins with a psychophysiological assessment (or "psychophysiological stress profile") that contains the components described below (Flor 2001; Andrasik and Flor 2003; Arena and Schwartz 2003).

Adaptation, to allow patients to become familiar with the setting and recording procedure, to minimize presession effects (for example, rushing to the appointment, or temperature and humidity differences between the office and outdoors), and to allow patients to become habituated to the orienting response. Patients are instructed merely to sit quietly during this period.

Baseline, to serve as the basis of comparison for subsequent assessment phases and for gauging progress in future treatment sessions. In clinical practice, the baseline period typically lasts for 1–5 minutes, during which time most responses will stabilize.

When the goal of biofeedback is generalized relaxation, therapists may collect a second baseline during which the patient is instructed as follows: "I would now like to see what happens when you try to relax as deeply as you can. Use whatever means you believe will be helpful. Please let me know when you are as relaxed as possible."

Reactivity, to assess responding to simulated stressors that are personally relevant or conditions that approximate real-world events that are associated with pain onset or exacerbation. Some examples of commonly used stimulus conditions are: (1) negative imagery, wherein a patient concentrates on a personally relevant unpleasant situation; (2) cold exposure or the cold pressor test (immersion of the hand in ice water, which serves as a general physical stressor); (3) movement, such as sitting, rising, bending, stooping, or walking; (4) load bearing, such as lifting or carrying an object; and (5) operation of a keyboard. Although baseline differences for EMG do not reliably characterize pain disorders (Flor and Turk 1989), certain pain conditions show more consistent symptom-specific responses to stimuli (see Flor 2001 for a review).

Recovery from stress, to assess how and when a patient's physiology returns to a value close to that observed prior to stimulus presentation (responses often do not return to their starting values).

The above components constitute the basic approach to psychophysiological assessment. Two additional components—muscle scanning and muscle discrimination—may be useful as well, but they are less common in practice.

Muscle scanning, which uses only two recording channels to quickly assess EMG activity from multiple sites. Two hand-held "post" electrodes provide brief, sequential bilateral recordings for approximately 2 seconds per site while the patient is sitting and standing. Normative databases are being developed to help determine which readings are abnormally high or low and identify any asymmetries (Cram 1990; Sella 1995). Differences between the right and left sides may suggest bracing or favoring of a position or posture. The goal of biofeedback is to return aberrant readings to a more normal state. Although seemingly straightforward, this approach is complex because several factors can influence the results, including the angle and force of sensor application, the amount of adipose tissue (fat acts as an insulator and dampens the signal), and the exactness of sensor placement.

Muscle discrimination, to assess a person's ability to perceive bodily states accurately. Flor and colleagues (1992, 1999) have shown that patients with chronic pain are unable to perceive muscle tension levels accurately in both affected and nonaffected muscles. When exposed to tasks requiring production of muscle tension, these patients overestimated physical symptoms, rated the task as more aversive, and reported greater pain. These findings point to a heightened sensitivity.

Muscle discrimination abilities can easily be assessed in a clinical setting (Flor 2001). Assessment involves: presenting the patient with a bar of varying height on a monitor; instructing the patient to tense a muscle to the level reflected in the height of the bar, which is varied from low to high; and correlating the EMG readings with the heights of the bars. Discrimination abilities with correlation coefficients ≥ 0.80 and ≤ 0.50 are considered "good" and "bad," respectively.

Examples of specific applications

Most research and practice has focused on the value of biofeedback as a general means of decreasing stress, tension, and pain. For patients with certain characteristics, more specific approaches are emerging as either alternative or preferred treatments. A few brief examples illustrate these approaches.

The studies used to support claims for efficacy of EMG biofeedback for recurrent headache (summarized in the concluding section) have monitored muscle activity almost exclusively from the forehead area, despite patient reports that other sites are central to their pain (such as occipital, temporal, neck, and shoulder areas). Support exists for using feedback from the upper trapezius muscles (Arena et al. 1995). A creative and novel approach, termed the frontal-posterior neck placement (Nevins and Schwartz 1985), seeks to monitor activity in the occipitalis area, which is a site of headache activity for certain tension-type headache patients. One active electrode is placed on the frontal area and a second is placed on the posterior neck on the same side. The summated electrical activity between these sites closely approximates that of the occipital area. This approach has been useful for determining headache activity in patients (Hudzynski and Lawrence 1988, 1990). For temporomandibular disorder, in addition to frontal sites, biofeedback is provided from the masseter and temporalis muscles (Glass et al. 1993; Crider and Glaros 1999; Glaros and Lausten 2003).

Sherman (1997) has helped to identify the most appropriate biofeedback treatment for patients experiencing phantom limb pain. Pain described as burning, throbbing, and tingling was associated with decreased temperature in the stump, while pain described as cramping was preceded by and associated with EMG changes. Targeting biofeedback accordingly led to the most successful outcome.

Finally, some researchers have turned their attention to the psychophysiological model of Travell and Simons (1983), who postulated that a large percentage of chronic muscle pain results from trigger points (hyperirritable spots that are painful when compressed). Hubbard (1996) has expanded upon their view using the following line of reasoning. Muscle tension and pain result from sympathetically mediated hyperactivity of muscle spindles, organs that are scattered throughout the muscle belly (hundreds within the trapezius muscle) and contain their own muscle fibers; although traditionally viewed as stretch sensors, they are now recognized to be pain and pressure sensors that can be activated by sympathetic stimulation. The pain associated with trigger points is thus thought to arise in the spindle capsule.

Support for this model comes from studies where indwelling electrode placements have detected high levels of EMG activity in the trigger points themselves, whereas nontender sites just 1 cm away are relatively silent (Hubbard and Berkoff 1993). Further, when the patient is exposed to a stressful stimulus, EMG activity increases at the trigger point but not at adjacent sites (McNulty et al. 1994). This work provides further evidence of the link between behavioral and emotional factors and mechanisms of muscle pain. As a result of this basic research, Gevirtz et al. (1996) have developed a comprehensive treatment program that uses EMG biofeedback to facilitate muscle tension awareness in sessions and in daily life activities so as to

identify stressors triggering increased tension and to assist patients in finding improved ways to cope with tension-producing situations.

INDIRECT APPROACH

The indirect approach to biofeedback, used more for clinical than empirical reasons (Belar and Kibrick 1986), can facilitate psychosomatic therapy.
Consider the example of the pain patient who steadfastly holds to a purely
somatic view of pain and refuses to accept the notion that emotional, behavioral, and environmental factors may be precipitating, perpetuating, or exacerbating pain and other symptoms. With this type of patient, a referral for
biofeedback is likely to be less threatening (it is construed as a "physical"
treatment for a "physical" problem) and can at least open the door for help.
As they acquire "physiological insight," such patients may begin to see the
interplay of physical and psychological factors. In fact, it is not uncommon
for a pain patient who denies psychological factors upon entering therapy to
make a request like the following after just a few sessions of biofeedback:
"Doc, how about turning off the biofeedback equipment today? I want to
talk about a few things." From this point on, session time is divided between
biofeedback and counseling.

SELECT TREATMENT CONSIDERATIONS

Patients beginning biofeedback (and relaxation and hypnosis) treatment
may feel anxious, depressed, and discouraged, are often confused about the
nature of their disorder, and often feel uncertain about their chances for
improvement. Brief instruction about factors underlying their condition, point-
ing out variables that patients can control, is often helpful in counteracting
initial feelings of helplessness and in mobilizing interest in treatment. These
introductory remarks are followed by a description of biofeedback, details
about the frequency and number of sessions and requirements for home
practice, and information about any ancillary treatment that may be used.
The explanation of biofeedback is best understood when accompanied by a
demonstration of the steps involved in measurement and provision of feedback. Education remains an integral part of treatment, as patients learn more
about the causes of their pain and discover new ways to react to it.

To facilitate general relaxation, initial sessions typically occur in a quiet,
dimly lit room with the patient semi-reclined in a comfortable chair that
supports the entire body. Most clinicians adopt a "coaching" model that
involves sharing observations for discussion, such as: "I noticed that your
EMG signal shot up. It seemed you might have been clenching your teeth

then. How about dropping your lower jaw and moving it just a bit forward? I wonder if anything particular might have been on your mind then?" The therapist should determine when breaks and encouragement might be needed, because early attempts to lower EMG or skin conductance or to raise hand temperature often produce the opposite effect, and this situation paradoxically worsens as patients try harder and harder. These occurrences can be of great therapeutic value by helping to demonstrate the relationship between thoughts and physiological functioning; explaining how and why this is happening helps to counteract frustration and get the patient back on track. The therapist should help patients to articulate and consolidate what they have learned. Biofeedback can be augmented with instruction in complementary relaxation approaches (see subsequent sections).

Biofeedback involves learning a skill that requires regular practice and eventually incorporating learned skills into day-to-day activities. Some patients become successful simply by concentrating on the feedback stimulus and becoming aware of corresponding sensations. Others engage in various mental games or attempt to empty their minds completely and think of nothing (Arena and Blanchard 1996). In early sessions, patients are encouraged to experiment with various techniques, but to remain with a given technique long enough to give it an ample trial period. The therapist is best viewed as a "coach," someone who has special skills the patient does not yet have, but who can impart these skills by properly timed guidance. With experience, the therapist learns when the patient needs uninterrupted time to practice biofeedback and when support and assistance would be valuable (Borgeat et al. 1980).

A typical treatment session begins with sensor attachment and time for adaptation, initial progress review, and establishment of a resting baseline (as discussed previously). "Self-control" baseline is defined as the patient's ability to regulate the target response in the desired direction once training has begun but in the absence of feedback (Blanchard and Epstein 1978). It provides an index of the ability to perform the biofeedback skills outside of the treatment setting. The core of the session includes 20–40 minutes of feedback (continuous or interrupted by breaks), followed by resting or self-control baseline to assess the extent of learning within the session, and a final progress review and homework assignment.

Each session should end with a review of the strategies explored and an appraisal of their effectiveness. Once the patient has shown some ability to regulate target physiological levels in the clinic, practice outside the office is encouraged. Initially patients should practice the technique in a setting maximally conducive to achieving a relaxed state or concentrating on the task at hand. Subsequently, they can practice during everyday, but low-stress, activities such as driving, shopping, standing in line, or taking a coffee break. The final goal is to employ learned biofeedback skills to counteract the buildup of stress and physiological arousal. Skills must be highly developed to be successful in this context.

Thus, the goals of biofeedback are for the patient to be able to learn when to control the target response, to effect the necessary change in the absence of feedback, to apply the skills in daily life, and to continue to use the skills over the long term. Therapists are concerned with the generalization and maintenance of learned skills. Lynn and Freedman (1979) have identified several procedures that help increase the durability of biofeedback training effects, such as overlearning the response (i.e., continuing to practice learned skills); incorporating booster treatments; fading or gradually removing feedback during treatment; training under stimulating or stressful conditions, such as during noise and distractions, or while engaged in a physical or mental task; employing multiple therapists, which is possible in group practices; varying the physical setting; providing patients with portable biofeedback devices for use in real-life situations; and augmenting biofeedback with other physiological interventions and with cognitive and behavioral procedures (for details see other chapters in this volume).

No firm criteria guide when to terminate biofeedback. In research investigations of biofeedback as a general relaxation technique, patients commonly receive a set number of treatments, typically ranging from 8–12 sessions. In practice, clinical response determines the number of sessions, as gauged by degree of symptom relief or adequacy of control of the target response. Skilled therapists come to sense when treatment has reached the point of diminishing returns or marginal utility (i.e., response reaches a plateau from which further effort brings no improvement). Some have advocated a physiological training criterion as a deciding factor, such as the ability to reduce and keep EMG levels below a certain value for a specified time, or the ability to raise hand temperature above a certain value within a specified period. This intuitive notion has great clinical appeal, but we are not yet at a point where it is possible to recommend a specific approach.

Few difficulties have been reported for using biofeedback as a general relaxation procedure. A small portion of clients may experience what has been termed "relaxation-induced anxiety," a sudden increase in anxiety during deep relaxation that can range from mild to moderate intensity and that can approach the level of a minor panic attack (Heide and Borkovec 1983). It is important for the therapist to remain calm, reassure the patient that the episode will pass, and, when possible, have the patient sit up for a few minutes or even walk about the office. With patients who are believed to be at risk for relaxation-induced anxiety, it may be helpful to instruct them to focus more on the somatic aspects as opposed to the cognitive aspects of training (Arena and Blanchard 1996). See Schwartz et al. (2003) for a discussion of other problems and solutions.

THE ESSENCE OF RELAXATION

Several procedures in addition to biofeedback can promote generalized relaxation. Chief among these are imagery, diaphragmatic breathing, autogenic training, and progressive muscle relaxation training. Many of the comments and clinical approaches described for biofeedback apply equally to relaxation therapy.

IMAGERY

The first and simplest imagery technique is to imagine a pleasant or relaxing scene, such as lying on a blanket at the beach while listening to the waves roll in and out, or walking through a pleasant meadow on a warm, sunny day. It is best that patients avoid images that involve sexual content or vigorous physical activity that can increase rather than decrease arousal. Images should include as many sensory modalities (touch, sound, smell) and details as possible (Arena and Blanchard 1996). It is recommended that patients practice using several different relaxing images, so that they can switch to another image if the selected one is not working at a given time. With practice, images can be recalled quickly and vividly and can be used effectively to provide mental escape when situations seem overwhelming.

DIAPHRAGMATIC BREATHING

Most patients find this procedure particularly useful because breathing can be readily brought under voluntary control and is an activity that is vital to survival. The notion of relaxed breathing is deceptively simple, so most patients need detailed instructions for correct use. Improper application can lead to blood gas imbalance and hyper- or hypoventilation. Also, patients whose initial respiration rate is high (greater than 30 breaths per minute) may feel strange as their breathing rate approaches the relaxed range. Such patients are instructed to pay no particular attention to these peculiar feelings and are informed that they will pass with time. Gevirtz and Schwartz (2003) provide an excellent discussion of the topic, which briefly reviews the physiology of breathing and provides instructions on how to teach patients to breathe slowly (to a target range of 5–8 breaths per minute), deeply (to full lung capacity), and evenly (to facilitate approximately the same rate for exhaling and for inhaling), while concentrating on the associated physiological sensations. Having the patient subvocalize a word associated with relaxation on each exhalation can help "cue" subsequent relaxation.

Various methods can promote the desired breathing pattern. Patients can practice breathing while holding their arms straight overhead (which minimizes chest movement). They can lie on a firm surface with a medium-weight book placed on the abdomen, and raise and lower it with each breath cycle. Or they can place one hand on the chest and the other just below the rib cage and breathe in a manner that limits movement of the hand on the chest and maximizes movement of the hand on the abdomen.

Gevirtz and Schwartz (2003) discuss other approaches for promoting more relaxed breathing, including paced respiration, breath meditation, breath mindfulness, rebreathing, pursed-lip breathing, and instrument-based approaches. These very portable procedures can easily be combined with other relaxation techniques.

AUTOGENIC TRAINING

A third form of relaxation borrows from the well-developed body of literature on autogenic training, a type of meditation with an extensive history. Patients passively concentrate on key words and phrases selected for their ability to promote desired somatic responses (Schultz and Luthe 1969). Clinicians who provide autogenic training in conjunction with thermal biofeedback typically select two methods that are generally considered the most effective of the six traditional components of autogenic training. Patients are instructed to focus on sensations of warmth and heaviness in the extremities, a technique that is believed to facilitate increased blood flow to the extremities and thus promote peripheral warming and a reduction in sympathetic nervous arousal. It is recommended that patients develop their own phrases and subvocalize them 50–100 times during each practice session to maximize the effects (Arena and Blanchard 1996).

PROGRESSIVE MUSCLE RELAXATION TRAINING

The fourth and final technique, progressive muscle relaxation training, has the most extensive empirical basis (see concluding section), but it is also the most complex. The patient engages in a systematic series of muscle tensing and releasing exercises designed to help discriminate various levels of muscle tension, which facilitates a generalized state of relaxation.

Andrasik (1986) describes a typical relaxation training regimen for headache patients, as outlined in Table I. The introductory sessions stress that relaxation training consists of systematic tensing and relaxing of major muscle groups, that tensing muscles even for a brief period results in a subsequent lower level of tension, and that experiencing a broad range of muscle tension levels enables patients to better discriminate when muscle tension is building. With improved discrimination abilities and acquisition of skills for rapidly relaxing muscles, patients can use this technique to counteract tension buildup as it occurs throughout the day (termed *applied relaxation*). Trainers emphasize that achieving a deep state of relaxation is a learned skill that requires regular practice, and that the procedure will first focus on all major muscle groups, but muscle groups will subsequently be combined to permit rapid relaxation.

The procedure begins with the patient sequentially tensing and relaxing 14 separate muscle groupings in the 18 steps indicated in Table II. Prior to formal instruction, the patient completes a few practice tension-release cycles to ensure that the tension generated is neither incomplete nor overly zealous and is confined to the target muscle group. Muscles that are very painful or that have been strained are omitted so as not to cause further problems. Target muscle groups are tensed for 5–7 seconds and then relaxed for 20–30 seconds, which constitutes a complete cycle. The patient is instructed to note the sensations associated with tension and relaxation during each cycle. It is acceptable to modify the sequence according to the patient's preference, but it is important that the patient adhere to the modified sequence. Patients may periodically need to mentally scan previously targeted muscle groups to identify any residual tension. If tension is detected, another tension-release cycle may be completed. Various procedures, all involving therapist suggestions, may also be used to deepen the sense of relaxation (for example, the therapist may count out loud backwards from 5 to 1 and instruct the patient

Table I
Outline of progressive muscle relaxation training program

Session	1	2	3	4	5	6	7	8	9	10
Week	1	1	2	2	3	3	4	5	6	8
Introduction	x									
Number of muscle groups	14	14	14	14	8	8	4	4	4	4
Deepening exercises	x	x	x	x	x	x	x	x	x	x
Breathing exercises	x	x	x	x	x	x	x	x	x	x
Relaxing imagery		x	x	x	x	x	x	x	x	x
Muscle discrimination training			x	x	x	x	x	x	x	x
Relaxation by recall						x	x	x	x	x
Cue-controlled relaxation								x	x	x

Source: Adapted from Andrasik and Walch (2003).

Table II
Fourteen initial muscle groups and procedures for tensing in 18 steps

1. Right hand and lower arm (have client make a fist, simultaneously tense lower arm).
2. Left hand and lower arm.
3. Both hands and lower arms.
4. Right upper arm (have client bring hand to shoulder and tense biceps).
5. Left upper arm.
6. Both upper arms.
7. Right lower leg and foot (have client point toe while tensing calf muscles).
8. Left lower leg and foot.
9. Both lower legs and feet.
10. Both thighs (have client press knees and thighs tightly together).
11. Abdomen (have client draw abdominal muscles in tightly, as if bracing to receive a punch).
12. Chest (have client take a deep breath and hold it).
13. Shoulders and lower neck (have client "hunch" shoulders or draw shoulders up toward the ears).
14. Back of the neck (have client press head back against headrest or chair).
15. Lips/mouth (have client press lips together tightly, but not so tight as to clench teeth, or have client place tip of tongue on roof of mouth behind upper front teeth).
16. Eyes (have client close the eyes tightly).
17. Lower forehead (have client frown and draw the eyebrows together).
18. Upper forehead (have client wrinkle the forehead area or raise the eyebrows).

Source: Andrasik and Walch (2003).

to experience a deeper level of relaxation with each successive count). Relaxed breathing and imagery are added early on, in the manner discussed previously. Once the patient has made adequate progress at tensing and relaxing the 14 major muscle groups, the therapist begins to combine various groups, first using eight muscle groupings, and then four (see Table III).

Muscle discrimination training can be added to facilitate abilities to detect even trace amounts of tension increases in the target areas (such as the head, neck, and shoulders for headache patients). To demonstrate this aspect, a patient is asked to engage in a complete tension-release cycle involving the hand and lower arm, then to tense these muscles by only half as much. Then follows a tension cycle involving only one-quarter as much force. Once the concept of differential tension is understood, the patient can apply differential tensing to the muscles most associated with pain. Final techniques concern relaxation by recall and cue-controlled relaxation. To implement relaxation by recall, the patient first recalls the sensations associated with relaxation and then attempts to reproduce these sensations, using tension and release cycles as needed to promote the desired somatic state. Practice outside the office is necessary to maximize effects; patients are

Table III
Abbreviated muscle groups

Eight Muscle Groups
1. Both hands and lower arms
2. Both legs and thighs
3. Abdomen
4. Chest
5. Shoulders
6. Back of neck
7. Eyes
8. Forehead
Four Muscle Groups
1. Arms
2. Chest
3. Neck
4. Face (with a particular focus on the eyes and forehead)

Source: Andrasik and Walch (2003).

typically instructed to practice techniques once or twice a day. Audiotapes, prepared commercially or by the therapist during a session with the patient, can facilitate home practice. See Andrasik (1986), Arena and Blanchard (1996), Lichstein (1988), and Smith (1990) for further information about relaxation in general.

THE ESSENCE OF HYPNOSIS

Spiegel (2003) asks, "Why ... would one contemplate utilizing a technique such as hypnosis, which is often thought to involve relinquishing control, in the treatment of a disorder that is better managed with enhanced control?" He describes hypnosis as a "normal state of highly focused attention, with a relative diminution in peripheral awareness" (Spiegel and Spiegel 1987; Spiegel and Maldonado 1999; Spiegel et al. 2000), and likens this state to being so caught up and so absorbed in a movie, play, or novel as to lose awareness of the present moment and to gain entry into an imaginary world. He states, paradoxically, that the same state that appears to promote a loss of control can in actuality enhance control (the unwanted pain sensations are displaced to the periphery of awareness, are altered in form, or ideally are eliminated). It differs, therefore, from the commonly used technique of distraction, which seeks to focus the patient's attention on external events or objects (Kuttner and Culbert 2003).

Hypnosis and related procedures are believed to operate through two primary mechanisms: muscle relaxation and perceptual alteration (Spiegel

2003). The mechanism of relaxation for pain management has been discussed earlier. Below I offer a few examples of the second mechanism, designed to encourage patients to imagine the affected body part as becoming numb or insensitive to pain.

PAIN SWITCH TECHNIQUE

Kuttner and Culbert (2003) provide an example of this technique for children. The child is first taught how the brain processes nerve signals from the body:

> Right now the nerves in your body are sending a lot of pain information about your ... broken wrist. Your brain instantly understands these nerve signals, and sends messages back to the body, that keeps you aware of the pain. Now, I'm going to teach you how to focus your attention on the switches in your brain that control those incoming pain signals so that you can turn them down. As you do that your body will receive weaker pain messages and therefore feel less pain. The more you practice this the better you'll get at turning the pain switches down more quickly. And you'll feel less pain and be in more control (p. 151).

The hypnotic induction is then used to create a trance state, wherein the patient is instructed to focus on the switch within the brain that controls the painful body part. With each breath, the patient is instructed to turn down the pain switch to the extent possible. Posthypnotic suggestion helps maintain lowered pain and reminds the patient that further relief will occur with sustained practice. The goal of the pain switch technique, Kuttner and Culbert remind us, is not necessarily to completely eliminate pain, but rather to provide sufficient relief and promote a sense of mastery of pain (enhanced coping).

OTHER TECHNIQUES

By drawing upon past experiences with procaine during dental procedures, a patient can reproduce the sensations experienced in the jaw and mouth and to move these sensations to the new pain location in attempts to "numb" the present pain. The patient can use thermal images to help cool or warm the affected body part by employing strategies similar to those used in thermal biofeedback. Pain and temperature sensations share the same sensory system, the lateral spinothalamic tract (Spiegel 2003), which may promote this transformation of pain. Patients can learn to view pain as a substance that can move around within the body or that can even flow completely out of the body. A final technique involves "controlled dissociation." An example is having the patient "step outside" the body and "visit" another location, leaving the pain behind or floating above the body.

A trained hypnotherapist attempts to tailor the technique to the patient, guided in part by the patient's ability and susceptibility. Various components of relaxation training discussed previously are regularly incorporated to enhance and deepen the hypnotic effects. All hypnotic techniques share common goals: shifting the focus from fearing and fighting to understanding and accepting pain, reducing the intensity of or creating distance from the pain, lessening the impact of the pain, and transforming the experience of pain to something that is more bearable, in a departure from the more dichotomous thinking of pain as being either present or absent (Kuttner and Culbert 2003; Spiegel 2003). Holroyd (1996) provides a comprehensive review of various mechanisms of hypnosis.

THE EVIDENCE BASE

Extensive research on the procedures described in this chapter has been evaluated by task forces conducting evidence-based reviews and by scientists conducting quantitative or meta-analytic reviews. The chapter closes by providing a brief summary of the literature.

Biofeedback has proven beneficial for headache management in adults and children (Blanchard et al. 1980; Holroyd et al. 1984; Holroyd and Penzien 1986; Andrasik and Blanchard 1987; Blanchard and Andrasik 1987; Bogaards and ter Kuile 1994; Hermann et al. 1995; Task Force on Promotion and Dissemination of Psychological Procedures 1995; Haddock et al. 1997; Goslin et al. 1999; Holden et al. 1999; Campbell et al. 2000; Sarafino and Goehring 2000; McCrory et al. 2001; Eccleston et al. 2002), for temporomandibular disorders (Crider and Glaros 1999), and for other forms of recurrent pain (Keefe and Hoelscher 1987; NIH Technology Assessment Panel on Integration of Behavioral and Relaxation Approaches into the Treatment of Chronic Pain and Insomnia 1996; Morley et al. 1999). Most of these sources provide a similar level of support for relaxation treatments. Finally, Montgomery et al. (2000), in the most extensive meta-analysis of hypnosis, found it effective for both patients and healthy volunteers and concluded that it compared favorably to alternative treatment procedures. Further inspection of the data supported the notion that effects were optimized when patients possessed high levels of suggestibility. These findings support an earlier quantitative analysis (Kirsch et al. 1995).

REFERENCES

Andrasik F. Relaxation and biofeedback for chronic headaches. In: Holzman AD, Turk DC (Eds). *Pain Management: A Handbook of Psychological Treatment Approaches.* New York: Pergamon, 1986, pp 213–329.

Andrasik F. Biofeedback. In: Mostofsky DI, Barlow DH (Eds). *The Management of Stress and Anxiety Disorders in Medical Disorders.* Boston: Allyn and Bacon, 2000, pp 66–83.

Andrasik F, Blanchard EB. The biofeedback treatment of tension headache. In: Hatch JP, Fisher JG, Rugh JD (Eds). *Biofeedback: Studies in Clinical Efficacy.* New York: Plenum, 1987, pp 281–321.

Andrasik F, Flor H. Biofeedback. In: Breivik H, Campbell W, Eccleston C (Eds). *Clinical Pain Management: Practical Applications and Procedures.* London: Arnold, 2003, pp 121–133.

Andrasik F, Walch SE. Headaches. In: Nezu AM, Nezu CM, Geller PA (Eds). *Health Psychology,* Comprehensive Handbook of Psychology, Vol. 9. New York: Wiley, 2003, pp 245–266.

Arena JG, Blanchard EB. Biofeedback and relaxation therapy for chronic pain disorders. In: Gatchel RJ, Turk DC (Eds). *Psychological Approaches to Pain Management: A Practitioner's Handbook.* New York: Guilford Press, 1996, pp 179–230.

Arena JG, Schwartz MS. Psychophysiological assessment and biofeedback baselines: a primer. In: Schwartz MS, Andrasik F (Eds). *Biofeedback: A Practitioner's Guide,* 3rd ed. New York: Guilford Press, 2003, pp 128–158.

Arena JG, Bruno GM, Hannah SL, Meador KJ. A comparison of frontal electromyographic biofeedback training, trapezius electromyographic biofeedback training, and progressive muscle relaxation therapy in the treatment of tension headache. *Headache* 1995; 35:411–419.

Basmajian JV. Facts versus myths in EMG biofeedback. *Biofeedback Self Regul* 1976; 1:369–371.

Belar CD, Kibrick SA. Biofeedback in the treatment of chronic back pain. In: Holzman AD, Turk DC (Eds). *Pain Management: A Handbook of Psychological Treatment Approaches.* New York: Pergamon Press, 1986, pp 131–150.

Blanchard EB, Andrasik F. Biofeedback treatment of vascular headache. In: Hatch JP, Fisher JG, Rugh JD (Eds). *Biofeedback: Studies in Clinical Efficacy.* New York: Plenum, 1987, pp 1–79.

Blanchard EB, Epstein LH. *A Biofeedback Primer.* Reading, MA: Addison-Wesley, 1978.

Blanchard EB, Andrasik F, Ahles TA, et al. Migraine and tension headache: a meta-analytic review. *Behav Ther* 1980; 14:613–631.

Bonica JJ. Management of myofascial pain syndromes in general practice. *JAMA* 1957; 164:732–738.

Bogaards MC, ter Kuile MM. Treatment of recurrent tension headache: a meta-analytic review. *Clin J Pain* 1994; 10:174–190.

Borgeat F, Hade B, Larouche LM, Bedwani CN. Effect of therapist's active presence on EMG biofeedback training of headache patients. *Biofeedback Self Regul* 1980; 5:275–282.

Boucsein W. *Electrodermal Activity.* New York: Plenum, 1992.

Cacioppo JT, Tassinary LG, Bernston GG (Eds). *Handbook of Psychophysiology,* 2nd ed. Cambridge: Cambridge University Press, 2000.

Campbell JK, Penzien DB, Wall EM. *Evidence-Based Guidelines for Migraine Headaches: Behavioral and Physical Treatments.* April 2000. Available via the Internet: www.aan.com.

Cram JR. EMG muscle scanning and diagnostic manual for surface recordings. In: Cram JR, et al. (Eds). *Clinical EMG for Surface Recordings,* Vol. 2. Nevada City, CA: Clinical Resources, 1990, pp 1–141.

Crider AB, Glaros AG. A meta-analysis of EMG biofeedback treatment of temporomandibular disorders. *J Orofac Pain* 1999; 13:29–37.

Eccleston C, Morley S, Williams A, Yorke L, Mastroyannopoulou K. Systematic review of randomised controlled trials of psychological therapy for chronic pain in children and adolescents, with a subset meta-analysis of pain relief. *Pain* 2002; 99:157–165.

Flor H. Psychophysiological assessment of the patient with chronic pain. In: Turk DC, Melzack R (Eds). *Handbook of Pain Assessment,* 2nd ed. New York: Guilford Press, 2001, pp 76–96.

Flor H, Turk DC. Psychophysiology of chronic pain: do chronic pain patients exhibit symptom-specific psychophysiological responses? *Psychol Bull* 1989, 105:219–259.

Flor H, Schugens MM, Birbaumer N. Discrimination of muscle tension in chronic pain patients and healthy controls. *Biofeedback Self Regul* 1992; 17:165–177.

Flor H, Fürst M, Birbaumer N. Deficient discrimination of EMG levels and overestimation of perceived tension in chronic pain patients. *Appl Psychophysiol Biofeedback* 1999; 24:55–66.

French DJ, Holroyd KA, Pinell C, et al. Perceived self-efficacy and headache-related disability. *Headache* 2000; 40:647–656.

Gevirtz RN, Schwartz MS. The respiratory system in applied psychophysiology. In: Schwartz MS, Andrasik F (Eds). *Biofeedback: A Practitioner's Guide,* 3rd ed. New York: Guilford Press, 2003, pp 212–244.

Gevirtz RN, Hubbard DR, Harpin RE. Psychophysiologic treatment of chronic lower back pain. *Prof Psychol Res Pr* 1996; 27:561–566.

Glaros AG, Lausten L. Temporomandibular disorders. In: Schwartz MS, Andrasik F (Eds). *Biofeedback: A Practitioner's Guide,* 3rd ed. New York: Guilford Press, 2003, pp 349–368.

Glass EG, Glaros AG, McGlynn FD. Myofascial pain dysfunction: treatments used by ADA members. *J Craniomandibular Pract* 1993; 11:25–29.

Goslin RE, Gray RN, McCrory DC, et al. *Behavioral Physical Treatments for Migraine Headache.* Technical Review 2.2. Agency for Health Care Policy and Research, February 1999. Available from the National Technical Information Service, NTIS Accession No. 127946.

Haddock CK, Rowan AB, Andrasik F, et al. Home-based behavioral treatments for chronic benign headache: a meta-analysis of controlled trials. *Cephalalgia* 1997; 17:113–118.

Hermann C, Kim M, Blanchard EB. Behavioral and prophylactic pharmacological intervention studies of pediatric migraine: an exploratory meta-analysis. *Pain* 1995; 60:239–256.

Heide FJ, Borkovec TD. Relaxation-induced anxiety: paradoxical anxiety enhancement due to relaxation training. *J Consult Clin Psychol* 1983; 51:171–182.

Holden EW, Deichmann MM, Levy JD. Empirically supported treatments in pediatric psychology: recurrent pediatric headache. *J Pediatr Psychol* 1999; 24:91–109.

Holroyd J. Hypnosis treatment of clinical pain: understanding why hypnosis is useful. *Int J Clin Exp Hypn* 1996; 44:33–51.

Holroyd KA, Penzien D. Client variables and the behavioral treatment of recurrent tension headache: a meta-analytic review. *J Behav Med* 1986; 9:515–536.

Holroyd KA, Penzien DB, Holm JE, Hursey KG. Behavioral treatment of tension and migraine headache: what does the literature say? *Headache* 1984; 24:167–168.

Hubbard D. Chronic and recurrent muscle pain: pathophysiology and treatment, and review of pharmacologic studies. *J Musculoskeletal Pain* 1996; 4:123–143.

Hubbard D, Berkoff G. Myofascial trigger points show spontaneous EMG activity. *Spine* 1993; 18:1803–1807.

Hudzynski LG, Lawrence GS. Significance of EMG surface electrode placement models and headache findings. *Headache* 1988; 28:30–35.

Hudzynski LG, Lawrence GS. EMG surface electrode normative data for muscle contraction headache and biofeedback therapy. *Headache Q* 1990; 1:224–229.

Keefe FJ, Hoelscher TJ. Biofeedback in the management of chronic pain syndromes. In: Hatch JP, Fisher JG, Rugh JD (Eds). *Biofeedback: Studies in Clinical Efficacy.* New York: Plenum, 1987, pp 211–253.

Kirsch I, Montgomery G, Sapirstein G. Hypnosis as an adjunct to cognitive-behavioral psychotherapy: a meta-analysis. *J Consult Clin Psychol* 1995; 63:214–220.

Kuttner L, Culbert T. Hypnosis, biofeedback, and self-regulation skills for children in pain. In: Breivik H, Campbell W, Eccleston C (Eds). *Clinical Pain Management: Practical Applications and Procedures.* London: Arnold, 2003, pp 148–162.

Lichstein KL. *Clinical Relaxation Strategies.* New York: Wiley and Sons, 1988.

Lynn SJ, Freedman RR. Transfer and evaluation of biofeedback treatment. In: Goldstein AP, Kanfer F (Eds). *Maximizing Treatment Gains: Transfer Enhancement in Psychotherapy.* New York: Academic Press, 1979, pp 445–484.

McCrory DC, Penzien DB, Hasselblad V, Gray RN. *Evidence Report: Behavioral and Physical Treatments for Tension-type and Cervicogenic Headache.* Des Moines: Foundation for Chiropractic Education and Research, 2001.

McNulty E, Gevirtz R, Hubbard D, Berkoff G. Needle electromyographic evaluation of trigger point response to a psychological stressor. *Psychophysiology* 1994, 31:313–316.

Montgomery GH, DuHamel KN, Redd WH. A meta-analysis of hypnotically induced analgesia: how effective is hypnosis? *Int J Clin Exp Hypn* 2000; 48:138–153.

Morley S, Eccleston C, Williams A. Systematic review and meta-analysis of randomized controlled trials of cognitive behaviour therapy and behaviour therapy for chronic pain in adults, excluding headache. *Pain* 1999; 80:1–13.

Neumann E, Blanton R. The early history of electrodermal research. *Psychophysiology* 1970; 6:453–475.

Nevins BG, Schwartz MS. An alternative placement for EMG electrodes in the study and treatment of tension headaches. *Biofeedback Self-Regul* 1985; 10:109.

NIH Technology Assessment Panel on Integration of Behavioral and Relaxation Approaches into the Treatment of Chronic Pain and Insomnia. Integration of behavioral and relaxation approaches into the treatment of chronic pain and insomnia. *JAMA* 1996; 276:313–318.

Peek CJ. A primer of biofeedback instrumentation. In: Schwartz MS, Andrasik F (Eds). *Biofeedback: A Practitioner's Guide,* 3rd ed. New York: Guilford Press, 2003, pp 43–87.

Sarafino EP, Goehring P. Age comparisons in acquiring biofeedback control and success in reducing headache pain. *Ann Behav Med* 2000; 22:10–16.

Sargent JD, Green EE, Walters ED. The use of autogenic training in a pilot study of migraine and tension headaches. *Headache* 1972; 12:120–124.

Schultz JH, Luthe W. *Autogenic Training,* Vol. 1. New York: Grune and Stratton, 1969.

Schwartz MS, Schwartz NM, Monastra VJ. Problems with relaxation and biofeedback-assisted relaxation, and guidelines for management. In: Schwartz MS, Andrasik F (Eds). *Biofeedback: A Practitioner's Guide,* 3rd ed. New York: Guilford Press, 2003, pp 251–264.

Schwartz NM, Schwartz MS. Definitions of biofeedback and applied psychophysiology. In: Schwartz MS, Andrasik F (Eds). *Biofeedback: A Practitioner's Guide,* 3rd ed. New York: Guilford Press, 2003, pp 27–39.

Sella G. *Neuro-muscular Testing with Surface EMG.* Martins Ferry, OH: Genmed, 1995.

Sherman R. *Phantom Pain.* New York: Plenum Press, 1997.

Smith JC. *Cognitive-Behavioral Relaxation Training: A New System of Strategies for Treatment and Assessment.* New York: Springer, 1990.

Spiegel D. Self-regulation skills training for adults, including relaxation. In: Breivik H, Campbell W, Eccleston C (Eds). *Clinical Pain Management: Practical Applications and Procedures.* London: Arnold, 2003, pp 113–119.

Spiegel D, Maldonado J. Hypnosis. In: Hales RE, Yudofsky S, Talbott J (Eds). *American Psychiatric Press Textbook of Psychiatry.* Washington, DC: American Psychiatric Press, 1999.

Spiegel H, Spiegel D. *Trance and Treatment: Clinical Use of Hypnosis.* Washington, DC: American Psychiatric Press, 1987.

Spiegel H, Greenleaf M, Spiegel D. Hypnosis. In: Sadock B, Sadock V (Eds). *Comprehensive Textbook of Psychiatry,* 7th ed. Philadelphia: Lippincott Williams and Wilkins, 2000, pp 2128–2146.

Stern RM, Ray WJ, Quigley KS. *Psychophysiological Recording*, 2nd ed. Oxford: Oxford University, 2001.

Surwit RS, Keefe FJ. Frontalis EMG-feedback training: an electronic panacea? *Behav Ther* 1978; 9:779–772.

Task Force on Promotion and Dissemination of Psychological Procedures. Training in and dissemination of empirically-validated psychological treatments: report and recommendations. *Clin Psychol* 1995; 48:3–23.

Travell J, Simons D. *Myofascial Pain and Dysfunction: The Trigger Point Manual.* New York: Williams and Wilkins, 1983.

Correspondence to: Frank Andrasik, PhD, Institute for Human and Machine Cognition, University of West Florida, 40 South Alcaniz Street, Pensacola, FL 32502, USA. Tel: 1-850-202-4460; Fax: 1-850-202-4440; email: fandrasik@ihmc.us.

Part IV
Complex Disorders

Psychosocial Aspects of Pain: A Handbook for Health Care Providers, Progress in Pain Research and Management, Vol. 27, edited by Robert H. Dworkin and William S. Breitbart, IASP Press, Seattle, © 2004.

14

Fibromyalgia: A Patient-Oriented Perspective

Dennis C. Turk

Department of Anesthesiology, University of Washington School of Medicine, Seattle, Washington, USA

Fibromyalgia syndrome (FMS) is a chronic condition that consists of a pervasive set of unexplained physical symptoms with generalized pain and hypersensitivity to palpation at specific body locations ("tender points") as the cardinal features. FMS sufferers report that although their pain fluctuates in intensity, it is nearly continuous. In addition, patients typically report a range of functional limitations and psychological dysfunctions including persistent fatigue (78.2%), sleep disturbance (75.6%), feelings of stiffness (76.2%), headaches (54.3%), depression and anxiety (44.9%), and irritable bowel disorder (35.7%) (Wolfe et al. 1990). Patients also report cognitive impairment and general malaise, sometimes referred to as "fibro fog" (Baumstark and Buckelew 1992). This pattern of symptoms has been reported under various names such as tension myalgia, psychogenic rheumatism, and fibromyositis since the early 19th century.

FMS is a prevalent condition, estimated to affect 3–6 million people in the United States (Goldenberg 1987). In general populations the prevalence of FMS is estimated to range from 0.66% to 10.5% (Schochat et al. 1994). A large-scale epidemiological study in Ontario, Canada (White et al. 1999) estimated that 5% of women and 1.6% of men are afflicted with FMS. Another large-scale study (Forseth and Gran 1992) in Norway suggests an annual incidence of 583 cases per 100,000 women.

FMS is more commonly observed in women, with a female-to-male ratio of persons seeking treatment of approximately 7 to 1. In community samples, however, the female-to-male ratio in those meeting the criteria for FMS is closer to 3 to 1. The number of persons diagnosed with FMS tends to increase from the second through the sixth decade of life. Although the syndrome seems relatively common in the general population, symptoms tend to be less severe and disabling in cases found in population-based samples compared to patients who seek treatment (Prescott et al. 1993).

FMS may have an insidious onset without any identifiable cause, may develop following a flu-like illness, or may rapidly develop following an identified trauma such as a motor vehicle accident or emotional distress (Turk et al. 1996a; Clauw and Chrousos 1997). The natural course of FMS symptoms seems to be chronic and nonprogressive, with fluctuations in symptom severity. There is no widely accepted biological marker to account for the set of symptoms reported. Radiographic and laboratory findings tend to be negative. Hypothesized plausible causal mechanisms include muscle fiber irregularities, neurotransmitter imbalances, and maladaptive psychological variables (Pillemer et al. 1997; Okifuji and Turk 1999). I will briefly describe these possible mechanisms below. There is no known cure for this syndrome.

There is little question that FMS adversely affects patients' lives. FMS patients report a lowered sense of physical well-being and greater health concerns, and are high utilizers of the health care system (Bombardier and Buchwald 1996; Wolfe et al. 1997). FMS sufferers rate the quality of their lives as significantly more compromised than do persons with other chronic illnesses such as rheumatoid arthritis (Burckhardt et al. 1993). Concurrent depression is diagnosed in a large proportion of FMS patients (Ahles et al. 1991; Walker et al. 1997).

CLASSIFICATION OF FMS

The proposed classification criteria for FMS are based on the American College of Rheumatology (ACR) multicenter study (Wolfe et al. 1990). The results of this study suggest that the only factors sensitive and specific for FMS are: (1) history of widespread pain of at least 3 months' duration and (2) report of pain on palpation of at least 11 of 18 specific tender points (see Fig. 1).

The procedures proposed to evaluate the ACR criteria are relatively broad and imprecise. MacFarlane and colleagues (1996) have suggested a specific coding system to refine the definition of "widespread pain" (i.e., pain in three of four body quadrants and along the midline). In an attempt to develop a reliable and standardized method to evaluate tender points, Okifuji et al. (1997) developed the Manual Tender Point Survey (MTPS), a protocol adapted from the ACR study (Wolfe et al. 1990) that includes detailed, step-by-step procedures (Table I). The MTPS specifies the order of palpation, patient response instructions, pressure application technique, precise locations of palpation sites, and patient and examiner position. The MTPS yields a

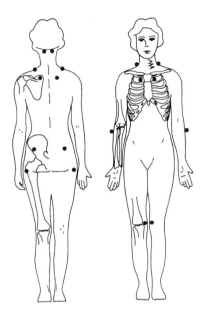

Fig. 1. Location of tender points in nine bilateral sites: *Occiput:* at the suboccipital muscle insertions. *Low cervical:* at the anterior aspects of the intertransverse spaces at C5–C7. *Trapezius:* at the midpoint of the upper border. *Supraspinatus:* at origins, above the scapula spine near the medial border. *Second rib:* at the second costochondral junctions, just lateral to the junctions on upper surfaces. *Lateral epicondyle:* at 2 cm distal to the epicondyles. *Gluteal:* in upper outer quadrants of buttocks in anterior fold of muscle. *Greater trochanter:* posterior to the trochanteric prominence. *Knee:* at the medial fat proximal to the joint line. Reprinted with permission from Okifuji et al. (1997).

pain rating score for each site, ranging from 0 (no pain at all) to 10 (worst pain ever experienced). This 11-point scale was included to permit greater sensitivity to detect changes in tenderness than simply the number of positive tender points; it can be used to evaluate changes over time or to assess the outcome of treatments. A videotape and a printed guide, developed to increase the consistency of performing the MTPS, are available from the authors (Okifuji et al. 1997).

MECHANISMS

The pathophysiological mechanisms underlying FMS are poorly understood. Numerous peripheral and central mechanisms have been proposed to explain the set of symptoms and signs observed in persons with FMS. I will highlight some of the most prominent theories; more detailed presentation is available elsewhere (e.g., Pillemer et al. 1997; Russell 2001).

Table I
Manual Tender Point Survey

General Procedures

1. The MTPS is performed at the beginning of the physical examination with the gowned patient seated on the front end of the examining table.
2. Read the explanation of the standard patient instructions to the patient.
3. Examine the survey sites in numerical order.
4. First locate the survey sites *visually and with light palpation.*
5. Use the thumb pad of your *dominant* hand throughout the exam. Apply thumb pad pressure perpendicularly at the site.
6. Press each survey site for 4 seconds *only once,* increasing the force by 1 kg per second.
7. Immediately record each response after the site is tested.

Procedure for Each Tender Point

1. Forehead (control site)
   Patient position: Seated; head in neutral position
   Examiner position: Front
   Procedure: (1) Support the back of the head with the nondominant hand; (2) press perpendicularly to the geographical center of the forehead

2 & 3. Occiput
   Patient position: Seated; head loosely flexed forward approximately 30 degrees
   Examiner position: Beside and behind
   Procedure: (1) Support the head with the nondominant hand on the forehead; (2) move the examining thumb up midline of the neck to the nuchal ridge, then laterally one thumb width to the insertion of the suboccipital muscles on the occiput; (3) press at this point just below the nuchal ridge

4 & 5. Trapezius
   Patient position: Seated; head in neutral position
   Examiner position: Beside and behind
   Procedure: (1) Identify the midpoint of the upper border of trapezius; (2) press down

6 & 7. Supraspinatus
   Patient position: Seated
   Examiner position: Beside and behind
   Procedure: Press immediately above the scapular spine, near the medial border of the scapula

8 & 9. Gluteal
   Patient position: Seated
   Examiner position: Beside and behind
   Procedure: Position the one hand (right for right side, left for left side) loosely on the iliac crest and place the space between the thumb and index finger on the mid-axillary line; the thumb falls naturally on the survey site on the gluteus medius, just anterior to the gluteus maximus. Press perpendicularly with the examining thumb.

Table I
Continued

---

10 & 11. Low cervical
  Patient position: Seated; head in neutral position
  Examiner position: Beside
  Procedure: (1) Identify the tip of the mastoid process and cricoid cartilage (C6) below the thyroid cartilage; (2) go straight down from the mastoid process to C5–C7 range (cricoid level); (3) support the other side of the neck; (4) press toward the opposite shoulder

12 & 13. Second rib
  Patient position: Seated
  Examiner position: Beside
  Procedure: (1) Find the sternal notch, move down to angle of Louis; (2) move to the 1st palpable rib (2nd rib), one thumb-width lateral to the manubrium sterni; (3) support the patient's back; (4) press the upper border

14 & 15. Lateral epicondyle
  Patient position: Seated; hands on lap
  Examiner position: Beside
  Procedure: (1) Support the forearm with the examiner's nondominant hand; (2) press the point 2 cm distal to the epicondyle

16. Right forearm (control site)
  Patient position: Seated
  Examiner position: Beside
  Procedure: (1) Support the forearm with the examiner's nondominant hand; (2) press at the junction of the distal and middle third of the forearm

17. Left thumb (control site)
  Patient position: Seated
  Examiner position: Beside
  Procedure: (1) Support the thumb with the examiner's nondominant hand; (2) press the entire nail area of the left thumb; (3) do not squeeze the thumb between the examiner's thumb and forefinger

18 & 19. Greater trochanter
  Patient position: Lying on opposite side; leg loosely fixed at the hip and knee
  Examiner position: Beside
  Procedure: Press perpendicularly one thumb-width posterior to the trochanteric prominence

20 & 21. Knee
  Patient position: Lying on back; feet slightly apart
  Examiner position: Beside
  Procedure: Press just above the joint line at the medial fat pad

---

Source: Okifuji et al. (1997).

MUSCULAR INVOLVEMENT

Given that myalgia is a primary complaint in FMS, possible pathophysiological mechanisms in muscle structures and metabolism are of interest. The earliest attempts to uncover the etiology of FMS assumed that reported pain was caused by demonstrable or occult physical abnormality, particularly related to muscle anatomy (Bengtsson et al. 1986), to physiological processes including oxygen availability and depletion (Bengtsson and Hendriksson 1989; Drewes et al. 1993), or to tension myalgia (Zidar et al. 1990).

Elevated muscle tension has been proposed as a potential contributing factor to persistent pain in FMS (Thompson 1990). The basic concept of tension myalgia considers chronic muscle pain as a primary symptom of a family of pain disorders. For example, FMS is a diagnostic classification that is distinct from myofascial pain syndrome. The primary feature that differentiates the two diagnostic entities is the presence of relatively localized *trigger points* with referred pain in myofascial pain syndrome in contrast to widespread pain with *point tenderness at specific locations throughout the body* in FMS. The tension myalgia model implies that sustained muscle tension, resulting from various reasons including spasms, overuse, and poor posture (Zidar et al. 1990), significantly contributes to the development and maintenance of myalgia. The model also implies that elevated muscle tension levels are pervasive and therefore present at all times. The available data, however, generally do not support the tension myalgia model. For example, the baseline tension levels of FMS patients are comparable to those of healthy controls (Zidar et al. 1990; Durette et al. 1991).

Despite various attempts to uncover a specific pathology underlying myalgia, no reliable muscle pathology has been identified (Lindh et al. 1995; Simms 1996). The accumulation of research suggests that the involvement of the peripheral pathology is nonspecific, cannot account for the diverse symptoms, and is unlikely to be primary; however, afferent input from the periphery might play a role as an initiator or maintenance factor of central nervous system (CNS) dysregulation in pain control (Bengtsson and Bengtsson 1988).

NEUROTRANSMITTER DYSREGULATION

Various neurochemical factors also have been studied in FMS patients, including dysregulation of the hypothalamic-pituitary-adrenal (HPA) axis (van Denderen et al. 1992; Crofford et al. 1996), serotonin imbalance (Wolfe et al. 1997), and low levels of insulin-like growth factor I (somatomedin C) (Bennett et al. 1992). However, to date, no definitive neurochemical basis for FMS has been identified. What is most notable in the studies examining various neuroendocrine substances in FMS is the large intragroup variability observed in any of the substances tested. Thus, although FMS patients may statistically be different from persons without FMS, the large individual differences within FMS patients make it difficult to interpret the results.

At present, none of the biomedical models appears to be adequate to explain the array of symptoms that characterize FMS. As is so often the case in medicine, when physiological explanations are unsatisfactory, attention turns to psychological models.

PSYCHOLOGICAL MECHANISMS

The failure to identify a direct association between physical pathology, coupled with the high degree of psychiatric comorbidity, have led some to suggest that FMS should be viewed as predominantly a psychogenic disorder. This view finds support in the fact that depression, stress, hypervigilance to sensory stimulation, and maladaptive appraisals and belief systems are prevalent in FMS sufferers.

Depression. Over half of patients diagnosed with FMS have a lifetime history of depression, and concurrent depression is diagnosed in 14–71% of FMS patients, a prevalence far exceeding that found in community populations (e.g., Ahles et al. 1991; Walker et al. 1997; Myers et al. 1984). Although the prevalence of depression in FMS is no higher than in rheumatoid arthritis (Ahles et al. 1991), some researchers hypothesize that the affective disorder is the primary mechanism underlying FMS (Hudson et al. 1985; Alfici et al. 1989). Clinical investigators who have observed the similarity and overlap of symptoms in FMS, chronic fatigue syndrome, irritable bowel syndrome, and temporomandibular disorders have proposed several overlapping "functional somatic syndromes" (Barsky and Borus 1999; Morriss et al. 1999). However, we lack empirical evidence in support of the psychogenic models.

Stress. Many FMS patients report that their symptoms began following physical or emotional stress (e.g., Turk et al. 1996b; Clauw and Chrousos 1997), which suggests that perception of stress may play a causal role. We must be cautious, however, in relying on retrospective reports that may be biased by the presence of symptoms and by the search for an explanation. Conversely, there is little doubt that living with FMS and related symptoms serves as an ongoing stressor. A large proportion of FMS patients report that stress is an aggravating factor for their condition. Thus stress may be both a causal and maintaining factor.

One possibility underlying the link between FMS and stress is that the syndrome is related to a disturbed stress-response system. Clinical observations suggest that many FMS patients exhibit dysregulation of the autonomic nervous system (ANS) and the HPA axis. Studies evaluating ANS regulation in FMS suggest that the syndrome is related to blunted sympathetic reactivity in response to stressors. For example, when isometric muscle stress is imposed, FMS sufferers display a lower level of sympathetic activity in the exercised muscle relative to healthy controls (Elam et al. 1992). During strenuous physical exercise, some FMS patients demonstrate lower levels of heart rate compared to healthy controls. Furthermore, despite a comparable pre-exercise level, the plasma cortisol level was significantly lower in FMS sufferers than in controls following exercise (Van Denderen et al. 1992).

Orthostatic examination suggests disturbed sympathovagal balance and reduced sympathetic activation upon postural challenge in FMS patients (Kelemen et al. 1998). Upright tilt-table testing also reveals a high prevalence of neurally mediated hypotension in patients with FMS, suggesting a hyporeactive sympathetic response to orthostatic stress (Bou-Holaigah et al. 1997). It is noteworthy that those who experience neurally mediated hypotension commonly report that modest levels of physical exertion (e.g., climbing stairs) trigger a hypotensive state with dizziness and light-headedness, fatigue, and abdominal discomfort (Low et al. 1995). These problems are frequently a part of FMS presentation. The central pathway for activating a vasovagal response descends from the corticohypothalamic centers to medullary cardiovascular centers (Van Lieshout et al. 1991). As a result, emotional and painful stressors can trigger sympathovagal activation in susceptible people.

Predispositional factors for neurally mediated hypotension are not well understood. However, genetic predisposition, physical deconditioning, and susceptibility to emotional stress are likely to contribute to the dysfunction. FMS patients tend to exhibit reduced physical conditioning (Bennett et al. 1989; Jacobsen and Holm 1992), although contrary results have been published (Sietsema et al. 1993; Norregaard et al. 1994), and many patients experience severe emotional distress such as depression and anxiety (Turk et al. 1996a; Celiker et al. 1997). These patients may be at risk of developing a hypofunctional sympathetic response to stressors.

To date, the accumulation of evidence from experiments testing FMS patients with physical, physiological, orthostatic, cold, and auditory stimulations fairly consistently supports the hypothesis that a hypofunctional stress system involving the ANS and the HPA axis plays a role in the pathophysiology of FMS. Further research is warranted to extend the available results. Several authors (e.g., Yunus 1992; Clauw 1995; Okifuji and Turk 1999) have proposed that FMS is related to dysregulated pain modulation in the CNS. Despite extensive research, however, no definitive organic pathology of FMS has been identified.

Hypervigilance. The diffused and generalized nature of FMS has led some investigators to consider impairment or dysfunction in information processing as a critical factor. Research investigating sensory processing of FMS patients has consistently demonstrated that they exhibit lower pain threshold than do age- and sex-matched healthy subjects (e.g., Kosek et al. 1996; McDermid et al. 1996). Based upon these results, Rollman and Lautenbacher (1993) proposed a hypervigilance model of FMS in which increased attention to somatosensory stimuli is a predisposing factor for developing the syndrome. Furthermore, vigilance to sensory information may not be limited to pain. Some data indicate that FMS patients are more sensitive to cold, noise, and environmental irritants (Norregaard et al. 1994; McDermid et al. 1996).

Cognitive beliefs and appraisals. Research has often demonstrated that cognitive factors such as beliefs and appraisals play an important part in determining adaptation to symptoms in chronic pain patients (e.g., Turk and Rudy 1986). As has been observed in many chronic pain syndromes, mal-adaptive thoughts and information processing seem to be closely associated with the functional limitations and affective distress observed in FMS. Cognitive factors are not generally considered to be etiological. However, research examining the effects of maladaptive cognition on the maintenance and aggravation of chronic pain suggests that physical pathology, which may have initiated the symptoms, plays a diminished role over time.

Perception and interpretation of the symptoms contribute to an internal representation of FMS. A dysfunctional representation is likely to facilitate an environment that supports "sick behaviors" and reduction of activities; in turn, patients experience decreased levels of social reinforcement and a diminished sense of accomplishment, along with progressive physical deconditioning, all of which facilitate further disability, distress, and pain. Other maladaptive cognitions such as catastrophizing and fear of movement may contribute to the depression (Hassett et al. 2000) and the physical disability (Martin et al. 1996; Vlaeyen et al. 1997) associated with FMS.

Several studies have shown that lower self-efficacy beliefs (beliefs in one's ability to control symptoms and related problems), in particular, relate to greater pain, disability, and depressive mood in FMS (Buckelew et al. 1995; Turk and Okifuji 1997). Among FMS patients who participated in a 6-week training intervention involving physical training and exercise, those with lower self-efficacy beliefs following treatment had lower post-treatment physical activity when compared to those with higher self-efficacy beliefs. Furthermore, improvements in self-efficacy during treatment were associated with lower tender point scores and less intense pain (Buckelew et al. 1996).

The specific role of psychological factors as causal agents in the development of FMS remains obscure. Significant research has demonstrated that psychological variables play an important role in the maintenance and exacerbation of symptoms and contribute to the disability that is prevalent in FMS. Although psychological factors may play a causal role, they are more likely to play a maintaining role in the disability and emotional distress that commonly accompany other FMS symptoms. Because FMS is a chronic disease and no cure is available, successful treatment should address psychological as well as physical factors. The failure of many pharmacological and physically based treatments may, in part, be attributed to the failure to concurrently address important psychological moderators and modulators.

TREATMENT

The lack of identification of a specific mechanism for FMS has resulted in treatment with a wide array of interventions. I will briefly review these and cite more detailed systematic reviews and meta-analyses for the interested reader. A significant drawback of the available studies, however, is the high dropout rate reported. At times the rates of attrition exceed 60%, with one study reporting a 95% dropout rate (Wysenbeek et al. 1985); a 30% rate of attrition is fairly typical. Rarely are intent-to-treat analyses reported when evaluating effectiveness. Although most of the trials required patients to adhere to the treatment recommendations, few studies have monitored or reported on the extent to which patients followed these recommendations. Moreover, the follow-up periods have been relatively short, ranging from an average of 8.7 weeks for treatment with antidepressants (O'Malley et al. 2000) to about 8 months for nonpharmacological treatments (Sim and Adams 2003). The samples were often small, ranging from 10 to 50 subjects, and many of the trials were nonrandomized. Although many studies report that the treatments provided statistically significant effects, the absolute improvements were often modest. For example, the relative improvements for antidepressant medication range from a high of 26% for pain to 45% for fatigue (O'Malley et al. 2000). Thus, the treatments have inconsistent benefits, with only a subset of patients making clinically significant improvements in pain and other symptoms.

Despite numerous efforts to treat FMS patients with diverse strategies, no universally effective treatments exist. Yet despite the limitations noted previously, there is moderate evidence that almost any treatment is better than no treatment. While no single strategy has been demonstrated to be effective, there is reasonably good evidence that multicomponent approaches that include education, exercise, and cognitive-behavioral therapy, delivered

Table II
Pharmacological treatments for fibromyalgia syndrome

Analgesics
  Ibuprofen (Yunus et al. 1989; Russell et al. 1991)
  Bromazepam (Quijada-Carrera et al. 1996)
  Carisoprodol (Vaeroy et al. 1989
  Naproxen (Goldenberg et al. 1986)
  Tenoxicam (Quijada-Carrera et al. 1996)
  Tiaprofenic acid (Donald and Molla 1980)
  Zolpidem (Moldofsky et al. 1996)
  Bromazepam + tenoxicam (Quijada-Carrera et al. 1996)
  Ibuprofen + alprazolam (Russell et al. 1991; Kravitz et al. 1994)
  Naproxen + amitriptyline (Goldenberg et al. 1986)
  Tramadol (Russell et al. 1997; Biasi et al. 1998)

Antidepressants
  Amitriptyline (e.g., Ginsberg et al. 1996; Drewes 1999)
  Clomipramine (Bibolotti et al. 1986)
  Citalopram (Anderberg et al. 2000; Norregaard et al. 1995)
  Cyclobenzaprine (Reynolds et al. 1991; Carette et al. 1994)
  Dothiepin (Caruso et al. 1987)
  Fluoxetine (Goldenberg et al. 1996; Arnold et al. 2002)
  Maprotiline (Bibolotti et al. 1986)
  Pirlindole (Ginsberg et al. 1998)
  S-adenosyl L-methionine (e.g., Di Benedetto et al. 1993; Volkmann et al. 1997)
  Venlafaxine (Dwight et al. 1998)
  Fluoxetine + amitriptyline (Goldenberg et al. 1996)

Hypnotic/Sedatives
  Alprazolam (Russell et al. 1991)
  Zopiclone (Drewes et al. 1991; Gronblad et al. 1993)

Steroids
  Prednisone (Clark et al. 1985)

Others
  Calcitonin (Bessette et al. 1998)
  5-Hydroxytryptophan (Caruso et al. 1990; Puttini and Caruso 1992)
  Gamma-hydroxybutyrate (Scharf et al. 1998)
  Growth hormone (IGF-1) (Bennett et al. 1998)
  Human interferon alpha (Russell et al. 1999)
  Lignocaine/lidocaine (intravenous) (Posner 1994; Bennett and Tai 1995)
  Ondansetron (5-hydroxytryptamine-type receptor antagonist) (Hrycaj et al. 1996)
  Regional sympathetic blockage with guanethidine (Backman et al. 1988)
  Super malic (malic acid and magnesium) (Russell et al. 1995)
  Tropisetron (Farber et al. 2000; Haus et al. 2000; Stratz et al. 2001)

Table III
Nonpharmacological treatments for fibromyalgia syndrome

Education (e.g., Nicassio et al. 1997; Buckelew et al. 1998)

Physical Modalities
 Acupuncture (e.g., Deluze et al. 1992; Berman et al. 1999)
 Balneotherapy (immersion in warm pool) (Yurtkuran and Celiktas 1996; Neumann et al. 2001)
 Chiropractic (Blunt et al. 1997)
 Exercise (e.g., Buckelew et al. 1998; Rooks et al. 2002)
 Feldenkrais intervention (Kendall et al. 2001)
 Light therapy (Parl et al. 1996)
 Hot packs (Samborski et al. 1992; Norregaard et al. 1997)
 Whole body cryotherapy (Samborski et al. 1992; Gutenbrunner et al. 1999)
 Hydrogalvanic therapy (electrotherapy) (Gunther et al. 1994)
 Massage (e.g., Blunt et al. 1997; Brattberg 1999)
 Musically fluctuating muscle vibration (Chesky et al. 1997)
 Magnetized mattress (Colbert et al. 1999)
 Neck support (Ambrogio et al. 1998)
 Sulfur mud bath (Ammer and Melnizky 1999)
 TENS* (Di Benedetto et al. 1993; Sunshine et al. 1996)
 Tender point injections (Reddy et al. 2000)
 Trigger point injections (Hong and Hsueh 1996)
 Laser therapy (Walker 1983)

Nutritional Supplements (Deuster and Jaffe 1998; Dykman et al. 1998; Merchant et al. 2001)

Psychological Modalities
 Biofeedback (Ferraccioli et al. 1987; Sarnoch et al. 1997)
 Hypnosis (Haanen et al. 1991)
 Relaxation (e.g., Buckelew et al. 1998; Keel et al. 1998)
 Stress management (Kaplan et al. 1993; Wigers et al. 1996)

Combined Therapies
 Education + exercise (Gowans et al. 1999; Mannerkorpi et al. 2000)
 Exercise + amitriptyline (Isomeri et al. 1993)
 Exercise + biofeedback (Buckelew et al. 1998)
 Exercise + coping skills (Sandstrom and Keefe 1998)
 Psychomotor therapy + marital counseling (de Voogd et al. 1993)

Multidisciplinary Rehabilitation (Keel et al. 1998; Turk et al. 1998a)

---

* Transcutaneous electrical nerve stimulation.

to groups of patients by a multidisciplinary team, are helpful for many FMS sufferers (Rossy et al. 1999; Sim and Adams 1999; Burckhardt 2001; Oliver et al. 2001). Even when receiving the most effective treatments, a large proportion of FMS patients continue to be symptomatic (see Okifuji and Turk 1999).

UNIDIMENSIONAL TREATMENTS

Various trials have investigated the effectiveness of a large number of pharmacological preparations including corticosteroids, nonsteroidal anti-inflammatory agents, benzodiazepines, and antidepressants (Table II; Rossy et al. 1999; Arnold et al. 2000; O'Malley et al. 2000; see Bennett 2001 for a general review). In addition to pharmacological agents, treatments include a diverse array of modalities that are listed in Table III (for extensive reviews of physical and nonpharmacological approaches see Rossy et al. 1999; Sim and Adams 1999, 2003; Karjalainen et al. 2000; Burckhardt 2001, 2002; Oliver et al. 2001).

Although many of the treatments for FMS have proven to have beneficial effects for some patients, none provides complete resolution of the symptoms, even for the subset of patients who derive some positive results. It is interesting to consider how it is possible for such a diverse set of interventions, including chiropractic manipulations, exercise, antidepressants, magnetic beds, cryotherapy, and light therapy, with very different putative mechanisms of action, to have positive effects on patients with the same disorder.

The results of unimodal treatment studies, in general, have led to pessimism and resignation among some clinicians about their ability to successfully treat FMS patients. Solomon and Liang (1997) have even questioned the appropriateness of rheumatologists continuing to treat FMS patients, given the limited results.

MULTIDISCIPLINARY TREATMENTS

In the past few decades, a growing number of investigators have emphasized the importance of addressing multiple factors associated with FMS (e.g., Bennett 1996; Okifuji and Turk 1999). Various types of multidisciplinary treatment programs that have been developed for FMS tend to include some common components including education, physical exercise, and some type of cognitive treatment to improve coping skills (e.g., Keel et al. 1998; Turk et al. 1998a,b).

In the absence of a cure, patients need to learn proper exercise techniques, to use relaxation to manage pain and stress, and to internalize new and adaptive cognitive and behavioral coping strategies. Nielson et al. (1992) developed a comprehensive inpatient program consisting of exercise, relaxation training, coping training, family education, and pacing exercises. The authors demonstrated that their program was effective in reducing pain, emotional distress, pain behaviors, and maladaptive cognitions. A subsequent study (White and Nielson 1995) reported on the maintenance of treatment benefits in emotional distress and pain behaviors at a 30-month follow-up of the patients treated in the 1992 study. Unfortunately, the authors did not assess typical FMS symptoms such as fatigue and sleep problems.

Other investigators have developed comprehensive outpatient programs consisting of cognitive-behavioral therapy, exercise, medication management, and activity pacing. The intensity and duration of these programs vary widely. For example, Bennett et al. (1996) provided weekly 90-minute sessions over 6 months. In contrast, Turk et al. (1998a) provided a similar treatment in six half-day sessions over a period of only 4 weeks. In both programs, patients reported significant improvements in various FMS-related areas including reductions in pain, fatigue, and distressed mood and enhancements in perceived functioning. The demonstrated efficacy of these multidisciplinary treatment programs suggests that the combination of medical, physical, and cognitive-behavioral therapy components should be the treatment of choice for all FMS patients. Certainly, the treatment effects on the average were statistically significant. However, the individual variation in treatment response was also considerable.

One way to view these discrepant results is to question whether the investigators failed to consider individual differences among patients. FMS patients are a heterogeneous group of people who may have similar symptoms but for whom the mechanisms producing the symptoms may vary. If this is the case, then the inconsistent results with diverse treatment approaches is understandable. Greater attention will be needed to identify the characteristics of subgroups of patients and match treatments to important differences (Flor and Turk 1988; Turk 1990).

HETEROGENEITY VS. HOMOGENEITY

Turk and Flor (1989) suggested that FMS might be a heterogeneous disorder consisting of several patient subgroups with different constellations of physical and psychological features. They argued that delineation of the relevant subgroups would facilitate the identification of the mechanisms underlying the symptoms of FMS and the development of treatments customized to address specific needs of different patient groups. Various studies have attempted to identify the characteristics of subgroups of FMS sufferers. Some studies have focused on differences depending on symptom onset, for example, idiopathic versus traumatic onset (Greenfield et al. 1992; Waylonis and Perkins 1994; Turk et al. 1996a).

Turk and Rudy (1988) suggested that multiple psychosocial and behavioral factors are important in understanding chronic pain patients and that these factors may be used to differentiate subgroups. They identified an empirically derived taxonomy of chronic pain patients based upon patients' responses to the West Haven-Yale Multidimensional Pain Inventory (MPI; Kerns et al. 1985), naming the subgroups Dysfunctional (DYS), Interpersonally Distressed (ID), and Adaptive Copers (AC). The characteristics of these three subgroups are described in Table IV. Turk et al. (1996b) subsequently determined that 87% of FMS patients could be classified into one of these three subgroups that previously had been established in diverse chronic pain populations (e.g., Turk and Rudy 1988, 1990; Turk et al. 1998c).

The distinct characteristics associated with each patient subgroup suggest that prescription of a uniform intervention for all patients might result in less than optimal outcomes because it would fail to address the specific

Table IV
Reports of pain and its impact in subgroups of chronic pain patients
based on the Multidimensional Pain Inventory

Dysfunctional Patients
   Higher levels of pain
   Higher levels of perceived interference of pain with their lives
   Higher levels of emotional distress
   Lower levels of perceived control over their lives
   Lower levels of activity

Interpersonally Distressed Patients
   Lower levels of perceived support
   Higher levels of negative (punishing) responses from significant others
   Lower levels of solicitous responses from significant others
   Lower levels of distracting responses from significant others

Adaptive Coper Patients
   Lower levels of pain (although still seeking treatment)
   Lower levels of perceived interference of pain with their lives
   Lower levels of emotional distress
   Higher levels of perceived control over their lives
   Higher levels of activity

Source: Turk and Rudy (1988).

needs of some patients. It may be more appropriate to customize treatment in order to meet individual patients' specific clinical needs (Turk 1990). For example, although the patients in both the DYS and ID groups were depressed, depression in the latter group may be closely related to marital and interpersonal problems. Meaningful improvement, therefore, may not be achieved without addressing interpersonal or marital issues for the ID group. Being able to prescribe specific treatments based upon patient characteristics, rather than using the more typical one-size-fits-all approach, is likely to benefit a greater number of patients and ultimately be more cost-effective. The value of customizing treatment to the three subgroups identified has recently been demonstrated in several studies (Turk et al. 1996c; Dahlstrom et al. 1997; Bergstrom et al. 2001; Talo et al. 2001).

Turk et al. (1998a) evaluated the effectiveness of a rehabilitation approach for FMS patients that consisted of six 4-hour sessions spaced over a period of 1 month. Three sessions were conducted during the first week, followed by one session during each of the next three weeks. Each session included information about FMS presented by a physician. In addition, a physical therapist focused on aerobic exercises, an occupational therapist explained activity pacing and body mechanics, and a psychologist used a cognitive-behavioral approach that focused on the role of stress and pain management techniques such as relaxation, attention diversion, and problem-solving. In general, this protocol was effective in reducing pain, depression, and disability at the end of treatment and at a 6-month follow-up for the total sample of patients. Careful examination of the results, however, revealed that the DYS patients responded quite well to the treatment and the AC patients somewhat less well. The ID patients, however, appeared to achieve no benefit from the treatment. The differential response to treatment among the different subgroups supports the need to reconsider the components of treatment provided. For example, ID patients are characterized by their perceptions of low levels of support from significant others. The comprehensive treatment's failure to directly address interpersonal problems or attempt to improve communication patterns may have impeded these patients from benefiting from the more general information, exercise, and pain coping strategies that were included.

Vlaeyen et al. (1997) also highlighted the importance of differences among FMS patients in response to treatment. These investigators developed a treatment based on reducing fear, which they believed to be an important factor in FMS patients' avoidance of activities. The treatment included education about psychosocial factors that influence pain and about ergonomic principles as applied to daily activities. One group received cognitive-behavioral therapy consisting of training in coping skills and applied relaxation skills in addition to the educational component. The authors found that patients who had lower levels of fear responded somewhat better to the treatment that included the cognitive component, whereas patients with high levels of fear showed somewhat better outcomes in response to the education and discussion alone.

To summarize, it is important to acknowledge that FMS patients are not a homogeneous group (Turk et al. 1996a). It is reasonable to assume that substantial individual differences existed prior to the development of FMS and that these differences persist or are magnified in response to the stress associated with a chronic condition. Thus, although the evolving processes may be present in all FMS patients, the degrees to which the processes become dysregulated may vary across individuals due to differences in predispositional factors (Okifuji and Turk 1999). Subgroups may respond to an identical intervention in different ways. Consequently, providing all FMS patients with the same treatment is unlikely to be effective (Bennett 2001). This heterogeneity among patients may explain why so many different treatments are helpful for subsets of patients. Identification of patients' characteristics and matching them to specific treatments may help maximize clinical efficacy.

It is equally plausible to postulate that there may be subgroups based on immunological, endocrinological, and ANS perturbations. Delineation of specific characteristics of subgroups of FMS patients may help us to determine group-specific pathophysiology and allow us develop optimal interventions for this prevalent, puzzling, and disabling disorder. To date, however, no studies have attempted to test the physiological heterogeneity hypothesis of FMS.

LIVING WITH FMS

Persons with FMS often look well despite the symptoms, and others may question the severity and seriousness of their condition. The lack of objective medical findings to confirm the diagnosis can result in confusion and frustration. Although they may feel relief when hearing that their symptoms reflect a "benign" and nonprogressive condition, patients often wonder, "How can I be in so much pain and yet look normal on all the tests?" Moreover, not only is the sufferer affected, but significant others are often confused and frustrated. Relationships can suffer as the costs of pain extend well beyond the physical and begin to affect the emotional, occupational, social, and recreational life of those afflicted.

To work effectively with FMS patients, it is important to appreciate their suffering and the difficulties associated with having a chronic condition for which no apparent physical cause can be identified. This appreciation is important in establishing rapport with patients and in understanding aspects of their behavior that might at times seem surprising.

GENERAL TREATMENT RECOMMENDATIONS

Given that greater success has been reported for more comprehensive, rehabilitation-oriented programs, health care providers may be able to treat patients effectively if they orient their approach to the person with FMS and not just the disease.

EDUCATION

Information and reassurance are essential in treating FMS patients. The lack of a definitive explanation for the symptoms often produces fears that something serious, but as yet unidentified, is causing the symptoms and that the symptoms will become progressively worse. Patients may anticipate the frustrating scenario of being told that nothing can be done, that the problems are all caused by psychological factors (i.e., "imaginary" and "all in their heads"), and that they must learn to live with their symptoms without being told how. Consequently, it is essential that treatment begin with information about the nature of FMS, the possible causes, and the contributions of emotional, behavioral, and cognitive variables, as well as physical factors.

Education should include a discussion of the distinction between acute pain and chronic pain. Acute pain is rightly seen as a signal of *harm* or potential damage or danger to the body. In the case of FMS, however, pain is no longer a signal of damage to the body. Thus, it is important to make the distinction between *hurt* and *harm*. Patients should be informed that they will need to increase physical activity and exercise. The clinician should acknowledge that a conditioning program is likely to cause some increase in the level of pain as muscles become sore after months or years of disuse, but that the exercises will cause no permanent damage.

ACCEPTANCE

The idea of acceptance, rather than cure, is often a wise course to follow with FMS patients. However, some patients view acceptance as synonymous with failure, that is, an admission that "I'll never be better." Acceptance is necessary before adopting significant lifestyle and behavior changes. Rather than viewing acceptance as "living with FMS," patients should consider "living *despite* FMS."

FOCUS ON FUNCTION RATHER THAN CURE

Rigid conviction that something is physically wrong and needs to be corrected can obstruct treatment because it reinforces a passive role that will impede acceptance of self-management. If patients and health care providers agree to embark on treatment, the emphasis should be on reducing emotional distress, making functional gains, and improving quality of life, rather than on completely eliminating the symptoms.

GOAL-SETTING

Clinicians should focus on goal-setting as a means to direct patients to work toward achievable, reinforcing objectives. Goal-setting achieves multiple purposes. First, patients with FMS need to have realistic goals. If a patient enters treatment with the goal of "being pain free" and "just like I was before I developed fibro" then the clinician must direct greater attention toward providing information about FMS. In addition, he or she should inform the patient that treatment will involve making significant lifestyle changes, pacing oneself, and maintaining these changes despite symptom flare-ups and remissions.

A second function of goal-setting is to evaluate the concordance between the patient's and the clinician's expectations. Clinicians must ensure that treatment goals are mutually understood and acceptable. Lack of acceptance will undermine patients' motivation and impede successful outcomes. Clinicians should emphasize a collaborative relationship. Together, the therapist and patient should work to identify achievable goals that are measurable and within the patient's control.

RELAXATION

Relaxation is an integral part of the self-management program for FMS sufferers. Many different methods that can help patients learn to relax include controlled breathing, progressive muscle relaxation, and warm baths. No method is universally superior, and different people will find different methods more appealing. Thus, the health care provider should work with each patient to help determine which methods may be most appropriate.

PACING AND INCREASING ACTIVITIES

Bennett et al. (1989) found that 80% of FMS patients were physically unfit. FMS sufferers often anticipate that physical activity will cause pain and further damage. They may avoid activities to prevent more pain, fatigue, and injury (Vlaeyen et al. 1997). Treatment should focus on breaking the association between activity and anticipated pain by encouraging patients to gradually increase the pace of their activity. The patient should be persuaded that a gradual increase in activity will increase endurance and reduce fatigue.

Pacing calls for patients to establish and follow a daily time quota for a particular activity. Patients should be asked to perform the activity for several days, up to the point where they are beginning to feel pain, fatigue, or any other sign that they have reached their limit. Using this level of activity as a baseline, the health care provider should help patients to create a manageable activity plan, with gradually increasing activity levels that they are likely to be able to maintain. Nonadherence is a significant problem, so the health care provider must explain the importance of a regular exercise regimen and the need for persistence even when the exercises cause some fatigue and pain. Over time, endurance should increase and pain should diminish.

IMPROVING SLEEP

A common symptom reported by FMS sufferers is poor sleep. The clinician should encourage patients to establish a sleep hygiene plan that consists of a standard wake-up time, getting out of bed during extended periods of being awake, avoiding sleep-incompatible behaviors in the bed, eliminating daytime napping, and avoiding consumption of caffeine or alcohol near bedtime as well as reducing other activities that might interfere with sleep.

ELIMINATING MALADAPTIVE THOUGHTS

Many persons with FMS subscribe to a number of negative and maladaptive thoughts about themselves and their plight. Clinicians should directly address the relationship between thoughts, feelings, behavior, and physiology. To assist in the discovery process, patients may be asked to complete a diary recording when their symptoms are worse, what they were doing, what they were thinking, how they felt, and how their thoughts and feelings affected what they did.

Clinicians may use an *ABCD* model to help the patient identify and alter maladaptive thoughts and behaviors, where *A* is an activating event or stressor, *B* is the belief system (thoughts and attitudes) about the stressful event, *C* represents the consequences of the activating event (feelings) and a way to change the above sequence of events, and *D* stands for disputing the negative thinking discovered in *B*, which can affect how badly people feel in *C*.

UNDERSTANDING THE ROLE OF STRESS

Many patients with FMS fail to see the relationship between stress and their physical health. Clinicians should help patients to identify stressors and distinguish between stressors they can and cannot control. Emphasis can be placed on modifying the stressors that patients can control and practicing other skills such as relaxation, time management, and effective communication to cope with stressors that they cannot control.

COPING WITH RELAPSE

FMS is a chronic condition in which symptoms will fluctuate between relative reductions and flare-ups, hence the emphasis on pacing oneself noted previously. As a consequence, a relapse prevention model is important. Clinicians should present this as a process where patients who find themselves relapsing can have recourse to their self-management plan. Patients must acknowledge that there will be good and bad days as everyone experiences "ups and downs." The key to consistent recovery is not the absence of symptoms but the willingness to reenter the process of recovery with independent action even after a flare-up of symptoms.

The challenge for patients is twofold—first, to recognize when they are relapsing, and second, to return to the use of their self-management skills. Patients can be asked to list the behaviors, thoughts, and feelings that act as cues or predictors that a relapse is likely to occur. They should then be asked to list the behaviors that have helped in the past and to develop a written plan for engaging in those behaviors. Patients can be encouraged to think of factors that might contribute to flare-ups and to identify *high-risk* circumstances. If they can identify such situations, they can attempt to alter them, avoid them, plan on how to respond to them, or accept them as inevitable and decide how they will accommodate their activities when flare-ups do occur.

COPING WITH INTERPERSONAL PROBLEMS

A high percentage of patients with FMS best fit an ID profile on the MPI (Turk et al. 1996a). People with such profiles show high levels of pain and depression and report low social support or high levels of negative responses from significant others. For these patients the clinician should spend some time on fostering effective communication skills (openness and honesty in communicating with significant others).

MEDICATIONS

Medication that targets key symptoms (fatigue, poor sleep, and depression) should also be considered as an adjunct to exercise and psychologically oriented treatments (Goldenberg et al. 1986; O'Malley et al. 2000). Providing some symptomatic relief may enable patients to sleep better and to engage in paced physical activities. In particular, antidepressant medication may work because it not only addresses depression itself, but may also be helpful in improving sleep quality or in somehow reducing pain severity, even at doses that are typically lower than those used for clinical depression. It is interesting to note that while low-dose tricyclic antidepressants can be effective with FMS, the newer selective serotonin reuptake inhibitors have had a less positive outcome. To my knowledge, no blinded, randomized, controlled trials with long-term follow-ups have evaluated the effectiveness of treatments combining medication with other modalities.

CONCLUDING COMMENTS

FMS is a prevalent and perplexing condition of unknown etiology and with no cure. Many treatments have some beneficial effects, but the syndrome remains a chronic problem. Like diabetes, asthma, or any chronic disease, successful treatment of FMS requires continuity of care and patient acceptance of responsibility for self-management. Research is needed to determine what set of FMS patients, with what characteristics, can benefit from what type of treatments. The failure of many patients to achieve and maintain positive outcomes indicates, most assuredly, that one size does not fit all.

ACKNOWLEDGMENTS

Preparation of this manuscript was supported in part by grants from the National Institute of Arthritis and Musculoskeletal and Skin Diseases (AR/AI44724, AR47298) and the National Institute of Child Health and Human Development/National Center for Medical Rehabilitation Research (HD33989).

REFERENCES

Ahles TA, Khan SA, Yunus MB, et al. Psychiatric status of patients with primary fibromyalgia, patients with rheumatoid arthritis and subjects without pain: a blind comparison of DSM III diagnoses. *Am J Psychiatry* 1991; 148:1721–1726.

Alfici S, Sigal M, Landau M. Primary fibromyalgia syndrome—a variant of depressive disorder. *Psychother Psychosom* 1989; 51:156–161.

Ambrogio N, Cuttiford J, Lineker S, et al. A comparison of three types of neck support in fibromyalgia patients. *Arthritis Care Res* 1998; 11:405–410.

Ammer K, Melnizky P. Medicinal baths for the treatment of generalized fibromyalgia. *Forsch Komplementarmed* 1999; 6:80–85

Anderberg UM, Marteinsdottir I, von Knorring L. Citalopram in patients with fibromyalgia—a randomized, double-blind, placebo controlled study. *Eur J Pain* 2000; 4:27–35.

Arnold LM, Keck PE Jr, Welge JA. Antidepressant treatment of fibromyalgia: a meta-analysis and review. *Psychosomatics* 2000; 41:104–113.

Arnold LM, Hess EV, Hudson JI, et al. A randomized, placebo-controlled, double-blind, flexible-dose study of fluoxetine in the treatment of women with fibromyalgia. *Am J Med* 2002; 112:191–197.

Backman E, Bengtsson A, Bengtsson M, et al. Skeletal muscle function in primary fibromyalgia. Effect of regional sympathetic blockage with guanethidine. *Acta Neurol Scand* 1988; 77:187–191.

Barsky AJ, Borus JF. Functional somatic syndromes. *Ann Intern Med* 1999; 130:910–921.

Baumstark KE, Buckelew P. Fibromyalgia: clinical signs, research findings, treatment implications, and future directions. *Ann Behav Med* 1992; 14:282–291.

Bengtsson A, Bengtsson M. Regional sympathetic blockade in primary fibromyalgia. *Pain* 1988; 33:161–167.

Bengtsson A, Henriksson KG. The muscle in fibromyalgia—a review of Swedish studies. *J Rheumatol* 1989; 19:144–149.

Bengtsson A, Henriksson KG, Larsson J. Muscle biopsy in primary fibromyalgia. Light-microscopical and histochemical findings. *Scand J Rheumatol* 1986; 15:1–6.

Bennett MI, Tai YM. Intravenous lignocaine in the management of primary fibromyalgia syndrome. *Int J Clin Pharmacol Res* 1995; 15:115–119.

Bennett RM. Multidisciplinary group programs to treat fibromyalgia patients. *Rheum Dis Clin North Am* 1996; 22:351–367.

Bennett R. Pharmacological treatment of fibromyalgia. *J Funct Syndromes* 2001; 1:79–92.

Bennett RM, Clark SR, Goldberg L, et al. Aerobic fitness in patients with fibrositis: a controlled study of respiratory gas exchange and I33-xenon clearance from exercising muscle. *Arthritis Rheum* 1989; 32:454–460.

Bennett RM, Clark SR, Campbell SM, Burckhardt CS. Low levels of somatomedin C in patients with the fibromyalgia syndrome. A possible link between sleep and muscle pain. *Arthritis Rheum* 1992; 35:1113–1116.

Bennett RM, Burckhardt CS, Clark SR, et al. Group treatment of fibromyalgia: a 6 month outpatient program. *J Rheumatol* 1996; 23:521–528.

Bennett RM, Clark SR, Walczyk J. A randomized, double-blind, placebo-controlled study of grown hormone in the treatment of fibromyalgia. *Am J Med* 1998;10:227–231.

Bergstrom G, Jensen IB, Bodin L, et al. The impact of psychologically different patient groups on outcome after a vocational rehabilitation program for long-term spinal pain patients. *Pain* 2001; 93:229–237.

Berman BM, Ezzo J, Hadhazy V, et al. Is acupuncture effective in the treatment of fibromyalgia? *J Fam Pract* 1999; 48:213–218.

Bessett L, Carette S, Fossel AH, et al. A placebo controlled crossover trial of subcutaneous salmon calcitonin in the treatment of patients with fibromyalgia. *Scand J Rheumatol* 1998; 27:112–116.

Biasi G, Manca S, Manganelli S, et al. Tramadol in the fibromyalgia syndrome: a controlled clinical trial versus placebo. *Int J Clin Pharmacol Res* 1998; 18:13–19.

Bibolotti E, Borghi C, Paculli E. The management of fibrositis: a double blind comparison of maprotiline, clomipramine, and placebo. *Clin Trials J* 1986; 23:269–280.

Blunt KL, Rajwani MH, Cuerriero R. The effectiveness of chiropractic management of fibromyalgia patients: a pilot study. *J Manipulative Physiol Ther* 1997; 20:389–399.

Bombardier CH, Buchwald D. Chronic fatigue, chronic fatigue syndrome, and fibromyalgia: disability and health care use. *Med Care* 1996; 34:924–930.

Bou-Holaigah I, Calkins H, Flynn JA, et al. Provocation of hypotension and pain during upright tilt table testing in adults with fibromyalgia. *Clin Exp Rheumatol* 1997; 15:239–246.

Brattberg G. Connective tissue massage in the treatment of fibromyalgia. *Eur J Pain* 1999; 3:235–245.

Buckelew SP, Murray SE, Hewett JE. Self-efficacy, pain, and physical activity among fibromyalgia subjects. *Arthritis Care Res* 1995; 8:43–50.

Buckelew SP, Huyser B, Hewett JE, et al. Self-efficacy predicting outcome among fibromyalgia subjects. *Arthritis Care Res* 1996; 9:97–104.

Buckelew SP, Conway R, Parker J, et al. Biofeedback/relaxation training and exercise interventions for fibromyalgia: a prospective trial. *Arthritis Care Res* 1998; 11:196–209.

Burckhardt CS. Non-pharmacological treatment of fibromyalgia syndrome. *J Funct Syndromes* 2001; 1:103–115.

Burckhardt CS. Nonpharmacologic management strategies in fibromyalgia. *Rheum Dis Clin NA* 2002; 28:291–304.

Burckhardt CS, Clark SR, Bennett RM. Fibromyalgia and quality of life: a comparative analysis. *J Rheumatol* 1993; 20:475–479.

Carrette S, Bell MV, Reynolds WJ. Comparison of amitriptyline, cyclobenzaprine, and placebo in the treatment of fibromyalgia: a randomized, double-blind clinical trial. *Arthritis Rheum* 1994; 37:32–40.

Caruso I, Sarzi-Puttini P, Boccassini L, et al. Double-blind study of dothiepin versus placebo in the treatment of primary fibromyalgia syndrome. *J Int Med Res* 1987; 15:154–159.

Caruso I, Sarzi-Puttini P, Cazzola M, et al. Double-blind study of 5-hydroxytryptophan versus placebo in the treatment of primary fibromyalgia syndrome. *J Int Med Res* 1990; 18:201–209.

Celiker R, Borman P, Oktem F, et al. Psychological disturbance in fibromyalgia: relation to pain severity. *Clin Rheumatol* 1997; 16:179–184.

Chesky KS, Russell IJ, Lopez Y, et al. Fibromyalgia tender point pain: a double-blind, placebo-controlled pilot study of music vibration using the music vibration table. *J Musculoskel Pain* 1997; 5:33–52.

Clark S, Tindall E, Bennett RM. A double blind crossover trial of prednisone versus placebo in the treatment of fibrositis. *J Rheumatol* 1985; 12:980–983.

Clauw DJ. The pathogenesis of chronic pain and fatigue syndromes, with special reference to fibromyalgia. *Med Hypotheses* 1995; 44:369–378.

Clauw DJ, Chrousos GP. Chronic pain and fatigue syndromes: overlapping clinical and neuroendocrine features and potential pathogenic mechanisms. *Neuroimmunomodulation* 1997; 4:134–153.

Colbert AP, Markov MS, Banerji M, et al. Magnetic mattress pad use in patients with fibromyalgia: a randomized double-blind pilot study. *J Back Musculoskel Rehabil* 1999; 13:19–31.

Crofford LJ, Engleberg NC, Demitrack MA. Neurohormonal perturbations in fibromyalgia. *Bailliere's Clin Rheumatol* 1996; 10:365–378.

Dahlstrom L, Widmark G, Carlsson SG. Cognitive-behavioral profiles among different categories of orofacial pain patients: diagnosis and treatment implications. *Eur J Oral Sci* 1997; 105:377–383.

DeLuze C, Bosia L, Zirbs A, et al. Electroacupuncture in fibromyalgia: results of a controlled trial. *BMJ* 1992; 305:1249–1252.

Deuster PA, Jaffe RM. A novel treatment for fibromyalgia improves clinical outcomes in a community-based study. *J Musculoskel Pain* 1998; 6:133–149.

De Voogd J, Knipping A, de Blecourt A, et al. Treatment of fibromyalgia syndrome with psychomotor therapy and marital counseling. *J Musculoskel Pain* 1993; 1:273–281.

Di Benedetto P, Iona LG, Zidarich V. Clinical evaluation of S-adenosyl-L-methionine versus transcutaneous electrical nerve stimulation in primary fibromyalgia. *Curr Ther Res* 1993; 53:222–229.

Donald JF, Molla AL. A comparative double-blind study of tiaprofenic acid and aspirin in the treatment of muscular rheumatism, fibrositis, sprains and soft tissue injuries in general practice. *J Int Med Res* 1980; 8:382–387.

Drewes AM. Pain and sleep disturbances. Clinical, experimental and methodological aspects with special reference to the fibromyalgia syndrome and rheumatoid arthritis. *Scand J Rheumatol* 1999; 28:126–134.

Drewes AM, Andreasen A, Jennum P, et al. Zopiclone in the treatment of sleep abnormalities in fibromyalgia. *Scand J Rheumatol* 1991; 20:288–293.

Drewes AM, Andreasen A, Schroder HD, et al. Pathology of skeletal muscle in fibromyalgia: a histo-immuno-chemical and ultrastructural study. *Br J Rheumatol* 1993; 32:479–483.

Durette MR, Rodriquez AA, Agre JC, et al. Needle electromyographic evaluation of patients with myofascial or fibromyalgic pain. *Am J Phys Med Rehabil* 1991; 70:154–156.

Dwight MM, Arnold LM, O'Brien H, et al. An open clinical trial of venlafaxine treatment of fibromyalgia. *Psychosomatics* 1998; 39:14–17.

Dykman KD, Tone C, Ford C, et al. The effects of nutritional supplements on the symptoms of fibromyalgia and chronic fatigue syndrome. *Integr Physiol Behav Sci* 1998; 33:61–71.

Elam M, Johansson G, Wallin BG. Do patients with primary fibromyalgia have an altered muscle sympathetic nerve activity? *Pain* 1992; 48:371–375.

Farber L, Stratz T, Bruckle W, et al. Efficacy and tolerability of tropisetron in primary fibromyalgia—a highly selective and competitive 5-HT$_3$ receptor antagonist. German Fibromyalgia Study Group. *Scand J Rheumatol* 2000; 113(Suppl):49–54.

Ferraccioli G, Ghirelli L, Scita F, et al. EMG-biofeedback training in fibromyalgia syndrome. *J Rheumatol* 1987; 14:820–825.

Flor H, Turk DC. Chronic back pain and rheumatoid arthritis: predicting pain and disability from cognitive variables. *J Behav Med* 1988; 11:251–265.

Forseth KO, Gran JT. The prevalence of fibromyalgia among women aged 20–49 in Arendal, Norway. *Scand J Rheumatol* 1992; 21:74–78.

Ginsberg F, Mancaux A, Joos E, et al. A randomized placebo-controlled trial of sustained-release amitriptyline in primary fibromyalgia. *J Musculoskel Pain* 1996; 4:37–47.

Ginsberg F, Joos E, Geczy J, et al. A pilot randomized placebo-controlled study of pirlindole in treatment of primary fibromyalgia *J Musculoskel Pain* 1998; 6:5–17.

Goldenberg D. Fibromyalgia syndrome. An emerging but controversial condition. *JAMA* 1987; 257:2782–2787.

Goldenberg DL, Felson DT, Dinerman H. A randomized, controlled trial of amitriptyline and naproxen in the treatment of patients with fibromyalgia. *Arthritis Rheum* 1986; 29:1371–1377.

Goldenberg D, Mayskiy M, Mossey C, et al. A randomized, double-blind, crossover trial of fluoxetine and amitriptyline in the treatment of fibromyalgia. *Arthritis Rheum* 1996; 39:1852–1859.

Gowans SE, de Hueck A, Voss S, et al. A randomized controlled trial of exercise and education for individual with fibromyalgia. *Arthritis Care Res* 1999; 12:120–128.

Greenfield S, Fitzcharles MA, Esdaile JM. Reactive fibromyalgia syndrome. *Arthritis Rheum* 1992; 35:678–681.

Gronblad M, Nykanem, Konttinen E, et al. The effect of zopiclone on sleep quality, morning stiffness, widespread tenderness and pain and general discomfort in primary fibromyalgia patients. A double blind randomized trial. *Clin Rheumatol* 1993; 12:186–191.

Günther V, Mur E, Kinigadner U, et al. Fibromyalgia—the effect of relaxation and hydrogalvanic bath therapy on the subjective pain experience. *Clin Rheumatol* 1994; 13:573–578.

Gutenbrunner C, Englert G, Neus-Lausen M, et al. Analgetic effects of natural sulfur baths and cold chamber expositions in fibromyalgia. *Phys Rehabil Kur Med* 1999; 9:56–62.

Haanen HCM, Hoenderdos HTW, van Roumunde LKJ, et al. Controlled trial of hypnotherapy in the treatment of refractory fibromyalgia. *J Rheumatol* 1991; 18:72–75.

Hassett AL, Cone JD, Sigal, LH. The role of catastrophizing in the pain and depression of women with fibromyalgia syndrome. *Arthritis Rheum* 2000; 43:2493–2500.

Haus U, Varga B, Stratz T, et al. Oral treatment of fibromyalgia with tropisetron given over 28 days: influence on functional and vegetative symptoms, psychometric parameters and pain. *Scand J Rheumatol* 2000; 113(Suppl):55–58.

Hong CZ, Hsueh TC. Difference in pain relief after trigger point injections in myofascial pain patients with and without fibromyalgia. *Arch Phys Med Rehabil* 1996; 77:1161–1166.

Hrycaj P, Stratz T, Mennet P, et al. Pathogenetic aspects of responsiveness to ondansetron (5-hydroxytryptamine type 3 receptor antagonist) in patients with primary fibromyalgia syndrome—a preliminary study. *J Rheumatol* 1996; 23:1418–1423.

Hudson JI, Hudson MS, Pliner LF, et al. Fibromyalgia and major affective disorder: a controlled phenomenology and family history study. *Am J Psychiatry* 1985; 142:441–466.

Isomeri R, Mikkelsson M, Latikka P, et al. Effects of amitriptyline and cardiovascular fitness training on pain patients with primary fibromyalgia. *J Musculoskel Pain* 1993; 1:253–260.

Jacobsen S, Holm B. Muscle strength and endurance compared to aerobic capacity in primary fibromyalgia syndrome. *Clin Exp Rheumatol* 1992; 10:419–420.

Kaplan KH, Goldenberg DL, Galvin-Nadeau M. The impact of a meditation-based stress reduction program on fibromyalgia. *Gen Hosp Psychiatry* 1993; 15:284–289.

Karjalainen K, Malmivaara AOV, van Tulder MW, et al. Multidisciplinary rehabilitation for fibromyalgia and musculoskeletal pain in working age adults. *Cochrane Database Syst Rev* 2000; 3:1–24.

Keel PJ, Bodoky C, Gerhard U, et al. Comparison of integrated group therapy and group relaxation training for fibromyalgia. *Clin J Pain* 1998; 14:232–238.

Kelemen J, Lang E, Balint G, et al. Orthostatic sympathetic derangement of baroreflex in patients with fibromyalgia. *J Rheumatol* 1998; 25:823–825.

Kendall SA, Ekselius L, Gerdle B, et al. Feldenkrais intervention in fibromyalgia patients: a pilot study. *J Musculoskel Med* 2001; 9:25–35.

Kerns RD, Turk DC, Rudy TE. The West Haven-Yale Multidimensional Pain Inventory (WHYMPI). *Pain* 1985; 23:345–356.

Kosek E, Ekholm J, Hansson P. Sensory dysfunction in fibromyalgia patients with implications for pathogenic mechanisms. *Pain* 1996; 68:375–383.

Kravitz HM, Katz RS, Helmke N, et al. Alprazolam and ibuprofen in the treatment of fibromyalgia—report of a double-blind placebo controlled study. *J Musculoskel Med* 1994; 2:3–27.

Lindh M, Johansson G, Hedberg M, et al. Muscle fiber characteristics, capillaries and enzymes in patients with fibromyalgia and controls. *Scand J Rheumatol* 1995; 24:34–37.

Low, PA, Opfer-Gehrking TL, McPhee BR, et al. Prospective evaluation of clinical characteristics of orthostatic hypotension. *Mayo Clin Proc* 1995; 70:617–22.

MacFarlane GJ, Croft PR, Schollum J, et al. Widespread pain: is an improved classification possible? *J Rheumatol* 1996; 23:1628–1632.

Mannerkorpi K, Nyberg B, Ahlmen M, et al. Pool exercise combined with an education program for patients with fibromyalgia syndrome: a prospective randomized study. *J Rheumatol* 2000; 27:2473–2478.

Martin MY, Bradley LA, Alexander RW, et al. Coping strategies predict disability in patients with primary fibromyalgia. *Pain* 1996; 68:45–53.

McDermid AJ, Rollman GB, McCain GA. Generalized hypervigilance in fibromyalgia: evidence of perceptual amplification. *Pain* 1996; 66:133–144.

Merchant RE, Andre CA, Wise CM. Nutritional supplementation with *Chlorella pyrenoidosa* for fibromyalgia syndrome: a double-blind, placebo-controlled, crossover study. *J Musculoskel Pain* 2001; 9:37–54.

Moldofsky H, Lue FA, Mously C, et al. The effect of zolpidem in patients with fibromyalgia: a dose ranging, double blind, placebo controlled, modified crossover study. *J Rheumatol* 1996; 23:529–533.

Morriss RK, Ahmed M, Wearden AJ, et al. The role of depression in pain, psychophysiological syndromes and medically unexplained symptoms associated with chronic fatigue syndrome. *J Affect Disord* 1999; 55:143–148.

Myers JK, Weissman MM, Tischler GL. Six-month prevalence of psychiatric disorders in three communities 1980 to 1982. *Arch Gen Psychiatry* 1984; 41:959–967.

Neumann L, Sukenik S, Bolotin A, et al. The effect of balneotherapy at the Dead Sea on the quality of life of patients with fibromyalgia syndrome *Clin Rheumatol* 2001; 20:15–19.

Nicassio PM, Radjovic V, Weisman MH, et al. A comparison of behavioral and educational interventions for fibromyalgia. *J Rheumatol* 1997; 24:2000–2007

Nielson WR, Walker C, McCain GA. Cognitive behavioral treatment of fibromyalgia syndrome: preliminary findings. *J Rheumatol* 1992; 19:98–103.

Norregaard J, Bülow PM, Mehlsen J, et al. Biochemical changes in relation to a maximal exercise test in patients with fibromyalgia. *Clin Physiol* 1994; 14:159–167.

Norregaard J, Volkman H, Danneskiold-Samsoe B. A randomized controlled trial of citalopram in the treatment of fibromyalgia. *Pain* 1995; 61:445–449.

Norregaard J, Lykkegaard JJ, Mehlsen J, et al. Exercise training in treatment of fibromyalgia. *J Musculoskel Pain* 1997; 5:71–79.

Okifuji A, Turk D. Fibromyalgia: search for mechanisms and effective treatments. In: Gatchel RJ, Turk DC (Eds). *Psychological Factors in Pain: Critical Perspectives.* New York: Guilford, 1999, pp 227–246.

Okifuji A, Turk DC, Sinclair JD, et al. A standardized manual tender point survey. I. Development and determination of a threshold point for the identification of positive tender points in fibromyalgia syndrome. *J Rheumatol* 1997; 24:377–383.

Oliver K, Cronan TA, Walen HR. A review of multidisciplinary interventions for fibromyalgia patients: where do we go from here? *J Musculoskel Pain* 2001; 9:63–80.

O'Malley PG, Balden E, Tomkins G, et al. Treatment of fibromyalgia with antidepressants: a meta-analysis. *J Gen Intern Med* 2000;15:659–666.

Parl SJ, Lue F, MacLean AW, et al. The effects of bright light treatment on the symptoms of fibromyalgia. *J Rheumatol* 1996; 23:896–902.

Pillemer S, Bradley LA, Crofford LJ, et al. The neuroscience and endocrinology of fibromyalgia. *Arthritis Rheum* 1997; 40:1928–1939.

Posner I. Treatment of fibromyalgia syndrome with intravenous lidocaine: a prospective, randomized pilot study. *J Musculoskel Pain* 1994; 2:55–65.

Prescott E, Jacobsen S, Kjoller M, et al. Fibromyalgia in the adult Danish population: I. Prevalent study. *Scand J Rheumatol* 1993; 22:238–242.

Puttini PS, Caruso I. Primary fibromyalgia syndrome and 5-hydroxy-L-tryptophan: a 90-day open study. *J Int Med Res* 1992; 20:182–189.

Quijada-Carrera J, Valenzuela-Costano A, Povdeano-Gomez J, et al. Comparison of tenoxicam and bromazepam in the treatment of fibromyalgia: a randomized, double-blind, placebo-controlled trial. *Pain* 1996; 65:221–225.

Reddy SS, Yunus MB, Inanici F, et al. Tender point injections are beneficial in fibromyalgia syndrome: a descriptive, open study. *J Musculoskel Pain* 2000; 8:7–18.

Reynolds WJ, Moldofsky H, Saskin P, et al. The effects of cyclobenzaprine on sleep physiology and symptoms in patients with fibromyalgia. *J Rheumatol* 1991; 18:452–454.

Rollman GB, Lautenbacher S. Hypervigilance effects in fibromyalgia: pain experience and pain perception. In: Vaeroy H, Merskey H (Eds). *Progress in Fibromyalgia and Myofascial Pain.* Amsterdam: Elsevier, 1993, pp 89–112.

Rooks DS, Silverman CB, Kantrowitz FG. The effects of progressive strength training and aerobic exercise on muscle strength and cardiovascular fitness in women with fibromyalgia: a pilot study. *Arthritis Rheum* 2002; 47:22–28.

Rossy LA, Buckelew SP, Dorr N, et al. A meta-analysis of fibromyalgia treatment interventions. *Ann Behav Med* 1999; 21:180–191.

Russell IJ. Fibromyalgia syndrome. In: Loeser JD, Butler SH, Chapman CR, et al. (Eds). *Bonica's Management of Pain*, 3rd ed. Philadelphia: Lippincott Williams & Wilkins, 2001, pp 543–556.

Russell IJ, Fletcher EM, Michalek JE, et al. Treatment of primary fibrositis/fibromyalgia syndrome with ibuprofen and alprazolam. A double-blind, placebo-controlled study. *Arthritis Rheum* 1991; 34:552–560.

Russell IJ, Michalekje Flechas JD, Abraham GD. Treatment of fibromyalgia syndrome with super malic, a randomized double blind placebo controlled crossover pilot study. *J Rhuematol* 1995; 22:953–958.

Russell IJ, Kamin M, Sager D, et al. Efficacy of Ultram™ [Tramadol HCL] treatment of fibromyalgia syndrome: preliminary analysis of a multi-center, randomized, placebo-controlled study. *Arthritis Rheum* 1997; 40:S214.

Russell IJ, Michalek JE, Kang AB, et al. Reduction of morning stiffness and improvement in physical function in fibromyalgia syndrome patients treated sublingually with low dose human interferon alpha. *J Interferon Cytokine Res* 1999; 19:961–968.

Samborski W, Stratz T, Sobieska M, et al. Intraindividual comparison of effectiveness of wholebody cold therapy and hot-pack therapy in patients with generalized tendomyopathy (fibromyalgia). *Z Rheumatol* 1992; 51:25–31.

Sandstrom MJ, Keefe FJ. Self-management of fibromyalgia: the role of formal coping skills training and physical exercise training programs. *Arthritis Care Res* 1998;11:432–447.

Sarnoch H, Adler F, Scholz OB. Relevance of muscular sensitivity, muscular activity, and cognitive variables on pain reduction associated with EMG biofeedback in fibromyalgia. *Percept Mot Skills* 1997; 84:1043–1050.

Scharf MB, Hauck M, Sover R, et al. Effect of Gamma-Hydroxybutyrate on pain, fatigue, and the alpha sleep anomaly in patients with fibromyalgia. Preliminary report. *J Rheumatol* 1998; 25:1986–1990.

Schochat T, Croft P, Raspe H. The epidemiology of fibromyalgia. *Br J Rheumatol* 1994; 33:783–786.

Sietsema KE, Cooper DM, Caro X, et al. Oxygen uptake during exercise in patients with primary fibromyalgia syndrome. *J Rheumatol* 1993; 20:860–865.

Sim J, Adams N. Physical and non-pharmacological interventions for fibromyalgia. *Balliere's Clin Rheumatol* 1999; 13:129–145.

Sim J, Adams N. Systematic review of randomized controlled trials of nonpharmacological interventions for fibromyalgia. *Clin J Pain* 2003; 18:324–336.

Simms RW. Is there muscle pathology in fibromyalgia syndrome? *Rheum Dis Clin North Am* 1996; 22:245–266.

Solomon DH, Liang MH. Fibromyalgia: scourge of humankind or bane of a rheumatologist's existence? *Arthritis Rheum* 1997; 40:1553–1555.

Stratz T, Farber L, Varga B, et al. Fibromyalgia treatment with intravenous tropisetron administration. *Drugs Exp Clin Res* 2001; 27:113–118.

Sunshine W, Field TM, Quintino O, et al. Fibromyalgia benefits from message therapy and transcutaneous electrical nerve stimulation. *J Clin Rheumatol* 1996; 2:18–22.

Talo S, Forssell H, Heikkonen S, et al. Integrative group therapy outcome related to psychosocial characteristics in patients with chronic pain. *Int J Rehabil Res* 2001; 24:25–33.

Thompson JM. Tension myalgia as a diagnosis at the Mayo Clinic and its relationship to fibrositis, fibromyalgia, and myofascial pain syndrome. *Mayo Clin Proc* 1990; 65:1237–1247.

Turk DC. Customizing treatment for chronic pain patients: who, what, and why. *Clin J Pain* 1990; 6:255–270.

Turk, DC, Flor H. Primary fibromyalgia is more than tender points: toward a multiaxial taxonomy. *J Rheumatol* 1989; 16:80–86.

Turk DC, Rudy TE. Assessment of cognitive factors in chronic pain: a worthwhile enterprise? *J Consult Clin Psychol* 1986; 54:760–768.

Turk DC, Rudy TE. Toward an empirically derived taxonomy of chronic pain states: integration of psychological assessment data. *J Consult Clin Psychol* 1988; 56, 233–238.

Turk DC, Rudy TE. The robustness of an empirically derived taxonomy of chronic pain patients. *Pain* 1990; 42:27–35.

Turk DC, Okifuji A. Evaluating the role of physical, operant, cognitive, and affective factors in the pain behaviors of chronic pain patients. *Behav Modif* 1997; 21:259–280.

Turk DC, Okifuji A, Sinclair JD, et al. Pain, disability, and physical functioning in subgroups of patients with fibromyalgia. *J Rheumatol* 1996a; 23:1255–1262.

Turk DC, Okifuji A, Starz TW, et al. Effects of type of symptom onset on psychological distress and disability in fibromyalgia syndrome patients. *Pain* 1996b; 68:423–430.

Turk DC, Rudy TE, Kubinski JA, et al. Dysfunctional TMD patients: evaluating the efficacy of a tailored treatment protocol. *J Consult Clin Psychol* 1996c; 64:139–146.

Turk DC, Okifuji A, Sinclair JD, et al. Interdisciplinary treatment for fibromyalgia syndrome: clinical and statistical significance. *Arthritis Care Res* 1998a; 11:186–195.

Turk DC, Okifuji A, Starz TW, et al. Differential responses by psychosocial subgroups of fibromyalgia syndrome patients to an interdisciplinary treatment. *Arthritis Care Res* 1998b; 11:397–404.

Turk DC, Sist TC, Okifuji A, et al. Adaptation to metastatic cancer pain, regional/local cancer pain and non-cancer pain: role of psychological and behavioral factors. *Pain* 1998c; 74:247–256.

Vaeroy H, Abrahamsen A, Forre O. Treatment of fibromyalgia (fibrositis syndrome): a double-blind trial with carisoprodol, paracetamol, and caffeine [Somadril comp[R]] versus placebo. *Clin Rheumatol* 1989: 8:245–250

Van Denderen JC, Boersma JW, Zeinstra P, et al. Physiological effects of exhaustive physical exercise in primary fibromyalgia syndrome (PFS): Is PFS a disorder of neuroendocrine reactivity? *Scand J Rheumatol* 1992; 21:35–37.

Van Lieshout J, Wieling W, Karemaker J, et al. The vasovagal response. *Clin Sci* 1991; 81:575–586.

Vlaeyen JWS, Nooyen-Haazen IWCJ, Boossens MEJB, et al. The role of fear in the cognitive-educational treatment of fibromyalgia. In: Jensen TS, Turner JA, Wiesenfeld-Hallin Z (Eds). *Proceedings of the 8th World Congress on Pain,* Progress in Pain Research and Management, Vol. 8. Seattle: IASP Press, 1997, pp 693–704.

Volkmann H, Norregaard J, Jacobsen S, et al. Double-blind, placebo-controlled cross-over study of intravenous S-adenosyl-L-methionine in patients with fibromyalgia. *Scand J Rheumatol* 1997; 26:206–211.

Walker EA, Keegan D, Gardner G, et al. Psychosocial factors in fibromyalgia compared with rheumatoid arthritis: I. Psychiatric diagnoses and functional disability. *Psychosom Med* 1997; 59:565–571.

Walker J. Relief from chronic pain by low power laser irradiation. *Neurosci Lett* 1983; 43:339–344.

Waylonis GW, Perkins RH. Post-traumatic fibromyalgia. A long-term follow-up. *Am J Phys Med Rehabil* 1994; 73:403–412.

White KP, Nielson WR. Cognitive behavioral treatment of fibromyalgia syndrome: a follow up assessment. *J Rheumatol* 1995; 22:717–721.

White KP, Speechley M, Hart M, et al. The London Fibromyalgia Epidemiology Study: the prevalence of fibromyalgia syndrome in London, Ontario. *J Rheumatol* 1999; 26:1570–1576.

Wigers SH, Stiles TC, Vogel PA. Effects of aerobic exercise versus stress management treatment in fibromyalgia. *Scand J Rheumatol* 1996; 25:77–86.

Wolfe F, Smythe HA, Yunus MB, et al. The American College of Rheumatology 1990 criteria for the classification of fibromyalgia: report of the multicenter criteria committee. *Arthritis Rheum* 1990; 36:160–172.

Wolfe F, Russell IJ, Vipraio G, et al. Serotonin levels, pain threshold, and fibromyalgia symptoms in the general population. *J Rheumatol* 1997; 24:555–559.

Wysenbeek AJ, Mor F, Lurie Y, et al. Imipramine for the treatment of fibrositis: a therapeutic trial. *Ann Rheum Dis* 1985; 44:753–753.

Yunus MB. Towards a model of pathophysiology of fibromyalgia: aberrant central pain mechanisms with peripheral modulation. *J Rheumatol* 1992; 19:846–850.

Yunus MB, Masi AT, Aldag JC. Short-term effects of ibuprofen in primary fibromyalgia syndrome: a double-blind, placebo-controlled trial. *J Rheumatol* 1989; 16:527–532.

Yurtkuran M, Celiktas M. A randomized controlled trial of balneotherapy in the treatment of patients with primary fibromyalgia syndrome. *Phys Med Rehabil Kurortmed* 1996; 6:109–112.

Zidar J, Backman B, Bengtsson A, et al. Quantitative EMG and muscle tension in painful muscle in fibromyalgia. *Pain* 1990; 40:249–254.

Correspondence to: Dennis C. Turk, PhD, Department of Anesthesiology, Box 356540, University of Washington, Seattle, WA 98195, USA. Email: turkdc@u.washington.edu.

Psychosocial Aspects of Pain: A Handbook for Health Care Providers, Progress in Pain Research and Management, Vol. 27, edited by Robert H. Dworkin and William S. Breitbart, IASP Press, Seattle, © 2004.

15

Complex Regional Pain Syndrome

Stephen Bruehl and Ok Yung Chung

Department of Anesthesiology, Vanderbilt University School of Medicine, Nashville, Tennessee, USA

Complex regional pain syndrome (CRPS) is the current diagnostic label for the syndrome historically referred to by various terms, including reflex sympathetic dystrophy (RSD), causalgia, Sudeck's atrophy, shoulder-hand syndrome, neuroalgodystrophy, and reflex neurovascular dystrophy. It is a neuropathic pain disorder characterized by significant involvement of the autonomic nervous system. CRPS is subdivided into CRPS-I (reflex sympathetic dystrophy) and CRPS-II (causalgia), reflecting the absence or presence of major nerve injury, respectively. Current diagnostic criteria for CRPS are presented in Table I (Merskey and Bogduk 1994).

The classic presentation of CRPS includes a seemingly non-anatomical stocking or glove pain distribution; severe pain in response to touch or temperature changes (allodynia); skin color changes and temperature asymmetry, edema, and altered sweating in the affected extremity, and often pronounced pain behavior (e.g., extreme guarding). Objective signs of CRPS such as skin temperature and color changes are often phasic rather than tonic in nature, resulting in patient-reported symptoms that may not be observed at the time of physical examination. Apparent spreading of CRPS to other extremities unaffected by the precipitating injury may occur with some frequency (Maleki et al. 2000). Moreover, CRPS patients are often described in the clinical literature as experiencing intense emotional distress (Bruehl and Carlson 1992). The often dramatic and unusual presentation of CRPS patients has been the impetus for some to consider it primarily a psychiatric (somatoform) condition (e.g., Ochoa and Verdugo 1995). Research has increasingly documented the pathophysiology underlying CRPS (Gracely et al. 1992; Woolf et al. 1992; Baron and Maier 1996; Birklein et al. 1998; Kurvers et al. 1998), underscoring that psychological factors alone do not account for this perplexing syndrome. Although the role of psychological

Table I
Diagnostic criteria for CRPS-I and associated signs and symptoms

Diagnostic Criteria

1) The presence of an initiating noxious event or a cause of immobilization.
2) Continuing pain, allodynia, or hyperalgesia with which the pain is disproportionate to any inciting event.
3) Evidence at some time of edema, changes in skin blood flow, or abnormal sudomotor activity in the region of pain.
4) This diagnosis is excluded by the existence of conditions that would otherwise account for the degree of pain and dysfunction.

Associated Signs and Symptoms

1) Atrophy of the hair, nails, and other soft tissues
2) Alterations in hair growth
3) Loss of joint mobility
4) Impairment of motor function, including weakness, tremor, and dystonia
5) Sympathetically maintained pain may be present

Source: Merskey and Bogduk (1994, pp. 41–42).

factors in the onset and maintenance of CRPS is not yet well understood, we propose that a psychophysiological model may be useful for understanding interactions between psychological factors and this challenging pain disorder.

This chapter will briefly summarize the pathophysiology of CRPS, with an emphasis on theoretical mechanisms by which psychological factors might interact with CRPS pathophysiology. We will then provide an overview of the research literature examining psychological factors in CRPS and conclude by examining the role of psychological factors in the clinical management of CRPS.

PATHOPHYSIOLOGY OF CRPS

Several pathophysiological mechanisms believed to contribute to CRPS may be relevant to understanding how psychological or behavioral factors could influence the syndrome. Fig. 1 displays hypothesized interactions between psychological or behavioral factors and a number of pathophysiological mechanisms that may underlie CRPS. Sympathetic hypofunction following peripheral nerve injury is believed to lead to upregulation of peripheral catecholaminergic receptors (Arnold et al. 1993; Harden et al. 1994; Birklein et al. 1998; Kurvers et al. 1998). This receptor upregulation produces a supersensitivity to circulating catecholamines that is associated with exaggerated vasoconstriction (Arnold et al. 1993; Baron and Maier 1996; Birklein et al. 1998), leading to the cool, bluish extremity characteristic of chronic CRPS. Nociceptive afferents also may become sensitive to adrenergic

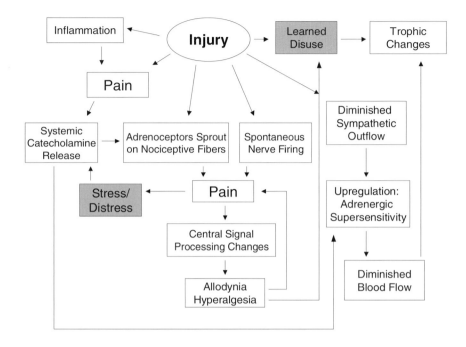

Fig. 1. Possible interactions between psychological/behavioral factors and pathophysiological mechanisms contributing to CRPS. Adapted from Bruehl and Chung (2003).

excitation following nerve injury, leading to increased firing in the presence of sympathetic discharge or circulating catecholamines (Harden et al. 1994; Drummond et al. 2001; Jänig and Baron 2001). This catecholamine-induced nociceptive firing contributes to the persistent nociceptive input that is believed to produce and maintain the altered spinal processing of afferent input underlying allodynia and hyperalgesia in CRPS (Gracely et al. 1992; Woolf et al. 1992). A vicious cycle may be created in which altered central processing leads to increased pain, which provokes catecholamine release that further stimulates the nociceptive input maintaining the central processing alterations. The presence of these central nervous system changes is also presumed to underlie spreading of CRPS to other extremities in some cases (Maleki et al. 2000).

Another important pathophysiological mechanism that may contribute to CRPS is the profound disuse of the affected extremity that often develops in an effort to avoid stimuli that may trigger hyperalgesic and allodynic responses. This possibility is supported by work suggesting that even in healthy individuals, prolonged disuse from wearing a cast may lead to temperature and color changes and hyperalgesia similar to those observed in CRPS patients (Butler 2001). Diminished active range of motion is common even in early CRPS (Schurmann et al. 1999), and the syndrome is associated with significantly reduced mobility and impaired use of the affected extremity (Kemler and de Vet 2000). Furthermore, the ability to carry out activities of daily living is inversely correlated with pain intensity in CRPS patients (Geertzen et al. 1998a). The findings above are all consistent with the proposition that CRPS patients may learn to avoid many normal activities of daily living because they trigger allodynia or increased spontaneous pain. The fact that activity avoidance is subject to the influence of operant conditioning (i.e., reduced activity is reinforced by the avoidance of pain) can sometimes result in extreme alterations in activity patterns. For example, some patients have reported being unwilling to leave their home or to socialize with others in order to avoid the possibility that their affected extremity might accidentally be touched during such activities, triggering allodynia. Because activity avoidance can be reinforced simply by the diminished anxiety accompanying avoidance of *feared* pain exacerbations (even if they never occur), learned activity avoidance can persist even when physical capabilities have improved through treatment. The tendency of significant others to assume responsibility for activities that appear to provoke increases in the patient's pain may further reinforce this learned disuse, even though it is intended to be a supportive response (Fordyce et al. 1973; Bruehl et al. 2001).

Operantly conditioned disuse of the affected extremity, whether reinforced by avoidance of actual pain, by reduced anxiety, or by the solicitous behavior of others, can prevent desensitization and eliminate the normal tactile and proprioceptive input from the extremity that may be necessary to restore normal central signal processing (Carlson and Watson 1988; Stanton-Hicks et al. 1998). Learned disuse may also impair the natural pumping action associated with movement that helps prevent accumulation of catecholamines and sensitizing neurochemicals in the affected extremity, which can exacerbate CRPS signs and symptoms (e.g., Drummond et al. 2001; Weber et al. 2001).

Pain-related learned disuse may therefore interact with other pathophysiological mechanisms to prevent the patient from ending the vicious cycle that maintains the primary features of CRPS (Bruehl 2001). Moreover, given the pathophysiological mechanisms described above, any psychological factor associated with altered catecholamine activity could directly affect pain intensity and vasomotor changes, and by exacerbating pain, could indirectly help maintain the central signal-processing changes that may underlie CRPS. In another important vicious cycle, the stress associated with increased pain severity is itself likely to increase catecholamine release, thereby further increasing pain and stress.

WHAT ROLE DO PSYCHOLOGICAL FACTORS PLAY IN THE ONSET AND MAINTENANCE OF CRPS?

Uncontrolled studies have often reported psychological factors to be an apparent contributor to the onset of CRPS (Bruehl and Carlson 1992). Few well-controlled studies have directly tested this clinical assumption, and the research that is available does not provide strong support for this assumed causative role (see Table II for a summary). Despite the absence of definitive studies, theoretical mechanisms exist through which psychological factors *might* affect the development and maintenance of CRPS. Life stress and dysphoric emotional states (anxiety, anger, and depression) are associated with altered catecholaminergic activity (e.g., Charney et al. 1990; Light et al. 1998), and through this mechanism could interact with the pathophysiological processes described above. Whether psychological factors do in some cases contribute to the onset of CRPS (in the context of physical injury), or help maintain the pathophysiology of the syndrome once it has developed, remains an open question.

Prospective studies are required to draw any conclusions regarding psychological causation, and due to the infrequency with which CRPS occurs even after major injury, such studies are rarely conducted. Although the results of one published prospective study suggest that personality factors (e.g., "sthenic," "unstable," and "ambitious") can predict the onset of CRPS following hand surgery with 91% accuracy (Zachariae 1964), the poorly defined nature of these psychological predictor variables argues against the reliability of these findings. In contrast to these positive results, unpublished results from our clinic indicated that baseline ratings of depression (on the Beck Depression Inventory) and anxiety (on the State Trait Anxiety Inventory) were not a significant predictor of CRPS-like symptoms 6 months following total knee replacement. No other prospective studies addressing this issue have been published.

One well-designed prospective study, while it did not address the role of psychological factors in the onset of CRPS, has convincingly demonstrated that psychological factors do affect the intensity of pain once CRPS has developed (Feldman et al. 1999). This study used time-series diary methodology, in which CRPS-I patients provided daily ratings of pain and mood for 28 days. Results indicated that daily variations in depressed mood, but not in angry or anxious mood, significantly predicted CRPS pain intensity on the following day. Not surprisingly, the results also indicated that increased pain on a given day predicted increased depressed, angry, and anxious mood on the following day. Results of this study suggest a potential vicious cycle

Table II

Published studies addressing psychological factors in CRPS patients

Study	Design	Sample	Results
Zachariae 1964	Prospective; preop. psychiatric interviews	47 Dupuytren's contracture	91% accuracy in using presurgical judgments of psychiatric risk factors to predict postsurgical CRPS-I-type symptoms
Van Houdenhove 1986	Uncontrolled case series	32 CRPS-I	Relationship between CRPS-I onset and contemporaneous emotional loss in all patients
Haddox et al. 1988	Case-control	21 CRPS-I, 21 radicular LBP	No significant differences in anxiety or personality profile on MMPI
Hardy and Merritt 1988	Case-control	9 CRPS-I, 8 non-CRPS pain	Elevated depression, anxiety, and interpersonal sensitivity in CRPS group
Zucchini et al. 1989	Case-control	13 CRPS-I, 23 brachial plexus lesion	More frequent elevations on MMPI scales 1–3 in the CRPS-I group
Egle and Hoffmann 1990	Uncontrolled case series	12 CRPS-I	One or more significant life stressors in the 6 months prior to CRPS-I onset in all patients
DeGood et al. 1993	Case-control	71 CRPS-I, 66 LBP, 51 headache	CRPS-I group the same or lower in distress on the SCL-90 compared to controls
Geertzen et al. 1994	Case-control	24 CRPS-I, 43 non-CRPS hand surgery	Female CRPS-I patients more anxious than non-CRPS patients; male CRPS-I patients more depressed than non-CRPS patients

Bruehl et al. 1996	Case-control	34 CRPS-1/SMP, 50 non-SMP limb pain, 165 LBP	Phobic anxiety, interpersonal sensitivity, and somatization higher in CRPS-I patients than LBP patients; stronger pain intensity/distress correlation in CRPS-I than LBP
Nelson and Novy 1996	Case-control	58 CRPS-I, 214 myofascial pain	CRPS-I patients scored lower on MMPI scales 1, 2, 3, and 7, but higher on scale 9
Ciccone et al. 1997	Case-control	25 CRPS-I, 21 local neuropathy, 44 LBP	CRPS-I patients had greater somatic symptoms of depression than neuropathy, but no differences from LBP patients
Geertzen et al. 1998	Case-control	24 CRPS-I, 42 non-CRPS hand surgery	Stressful life events significantly more common among CRPS patients in the 2 months prior to or 1 month after the initiating physical trauma
Monti et al. 1998	Structured psychiatric diagnostic interview	25 CRPS-I, 25 radicular LBP	24% prevalence of Axis I psychiatric disorders in CRPS patients; no difference from LBP group
Feldman et al. 1999	Prospective time series	109 CRPS-I	Increases in daily depressed mood predicted greater pain intensity the following day; greater daily pain intensity predicted increased depressed, angry, and anxious mood the following day
Rommel et al. 2001	Structured psychiatric diagnostic interview	37 CRPS-I	46% diagnosed with major or minor depression, 27% met criteria for an anxiety disorder

Source: Modified from Bruehl (2001, p. 283).
Note: Studies are listed by date of publication; LBP = low back pain; MMPI = Minnesota Multiphasic Personality Inventory; SCL-90 = Symptom Checklist-90; SMP = sympathetically maintained pain.

in which increased CRPS pain intensity results in more depressed mood, which in turn produces further increases in pain intensity. The notion that this apparent vicious cycle might conform to the psychophysiological model proposed earlier is supported indirectly by experimental evidence that depressed mood in CRPS patients is associated with increased plasma epinephrine levels (R.N. Harden et al., unpublished manuscript), and by evidence that sympathetic arousal increases pain in CRPS patients (Drummond et al. 2001).

The primary limitation of the Feldman et al. (1999) study is that no non-CRPS chronic pain group was available for comparison regarding these mood-pain interactions. However, one cross-sectional study suggests that the relationship between mood and pain intensity may be stronger in CRPS patients than in non-CRPS chronic pain patients. Bruehl et al. (1996) found a significantly stronger correlation between emotional distress and pain intensity among a series of 34 CRPS patients with sympathetically maintained pain than was found in a comparison group of 165 low back pain patients. While these findings are correlational and do not show causality, they are consistent with Feldman et al.'s results and would support the possibility of a greater role for emotional distress in determining CRPS pain intensity.

All other studies that have examined the role of psychological factors in CRPS have been limited to case-series descriptions or cross-sectional psychological comparisons between CRPS patients and non-CRPS chronic pain patients. For example, one uncontrolled retrospective study reported a strong relationship between onset of CRPS and a contemporaneous emotional loss (e.g., death of a loved one or divorce) among a series of 32 CRPS patients (Van Houdenhove 1986). Egle and Hoffmann (1990) similarly reported that among a series of 12 CRPS patients, one or more significant life stressors were identified retrospectively as occurring in the 6 months prior to the onset of CRPS. Both of these uncontrolled case series suffer from serious methodological limitations that prevent any conclusions from being drawn.

The only controlled study regarding the role of life stress in CRPS onset found results similar to the case series above. Geertzen et al. (1998b) compared 24 CRPS patients to 42 patients without CRPS who were scheduled to undergo elective hand surgery. Results indicated that 80% of the CRPS group recalled a stressful life event in the time period immediately preceding or following the initiating physical trauma, in contrast to only 20% of the control group. Although these findings suggest that stressful life events may contribute to development of CRPS following physical trauma, no prospective tests of this hypothesis have been published.

Psychological factors such as comorbid depression, anxiety, and personality dysfunction have also been hypothesized to be of relevance in understanding the onset or maintenance of CRPS. Two controlled studies have reported on the prevalence of psychiatric comorbidity in CRPS patients based on structured diagnostic interviews. Monti et al. (1998) reported a prevalence of 24% for DSM-IV Axis I disorders (predominantly depression) in a sample of CRPS patients, a rate not significantly different from that observed in a control group of non-CRPS chronic pain patients. More recently, Rommel et al. (2001) reported that in a sample of CRPS-I patients, 46% met criteria for a depressive disorder and 27% met criteria for an anxiety disorder, although no non-CRPS group was available for comparison. This apparently wide variability in prevalence of Axis I disorders among CRPS patients across samples highlights the likely impact of referral patterns on the results of such studies. Neither of the above studies documented psychiatric status *prior to* CRPS onset, and therefore neither can address the issue of causality. At present, there is no evidence that CRPS patients suffer from diagnosable psychiatric disorders at a higher rate than do other chronic pain patients.

If psychological factors such as depression are more directly involved in the onset or maintenance of pain in CRPS than in other types of chronic pain as suggested by the psychophysiological model above, emotional distress might be expected to be more common and more intense among CRPS patients than among comparable non-CRPS pain patients. In accordance with this hypothesis, several cross-sectional studies have reported that CRPS patients are more emotionally distressed than non-CRPS pain patients. Geertzen et al. (1994) compared patients with upper-extremity CRPS to non-CRPS patients awaiting elective hand surgery. Male CRPS patients were more anxious than their non-CRPS counterparts, and female CRPS patients were more depressed than their non-CRPS counterparts (Geertzen et al. 1994). Hardy and Merritt (1988) also found elevated symptoms of depression, anxiety, and interpersonal sensitivity in a small sample of CRPS patients relative to a comparison group of non-CRPS chronic pain patients. Results of work examining CRPS patients with sympathetically maintained pain (i.e., pain responsive to pharmacological sympathetic blockade) similarly found greater phobic anxiety and depression among CRPS patients compared to low back pain patients (Bruehl et al. 1996). Recent unpublished findings from our clinic are consistent with the studies above. Patients displaying signs and symptoms of CRPS 6 months after total knee replacement showed significantly higher levels of anxiety compared to patients without CRPS, despite the fact that both groups were continuing to experience at least some degree of pain. As noted previously, *baseline* anxiety and depression did not predict CRPS status at 6 months, suggesting that the observed elevations in psychological distress were a result of CRPS pain rather than a cause. In light of these findings, one possible explanation for elevated distress in CRPS patients relative to non-CRPS chronic pain patients might be that the unusual and sometimes dramatic symptomatology of CRPS (e.g., allodynia, hyperalgesia, vasomotor changes, significant edema, and motor changes) is more distressing than experiencing more common forms of chronic pain.

While the above results are intriguing, support for the proposition that CRPS patients are more distressed than comparable non-CRPS chronic pain patients is weakened by inconsistent findings from other studies. For example, work by Ciccone and colleagues (1997) provides only partial support for this hypothesis, finding that CRPS patients reported more somatic symptoms of depression than did patients with local neuropathy, but displayed no emotional differences relative to low back pain patients. Other studies have found no evidence of elevated distress among CRPS patients compared to radiculopathy patients (Haddox et al. 1988) or headache and low back pain patients (DeGood et al. 1993). Although exact reasons for these differences across studies are unclear, variations in sample selection, pain duration, clinic referral patterns, and specific psychometric measures used may account for these mixed results. In the absence of additional well-controlled studies, it remains unclear whether the findings suggesting uniquely elevated distress in CRPS patients are an artifact of sample selection.

The few studies comparing CRPS to other pain patients using validated personality measures have not demonstrated any consistent evidence of unique personality functioning in CRPS patients. Zucchini and colleagues (1989) reported that CRPS patients displayed more frequent elevations on scales 1–3 of the Minnesota Multiphasic Personality Inventory (MMPI) compared to a group of non-CRPS brachial plexus injury patients. In contrast, Nelson and Novy (1996) reported that CRPS patients scored *lower* on scales 1 (hypochondriasis), 2 (depression), 3 (hysteria), and 7 (psychasthenia) of the MMPI compared to myofascial pain patients, but scored higher than this comparison group on scale 9 (mania). These opposing results do not support consistent personality influences on the development or maintenance of CRPS.

In summary, there is no evidence to suggest unequivocally that psychological factors are involved in the onset or maintenance of CRPS, although such connections would not be theoretically implausible. Evidence is mixed regarding whether CRPS patients experience relatively greater life stress or emotional distress than other types of chronic pain patients, although several studies suggest that this may be the case. Existing work does support the proposition that psychological distress affects CRPS pain intensity, with one study raising the possibility that the distress-pain relationship may be stronger in CRPS than in non-CRPS pain conditions (Bruehl et al. 1996). Such differences would presumably be due to relationships between emotional distress and catecholamines, and to the relatively greater role of catechola-minergic mechanisms in determining symptomatology in CRPS patients.

THE ROLE OF PSYCHOLOGICAL FACTORS
IN CRPS MANAGEMENT

Consensus reports by expert clinicians and researchers have emphasized the importance of integrated multidisciplinary care for CRPS, with a primary focus of treatment being the restoration of normal use of the affected extremity (Stanton-Hicks et al. 1998, 2002). Whether or not psychological factors directly influence CRPS through the psychophysiological interactions described above, several psychological and behavioral factors are potential barriers to achieving this goal of renormalized use. As described previously, learned avoidance behavior may play a significant role in the disuse phenomena often seen in CRPS patients. Providing physical and occupational therapy (PT/OT) without addressing these learned barriers to normal use is likely to result in continued dysfunction in daily life even if functional *capabilities* are objectively improved during treatment sessions. Lack of motivation related to comorbid major depression may impair patients' ability to follow through on home therapy exercises, and again, inhibit functional progress in PT/OT. Cognitive factors may be important to consider as well. For example, an unrealistic focus on invasive procedures (e.g., sympathetic blocks) as curative, failure to adopt an active self-management focus in treatment, excessive fears that pain associated with use of the extremity signals tissue damage, and unfounded beliefs that CRPS is inherently a progressive and deteriorating condition can all interfere with motivation to engage in optimal treatment. As in other types of chronic pain, habitual engagement in catastrophic and other maladaptive cognitions can also be problematic ("This is awful—I can't handle this," "I can't do that—it will make my CRPS worse," "I've done treatment before—it doesn't work"). It is imperative to address these dysfunctional cognitions and find a means of enhancing patients' perceived level of control over their condition (e.g., using psychological pain management techniques), even if such control is limited in scope.

Controlled studies suggest that the psychological component of CRPS management may play an important role in overall progress in multidisciplinary treatment. Quantitative reviews of randomized trials regarding efficacy of psychologically based chronic pain treatments have shown that they are effective for reducing pain intensity and pain behavior and for improving pain coping (e.g., Flor et al. 1992; Morley et al. 1999). Studies included in these reviews have reflected samples with heterogeneous chronic pain diagnoses. Based on clinical experience, similar efficacy would seem likely for CRPS patients as well, although to date only one published randomized trial has specifically evaluated psychological interventions in CRPS patients. Fialka et al. (1996) randomized 18 CRPS patients to receive either home physical therapy (PT) or home PT plus once-weekly autogenic relaxation training for 10 weeks. Both groups showed improved pain, range of motion, and edema, with no significant differences between groups. However, patients receiving both PT and autogenic training demonstrated significantly greater improvements in limb temperature compared to those receiving PT alone. Although the small sample size limited statistical power for testing intervention efficacy, these results suggest that relaxation-based interventions may have some benefit in the management of CRPS. Results of several published case studies and small case series further suggest that the pain of CRPS may be reduced through use of techniques including hypnotherapy, imagery, progressive muscle relaxation, autogenic training, and thermal biofeedback (Blanchard 1979; Alioto 1981; Barowsky et al. 1987; Kawano et al. 1989; Gainer 1992). For example, Blanchard (1979) described a CRPS-I patient who had demonstrated no reduction in symptoms after several months of medication and sympathetic blocks. A series of 18 thermal biofeedback sessions resulted in the patient's ability to raise finger temperature by 1.5°C, coinciding with a nearly complete resolution of CRPS pain that was maintained at 1-year follow-up. While not representing a controlled trial, these results suggest the potential efficacy of psychologically based pain control techniques in CRPS patients.

Other research has addressed the multidisciplinary aspects of treatment, suggesting that integration of psychological methods with medical and physical therapy may assist in the successful management of CRPS (Oerlemans et al. 1999, 2000; Sherry et al. 1999). Among a prospective case series of 103 primarily adolescent CRPS patients, treatment incorporating conservative medication management, regular active physical therapy, and psychological counseling reportedly resulted in 92% of the sample achieving symptom-free status (Sherry et al. 1999). Results of the only other randomized trials of nonmedical interventions for CRPS are also notable, indicating that an intervention combining passive physical therapy, pain coping skills, and relaxation training resulted in significantly improved pain, active range of motion, and impairment levels compared to a social work control group (Oerlemans et al. 1999, 2000).

In summary, randomized controlled studies of psychological interventions for CRPS, alone or in the multidisciplinary context, are almost entirely absent from the literature. The clinical studies available, however, do suggest that psychological interventions are likely to be a useful part of a comprehensive multidisciplinary treatment package for CRPS. Referral for appropriate psychological pain management treatment should be routinely made once CRPS patients have moved beyond the acute phase without substantial resolution of symptoms (approximately 8 weeks). This treatment should include relaxation and imagery training assisted with biofeedback, as well as cognitive and behavioral components (see Bruehl and Chung, in press for additional details). Inclusion of family members in this treatment may be helpful given that their solicitous responses to the patient's pain behavior may contribute to disuse phenomena.

CONCLUSIONS

Some experts have argued that CRPS is primarily a psychiatric disturbance (Ochoa and Verdugo 1995). Lack of treatment progress, dramatic pain behavior and complaints, and confusing symptom reports are often reasons for adopting this psychogenic viewpoint. While a patient presenting with CRPS-like complaints might on rare occasions be suffering from a somatoform psychiatric disorder rather than a true chronic pain syndrome, data do not support the argument that all CRPS patients are experiencing a psychiatrically based pain disorder. This clinical assumption ignores the growing body of research documenting the pathophysiology of CRPS, and may prevent serious rehabilitative efforts from being undertaken despite real prospects for improved management of the condition.

An alternative view of psychological stress and emotional distress as factors that at a minimum exacerbate CRPS pain is supported by experimental evidence. A significant correlation between emotional distress and pain intensity has been convincingly shown in CRPS patients (Bruehl et al. 1996; Feldman et al. 1999). In fact, it would be surprising if such relationships were not observed in CRPS, given evidence that dysphoric mood states directly exacerbate pain intensity in various other chronic pain syndromes (e.g., Arena et al. 1990; Affleck et al. 1992).

The question of whether psychological factors are more directly involved in the onset and maintenance of CRPS remains to be answered. No well-controlled prospective studies have addressed this issue, although the neurochemical sequelae of psychological stress and emotional distress could in theory interact with the pathophysiological mechanisms underlying CRPS to produce or maintain the syndrome. Cross-sectional studies have often reported CRPS patients to be more psychologically distressed than comparable non-CRPS pain patients, although results have sometimes been inconsistent. While none of the available research conclusively demonstrates that psychological factors are involved in the development or maintenance of CRPS, we have sufficient experimental data and theoretical reasons to justify considering this possibility further.

Regardless of whether psychological factors are directly intertwined with the pathophysiology of CRPS, the syndrome is most appropriately viewed as a complex biopsychosocial problem that should be treated using an aggressive multidisciplinary approach. Close integration of psychological assessment and cognitive-behavioral pain management treatment with medical therapy, physical therapy, and occupational therapy is likely to optimize treatment outcomes (Stanton-Hicks et al. 1998, 2002; Bruehl et al. 2001). Although CRPS is aptly termed a complex pain syndrome, clinical experience indicates that coordinated and intensive multidisciplinary care can produce positive outcomes in these patients even when the condition has become chronic.

REFERENCES

Affleck G, Urrows S, Tennen H, et al. Daily coping with pain from rheumatoid arthritis: patterns and correlates. *Pain* 1992; 51:221–229.

Alioto JT. Behavioral treatment of reflex sympathetic dystrophy. *Psychosomatics* 1981; 22:539–540.

Arena JG, Sherman RA, Bruno GM, Smith JD. The relationship between situational stress and phantom limb pain: cross-lagged correlational data from six month pain logs. *J Psychosom Res* 1990; 34:71–77.

Arnold JMO, Teasell RW, MacLeod AP, Brown JE, Carruthers SG. Increased venous alpha-adrenoceptor responsiveness in patients with reflex sympathetic dystrophy. *Ann Intern Med* 1993; 118:619–621.

Baron R, Maier C. Reflex sympathetic dystrophy: skin blood flow, sympathetic vasoconstrictor reflexes, and pain before and after surgical sympathectomy. *Pain* 1996; 67:317–326.

Barowsky EI, Zweig JB, Moskowitz J. Thermal biofeedback in the treatment of symptoms associated with reflex sympathetic dystrophy. *J Child Neurol* 1987; 2:229–232.

Birklein F, Riedl B, Claus D, Neudorfer B. Pattern of autonomic dysfunction in time course of complex regional pain syndrome. *Clin Autonom Res* 1998; 8:79–85.

Blanchard EB. The use of temperature biofeedback in the treatment of chronic pain due to causalgia. *Biofeed Self-Regul* 1979; 4:183–188.

Bruehl S. Do psychological factors play a role in the onset and maintenance of CRPS? In: Harden RN, Baron R, Jänig W (Eds). *Complex Regional Pain Syndrome,* Progress in Pain Research and Management, Vol. 22. Seattle: IASP Press, 2001.

Bruehl S, Carlson CR. Predisposing psychological factors in the development of reflex sympathetic dystrophy: a review of the empirical evidence. *Clin J Pain* 1992; 8:287–299.

Bruehl S, Chung OY. Complex regional pain syndrome. In: Aminoff MJ, Daroff RB (Eds). *Encyclopedia of the Neurological Sciences*. San Diego: Academic Press, 2003, pp 749–754.

Bruehl S, Chung OY. Psychological and behavioral aspects of CRPS management. *Clin J Pain;* in press.

Bruehl S, Husfeldt B, Lubenow T, et al. Psychological differences between reflex sympathetic dystrophy and non-RSD chronic pain patients. *Pain* 1996; 67:107–114.

Bruehl S, Steger HG, Harden RN. Assessment of complex regional pain syndrome. In: Turk DC, Melzack R (Eds). *Handbook of Pain Assessment,* 2nd ed. New York: Guilford Press, 2001.

Butler S. Disuse and complex regional pain syndrome. In: Harden RN, Baron R, Jänig W (Eds). *Complex Regional Pain Syndrome,* Progress in Pain Research and Management, Vol. 22. Seattle: IASP Press, 2001.

Carlson LK, Watson HK. Treatment of reflex sympathetic dystrophy using the stress-loading program. *J Hand Ther* 1988; July–September:149–153.

Charney DS, Woods SW, Nagy LM, et al. Noradrenergic function in panic disorder. *J Clin Psychiatry* 1990; 51(Suppl A):5–10.

Ciccone DS, Bandilla EB, Wu W. Psychological dysfunction in patients with reflex sympathetic dystrophy. *Pain* 1997; 71:323–333.

DeGood DE, Cundiff GW, Adams LE, Shutty MS. A psychosocial and behavioral comparison of reflex sympathetic dystrophy, low back pain, and headache patients. *Pain* 1993; 54:317–322.

Drummond PD, Finch PM, Skipworth S, Blockey P. Pain increases during sympathetic arousal in patients with complex regional pain syndrome. *Neurology* 2001; 57:1296–1303.

Egle UT, Hoffmann SO. Psychosomatische Zusammenhänge bei sympathischer Reflexdystrophie (Morbus Sudeck). *Psychother Med Psychol* 1990; 40:123–135.

Feldman SI, Downey G, Schaffer-Neitz R. Pain, negative mood, and perceived social support in chronic pain patients: a daily diary study of people with reflex sympathetic dystrophy syndrome. *J Consult Clin Psychol* 1999; 67:776–785.

Fialka V, Korpan M, Saradeth T, et al. Autogenic training for reflex sympathetic dystrophy: a pilot study. *Complement Ther Med* 1996; 4:103–105.

Flor H, Fydrich T, Turk DC. Efficacy of multidisciplinary pain treatment centers: a meta-analytic review. *Pain* 1992; 49:221–230.

Fordyce WE, Fowler RS, Lehmann JF, et al. Operant conditioning in the treatment of chronic pain. *Arch Phys Med Rehabil* 1973; 54:399–408.

Gainer MJ. Hypnotherapy for reflex sympathetic dystrophy. *Am J Clin Hypn* 1992; 34:227–232.

Geertzen JHB, de Bruijn H, de Bruijn-Kofman AT, Arendzen JH. Reflex sympathetic dystrophy: early treatment and psychological aspects. *Arch Phys Med Rehabil* 1994; 75:442–446.

Geertzen JHB, Dijkstra PU, Groothoff JW, van ten Duis H, Eisma WH. Reflex sympathetic dystrophy of the upper extremity–a 5.5 year follow-up. *Acta Orthop Scand* 1998a; 279(Suppl):12–18.

Geertzen JHB, de Bruijn-Kofman AT, de Bruijn HP, et al. Stressful life events and psychological dysfunction in complex regional pain syndrome type I. *Clin J Pain* 1998b; 14:143–147.

Gracely RH, Lynch SA, Bennett GJ. Painful neuropathy: altered central processing maintained dynamically by peripheral input. *Pain* 1992; 51:175–194.

Haddox JD, Abram SE, Hopwood MH. Comparison of psychometric data in RSD and radiculopathy. *Reg Anesth* 1988; 13:27.

Harden RN, Duc TA, Williams TR, et al. Norepinephrine and epinephrine levels in affected versus unaffected limbs in sympathetically maintained pain. *Clin J Pain* 1994; 10:324–330.

Hardy MA, Merritt WH. Psychological evaluation and pain assessment in patients with reflex sympathetic dystrophy. *J Hand Ther* 1988; July–September:155–164.

Jänig W, Baron R. The role of the sympathetic nervous system in neuropathic pain: clinical observations and animal models. In: Hansson PT, Fields HL, Hill RG, Marchettini P (Eds). *Neuropathic Pain: Pathophysiology and Treatment,* Progress in Pain Research and Management, Vol. 21. Seattle: IASP Press, 2001.

Kawano M, Matsuoka M, Kurokawa T, et al. Autogenic training as an effective treatment for reflex sympathetic dystrophy: a case report. *Acta Paediatr Jpn* 1989; 31:500–503.

Kemler MA, de vet HCW. Health-related quality of life in chronic refractory reflex sympathetic dystrophy (complex regional pain syndrome type I). *J Pain Symptom Manage* 2000; 20:68–76.

Kurvers H, Daemen M, Slaaf D, et al. Partial peripheral neuropathy and denervation induced adrenoceptor supersensitivity. *Acta Orthop Belg* 1998; 64:64–70.

Light KC, Kothandapani RV, Allen MT. Enhanced cardiovascular and catecholamine responses in women with depressive symptoms. *Int J Psychophysiol* 1998; 28:157–166.

Maleki J, LeBel AA, Bennett GJ, Schwartzman RJ. Patterns of spread in complex regional pain syndrome, type I (reflex sympathetic dystrophy). *Pain* 2000; 88:259–266.

Merskey H, Bogduk N. *Classification of Chronic Pain: Descriptions of Chronic Pain Syndromes and Definitions of Pain Terms,* 2nd ed. Seattle: IASP Press, 1994.

Monti DA, Herring CL, Schwartzman RJ, Marchese M. Personality assessment of patients with complex regional pain syndrome type I. *Clin J Pain* 1998; 14:295–302.

Morley S, Eccleston C, Williams A. Systematic review and meta-analysis of randomized controlled trials of cognitive behaviour therapy and behaviour therapy for chronic pain in adults, excluding headache. *Pain* 1999; 80:1–13.

Nelson DV, Novy DM. Psychological characteristics of reflex sympathetic dystrophy versus myofascial pain syndromes. *Reg Anesth* 1996; 21:202–208.

Ochoa JL, Verdugo RJ. Reflex sympathetic dystrophy: a common clinical avenue for somatoform expression. *Neurol Clin* 1995; 13:351–363.

Oerlemans HM, Oostendorp RAB, de Boo T, Goris RJA. Pain and reduced mobility in complex regional pain syndrome I: outcome of a prospective randomized controlled clinical trial of adjuvant physical therapy versus occupational therapy. *Pain* 1999; 83:77–83.

Oerlemans HM, Oostendorp RAB, de Boo T, et al. Adjuvant physical therapy versus occupational therapy in patients with reflex sympathetic dystrophy/complex regional pain syndrome type I. *Arch Phys Med Rehabil* 2000; 81:49–56.

Rommel O, Malin JP, Zenz M, Jänig W. Quantitative sensory testing, neurophysiological and psychological examination in patients with complex regional pain syndrome and hemisensory deficits. *Pain* 2001; 93:279–293.

Schurmann M, Gradl G, Andress HJ, Furst H, Schildberg FW. Assessment of peripheral sympathetic nervous function for diagnosing early post-traumatic complex regional pain syndrome type I. *Pain* 1999; 80:149–159.

Sherry DD, Wallace CA, Kelley C, Kidder M, Sapp L. Short- and long-term outcomes of children with complex regional pain syndrome type I treated with exercise therapy. *Clin J Pain* 1999; 15:218–223.

Stanton-Hicks M, Baron R, Boas R, et al. Complex regional pain syndromes: guidelines for therapy. *Clin J Pain* 1998; 14:155–166.

Stanton-Hicks MD, Burton AW, Bruehl SP, et al. An updated interdisciplinary clinical pathway for CRPS: report of an expert panel. *Pain Practice* 2002; 2:1.

Van Houdenhove B. Neuro-algodystrophy: a psychiatrist's view. *Clin Rheumatol* 1986; 5:399–406.

Weber M, Birklein F, Neundorfer B, Schmelz M. Facilitated neurogenic inflammation in complex regional pain syndrome. *Pain* 2001; 91:251–257.

Woolf CJ, Shortland P, Coggeshall RE. Peripheral nerve injury triggers central sprouting of myelinated afferents. *Nature* 1992; 355:75–78.

Zachariae L. Incidence and course of posttraumatic dystrophy following operation for Dupuytren's contracture. *Acta Chir Scand* 1964; (Suppl)336:7–51.

Zucchini M, Alberti G, Moretti MP. Algodystrophy and related psychological features. *Funct Neurol* 1989; 4:153–156.

Correspondence to: Stephen Bruehl, PhD, Department of Anesthesiology, Vanderbilt University School of Medicine, 504 Oxford House, 1313 Twenty-First Avenue South, Nashville, TN 37232-4125, USA. Tel: 615-936-1821; Fax: 615-936-2801; email: stephen.bruehl@vanderbilt.edu.

Psychosocial Aspects of Pain: A Handbook for Health Care Providers, Progress in Pain Research and Management, Vol. 27, edited by Robert H. Dworkin and William S. Breitbart, IASP Press, Seattle, © 2004.

16

Irritable Bowel Syndrome and Chronic Pelvic Pain

Leslie J. Heinberg,[a] Robert R. Edwards,[b] and Jennifer A. Haythornthwaite[b]

[a]Department of Psychiatry, Case Western Reserve University School of Medicine, Cleveland, Ohio, USA; [b]Department of Psychiatry and Behavioral Sciences, Johns Hopkins University School of Medicine, Baltimore, Maryland, USA

Psychological factors predicting the onset, maintenance, and treatment outcome of chronic pain have long been established. However, much of the psychological literature in chronic pain focuses on circumscribed pain disorders such as low back pain, headache, and arthritis. More recently, a significant literature has developed examining psychological variables in both abdominal and pelvic pain. Although remarkably common in the general population, particularly among women, both pain subtypes are notably broad and oftentimes poorly defined. Psychological variables are important in both abdominal and pelvic pain. A brief overview of each disorder will be followed by a discussion of known psychological and psychiatric comorbidity, psychological factors associated with the disorders, and psychological treatments. We focus primarily on irritable bowel syndrome (IBS), given that it is the most common and well-researched type of chronic abdominal pain in adults. Similarly, we will review studies that examine a broad diagnosis of pelvic pain related to menstruation or the reproductive organs. A separate literature has developed examining vulvodynia, or chronic vulvar discomfort. Many similarities exist between vulvodynia and chronic pelvic pain (CPP); for example, both are associated with significant interference in sexual functioning. However, vulvodynia is better defined, with five distinct subtypes, is less common, and has distinct theories of etiology implicating candidiasis, neurological or hormonal factors, and allergy (Masheb et al. 2000). Perhaps because of the broader focus of pelvic pain and its enigmatic and frustrating nature, there has been greater focus in the literature on its psychological aspects. Thus, this chapter will concentrate on nonvulvar pelvic pain except for studies that compare the two.

Discussion of the literature on psychiatric and psychological comorbidity in IBS and CPP should begin with an important caveat. While most studies of IBS and CPP are conducted on samples of patients seeking treatment or referred for treatment at tertiary care clinics, symptoms of these disorders are extremely common in the general population. For example, the majority (75–90%) of individuals who meet criteria for IBS do not see physicians for treatment (Drossman 1999a; Camilleri 2001). Drossman and his colleagues, as well as several other groups of investigators, have compared samples of patients with IBS referred for treatment ("consulters") to demographically matched samples of individuals in the community meeting criteria for IBS but not seeking treatment for their symptoms ("nonconsulters"; see Drossman 1999a). Collectively, the findings suggest that distress, rather than the severity of gastrointestinal (GI) symptomatology, differentiates treatment-seeking IBS patients from nonconsulters (Drossman et al. 1988; Whitehead et al. 1988; Drossman 1999a). In general, nonconsulters with IBS do not differ from normal controls on measures of psychological symptomatology, while IBS patients seeking treatment show higher rates of depression, anxiety, and severe life stress. Although not as thoroughly studied, CPP nonconsulters have been shown to be similar in general health, pain severity, and measures of pain-related functioning to women with dysmenorrhea alone, whereas consulters have greater pain, pain-related disability, and sleep disturbance and poorer general health status (Zondervan et al. 2001). Thus, the majority of the psychological literature, in focusing primarily on treatment-seeking patients, will be biased in favor of finding differences between individuals with IBS and controls.

IRRITABLE BOWEL SYNDROME

OVERVIEW

IBS is a functional disorder of the lower GI tract whose symptoms most likely derive from dysregulation of communication between the brain and GI tract (Ringel et al. 2001). This bidirectional communication system is clearly influenced by psychological factors and environmental events (Mayer et al. 2001). Three sets of diagnostic criteria for IBS have been widely used, all of which emphasize recurrent abdominal pain or discomfort and alterations in bowel habits (Blanchard and Scharff 2002). The most recent is the set of "Rome II" criteria, which require for a positive diagnosis that an individual has had 12 weeks or more, within the past year, of abdominal pain or discomfort that is not explained by structural or metabolic abnormalities, and that has two of the following three features: (1) it is relieved with defecation, (2) the onset is associated with a change in stool frequency, or (3) the onset is associated with a change in stool form (Drossman 1999b). Using a variety of diagnostic criteria, epidemiological studies have provided a range of prevalence estimates from 8% to 23% (Camilleri 2001; Ringel et al. 2001), with women outnumbering men by approximately two to one in most studies. IBS shows substantial comorbidity with a number of other chronic pain syndromes (Burke et al. 1999), including fibromyalgia (33%), chronic fatigue syndrome (50%), CPP (35%), temporomandibular disorders (20%), headaches (50%), and back pain (30–60%) (Whitehead et al. 2002). IBS patients with one or more of these comorbid conditions are more anxious, depressed, somatically focused, and pain-sensitive than are IBS patients without such comorbidities. Overall, IBS is a highly prevalent syndrome with substantial social and personal costs. IBS patients make twice as many health care visits as do controls (Whitehead et al. 2002), and the syndrome is associated with substantial disability, lost productivity, and numerous deleterious psychological sequelae (Whitehead et al. 2002).

PSYCHIATRIC AND PSYCHOLOGICAL COMORBIDITY IN IBS

Most studies of psychiatric comorbidity in IBS find that a large percentage, from roughly 50% to over 90%, of IBS patients meet the American Psychiatric Association's *Diagnostic and Statistical Manual of Mental Disorders* (DSM) criteria for at least one Axis I diagnosis (i.e., a psychological disorder such as major depressive disorder or panic disorder) (Whitehead et al. 2002). Whitehead and colleagues (2002) conclude that over 90% of IBS patients seen for treatment, compared to 20% of nonconsulters, have one or more Axis I diagnoses. The proportion of IBS patients with an Axis I diagnosis is generally higher than the rates observed for either healthy controls or patients with other GI diseases (Trikas et al. 1999), with 40–60% of clinic patients with IBS having either a mood or anxiety disorder (Creed 1999). Interestingly, the predominance of anxious or depressive symptoms may vary across IBS samples. Creed (1999) suggests that, while patients with first-time referrals to a GI clinic are typically anxious, depression predominates over anxiety disorders (39% vs. 10%, respectively) among chronic clinic attenders (Guthrie et al. 1992).

Questionnaire-based studies suggest that IBS patients nearly always report significantly higher levels of anxiety, depression, neuroticism, and life stress compared to healthy controls, and often when compared to samples of patients with organic GI disease as well (Luscombe 2000). A recent review of the literature on health-related quality of life (HRQOL) indicated that IBS patients demonstrate lower HRQOL scores than healthy controls across all age groups (Luscombe 2000). In addition, IBS patients report lower scores on many subscales of the Medical Outcome Study Short-Form General Health Survey (SF-36) relative to patients with inflammatory bowel disease, gastroesophageal reflux disease, diabetes, hypertension, end-stage renal disease, and acute myocardial infarction (Gralnek et al. 2000; Luscombe 2000). Additional domains of HRQOL that may be impaired by IBS include sleep, dietary choices, and sexual function; indeed, one study found that over 80% of female IBS patients reported abdominal or vaginal pain associated with sexual intercourse.

ASSOCIATION OF PSYCHOLOGICAL FACTORS WITH GI SYMPTOMS

Cross-sectional studies report significant relationships between the severity of IBS symptoms and psychological factors such as depression and anxiety (Blanchard and Scharff 2002), neuroticism and indices of inhibited aggression (Tanum and Malt 2001), poorer physical functioning, more maladaptive coping strategies, and greater health care utilization (Drossman et al. 2000b). Certain beliefs are also associated with symptom severity; patients who believe that their GI symptoms are indicative of serious underlying pathology report more severe IBS (Drossman et al. 1999).

Psychological factors may also predict the onset and longitudinal course of the illness. A prospective study of post-infectious IBS (Gwee et al. 1996) followed 75 patients with acute gastroenteritis; 6 months later, 22 patients had persistent symptoms of IBS. Baseline anxiety and depression scores were significant predictors of IBS onset; the odds of developing IBS increased by a factor of 1.4 for every unit of increase in the score on the Hospital Anxiety and Depression checklist. Fowlie and colleagues (1992) followed IBS patients over 5 years and found that higher anxiety at baseline was associated with worsening symptoms over the course of the study, while no baseline disease-related factors (i.e., symptom severity or duration) predicted changes in IBS symptomatology. In addition to baseline anxiety, chronic social stress is a predictor of IBS outcome (Bennett et al. 1998). High levels of catastrophizing and low self-efficacy predicted poorer health-related outcomes 12 months later in women referred to a GI clinic (Drossman et al. 2000a).

Effects of stress on IBS. It is widely accepted that life stress is associated with the onset of IBS and other functional GI disorders. The diagnosis of IBS is often preceded by significant increases in negative, stressful life events (Creed 1999). Moreover, stressful events that threaten an individual's security are prospectively associated with symptom exacerbations (Bennett et al. 1998). Drossman (1999a) suggested that psychosocial factors, particularly life stress, may directly affect mucosal inflammation, visceral function, visceral sensation, and central modulation of afferent visceral input. Stress appears to have both immediate and delayed adverse effects on GI symptoms such as pain and altered bowel habits (Greene and Blanchard 1994). Investigators have documented strong cross-sectional relationships between stress and GI symptoms, as well as an effect of the previous days' and month's stress on current GI symptoms (Greene and Blanchard 1994; Dancey et al. 1998).

A detailed depiction of the neurobiology of stress is beyond the scope of this chapter, but several excellent recent reviews are available (Mayer 2000b; Mayer et al. 2001). Four pathways by which different types of stress may cause GI symptoms have been proposed (Mayer 2000b; Mayer et al. 2001). Early life stress and trauma in the form of abuse or loss, as well as acute, life-threatening stress in adulthood (e.g., rape or other types of assault) may permanently enhance stress responsiveness and predispose individuals to develop functional GI disorders. Other physical stressors such as infections, trauma, or surgery may act as trigger factors in vulnerable individuals. Minor daily life stressors and symptom-related anxiety affect GI symptoms on a day-to-day basis. Finally, a positive feedback loop is proposed in which conditioned anxiety responses to interoceptive stimuli provoke further stress responses, which in turn exacerbate GI symptoms, thus contributing to symptom chronicity in IBS patients (Mayer 2000b).

Psychophysiological studies have examined relationships between psychological stress and GI-related physiological responses. In healthy subjects, strong emotion and environmental stress are associated with increased motility in the stomach, small intestine, and colon (Mayer et al. 2001). These physiological responses to stress are exaggerated in functional GI disorders such as IBS, although such motor responses show inconsistent relationships with GI symptoms and may not be sufficient to explain the chronic recurrent abdominal pain experienced by IBS patients (Drossman 1999a).

Family history and social learning. Individuals with both IBS and recurrent abdominal pain (RAP) have a family history of GI disorder in approximately 50% of cases, a significantly higher percentage than that found in control samples of subjects without either disorder. IBS patients are also more likely than controls to report childhood losses and separations and unsatisfactory family relationships (Burke et al. 1999). Further, parental behaviors, attitudes, and modeling and reinforcement of GI-related illness

behavior might potentially play an etiological role in the development of
IBS (Whitehead et al. 1994) and in health-care-seeking behavior (Levy et al.
2000). Childhood learning of illness behavior appears to be symptom-
specific; parental modeling of GI-related illness behavior does not seem to
affect subsequent manifestations of menstrual or cold-related symptoms but
does affect subsequent displays of GI-related illness behavior (Whitehead
and Palsson 1998; Burke et al. 1999).

Physical and sexual abuse and IBS. It is important to note that methodological limitations of the available studies include variability in the definition of abuse, different methods used to identify abuse history (e.g., an
unstructured or structured interview, a single question in a questionnaire, a
validated multi-item measure, or court records), and use of retrospective
cross-sectional designs. Indeed, one recent study (Raphael et al. 2001) reported relationships between pain and self-reported abuse history but not
between pain and documented abuse history, suggesting that important biases may influence the reporting of both abuse and pain symptoms. History
of sexual or physical abuse is one of the more potent predictors of physical
and mental health among patients seeking treatment for GI symptoms
(Leserman et al. 1998). Elevated rates of abuse among IBS patients seeking
treatment have been found in a variety of studies, with rates ranging from
22% to 82% (Scarinci et al. 1994; Talley et al. 1995; Blanchard and Scharff
2002). These rates are higher than those seen in other painful conditions
such as inflammatory bowel disease (Delvaux et al. 1997; Drossman 1999a),
Crohn's disease (Reilly et al. 1999), and noncardiac chest pain (Scarinci et
al. 1994), although this was not the case in all studies (Talley et al. 1994;
Hobbis et al. 2002). Abuse history independently contributes to elevations in
psychological distress, dysfunction, and medical symptoms, and contributes
to higher health care utilization among women seeking treatment for IBS
(Talley et al. 1994; Leserman et al. 1996, 1998). Cross-sectional studies of
patients with severe IBS suggest that a history of sexual abuse is not associated with disability due to health problems or with health care costs (Creed
et al. 2001). However, in a longitudinal study of women referred to a GI
clinic, abuse severity independently predicted a variety of health outcomes,
including pain, distress, dysfunction, disability days in bed, physician visits,
and number of surgeries and procedures, over a 12-month period (Drossman
et al. 2000a). Most studies focus on a history of abuse, but ongoing partner
violence is also associated with high rates of abdominal and pelvic pain
(Campbell et al. 2002).

A recent prospective study contradicts much of the literature, suggesting
that a history of abuse places individuals at risk for pain problems (Raphael
et al. 2001). This carefully conducted follow-up of court-documented cases

of abuse in children before the age of 11 years found no consistent relationship between a documented history of abuse and the report of medically explained or unexplained pain complaints. However, self-reported history of abuse was associated with all pain complaints (Raphael et al. 2001) and specifically with abdominal pain complaints in adulthood (K.G. Raphael, personal communication).

Responses to standardized noxious stimuli. Whitehead and Palsson (1998) reviewed the growing literature on pain sensitivity in IBS and noted that relative to healthy controls, IBS patients demonstrate hyperalgesia to balloon distension of the rectum or lumen of the bowel. Similar findings were obtained for children with RAP, and one recent investigation reported that children with either RAP or IBS show visceral hyperalgesia in both the stomach and the rectum relative to healthy controls (Di Lorenzo et al. 2001). Somatization, or hypervigilance to somatic and visceral sensations, has been proposed to account for IBS patients' visceral hyperalgesia. IBS patients have higher monitoring and lower blunting scores on the Miller Behavioral Style Scale (suggesting a hypervigilant perceptual style; Cheng et al. 2000), demonstrate an increased attentiveness to GI-related stimuli (Gibbs-Gallagher et al. 2001), and show hyper-reactivity to auditory stimuli as assessed by event-related potentials (Blomhoff et al. 2000). Enhanced attention to noxious stimulation is associated with greater pain report for GI and other stimuli (Accarino et al. 1997), and the possibility that a hypervigilant perceptual style accounts for some of the increased pain sensitivity in IBS appears promising.

Conditioned fear to interoceptive cues, similar to that observed in panic disorder, has also been suggested to be a contributor to IBS patients' hypersensitivity to visceral stimuli. Mayer (2000a) hypothesized that sensations of fullness or urgency provoke physiological fear responses in individuals with IBS and that these responses enhance hypervigilance and impair pain modulation. At least seven studies suggest that IBS is associated with hypersensitivity throughout the GI tract, from colon to rectum, and with a heightened perception of normal, nonpainful intestinal contractions (Mayer et al. 2001). Consistent with this theory, women with IBS, gastroesophageal reflux disease, or noncardiac chest pain who reported a history of sexual or physical abuse showed lower pain thresholds in response to finger pressure stimuli in comparison to women without a history of abuse (Scarinci et al. 1994). Differences in pain threshold were attributed to lower standards for labeling a sensation as painful rather than to alterations in the ability to discriminate stimuli of varying intensity (Scarinci et al. 1994). In attempting to understand whether the lowered pain thresholds seen in IBS are attributable to a history of abuse, Whitehead et al. (1997) compared pain thresholds to rectal distension in three groups of women: those with a history of sexual abuse and IBS, those with IBS and no abuse history, and those with no IBS and no abuse history. Although the expected lower pain threshold was observed in the women with IBS, a history of sexual abuse was not associated with lowered pain thresholds to rectal distension. Rather than attributing the lowered pain thresholds seen in IBS to abuse history, these authors proposed other psychological influences on the labeling of painful stimuli (Whitehead et al. 1997).

In general, responses to standardized noxious stimuli administered in a laboratory show relationships to clinical symptoms. In a recent study of IBS patients and healthy controls (Verne et al. 2001), state anxiety and somatic focus correlated with ratings of noxious thermal stimuli applied to the hands and feet, although group differences in anxiety and somatic focus did not account for group differences in pain sensitivity. Distraction elevates sensory thresholds (Davis et al. 1978) for GI sensations, including pain, while attention to pain appears to enhance sensitivity (Accarino et al. 1997; Whitehead et al. 2002). Stress is associated with increased abdominal pain and bowel symptoms, as well as decreased pain thresholds (Mayer 2000a,b; Mayer et al. 2001). This effect may be mediated either by an increase in smooth muscle tone in the GI tract or by an enhancement of selective attention to pain and GI-related symptoms; such symptoms are relieved by stress reduction (Mayer et al. 2001; Mayer 2000a). Somatization also correlates with visceral pain thresholds in IBS (Whitehead et al. 2002), although other psychological variables such as depression and neuroticism show inconsistent relationships with laboratory-derived estimates of pain thresholds (Whitehead and Palsson 1998). According to Whitehead and Palsson, selective attention and disease attribution are the primary psychological factors influencing both pain sensitivity and GI symptomatology in IBS.

PSYCHOLOGICAL AND PSYCHIATRIC TREATMENTS IN IBS

Over the past several decades, as interest in a biopsychosocial model of IBS has grown, a number of studies have assessed the impact of psychological treatments for IBS, as well as the psychological factors that predict treatment outcome in patients with IBS (Blanchard and Scharff 2002). Drossman and colleagues (1999), reviewing the treatment literature for IBS, indicated that of nine studies with follow-up data of at least 9 months, eight demonstrate superiority of psychological treatment to conventional medical treatment. Overall, Blanchard and Scharff (2002) suggest that hypnotherapy and cognitive therapy have the strongest support as psychological interventions for IBS. Each has at least three separate randomized controlled trials supporting its efficacy in reducing symptomatology and improving quality of life. While hypnosis may not be a feasible option for most practicing physicians, audiotapes employing hypnotic induction techniques, a less time-intensive alternative, may provide benefits as well (Forbes et al. 2000). Cognitive-behavioral therapies are widely used in management of a variety of chronic pain syndromes (see Waters et al., this volume), and they show promise in IBS as well. For example, the addition of multicomponent behavioral therapy (including information and training in progressive muscle relaxation, coping strategies, and problem-solving) to standard treatment resulted in greater reductions of IBS symptoms and larger increases in quality of life, while rectovisceral perception remained unchanged (Heymann-Monnikes et al. 2000). Group cognitive-behavioral therapy reduced pain and GI symptoms, increased the use of successful coping strategies, and decreased avoidance behavior among IBS patients followed for a period of up to 4 years (van Dulmen et al. 1996). Both progressive muscle relaxation training (Blanchard et al. 1993) and cognitive therapy (Greene and Blanchard 1994) reduced GI symptoms more than self-help control interventions. Group psychotherapy and low-dose amitriptyline (25 mg) effected similar improvements in GI symptoms, though only drug treatment increased rectal pain thresholds (Bouin et al. 2002).

Changes in psychological distress appear to parallel changes in GI symptoms during treatment. IBS patients successfully treated with cognitive-behavioral therapy show significant reductions in symptoms of depression and anxiety, whereas those with no reductions in GI symptoms do not (Blanchard and Scharff 2002). In addition, several studies suggest that direct pharmacological treatment of comorbid Axis I psychiatric disorders in IBS patients improves GI symptoms concurrently with psychiatric symptoms (Lydiard and Falsetti 1999). Moreover, the benefits of psychologically based therapies may increase over time. Following a cognitive therapy treatment (Greene and Blanchard 1994), improvements in GI symptoms were maintained and even increased at 3-month follow-up (Payne and Blanchard 1995). Significant additional reductions in pain and bloating were noted at 3- to 12-month follow-up (Keefer and Blanchard 2002). Patients also showed significant reductions in depression and anxiety (Payne and Blanchard 1995), and GI symptom reductions were associated with increases in positive automatic thoughts and decreases in negative ones (Greene and Blanchard 1994).

PSYCHOLOGICAL FACTORS PREDICTING
TREATMENT OUTCOME FOR IBS

The literature is not extensive on psychosocial factors as predictors of treatment outcomes in IBS. Tanum and Malt (2000) studied 26 IBS patients treated with the tetracyclic antidepressant mianserin and noted that higher pretreatment levels of neuroticism, negativism, and depressive personality style predicted less treatment-associated improvement in pain. These personality factors were stronger predictors of treatment outcome than serotonergic sensitivity. Blanchard and colleagues (1988) found that the single best predictor of poor treatment outcome was trait anxiety. Similarly, the pretreatment presence of a diagnosable Axis I psychiatric disorder was associated with more modest improvement from cognitive and behavioral treatment among 90 IBS patients (Blanchard et al. 1992). Other psychological factors, including personality variables assessed by the Minnesota Multiphasic Personality Inventory, Beck Depression Inventory scores, and anxiety scores, failed to predict outcome. In Guthrie and colleagues' (1993) study of psychotherapy for treatment of IBS, subjects who improved with treatment, relative to those who did not improve or worsened, had greater social support, fewer psychiatric symptoms, and less worry about their illness. Similar findings have been reported in other conditions such as low back pain (Linton 2000; Pincus et al. 2002), in which psychological factors predict the onset and course of the pain condition. Thus, IBS studies emphasizing the potential importance of psychological and psychiatric variables in formulating treatment and predicting treatment success appear to parallel findings for other chronic pain syndromes.

SUMMARY

IBS is a highly prevalent functional GI disorder with many costly and deleterious sequelae. A variety of psychosocial factors, including depression, anxiety, life stress, somatization, hypervigilance, coping style, learning history, and abuse history, are involved in the onset, course, and treatment of IBS. Studies have documented relationships between these factors and such IBS-related variables as reported GI symptomatology, treatment-seeking behavior, health care utilization, pain sensitivity, and GI function. Given these relationships, it is not surprising that interest in psychologically based treatments for IBS appears to be growing. Indeed, the efficacy of both hypnosis and cognitive therapy has been demonstrated in multiple randomized, controlled trials. Furthermore, documented relationships between baseline psychological factors and treatment outcome in several IBS studies suggest that the addition of psychological components to other elements of IBS management may improve treatment effectiveness and enhance quality of life for those with IBS.

CHRONIC PELVIC PAIN

Almost exclusively, articles focusing on CPP open by commenting on the frequency of the problem followed by the challenge it presents to physicians, patients, and their families. Indeed, CPP can be considered a predominant issue in women's health, affecting approximately one in seven U.S. women (Mathias et al. 1996). Nevertheless, remarkably little is known about its pathophysiology or effective treatments (Moore and Kennedy 2000). Although CPP has been mentioned in men (Hakenberg and Wirth 2002), the following review will focus exclusively on women to reflect the preponderance of the literature.

OVERVIEW

The most commonly utilized definition of CPP—recurrent or constant pain in the lower abdominal region that has lasted for at least 6 months—does not consider etiology (Zondervan and Barlow 2000). More specifically, the International Association for the Study of Pain has provided the following delineated definition for CPP without obvious pathology (CPPWOP): "Chronic or recurrent pelvic pain that apparently has a gynecological origin but for which no definite lesion or cause is found" (Merskey and Bogduk 1994, p. 170). Other researchers have used terms such as "pelvalgia" and "pelvic pain syndrome" (Fry et al. 1997) synonymously with CPPWOP. However, such terms have been criticized for making an artificial dichotomy between organic and functional pain (Grace 2000) and for assuming that the underlying pathology of CPP can be known with certainty (Zondervan and Barlow 2000). Thus, studies examining psychological aspects of CPP will be reviewed independently of etiology.

Epidemiological studies examining CPP indicate a community prevalence of 15% in randomly selected, representatively sampled women aged 18–50 years (Mathias et al. 1996). In a study querying women in gynecologists' offices, 39% of women aged 18–45 years endorsed CPP, with 20% of women reporting CPP of at least 1 year's duration and greater prevalence noted in younger women (aged 26–30 years) and African-Americans (Jamieson and Steege 1996). Other studies have projected CPP's 3-month prevalence to be 24% (Zondervan et al. 2001), and the lifetime occurrence has been estimated at 33% (Walker et al. 1991). In the United Kingdom, annual prevalence in primary care is considered comparable to asthma and back pain (Zondervan et al. 1999). Other studies suggest that CPP accounts for 10–15% of new referrals to gynecologists and is the indication for 25–35% of laparoscopies and for 10–15% of hysterectomies performed in the United States (Savidge and Slade 1997; Reiter 1998). In the mid-1990s, total annual direct costs due to CPP in the United States were estimated to be $2.8 billion (Mathias et al. 1996).

The etiology of CPP is quite variable and can include gynecological, urinary, musculoskeletal, neuropathic, and gastrointestinal factors (McQuay et al. 1996). Quite commonly (in 61% of cases), the cause of CPP is unknown (Mathias et al. 1996). There is often little correlation between diagnostic signs and symptoms, and as a result, women with CPP are often suspected of having a psychological etiology to their illness (Grace 2000). More commonly, women report feeling demoralized, dismissed, and frustrated due to multiple physician visits, diagnostic studies, and surgical exploration without significant pain reduction or a definitive diagnosis (McDonald 1993). Perhaps this dissatisfaction contributes to the large number of studies examining psychological factors in CPP.

PSYCHOLOGICAL AND PSYCHIATRIC COMORBIDITY IN CPP

Failure to identify clear organic precipitants to CPP has led to an extensive literature about the influence of psychological factors, which has demonstrated a number of consistent findings (Fry et al. 1997; Savidge and Slade 1997; McGowan et al. 1998). For example, the lifetime prevalence of major depression in women with CPP has been reported at 64% compared to 17% of gynecological controls (women consulting gynecologists for reasons other than CPP), and a current incidence of depression for 28% of CPP patients versus 3% of gynecological controls (Harrop-Griffiths et al. 1988). Further, 73% of women with idiopathic CPP met diagnostic criteria for somatoform pain disorder in a study using structured interviews (Ehlert et al. 1999). Of note, somatoform pain disorder indicates that psychological factors (with or without a medical condition) play a major role in the onset, severity, exacerbation, and maintenance of pain.

In addition to rates of psychiatric comorbidity, numerous other studies have examined negative emotions in CPP. Women both with and without obvious pathology to their CPP had higher scores on the Beck Depression Inventory than did gynecological patients presenting for sterilization or women being treated for infertility (Waller and Shaw 1995). However, all groups were equivalent on a measure of state and trait anxiety. Other investigators demonstrated that women with abdominal pelvic pain reported significantly greater anxiety, depression, hostility, and somatic symptoms compared to gynecological controls (Slocumb et al. 1989). Despite these high rates of comorbidity, other data indicate that the CPP group is heterogeneous. For example, 56% of women with CPP scored within normal limits on measures of depression and anxiety (Slocumb et al. 1989).

Researchers have also examined, with mixed results, whether there are psychiatric and psychological factors that distinguish women with pelvic pain identified as having "organic disorders" versus those for whom a cause cannot be identified. A recent meta-analysis of 22 studies found no significant differences between the two groups on measures of depression, anxiety, neuroticism, and psychopathology (McGowan et al. 1998; Bush et al. 1999). This meta-analysis concluded that studies consistently find significant differences on these same domains when compared to pain-free controls but that these differences are most likely due to the presence of chronic pain rather than something specific to CPP (McGowan et al. 1998).

Only a handful of studies have examined pelvic pain patients in comparison to other patients with painful conditions, rather than pain-free gynecological controls. In a comparison of women with painful endometriosis to those with unexplained CPP, no differences were found in mood symptoms or personality characteristics, although women with endometriosis reported greater pain severity (Peveler et al. 1996). Similarly, Fry et al. (1997) compared pelvic pain patients with and without pelvic venous congestion, a condition characterized by engorged pelvic veins and impaired venous blood flow in the pelvic region. A higher incidence of childhood sexual abuse, more paternal overprotection, and more inwardly directed hostility were noted among those with pelvic venous congestion. No differences were found on measures of self-esteem, anxiety, depression, or psychosomatic symptomatology.

What is even less clear is whether women with pelvic pain are somehow different from other patients with other chronically painful conditions because of the site of their pain complaints. Location of pain may be a significant predictor for appraisals of pain, affective response, and disclosure of pain complaints (Wesselmann et al. 1997). In one study, subjects asked to imagine genital pain appraised themselves as being more ill and more likely to be experiencing an emergency than when asked to imagine chest, stomach, head, or mouth pain (Klonoff et al. 1993). Further, subjects believed that they would experience greater irritability with pain in the genitals and head than in other areas, and that they would be more worried, depressed, and embarrassed by pain in the genitals than in all other areas. Although this was an analogue study (i.e., subjects only imagined being in pain), these results suggest that previous data examining chronic pain in various locations may not be generalizable to urogenital pain disorders.

In order to better illuminate the influence of body site on the experience of chronic pain, recent studies have compared women with CPP to women with vulvar vestibulitis. Women with vulvar vestibulitis had lower scores on the McGill Pain Questionnaire (Haefner et al. 2000), less depression and emotional instability (Bodden-Heidrich et al. 1999), and less frequent abuse histories, diagnoses of depression, work absences, and somatic complaints (Reed et al. 2000). Our research group recently examined women with pelvic pain in comparison to men with urogenital pain complaints (L.J. Heinberg et al., unpublished manuscript). In addition, women and men with low back pain were included in order to assess the role of gender and site of pain on depression and disability related to pain and coping. It was hypothesized that patients with urogenital pain complaints would show greater depression than patients with low back pain. It was further hypothesized that this main effect of site would be explained by an interaction between site and gender. Specifically, women with CPP were expected to report the greatest levels of depression. Similar main effects and interactions were hypothesized for pain-related disability, with CPP women expected to report the highest levels of disability. However, no gender effects were found, and few site by gender interactions were significant. When compared to appropriate controls, women with CPP did not score higher on a measure of depression, did not report more pain-related disability, and did not exhibit unique or different coping strategies. Although pain severity ratings were higher in women with CPP as compared to men with chronic urogenital pain, their ratings were not significantly different from women or men with low back pain. These more recent studies suggest that selection of appropriate comparison groups are important to further understand psychological risk factors and sequelae in women with CPP.

ASSOCIATION OF PSYCHOLOGICAL FACTORS WITH CPP

Various nonmedical risk factors for CPP have been identified in the literature. One of the most frequently investigated, a history of abuse, will be reviewed in the next section. Other risk factors include the number of past sexual partners (Reed et al. 2000; Reiter and Gambone 1990), a history of nongynecological surgery (Reiter and Gambone 1990), and lower educational achievement (Roth et al. 2001).

As is the case in many chronic pain conditions, women with CPP demonstrate diminished quality of life, with a significant relationship between pain severity and functioning (Rannestad et al. 2000; Stones et al. 2000). Studies suggest that women with endometriosis as the cause for their CPP describe poorer health, greater interference in activities, and greater pain during intercourse after adjusting for age, education, and income compared to women with no diagnosis or other gynecological and nongynecological complaints (Mathias et al. 1996). Although women with CPP describe much of the pain-related interference reviewed in other chapters, pain during intercourse, and the resulting sexual interference, appear to be a particularly significant problem in this population. Eighty-eight percent of CPP respondents described having pain during or after intercourse some, most, or all of the time in the past month (Mathias et al. 1996). Reports of sexual interference were similar in women with CPP and in women with vulvodynia and were significantly greater than in normal controls (Reed et al. 2000) and in women presenting for sterility or infertility (Waller and Shaw 1995). However, studies have yet to fully examine the impact of this sexual interference, particularly in relationship to marital relationships, or whether psychological interventions focusing on pain management, interpersonal relationships, or sex therapy may be beneficial for this population.

Sexual and physical abuse and chronic pelvic pain. It has been hypothesized that a history of abuse may be etiological to women's complaints of both pelvic pain and psychiatric morbidity (Ehlert et al. 1999). However, a comprehensive review of the literature linking sexual abuse to CPP concluded that the available data do not permit clear conclusions regarding the specificity of childhood sexual abuse as a risk factor for CPP (Fry et al. 1997). Methodological limitations in existing studies include retrospective cross-sectional designs in which physical complaints were recorded at the same time as abuse history, variability in the recall of sexual contact across individuals, the fact that sexual abuse may reflect a disordered childhood environment, and methods used to identify "cases" by using nonstandardized screening questions or lacking an operational definition of abuse (Walker and Stenchever 1993). Although fewer studies with poorer methodologies have been completed in CPP as compared to IBS, a similar pattern is seen across most studies. Patients with CPP do appear to show elevated rates of sexual and physical abuse histories (Jacobsen et al. 1990; Walker et al. 1992, 1995; Walker and Stenchever 1993; M.K. Walling et al., unpublished manuscript). In most controlled studies, the prevalence of childhood sexual victimization of patients with CPP has been rated at around 50–60%, as compared to 20–30% for gynecological or pain controls (Walker et al. 1988; Walker and Stenchever 1993; Waller et al. 1993; Fry et al. 1997; Reed et al. 2000). Women with pelvic pain reported higher lifetime rates of major sexual abuse—involving penetration or other genital or anal contact—than did women who experienced chronic headaches or were pain-free (Walling et al. 1994a), and the rate of sexual abuse prior to the 15th birthday was higher in CPP patients as compared to low back pain patients or healthy controls

(Lampe et al. 2000). Lifetime rates of physical abuse also were elevated in CPP patients as compared to pain-free controls (Walling et al. 1994b; Lampe et al. 2000), although an older study found a higher prevalence of physical abuse in general chronic pain patients than in CPP patients (Jacobsen et al. 1990). In addition to these rates of abuse, recent data suggest that histories of emotional neglect in childhood may also be more common in CPP patients as compared to low back pain patients and pain-free controls (Lampe et al. 2000). The elevated rates of abuse, particularly childhood sexual abuse, increase the likelihood that a CPP patient will experience psychiatric comorbidity and negative emotions such as depression, anxiety, and somatization (Walling et al. 1994a).

Pain sensitivity. Unlike the situation for IBS, few laboratory studies have examined psychological aspects of pain sensitivity in CPP. Two studies in non-CPP gynecological populations may be informative. Recently, Granot and colleagues (2001) examined pain perception in women with dysmenorrhea compared to nondysmenorrheic women across the menstrual cycle. They found significant differences between the two groups at four time-points in the menstrual cycle. Dysmenorrheic women were more anxious, had longer latencies of pain-evoked potentials, and had higher estimations of suprathreshold pain. The authors concluded that dysmenorrhea might be due to enhanced pain perceptions as well as organ involvement. Similar findings were demonstrated in women with vulvar vestibulitis compared to healthy controls (Granot et al. 2002; Pukall et al. 2002). Women with vulvar vestibulitis had greater anxiety, lower pain thresholds, lower unpleasantness thresholds, higher estimations of suprathreshold pain, higher increases in blood pressure during pain stimuli (Granot et al. 2002), and systemic hypersensitivity to tactile and pain stimuli (Pukall et al. 2002). Similar studies should be conducted in CPP populations to evaluate possible treatments focusing on lowering generalized pain perception and anxiety.

PSYCHOLOGICAL AND PSYCHIATRIC TREATMENTS

The CPP literature has been criticized for its dearth of methodologically sound, randomized, controlled treatment trials (Howard 2000; Stones et al. 2000). Indeed, although concurrent psychological assessment and treatment are frequently recommended for CPP (Ling and Slocumb 1993; Grace 1998; Reiter 1998; Price and Blake 1999; Moore and Kennedy 2000), very few studies have examined the efficacy of psychological or psychiatric interventions in comparison to a control group.

Tricyclic antidepressants (TCAs) have been repeatedly shown in other pain disorders to improve pain tolerance, restore normal sleep, and reduce depressive symptoms (McQuay et al. 1995, Salerno et al. 2002). Open-label trials (Walker et al. 1991) and clinical reviews (Reiter 1998) suggest that the use of TCAs may be helpful for women with CPP, although the dropout rate tends to be high. Randomized, double-blind trials of TCAs as a treatment for CPP have yet to be completed. A more recent, small ($n = 23$), randomized, double-blind crossover trial of sertraline (Harel et al. 1995) revealed no significant improvement in pain or disability between women with CPP receiving sertraline versus placebo (Engel et al. 1998). Larger clinical trials examining the efficacy of antidepressants in this population are clearly needed. Biofeedback has shown impressive results for women with vulvodynia, with an 83% reduction in pain intensity, allowing 78% of participants to resume sexual intercourse (Glazer et al. 1995), and improvements in psychological adjustment (Bergeron et al. 2001). Studies should examine whether biofeedback is also helpful for women with CPP.

The multidisciplinary care protocol that consistently been successful in treating other chronic pain conditions (Flor et al. 1992; Serrao et al. 1992) has been adapted for the treatment of CPP. This approach was first piloted by Rapkin and Kames (1987) and has since proven superior to standard care in a randomized clinical trial. Peters et al. (1991) demonstrated that significantly more women randomized to receive an integrated approach of combined medical evaluation, psychological treatment, and physical therapy improved with regard to general pain, disturbance in daily activities, and symptoms associated with CPP compared to those receiving standard care. Surprisingly, however, randomized clinical trials have not continued to examine psychological interventions for CPP or its combination with other treatment modalities.

SUMMARY

Like IBS, CPP is highly prevalent, costly, and devastating, with often elusive etiologies and cures. CPP has long been associated clinically with psychiatric comorbidity, a history of sexual abuse, and severe psychological sequelae. Although carefully controlled studies do seem to indicate a higher prevalence of physical and sexual abuse history, more recent studies comparing women with CPP to appropriate control groups indicate that those with known versus unknown etiologies do not differ with regard to psychological functioning, and that women with CPP are analogous to women with other chronic pain conditions with regard to psychiatric comorbidity and psychosocial adjustment. Unlike the IBS literature, fewer studies have examined the efficacy of psychological interventions for women with CPP. Although preliminary work and randomized controlled studies in similar populations are promising, future work must examine the efficacy of multidisciplinary care, psychological intervention, and biofeedback in comparison to a control group.

REFERENCES

Accarino AM, Azpiroz F, Malagelada JR. Attention and distraction: effects on gut perception. *Gastroenterology* 1997; 113:415–422.

Bennett EJ, Tennant CC, Piesse C, Badcock CA, Kellow JE. Level of chronic life stress predicts clinical outcome in irritable bowel syndrome. *Gut* 1998; 43:256–261.

Bergeron S, Binik YM, Khalife S, et al. A randomized comparison of group cognitive-behavioral therapy, surface electromyographic biofeedback, and vestibulectomy in the treatment of dyspareunia resulting from vulvar vestibulitis. *Pain* 2001; 91:297–306.

Blanchard EB, Scharff L. Psychosocial aspects of assessment and treatment of irritable bowel syndrome in adults and recurrent abdominal pain in children. *J Consult Clin Psychol* 2002; 70:725–738.

Blanchard EB, Schwarz SP, Neff DF, Gerardi MA. Prediction of outcome from the self-regulatory treatment of irritable bowel syndrome. *Behav Res Ther* 1988; 26:187–190.

Blanchard EB, Scharff L, Payne A, et al. Prediction of outcome from cognitive-behavioral treatment of irritable bowel syndrome. *Behav Res Ther* 1992; 30:647–650.

Blanchard EB, Greene B, Scharff L, Schwarz-McMorris SP. Relaxation training as a treatment for irritable bowel syndrome. *Biofeedback Self Regul* 1993; 18:125–132.

Blomhoff S, Jacobsen MB, Spetalen S, Dahm A, Malt UF. Perceptual hyperreactivity to auditory stimuli in patients with irritable bowel syndrome. *Scand J Gastroenterol* 2000; 35:583–589.

Bodden-Heidrich R, Kuppers V, Beckmann MW, et al. Psychosomatic aspects of vulvodynia: comparison with the chronic pelvic pain syndrome. *J Reprod Med* 1999; 44:411–416.

Bouin M, Plourde V, Boivin M, Riberdy M, Lupien F. Rectal distention testing in patients with irritable bowel syndrome: sensitivity, specificity, and predictive values of pain sensory thresholds. *Gastroenterology* 2002; 122:1771–1777.

Burke P, Elliott M, Fleissner R. Irritable bowel syndrome and recurrent abdominal pain: a comparative review. *Psychosomatics* 1999; 40:277–285.

Bush EG, Rye MS, Brant CR, et al. Religious coping with chronic pain. *Appl Psychophysiol Biofeedback* 1999; 24:249–260.

Camilleri M. Management of the irritable bowel syndrome. *Gastroenterology* 2001; 120:652–668.

Campbell J, Jones AS, Dienemann J, Kub J, Schollenberger J. Intimate partner violence and physical health consequences. *Arch Intern Med* 2002; 162:1157–1163.

Cheng C, Hui W, Lam S. Perceptual style and behavioral pattern of individuals with functional GI disorders. *Health Psychol* 2000; 19:146–154.

Creed F. The relationship between psychosocial parameters and outcome in irritable bowel syndrome. *Am J Med* 1999; 107:74S–80S.

Creed F, Ratcliffe J, Fernandez L, et al. Health-related quality of life and health care costs in severe, refractory irritable bowel syndrome. *Ann Intern Med* 2001; 134:860–868.

Dancey CP, Taghavi M, Fox RJ. The relationship between daily stress and symptoms of irritable bowel: a time-series approach. *J Psychosom Res* 1998; 44:537–545.

Davis G, Buchsbaum M, Bunney W. Naloxone decreases diurnal variation in pain sensitivity and somatosensory evoked potentials. *Life Sci* 1978; 23:1449–1460.

Delvaux M, Denis P, Allemand H. Sexual abuse is more frequently reported by IBS patients than by patients with organic digestive diseases or controls: results of a multicentre inquiry. French Club of Digestive Motility. *Eur J Gastroenterol Hepatol* 1997; 9:345–352.

Di Lorenzo C, Youssef NN, Sigurdsson L, et al. Visceral hyperalgesia in children with functional abdominal pain. *J Pediatr* 2001; 139:838–843.

Drossman DA. Do psychosocial factors define symptom severity and patient status in irritable bowel syndrome? *Am J Med* 1999a; 107:41S–50S.

Drossman DA. The functional gastrointestinal disorders and the Rome II process. *Gut* 1999b; 45(Suppl 2):II1–II5.

Drossman DA, McKee DC, Sandler RS, Mitchell CM, Cramer EM. Psychosocial factors in the irritable bowel syndrome: a multivariate study of patients and nonpatients with irritable bowel syndrome. *Gastroenterology* 1988; 95:701–708.

Drossman DA, Creed FH, Olden KW, Svedlund J, Toner BB. Psychosocial aspects of the functional gastrointestinal disorders. *Gut* 1999; 45(Suppl 2):II25–II30.

Drossman DA, Lesserman J, Li Z. Effects of coping on health outcomes among women with GI disorders. *Psychosom Med* 2000a; 62:309–317.

Drossman DA, Whitehead WE, Toner BB. What determines severity among patients with painful functional bowel disorders? *Am J Gastroenterol* 2000b; 95:974–980.

Ehlert U, Heim C, Hellhammer DH. Chronic pelvic pain as a somatoform disorder. *Psychother Psychosom* 1999; 68:87–94.

Engel CC Jr, Walker EA, Engel AL, Bullis J, Armstrong A. A randomized, double-blind crossover trial of sertraline in women with chronic pelvic pain. *J Psychosom Res* 1998; 44:203–207.

Flor H, Fydrich T, Turk DC. Efficacy of multidisciplinary pain treatment centers: a meta-analytic review. *Pain* 1992; 49:221–230.

Forbes A, MacAuley S, Chiotakakou-Faliakou E. Hypnotherapy and therapeutic audiotape: effective in previously unsuccessfully treated irritable bowel syndrome? *Int J Colorectal Dis* 2000; 15:328–334.

Fowlie S, Eastwood MA, Prescott R. Irritable bowel syndrome: assessment of psychological disturbance and its influence on the response to fibre supplementation. *J Psychosom Res* 1992; 36:175–180.

Fry RP, Beard RW, Crisp AH, McGuigan S. Sociopsychological factors in women with chronic pelvic pain with and without pelvic venous congestion. *J Psychosom Res* 1997; 42:1–15, 71–85.

Gibbs-Gallagher N, Palsson OS, Levy RL, et al. Selective recall of gastrointestinal-sensation words: evidence for a cognitive-behavioral contribution to irritable bowel syndrome. *Am J Gastroenterol* 2001; 96:1133–1138.

Glazer HI, Rodke G, Swencionis C, Hertz R, Young AW. Treatment of vulvar vestibulitis syndrome with electromyographic biofeedback of pelvic floor musculature. *J Reprod Med* 1995; 40:283–290.

Grace VM. Mind/body dualism in medicine: the case of chronic pelvic pain without organic pathology: a critical review of the literature. *Int J Health Serv* 1998; 28:127–151.

Grace VM. Pitfalls of the medical paradigm in chronic pelvic pain. *Baillieres Best Pract Res Clin Obstet Gynaecol* 2000; 14:525–539.

Gralnek IM, Hays RD, Kilbourne A, Naliboff B, Mayer EA. The impact of irritable bowel syndrome on health-related quality of life. *Gastroenterology* 2000; 119:654–660.

Granot M, Yarnitsky D, Itskovitz-Eldor J, et al. Pain perception in women with dysmenorrhea. *Obstet Gynecol* 2001; 98:407–411.

Granot M, Friedman M, Yarnitsky D, Zimmer EZ. Enhancement of the perception of systemic pain in women with vulvar vestibulitis. *BJOG* 2002; 109:863–866.

Greene B, Blanchard EB. Cognitive therapy for irritable bowel syndrome. *J Consult Clin Psychol* 1994; 62:576–582.

Guthrie E, Creed FH, Whorwell PJ. Outpatients with IBS: a comparison of first time and chronic attenders. *Gut* 1992; 33:361–363.

Guthrie E, Creed F, Dawson D, Tomenson B. A randomised controlled trial of psychotherapy in patients with refractory irritable bowel syndrome. *Br J Psychiatry* 1993; 163:315–321.

Gwee KA, Graham JC, McKendrick MW, Collins SM, Marshall JS. Psychometric scores and persistence of irritable bowel after infectious diarrhoea. *Lancet* 1996; 347:150–153.

Haefner HK, Khoshnevisan MH, Bachman JE, et al. Use of the McGill Pain Questionnaire to compare women with vulvar pain, pelvic pain and headaches. *J Reprod Med* 2000; 45:665–671.

Hakenberg OW, Wirth MP. Chronic pelvic pain in men. *Urol Int* 2002; 68:138–143.

Harel Z, Biro FM, Tedford WL. Effects of long term treatment with sertraline (Zoloft) simulating hypothyroidism in an adolescent. *J Adolesc Health* 1995; 16:232–234.

Harrop-Griffiths J, Katon W, Walker E, et al. The association between chronic pelvic pain, psychiatric diagnoses, and childhood sexual abuse. *Obstet Gynecol* 1988; 71:589–594.

Heymann-Monnikes I, Arnold R, Florin I, et al. The combination of medical treatment plus multicomponent behavioral therapy is superior to medical treatment alone in the therapy of irritable bowel syndrome. *Am J Gastroenterol* 2000; 95:981–994.

Hobbis IC, Turpin G, Read NW. A re-examination of the relationship between abuse experience and functional bowel disorders. *Scand J Gastroenterol* 2002; 37:423–430.

Howard FM. An evidence-based medicine approach to the treatment of endometriosis-associated chronic pelvic pain: placebo-controlled studies. *J Am Assoc Gynecol Laparosc* 2000; 7:477–488.

Jacobsen PB, Manne SL, Gorfinkle K, et al. Analysis of child and parent behavior during painful medical procedures. *Health Psychol* 1990; 9:559–576.

Jamieson DJ, Steege JF. The prevalence of dysmenorrhea, dyspareunia, pelvic pain, and irritable bowel syndrome in primary care practices. *Prim Care* 1996; 87:55–58.

Keefer L, Blanchard EB. A one year follow-up of relaxation response meditation as a treatment for irritable bowel syndrome. *Behav Res Ther* 2002; 40:541–546.

Klonoff EA, Landrine H, Brown M. Appraisal and response to pain may be a function of its bodily location. *J Psychosom Res* 1993; 37:661–670.

Lampe A, Solder E, Ennemoser A, et al. Chronic pelvic pain and previous sexual abuse. *Obstet Gynecol* 2000; 96:929–933.

Leserman J, Drossman DA, Li Z, et al. Sexual and physical abuse history in gastroenterology practice: how types of abuse impact health status. *Psychosom Med* 1996; 58:4–15.

Leserman J, Li Z, Drossman DA. How multiple types of stressors impact on health. *Psychosom Med* 1998; 60:175–181.

Levy RL, Whitehead WE, Von Korff MR, Feld AD. Intergenerational transmission of gastrointestinal illness behavior. *Am J Gastroenterol* 2000; 95:451–456.

Ling FW, Slocumb JC. Use of trigger point injections in chronic pelvic pain. *Obstet Gynecol Clin North Am* 1993; 20:809–815.

Linton SJ. A review of psychological risk factors in back and neck pain. *Spine* 2000; 25:1148–1156.

Luscombe FA. Health-related quality of life and associated psychosocial factors in irritable bowel syndrome: a review. *Qual Life Res* 2000; 9:161–176.

Lydiard RB, Falsetti SA. Experience with anxiety and depression treatment studies: implications for designing irritable bowel syndrome clinical trials. *Am J Med* 1999; 107:65S–73S.

Masheb RM, Nash JM, Brondolo E, Kerns RD. Vulvodynia: an introduction and critical review of a chronic pain condition. *Pain* 2000; 86:3–10.

Mathias SD, Kuppermann M, Liberman RF, et al. Chronic pelvic pain: prevalence, health-related quality of life, and economic correlates. *Obstet Gynecol* 1996; 87:321–327.

Mayer EA. Spinal and supraspinal modulation of visceral sensation. *Gut* 2000a; 47(Suppl 4):69–72.

Mayer EA. The neurobiology of stress and gastrointestinal disease. *Gut* 2000b; 47:861–869.

Mayer EA, Naliboff BD, Chang L, Coutinho SV, V. Stress and irritable bowel syndrome. *Am J Physiol Gastrointest Liver Physiol* 2001; 280:G519–G524.

McDonald JS. Management of chronic pelvic pain. *Obstet Gynecol Clin North Am* 1993; 20:817–838.

McGowan L, Clark-Carter DD, Pitts MK. Chronic pelvic pain: a meta-analytic review. *Psychol Health* 1998; 13:937–951.

McQuay H, Carroll D, Jadad AR, Wiffen P, Moore A. Anticonvulsant drugs for management of pain: a systematic review. *BMJ* 1995; 311:1047–1052.

McQuay HJ, Tramer M, Nye BA, et al. A systematic review of antidepressants in neuropathic pain. *Pain* 1996; 68:217–227.

Merskey H, Bogduk N. *Classification of Chronic Pain: Descriptions of Chronic Pain Syndromes and Definitions of Pain Terms,* 2nd ed. Seattle: IASP Press, 1994.

Moore J, Kennedy S. Causes of chronic pelvic pain. *Baillieres Best Pract Res Clin Obstet Gynaecol* 2000; 14:389–402.

Payne A, Blanchard EB. A controlled comparison of cognitive therapy and self-help support groups in the treatment of irritable bowel syndrome. *J Consult Clin Psychol* 1995; 63:779–786.

Peters AAW, van Dorst E, Jellis B, et al. A randomized clinical trial to compare two different approaches in women with chronic pelvic pain. *Obstet Gynecol* 1991; 77:740–744.

Peveler R, Edwards J, Daddow J, Thomas E. Psychosocial factors and chronic pelvic pain: a comparison of women with endometriosis and with unexplained pain. *J Psychosom Res* 1996; 40(3):305–315.

Pincus T, Vlaeyen JW, Kendall NA, et al. Cognitive-behavioral therapy and psychosocial factors in low back pain: directions for the future. *Spine* 2002; 27:E133–E138.

Price JR, Blake F. Chronic pelvic pain: the assessment as therapy. *J Psychosom Res* 1999; 46:7–14.

Pukall CF, Binik YM, Khalife S, Amsel R, Abbott FV. Vestibular tactile and pain thresholds in women with vulvar vestibulitis syndrome. *Pain* 2002; 96:163–175.

Rannestad T, Eikeland OJ, Helland H, Qvarnstrom U. Quality of life, pain, and psychological well-being in women suffering from gynecological disorders. *J Womens Health Gend Based Med* 2000; 9:897–903.

Raphael KG, Widom CS, Lange G. Childhood victimization and pain in adulthood: a prospective investigation. *Pain* 2001; 92:283–293.

Rapkin AJ, Kames LD. The pain management approach to chronic pelvic pain. *J Reprod Med* 1987; 32:323–327.

Reed BD, Haefner HK, Punch MR, et al. Psychosocial and sexual functioning in women with vulvodynia and chronic pelvic pain: a comparative evaluation. *J Reprod Med* 2000; 45:624–632.

Reilly J, Baker GA, Rhodes J, Salmon P. The association of sexual and physical abuse with somatization: characteristics of patients presenting with irritable bowel syndrome and non-epileptic attack disorder. *Psychol Med* 1999; 29:399–406.

Reiter RC. Evidence-based management of chronic pelvic pain. *Clin Obstet Gynecol* 1998; 41:422–435.

Reiter RC, Gambone JC. Demographic and historic variables in women with idiopathic chronic pelvic pain. *Obstet Gynecol* 1990; 75:428–432.

Ringel Y, Sperber AD, Drossman DA. Irritable bowel syndrome. *Annu Rev Med* 2001; 52:319–338.

Roth RS, Punch MR, Bachman JE. Educational achievement and pain disability among women with chronic pelvic pain. *J Psychosom Res* 2001; 51:563–569.

Salerno SM, Browning R, Jackson JL. The effect of antidepressant treatment on chronic back pain: a meta-analysis. *Arch Intern Med* 2002; 162:19–24.

Savidge CJ, Slade P. Psychological aspects of chronic pelvic pain. *J Psychosom Res* 1997; 42:433–444.

Scarinci IC, McDonald-Haile J, Bradley LA, Richter JE. Altered pain perception and psychosocial features among women with gastrointestinal disorders and history of abuse: a preliminary model. *Am J Med* 1994; 97:108–118.

Serrao JM, Marks RL, Morley SJ, Goodchild CS. Intrathecal midazolam for the treatment of chronic mechanical low back pain: a controlled comparison with epidural steroid in a pilot study. *Pain* 1992; 48:5–12.

Slocumb JC, Kellner R, Rosenfeld RC, Pathak D. Anxiety and depression in patients with the abdominal pelvic pain syndrome. *Gen Hosp Psychiatry* 1989; 11:48–53.

Stones RW, Selfe SA, Fransman S, Horn SA. Psychosocial and economic impact of chronic pelvic pain. *Baillieres Best Pract Res Clin Obstet Gynaecol* 2000; 14 :415–431.

Talley NJ, Fett SL, Zinsmeister AR, Melton III LJ. Gastrointestinal tract symptoms and self-reported abuse: a population-based study. *Gastroenterology* 1994; 107:1040–1049.

Talley NJ, Fett SL, Zinsmeister AR. Self-reported abuse and gastrointestinal disease in outpatients: association with irritable bowel-type symptoms. *Am J Gastroenterol* 1995; 90:366–371.

Tanum L, Malt UF. Personality traits predict treatment outcome with an antidepressant in patients with functional gastrointestinal disorder. *Scand J Gastroenterol* 2000; 35:935–941.

Tanum L, Malt UF. Personality and physical symptoms in nonpsychiatric patients with functional gastrointestinal disorder. *J Psychosom Res* 2001; 50:139–146.

Trikas P, Vlachonikolis I, Fragkiadakis N. Core mental state in IBS. *Psychosom Med* 1999; 61:781–788.

van Dulmen AM, Fennis JF, Bleijenberg G. Cognitive-behavioral group therapy for irritable bowel syndrome: effects and long-term follow-up. *Psychosom Med* 1996; 58:508–514.

Verne GN, Robinson ME, Price DD. Hypersensitivity to visceral and cutaneous pain in the irritable bowel syndrome. *Pain* 2001; 93:7–14.

Walker EA, Stenchever MA. Sexual victimization and chronic pelvic pain. *Obstet Gynecol Clin North Am* 1993; 20:795–807.

Walker E, Katon W, Harrop-Griffiths J, et al. Relationship of chronic pelvic pain to psychiatric diagnoses and childhood sexual abuse. *Am J Psychiatry* 1988; 145:75–80.

Walker EA, Roy-Byrne PP, Katon WJ, Jemelka R. An open trial of nortriptyline in women with chronic pelvic pain. *Int J Psychiatry Med* 1991; 21:245–252.

Walker EA, Katon WJ, Neraas K, Jemelka RP, Massoth D. Dissociation in women with chronic pelvic pain. *Am J Psychiatry* 1992; 149:534–537.

Walker EA, Katon WJ, Hansom J, et al. Psychiatric diagnoses and sexual victimization in women with chronic pelvic pain. *Psychosomatics* 1995; 36:531–540.

Waller G, Hamilton K, Rose N, Sumra J, Baldwin G. Sexual abuse and body-image distortion in the eating disorders. *Br J Clin Psychol* 1993; 32:350–352.

Waller KG, Shaw RW. Endometriosis, pelvic pain, and psychological functioning. *Fertil Steril* 1995; 63:796–800.

Walling MK, O'Hara MW, Reiter RC, et al. Abuse history and chronic pain in women: II. A multivariate analysis of abuse and psychological morbidity. *Obstet Gynecol* 1994; 84:200–206.

Walling MK, Reiter RC, O'Hara MW, et al. Abuse history and chronic pain in women: I. Prevalences of sexual abuse and physical abuse. *Obstet Gynecol* 1994; 84:193–199.

Wesselmann U, Burnett AL, Heinberg LJ. The urogenital and rectal pain syndromes. *Pain* 1997; 73:269–294.

Whitehead WE, Palsson OS. Is rectal pain sensitivity a biological marker for irritable bowel syndrome: psychological influences on pain perception. *Gastroenterology* 1998; 115:1263–1271.

Whitehead WE, Bosmajian L, Zonderman AB, Costa PT Jr, Schuster MM. Symptoms of psychologic distress associated with irritable bowel syndrome: comparison of community and medical clinic samples. *Gastroenterology* 1988; 95:709–714.

Whitehead WE, Crowell MD, Heller BR, et al. Modeling and reinforcement of the sick role during childhood predicts adult illness behavior. *Psychosom Med* 1994; 56:541–550.

Whitehead WE, Crowell MD, Davidoff AL, Palsson OS, Schuster MM. Pain from rectal distension in women with irritable bowel syndrome: relationship to sexual abuse. *Dig Dis Sci* 1997; 42:796–804.

Whitehead WE, Palsson O, Jones KR. Systematic review of the comorbidity of irritable bowel syndrome with other disorders: what are the causes and implications? *Gastroenterology* 2002; 122:1140–1156.

Zondervan K, Barlow DH. Epidemiology of chronic pelvic pain. *Baillieres Best Pract Res Clin Obstet Gynaecol* 2000; 14:403–414.

Zondervan KT, Yudkin PL, Vessey MP, et al. Prevalence and incidence of chronic pelvic pain in primary care: evidence from a national general practice database. *Br J Obstet Gynaecol* 1999; 106:1149–1155.

Zondervan KT, Yudkin PL, Vessey MP, et al. The community prevalence of chronic pelvic pain in women and associated illness behaviour. *Br J Gen Pract* 2001; 51:541–547.

Correspondence to: Jennifer A. Haythornthwaite, PhD, Johns Hopkins Hospital, 218 Meyer, 600 N. Wolfe Street, Baltimore, MD 21287-7218, USA. Tel: 410-614-9850; Fax: 410-614-3366; email: jthaythor@jhmi.edu.

Psychosocial Aspects of Pain: A Handbook for Health Care Providers, Progress in Pain Research and Management, Vol. 27, edited by Robert H. Dworkin and William S. Breitbart, IASP Press, Seattle, © 2004.

17

Recurrent Headache Disorders

Kenneth A. Holroyd

Psychology Department, Ohio University, Athens, Ohio, USA

This chapter provides a brief clinical guide to psychosocial aspects of headache and psychological treatments for headache disorders. Following a brief review of the epidemiology and impact of migraine and tension-type headache and a description of the clinical characteristics and the psychosocial correlates of these two headache disorders, the chapter presents the basics of psychosocial treatment, emphasizing simple yet effective headache management skills that a variety of health care providers can teach.

EPIDEMIOLOGY AND IMPACT OF HEADACHE

Migraine affects 18% of women and 6% of men (e.g., 28 million individuals in the United States; Lipton et al. 2001a). About 30% of people in developed nations have tension-type headaches at least once a month and about 3% experience them more than 15 days per month (Rasmussen et al. 1991; Schwartz et al. 1998). As the frequency and severity of migraine or tension-type headaches increases, the impact of headaches on daily functioning is correspondingly greater (Schwartz et al. 1998; Holroyd et al. 2000). Almost a third of migraine sufferers miss work, and between one-half and three-quarters of migraine sufferers discontinue normal household activities or cancel family and social activities because of headaches (Lipton et al. 2001a).

CLINICAL CHARACTERISTICS

The majority of headache sufferers (probably over 95%) have benign, idiopathic headaches such as migraine and tension-type headache. These headaches are classified as episodic if they occur on fewer than 15 days per month, and chronic if they occur more frequently. Chronic headaches may also result from the overuse of acute headache medications.

MIGRAINE

Migraines are characterized by pulsating pain of moderate to severe intensity sufficient to inhibit or prohibit daily activities. A migraine episode lasts 4 to 72 hours, is accompanied by nausea, vomiting, or both, and by a heightened sensitivity to light and sound, and is aggravated by routine physical activities (e.g., climbing stairs). Head pain may be unilateral and frequently originates behind or around the eyes and then radiates to the frontal and temporal regions; it may progress to encompass the entire head. Thought, memory, and concentration may be impaired, and the sufferer may experience light-headedness, irritability, anorexia, diarrhea, and scalp tenderness. For the minority of headache sufferers who experience migraine with aura, the pain is preceded by temporary focal neurological symptoms that most often are visual disturbances (e.g., bright or blind spots, stars, wavy lines), but may include sensory disturbances (e.g., tingling or numbness), muscle weakness, or faintness.

TENSION-TYPE HEADACHE

Tension-type headaches are characterized by bilateral, nonthrobbing (pressing or tightening, dull, band-like, or cap-like) pain of mild to moderate intensity that may inhibit, but not prohibit daily activities. The pain is typically located in the forehead, neck, and shoulder areas. The typical tension-type headache may last 30 minutes to 7 days, is not aggravated by routine activities, is not accompanied by vomiting (nausea occurs only in the chronic form) or by acute sensitivity to light or sound, and is not preceded by focal neurological symptoms.

HEADACHE ASSOCIATED WITH SUBSTANCES
OR THEIR WITHDRAWAL

Individuals with medication overuse headaches (often referred to as "rebound headaches") are seldom pain-free and may have periods of severe headache superimposed on a nearly continuous headache of mild or moderate severity. Headaches are likely to resemble chronic tension-type or chronic migraine headaches; however, it is the frequent use of prescription or non-prescription analgesic medications or abortive medications (combination analgesics, opioids, nonopioid analgesics, barbiturates, ergots, and other abortive agents including triptans) that is worsening the original tension-type or migraine headaches (Limmroth et al. 2002). Medication overuse headache is estimated to occur in at least 30% of people treated in headache centers (Diener 2000) and should be suspected when acute medications are used for 20 days per month for at least a 3-month period. Medication overuse headaches can only be managed effectively if the use of the offending medications is reduced or eliminated (Diener 2000; Silberstein and Dongmei 2002).

PSYCHOSOCIAL ISSUES

DISABILITY

Diagnosis provides little information about the psychosocial impact of headaches; migraines or tension-type headaches may vary greatly in their impact on work, family, and social functioning. Information about the psychosocial impact of a headache disorder is important in assessing the severity of headaches and in planning treatment. This information can be obtained by asking questions about the impact of headaches on work, family, and social activities, or from easily administered questionnaires. The five-item Migraine Disability Assessment (MIDAS) questionnaire (Lipton et al. 2001b) and the six-item Headache Impact Test (Ware et al. 2000) allow rapid assessment of the impact of headaches on functioning. The MIDAS tool also allows headaches to be categorized into one of four severity or headache impact levels. The 25-item Headache Disability Inventory (Jacobson et al. 1994) assesses not only the direct impact of headaches on functioning, but also the individual's avoidance of activities when a headache is anticipated, and the amount of affective distress associated with headaches.

COMORBID PSYCHIATRIC DISORDERS

Epidemiological studies (Merikangas et al. 1990, 1993; Breslau and Davis 1993; Breslau et al. 1994a) confirm that the prevalence of mood and anxiety disorders is elevated in migraine sufferers (relative risk is typically between 2 and 3; i.e., the prevalence of such disorders is 2 to 3 times higher in migraine sufferers than in individuals without migraine). Longitudinal data further argue that the association between mood disorders and migraine is bidirectional: for example, Breslau and colleagues (1994a,b) found that migraine increased the risk of a *subsequent* episode of major depression (adjusted relative risk = 4.8), but the presence of major depression also increased the risk of *subsequently* developing migraine (adjusted relative risk = 3.3).

The prevalence of both anxiety and mood disorders also appears to be elevated in chronic tension-type headache, at least in clinical samples. Over 40% of chronic tension-type headache sufferers in primary care settings, and even higher percentages of chronic tension-type headache sufferers seen in specialty settings, receive a diagnosis of either an anxiety disorder or a mood disorder (Goncalves and Monteiro 1993; Guidetti et al. 1998; Puca et al. 1999; Holroyd et al. 2000).

A comorbid anxiety or mood disorder appears to increase the disability associated with headaches, so effective management of psychiatric disorders may improve functioning (Holroyd et al. 2000; Lipton et al. 2000). A number of instruments can be helpful in identifying psychiatric disorders or high levels of psychiatric distress. The PRIME-MD (Spitzer et al. 1994, 1999) is a brief, user-friendly, 5–10-minute interview or patient questionnaire that guides diagnosis of commonly encountered psychiatric disorders. The Beck Depression Inventory assesses the severity and symptoms of depression, while the Beck Anxiety Inventory and State-Trait Anxiety Inventory assess the symptoms and severity of anxiety (Spielberger et al. 1970; Beck et al. 1997).

EXPECTANCIES AND BELIEFS

Counter-therapeutic beliefs or unrealistic expectancies about treatment can undermine motivation to learn headache management skills. The rigid attribution of headaches to a single, stable, uncontrollable cause (e.g., "It's just the weather," or "There's nothing I can do because it runs in my family") is likely to defeat the aims of behavioral treatment (Martin et al. 1993). Similarly, individuals who adopt a passive stance in treatment because they assume that only the health care provider or only medication can help are unlikely to put forth the effort necessary to learn headache management skills (French et al. 2000). Patients who expect complete or immediate relief, or who are sufficiently motivated to use headache management skills only by a severe headache that is unlikely to respond to self-management efforts, will most likely become disillusioned and discontinue treatment. It is thus necessary to identify and challenge these counter-therapeutic beliefs prior to teaching headache management skills.

Self-efficacy refers to the belief that one can take action to influence the occurrence or severity of headaches and to enhance one's ability to function during headache episodes (Bandura 1997). A sense of personal self-efficacy can enhance adaptation to pain problems, whereas a sense of personal inefficacy can undermine efforts to adapt to pain. Perceptions of personal efficacy are associated with positive coping responses, with active efforts to prevent and manage pain, and with increased pain tolerance (French et al. 2000).

Self-efficacy can be roughly gauged by asking the question: "Are there things you can do to prevent headaches or to reduce their severity?" The 25-item Headache Specific Self-Efficacy Scale (French et al. 2000) can be used for more comprehensive assessment. Increases in self-efficacy during behavioral treatment predict a positive response to treatment whereas the failure to observe increases in self-efficacy predicts a negative response to treatment.

EVALUATION

MEDICAL EVALUATION

Prior to starting behavioral treatment, patients must undergo a medical evaluation to rule out headaches secondary to a disease state or structural abnormality. Secondary headaches often are associated with one or more of the following "red flags": (1) recent or sudden onset ("first or worst headache"); (2) recent head trauma; (3) changing or progressive symptoms, or accompanying neurological symptoms (other than the focal neurological symptoms associated with migraine aura); (4) fever or other signs of infection; (5) new onset at age 50 or over; or (6) onset in an individual with cancer or human immunodeficiency virus. Appearance of a "red flag" at any point during treatment is cause for referral for medical revaluation. Additional information can be found in Diamond and Dalessio (1992), Silberstein et al. (1998, 2001).

HEADACHE DIARIES AND SELF-MONITORING RECORDS

Information from a headache diary can facilitate the identification of patterns in headache activity, headache triggers, headache warning signs, and problems encountered in learning headache management skills. Daily diaries also provide the best measure of headache activity and medication consumption for use in assessing treatment outcome. Typically headache activity and medication use are recorded four times a day (upon arising and at lunchtime, dinnertime, and bedtime). A headache diary is completed for about a month prior to treatment (if possible), throughout treatment, for about a month after treatment, and at any follow-up evaluation. At relevant points in treatment, it is helpful to have patients also record other relevant information such as relaxation practice, headache precipitants, or thoughts and behavior in stressful situations. At each clinic visit, headache diaries and any self-monitoring forms are reviewed to gather information useful in treatment.

BEHAVIORAL TREATMENT

EFFICACY

Numerous qualitative and meta-analytic reviews have concluded that behavioral treatment yields a 40–60% reduction in migraine or tension-type headaches in adults (e.g., Holroyd and Penzien 1990; Bogaards and ter Kuile 1994; Rowan and Andrasik 1996; Haddock et al. 1997; Holroyd 2002). Children and adolescents may show somewhat better outcomes than adults (Hermann et al. 1995).

The U.S. Headache Consortium is a collaborative effort of the American Academy of Family Physicians, the American Academy of Neurology, the American Headache Society, the American College of Emergency Physicians, the American College of Physicians, the American Osteopathic Association, and the National Headache Foundation. Drawing on comprehensive evidence reports commissioned by the Agency for Health Care Research and Quality (AHCRQ; previously the Agency for Health Care Policy and Research) (Goslin et al. 1999), the consortium included relaxation training, thermal biofeedback combined with relaxation training, electromyographic (EMG) biofeedback, and cognitive-behavioral therapy as empirically supported treatments in its clinical practice guidelines for the management of migraine (Campbell et al. 2000; Silberstein and Rosenberg 2000). Similar guidelines have yet to be developed for tension-type headache, but the initial step of evaluating the evidence base for the use of behavioral treatments has been completed (McCrory et al. 2001).

TREATMENT FORMATS

Treatment can be administered either individually or in a group, in either a clinic-based or home-based format.

Clinic-based treatment. Clinic-based treatment typically involve 6 to 12 weekly sessions, 45–60 minutes in length if treatment is administered individually, and 60–120 minutes in length if treatment is administered in a group setting. This treatment format provides more clinician time and attention and allows the clinician greater opportunity to directly observe the patient than does a home-based treatment format, but it requires the patient to travel more frequently to the clinic and is more costly. Descriptions of clinic-based treatment are provided by Blanchard and Andrasik (1985) for individual treatment, and by Scharff and Marcus (1994) for group treatment with complicated headache problems.

Home-based treatment. Home-based or minimal-contact treatment involves three to four monthly treatment sessions 45–60 minutes in length for individual sessions, or 60–120 minutes in length for group sessions. Clinic visits introduce headache management skills and address problems encountered in acquiring or implementing these skills (see Table I). Patient manuals and audiotapes guide the learning and refinement of headache management skills at home. Lipchik et al. (2002) and Blanchard and Andrasik (1985) provide more detailed descriptions of home-based treatment.

SESSION STRUCTURE

With either treatment format, clinic sessions typically involve: (1) a review of self-monitoring forms and homework, (2) a discussion of any difficulties encountered in learning and applying headache management skills, (3) the presentation of the rationale for the new headache management skill that will be focus of the present session, (4) instruction and practice in this new skill, (4) formulation of a homework assignment, and (5) a summary.

OVERVIEW OF TREATMENT

Basic headache management skills will suffice for many individuals (see Table I). Advanced headache management skills include stress management using cognitive-behavioral therapy (see Waters et al., this volume) or thermal biofeedback training, which may need to be administered by specially trained psychologists, counselors, or biofeedback technicians. The basic headache management skills presented in this chapter can more easily be incorporated into general clinical practice.

Migraine. Basic migraine management skills include relaxation training, recognition of headache triggers and early warning signs, effective use of headache medications, pain management, and the development of a RESCUE plan to respond to migraine triggers and warning signs (see Table I; the acronym is explained below in the section "Responding to early warning signs and triggers"). As part of the RESCUE plan, the health care provider and client develop a plan for the effective use of both migraine medications and behavioral headache management strategies. In the third month, treatment continues to focus on the application and refinement of these "basic" migraine management skills or, if advanced migraine management skills are introduced, the focus shifts to the introduction of either (1) training in stress management (cognitive-behavioral therapy) or (2) thermal (hand-warming) biofeedback skills. The final treatment session emphasizes integrating the headache management skills that have proven effective for a given patient into an individualized headache management plan, as well as further refinement of these skills and relapse prevention.

Table I

The structure of behavioral treatment

Week	Contact with Therapist	Migraine	Tension-Type Headache
1	1st clinic visit	Orient patient to self-management of headaches Explain treatment Introduce progressive muscle relaxation, deep breathing, muscle stretches, imagery	Same Same Same
2	No contact	Introduce brief forms of relaxation Begin monitoring migraine triggers/warning signs	Same Begin monitoring headache warning signs and headache-related stressors
3	Phone contact	Address difficulties with home practice Introduce cue-controlled relaxation, relaxation by recall, autogenic phrases	Same Same
4	No contact	Application of quick relaxation skills to daily activities	Same
5	2nd clinic visit	Address problems in using relaxation skills Identify headache triggers and warning signs Explain effective use of migraine medications Review pain management Develop RESCUE* plan for responding to warning signs and migraines	Same Identify headache-related warning signs and stresses Continue refinement of basic relaxation skills *or* introduce advanced stress-management skills Review pain management
6	No contact	Apply and refine RESCUE plan	Apply and refine relaxation or stress-management skills

7	Phone contact	Address problems and refine RESCUE plan	Address problems in the application of relaxation skills or stress-management skills
8	No contact	Continue to evaluate and refine RESCUE plan	Continue to develop and refine relaxation or stress-management skills
9	3rd clinic visit	Continue with basic headache management skills *or* introduce either (1) stress-management or (2) thermal (hand-warming) biofeedback training skills	Identify most useful headache management skills for this patient
			Develop a long-term headache management plan, including coping with anticipated problems following treatment and relapse prevention
10	No contact	Practice and refine chosen activity	
11	Phone contact	Address difficulties in application of chosen headache management skill	
12	No contact	Apply and evaluate preferred headache management skills	
13		Identify most useful headache management activities for this patient	
		Develop long-term headache management plan, including coping with anticipated problems following treatment and relapse prevention	

Note: Health care professionals may request a copy of the patient manuals and audiotapes that are used in treatment from Kenneth A. Holroyd. The migraine materials are in a 13-chapter manual and 10 audiotape sides; the tension-type headache materials are in an 8-chapter manual and 8 audiotape sides.

* RESCUE = acronym for headache management plan incorporating basic headache management skills (see explanation in text).

Tension-type headache. Basic tension-type headache management skills focus on relaxation training and the application of relaxation and pain management skills (see Table I). The optional advanced headache management skill, introduced in the second month, is stress management.

BASIC HEADACHE MANAGEMENT SKILLS

Patient education

It is critical to insure that the patient understands behavioral treatment. In our clinic we use the initial part of the first treatment session to inform patients about this treatment approach, how they will participate in their treatment, and what they can expect in terms of outcome.

1. Structure of behavioral treatment. Orientation begins with an overview of the structure of behavioral treatment, including a brief discussion of the treatment components (e.g., relaxation, identification of migraine triggers and warning signs) and an outline of the schedule and length of sessions and telephone contacts.

2. Rationale for behavioral treatment. A clear rationale for behavioral treatment of headache should be provided. We present a biopsychosocial model that conceptualizes headaches as a biological disorder in which multiple environmental, social, physical, and psychological factors play a role in the onset, course, and maintenance of headaches (see also Flor and Hermann, this volume). This model helps patients to understand the relevance of psychological and behavioral interventions, without conceptualizing their headaches as a psychological problem. Relaxation training is introduced as a method for reducing the physical arousal and muscle tension that may both precipitate and result from headaches. The overall rationale for behavioral treatment is explained during the initial treatment session; at each subsequent session, a more specific rationale is provided for the interventions that will be introduced in that session.

3. Treatment requires an active patient. Patients may enter treatment assuming they will be passive recipients, with attendance at scheduled appointments as their only responsibility. This belief will interfere with treatment adherence and is best addressed at the beginning of treatment. It is essential to orient patients to the collaborative process, explaining that successful treatment requires the active involvement of both the health care provider and the patient. We explain that the role of the health care provider is not to take responsibility for fixing the headaches, but to provide tools for the patient to learn to better manage headaches.

4. Homework. We stress that clinic visits are a small part of treatment. We want patients to understand that it is essential to maintain headache diaries and fill out self-monitoring forms. The benefits of behavioral head-ache management depend upon the patient's commitment to practice at home the headache management skills learned in clinic sessions.

5. *Encouraging realistic expectations for treatment outcome.* We ex-plain that a "cure" is unlikely. We tell patients that by applying skills and making lifestyle changes, they are likely to experience moderate reductions in headache activity; a reduced need for drug therapy; improvements in affective distress, quality of life, and functioning; and a restored sense of personal control over headaches. We explain that we cannot know in ad-vance who will benefit from headache management training, or predict the exact benefit a particular patient will receive. We also warn that improve-ment is not likely to be observed until headache management skills have been used for a number of months. Although we acknowledge that headache management skills may mitigate the duration and severity of headache epi-sodes, we emphasize that behavioral treatments are to be used regularly with the aim of *preventing* headache episodes.

Attitude

Because patients' confidence in their ability to manage their headaches may be more important than their ability to regulate specific physiological responses (Holroyd et al. 1984; Blanchard et al. 1993), it is important for the health care provider to attend to patients' perceptions of their performance, as well as to their actual performance during skills training. Initially, we magnify small successes and normalize any problems as an expected phase of treatment. We encourage patients to take credit for their successes through-out treatment. We remind them that the clinician serves primarily as a teacher and a coach, while the patients do the more difficult work of experimenting with and refining the various headache management techniques.

RELAXATION SKILLS

Orientation

We explain that relaxation skills may enable patients to decrease their overall level of muscle tension and autonomic arousal and to recognize subtle signs of tension so that they can apply quick relaxation skills to prevent the buildup of additional muscle tension and to lower tension levels following periods of stress.

Relaxation training includes abbreviated progressive muscle relaxation (PMR) training and "quick relaxation" techniques that we encourage pa-tients to use throughout the day. We teach a variety of "quick relaxation" skills including abdominal breathing, relaxation by recall, cue-controlled relaxation, and the use of autogenic phrases (see below). Patients typically do not become proficient in all of these strategies, and it is not necessary for them to incorporate all of them into their repertoire. Instead, we encourage patients to try each of the strategies before deciding which ones they want to build into their regular routine. Full scripts of relaxation sessions with instructions for health care providers have been presented elsewhere (Bernstein and Borkovec 1973; Blanchard and Andrasik 1985; Bernstein and Carlson 1993). These resources also provide instructions for teaching the "quick relaxation" skills we use (see also Andrasik, this volume).

Instruction

Prior to initiating PMR training, the clinician introduces abdominal breathing (see "Muscle scanning and quick relaxation" below) and patients are instructed to practice abdominal breathing periodically during the PMR training session. Throughout the training session, we monitor behavioral signs of relaxation (see Table II) and repeat a tension-release cycle if we notice that a particular muscle group has not relaxed.

PMR training begins with tension-release cycles in 12 muscle groups to relax the entire body. However, muscles of the shoulders, neck, and face receive the greatest attention because they are most likely involved in headaches. We pay particular attention to problems commonly encountered during relaxation training and possible therapeutic responses (see Table III). At the end of PMR training, an image, selected by the patient prior to PMR practice, is used to demonstrate the use of relaxation through guided imagery (see "Muscle scanning and quick relaxation" below).

We suggest that patients practice PMR at least once, and preferably twice a day, in the morning and in the afternoon or evening. We ask patients to keep records or logs of their home practice. The log includes the date of practice and relaxation ratings before and after practice using a rating scale from 0 (no tension, or most relaxed you can imagine) to 100 (extremely tense, or the most tense you can remember).

When patients have mastered the initial muscle relaxation procedure, they are encouraged to practice a briefer relaxation technique tensing and releasing activity in a smaller number muscle groups using the audiotapes that are provided. The needs of each patient determine progress. Once a variety of brief relaxation techniques have been mastered, the focus shifts to incorporating brief relaxation skills into daily living. Even moderate levels of muscle tension, or a situation that has been associated with tension in the past, becomes a cue to use brief relaxation skills.

Table II
Relaxed behaviors based on Poppen's behavioral relaxation scale

1	Head: supported by chair; not tilted; nose in midline of the body; no motion
2	Eyes: eyelids lightly closed with smooth appearance; no motion under eyelids
3	Mouth: lips parted slightly at the center of the mouth; front teeth slightly parted; no tongue movement
4	Throat: no motion (e.g., swallowing, other larynx action, twitches)
5	Shoulders: slightly rounded, transecting the same horizontal plane and resting against chair; no motion
6	Body: torso, hips, legs are symmetrical around midline and resting on chair; no movement
7	Hands: resting on armrest or lap with palms down and fingers slightly curled in a claw-like fashion
8	Feet: pointed away from each other at a 60–90° angle; feet not crossed at ankle; no movement
9	Quiet: no vocalizations or loud respiratory sounds (no talking, sighing, laughing, gasping, or coughing)
10	Breathing: breath frequency less than observed at beginning of session; no breathing irregularities that interrupt the regular rhythm of breathing (e.g., coughing, sneezing, or yawning)

Note: Based on Poppen (1988).

Muscle stretching. Muscle-stretching exercises gently lengthen sore and tight neck and shoulder muscles. Gentle neck and shoulder stretches using sideways turns of the head, forward bends, and diagonal bends of the neck and head are demonstrated (e.g., DeGood 1997). The patient with a head-forward posture is instructed to monitor head and neck posture and to use chin tucks throughout the day to change this postural habit. The patient is instructed to perform brief gentle stretches intermittently throughout the day, as well as immediately prior to practicing PMR. We explain that as they progress, they will be more aware of muscles that tighten prior to, or early in, a headache episode. This awareness will allow patients to stretch or relax muscles strategically, preventing muscle tension from developing into a full-blown headache. Muscle-stretching exercises should be done gently so that already constricted shoulder and neck muscles are not extended so far as to induce pain or injury.

Muscle scanning and quick relaxation. Quick relaxation techniques enable the patient to rapidly produce the relaxation response that was learned during PMR training. Therefore, before attempting quick relaxation it is important that the patient is able to relax deeply when practicing the full version of PMR.

To help determine when to use quick relaxation techniques, patients are asked to periodically "scan" or monitor sensations of muscle tension,

Table III
Relaxation training: problems and solutions

Problems	Solutions
A. *Patient's Attitude*	
1. Patient is self-critical or hesitant during training.	Identify self-critical thoughts and help patient to challenge them. Offer reassurance.
2. Patient is overly concerned about performance.	Suggest that trying hard is counterproductive; instruct patient in alternative attitude of passive volition.
3. Patient is hesitant to relinquish control.	Discuss fears about loss of control; explain that novelty of sensations of relaxation may be triggering anxiety.
B. *Learning the Skill*	
1. Patient's concentration is disturbed by distracting thoughts or feelings. This is the most common problem; discuss it with patient prior to practice.	Encourage patient *not* to fight these thoughts, but to let them pass through mind. Remind patient that these will lessen as he/she gets better at relaxation. Use imagery techniques (e.g., placing interfering thoughts in an imaginary trunk, seeing thoughts floating by on clouds) or autogenic phrases (e.g., peaceful, calm) to focus attention. If distracting thoughts continue, and are severe, try thought stopping.
2. Patient falls asleep when practicing relaxation.	Do not schedule relaxation practice just after meals or just before bedtime. Have patient practice seated rather than lying down.
3. Patient has difficulty detecting the difference between sensations of tension and relaxation.	Have patient place one hand on muscle while tensing or relaxing muscle. Introduce alternate tensing techniques. Use partial tensing of muscles (discrimination training) to help patient identify subtle cues of tension and relaxation.
4. Certain muscles are difficult to relax.	Repeat tensing-relaxing sequence with specific muscles; use muscle-stretching exercises prior to relaxation practice.
C. *Maintenance and Generalization*	
1. Patient reports no carry-over effect after relaxation.	Introduce brief cue-controlled relaxation techniques to use periodically throughout the day. Identify thoughts or situations that evoke arousal.
2. Patient has difficulty detecting the difference between sensations of tension and relaxation in daily situations.	Ask patient to discuss a recently stressful situation and note any muscle tension, such as clenched jaws or fists, furrowed brows, tightened shoulders.

particularly in the shoulders, neck, and face, during the day. Scanning increases awareness of even low levels of muscle tension. The identification of low levels of tension then provides a cue for the early use of one of the quick relaxation techniques. This will help to *prevent* muscle tension from building to a headache. Patients are also encouraged to use specific environmental cues such as a change of work tasks, the alarm on their wristwatch or computer, or self-adhesive colored dots placed in strategic locations to signal them to use quick relaxation skills. The goal is to integrate muscle scanning and preferred quick relaxation techniques into patients' daily routines.

Abdominal breathing. Abdominal or diaphragmatic breathing brings air to the base of the lungs, where oxygen is efficiently transferred to the bloodstream. Abdominal deep breathing involves slow deep breaths (about 10 breaths per minute), with exhalation lasting longer than inhalation. Initially, we ask patients to practice abdominal breathing for 5–10 minutes twice daily. We also ask patients to say to themselves the word "relax" with each exhalation, as they attend to the rhythm of their breathing. In time, the word "relax" comes to serve as a cue to trigger a quick relaxation response (see "Relaxation by recall/cue-controlled relaxation" below).

Guided imagery. In guided imagery, patients call a pleasant, relaxing image to mind and focus their attention on the sensory details of the image (e.g., sensations of light, color, sound, temperature, texture, and physical activity). Using imagery can be helpful in evoking a quick relaxation response, as well as in providing a brief respite from a stressful situation. We incorporate instructions for guided imagery into the PMR protocol to deepen relaxation. Most likely not all patients will have the ability to develop an image or use imagery as a quick relaxation strategy.

Relaxation by recall/cue-controlled relaxation. In relaxation by recall, the relaxation response is produced without tensing muscles, but instead by mentally evoking sensations of relaxation in specific muscle groups. The patient first identifies sensations of tension in specific muscle groups (e.g., by muscle scanning) and then mentally recalls sensations of relaxation, maintaining these sensations for 30–40 seconds. Typically, a cue or signal (e.g., the word "relax") that has been repeatedly paired with the relaxation response during PMR practice is used to evoke the relaxation response.

Autogenic training. Autogenic training is a set of self-regulation techniques in which the patient holds in thought phrases such as "my forehead is cool," "my arms feel heavy and warm," or "I feel relaxed and at peace" while concentrating on his or her body sensations (Schultz and Luthe 1959). We instruct patients to become aware of random background thoughts and images, and suggest that they use autogenic phrases to counteract this "mental traffic" and facilitate deep relaxation.

IDENTIFYING EARLY WARNING SIGNS
AND HEADACHE PRECIPITANTS

Orientation

If common migraine triggers and prodromal symptoms are described and recorded prospectively, most patients can learn to identify early warning signs they previously might not have noticed. This information is valuable because it often allows patients to take effective action to prevent or manage migraines, prompting them to use behavioral headache management skills or, where appropriate, to take medication to abort a headache episode. Even patients who experience aura typically will not experience it with every migraine, and thus will benefit from learning to identify more subtle prodromal symptoms.

Instruction

We assist patients in systematically recording early warning signs and in evaluating their significance. Such signs can be psychological, neurological, constitutional, or autonomic. Psychological symptoms include irritability, depression, moodiness, euphoria, restlessness, hyperactivity, fatigue, and drowsiness. Neurological symptoms include photophobia, phonophobia, hyperosmia, yawning, dysphasia, and difficulty concentrating. Other symptoms can include stiff neck, food cravings, feeling cold, anorexia, increased thirst, fluid retention, frequent urination, diarrhea, constipation, or sluggishness. These symptoms will differ among individuals, but each patient will have a consistent pattern.

Although prodromal symptoms may initially be difficult to link to migraine episodes, it is helpful for patients to identify them so that they can learn to predict an attack. To help identify prodromal symptoms, we ask patients to record any "odd" or "just not right" sensations they experienced prior to the onset of the migraine. Next, we ask patients to identify how often these symptoms occur when they do not develop a migraine. This step enables patients to determine whether a symptom is truly a reliable early warning sign.

We also assist patients in systematically recording possible headache triggers. Many triggers are relevant for both migraine and tension-type headache. General population studies indicate that stress, sleep difficulties, and hormonal factors (relevant specifically for migraine) are the triggers most frequently identified by headache suffers (Rasmussen 1993). Headache triggers are ordered according to the strength of supporting evidence in Table IV.

We explain that headache triggers are not universal and do not necessarily precipitate an attack on every exposure. Headaches may occur hours after exposure to a headache trigger. Several triggers occurring within close proximity are more likely to start a migraine than a single precipitant. Patients begin by noting whether particular settings, times of the day or week, or activities are associated with headache onset. They also review the 12 hours or so prior to each headache onset for possible headache triggers to see whether a pattern emerges. Prospective monitoring often identifies triggers they had overlooked.

Stress. Stress is the most frequently identified headache precipitant for both migraine and tension-type headache (Rasmussen 1993). Headaches may be triggered by stress or by relaxation following a period of stress ("letdown headaches"). Relaxation and stress management interventions address headaches that occur in response to stress.

Table IV
Commonly reported headache triggers and empirical support
for reported triggers

Trigger Factor	Migraine	Headache
*Strong Evidence**		
Stress	Yes	Yes
Menstruation	Yes	Yes
Caffeine withdrawal	Unknown	Yes
Visual stimuli (e.g., lights)	Yes	Yes
Weather changes	Yes	Yes
Moderate Evidence		
Nitrates	Yes	Yes
Fasting	Probable	Yes
Sleep disturbances	Possible	Yes
Wine	Yes	Yes
Monosodium glutamate	Unknown	Yes
Aspartame	Yes	Yes
Limited Evidence		
Smoking	Not proven	Unknown
Odors	Not proven	Not proven
Chocolate	Not proven	Not proven
Tyramine (e.g., aged cheeses)	Not proven	Not proven

Source: Adapted from Martin and Behbehani (2002).
* Strength of evidence is defined as follows: Strong: at least two prospective, randomized, controlled or diary studies confirming an association with no dissenting studies. Moderate: at least one randomized, controlled trial or a prospective diary study confirming an association with no dissenting studies or a prospective diary study confirming an association with no dissenting studies, or two supporting studies with one dissenting study.

Sleep. Sleep difficulties are commonly identified as a headache trigger, with insufficient sleep, oversleeping, or an irregular sleep schedule identified as the most common sleep precipitants (Sahota and Dexter 1990; Rasmussen 1993). Patients can be instructed in sleep hygiene and advised to maintain a regular sleep schedule. Practicing relaxation techniques prior to bedtime may facilitate sleep onset.

Hormonal factors. Fluctuations in reproductive hormones, whether due to menarche, menstruation, pregnancy, menopause, or hormone replacement therapy, are associated with headache disorders, particularly migraine (for a review, see Silberstein and Merriman 1997).

Meal schedules and dietary factors. Close to 30% of people with headaches, primarily those with migraine, report that dietary factors, such as skipping or delaying meals or ingesting specific foods, beverages, or ingredients sometimes trigger their headaches (Robbins 1994). Few double-blind studies of dietary triggers have been conducted, and clinical opinions differ regarding the benefits from dietary alterations (Martin and Behbehani 2002). Most people with headaches do not require severely restricted diets, but should avoid foods or additives that appear to trigger headaches. Generally, it is advised that people with migraine consume alcohol, particularly red wine, with caution. People with migraine may also benefit from a trial of limiting or eliminating monosodium glutamate, aspartame, and nitrites, because these substances may trigger migraines in susceptible individuals (Martin and Behbehani 2002). They should be cautioned that missing or delaying meals also might trigger headaches.

The role of caffeine as a potential precipitant may needs to be explored if individuals with migraine regularly consume more than 300 milligrams of caffeine a day (approximately the amount found in two strong cups of coffee), because this amount of caffeine may precipitate headaches in sensitive individuals, either through the rebound effect or through caffeine sensitivity. Caffeine in medications should be included in calculations of caffeine intake. Prospective monitoring may help to determine whether caffeine intake or withdrawal are headache triggers for a particular patient.

Environmental factors. Headache patients should be assisted in avoiding or restricting their exposure to various environmental factors (e.g., glare or chemical odors) that they have identified as headache triggers. Avoiding or restricting exposure to environmental precipitants often can be accomplished with little lifestyle disruption.

EFFECTIVE USE OF MIGRAINE MEDICATIONS

Orientation

The effective use of headache medications may require the application of complex decision rules; thus, making these rules explicit enables patients to use their medications most effectively. We help the patient develop and effectively apply optimal decision rules to guide the use of symptomatic and abortive medications, as well as relaxation, cognitive, and other psychological headache management techniques. The goal is both to prevent medication overuse and to maximize the effectiveness of headache medications. In order to assist patients in effectively using migraine medications, the health care provider must be knowledgeable about headache medications and work closely with the prescribing physician.

Headache medications

Below is a synopsis of four types of migraine medication. Detailed discussions of these medications can be found in Robbins (2000), Silberstein et al. (2001), and Davidoff (1995). Holroyd et al. (1998) present guidelines for the integration of medication and behavioral treatment.

Symptomatic medications include analgesics prescribed primarily to reduce pain such as nonsteroidal anti-inflammatory drugs (NSAIDs), including cyclooxygenase-2 (COX-2) inhibitors; mixed analgesics containing barbiturates (e.g., butalbital) or opioids (codeine); and opioids (oxycodone). Effective symptomatic therapy should reduce pain from mild to none or from moderate to mild within 1–2 hours. The use of opioid and mixed analgesics must be limited because overuse can cause rebound headaches and even dependence. NSAIDs are probably less likely to induce rebound headaches, but should be used in moderation.

Migraine-specific medications today typically are serotonin receptor agonists (triptans such as sumatriptan, rizatriptan, naratriptan, zolmitriptan, almotriptan, eletriptan, and frovatriptan). Effective treatment should prevent migraine pain from becoming moderate or severe if taken when pain is mild, or reduce severe or moderate pain to mild or no pain within 2 hours. These agents should be used no more than two to three days per week to avoid rebound headaches.

Antiemetics (e.g., prochlorperazine, metoclopramide) are used to treat the nausea and vomiting associated with migraines. The goal of antiemetic therapy is to reduce nausea within 1–2 hours and control vomiting most of the time. Antiemetics also improve the absorption of some oral medications, including analgesics, and may have anti-migraine effects themselves. Patients who experience nausea and vomiting are instructed to take an antiemetic before or along with their analgesic.

Preventive or prophylactic medications for migraine include beta-blockers, anticonvulsants, antidepressants (tricyclic, serotonin reuptake inhibitors, and monoamine oxidase inhibitors), calcium channel blockers, and NSAIDs. Antidepressants (for the most part tricyclics) are the primary preventive medications for tension-type headache (Holroyd et al. 1998, 2001b). The goal of preventive therapy is to reduce the frequency of headaches by 50% or more.

Instruction

The symptomatic and migraine-specific medications receive the greatest attention because their effective use may require complex decisions based on the limits on the use of the medication, patients' headache symptoms (e.g., do these symptoms predict a moderate to severe migraine?), and previous empirical observations of patients' responses to specific medications. For example, for one headache sufferer, analgesics, NSAIDs, or a single triptan dose may effectively abort a migraine when taken early on, but the same medication will be much less effective, even in multiple doses, when taken later in an episode. In this case, overall medication use per episode can be reduced and the efficacy of the medication improved by implementing a judicious plan to initiate treatment early. Another person may not be able to confidently predict if a mild headache will develop into a severe migraine; attempting to initiate treatment early in an episode, the person not only may fail to reduce medication consumption but may be tempted to overuse medications. Thus, effective use of medications in the acute treatment of migraine requires a systematic plan that takes into account multiple factors in each decision to treat. Decision rules also must be refined as the patient collects data by experimenting with different possible treatment options. We assist the patient in formulating decision rules for medication use that are consistent with medical advice and help the patient devise "experiments" to test different treatment options and evaluate data from such "experiments."

RESPONDING TO EARLY WARNING SIGNS AND TRIGGERS

Orientation

Information collected about early headache warning signs and headache triggers is now used to develop an action plan directed at preventing and managing headaches. The prodromal symptoms and aura symptoms the patient has identified serve as signals to take actions to abort or reduce the severity of the anticipated migraines. Headache triggers provide information that can help the patient take actions to prevent or manage headaches. The goal is to replace the sense of dread, anxiety, and helplessness many individuals feel when anticipating a headache with a sense of self-efficacy and a plan of action.

Instruction

Decisions about effective medication use and about the use of relaxation skills are integrated in an action plan that incorporates this new knowledge about early warning signs and triggers. For example, specific early warning signs that reliably signal the onset of a migraine may now serve as a cue for a patient to use a triptan medication, apply quick relaxation skills, and limit exposure to possible triggers. This tentative action plan is then further refined on the basis of subsequent experience. We use the RESCUE acronym below to remind patients of the general underlying principles, but we develop a specific plan for each person.

Remain calm. Worrying about how to work around a migraine or denying that it might occur usually makes it more long-lasting and severe.

Escape from known triggers. Your body may be more susceptible to triggers during the preheadache (or prodromal) phase. Avoid or minimize triggers wherever possible.

Stay away from stress or stressful situations. Avoid taking on extra work. Let go of things that do not have to be completed right now. Be extra kind to yourself.

Carry your migraine medications with you at all times. Make sure you have quick and easy access to your medications wherever you go. Always be prepared.

Use relaxation exercises. Concentrate on the exercises you find most useful. Remember that relaxation may help control some of the physical changes associated with migraine.

Eat and sleep on schedule. This is not the time to skip meals or go without sleep. Do not try to finish everything you think you have to do before the migraine begins.

ADVANCED HEADACHE MANAGEMENT SKILLS

By mastering and employing basic headache management skills, many individuals who experience episodic rather than chronic headaches will achieve clinically significant improvements in headache activity and reductions in disability and affective distress. However, some individuals will only benefit, and others will show additional benefit, from the addition of "advanced" headache management skills such as stress management therapy, or thermal biofeedback training for migraine, although empirical support for this contention is limited. The use of stress management therapy and thermal biofeedback training in the treatment of headaches is described by Blanchard and Andrasik (1985), Holroyd et al. (1998, 2001a), and Lipchik et al. (2002).

MAINTENANCE OF SELF-MANAGEMENT

Orientation

The goal of treatment is long-term headache management. At the final treatment session we explain to patients that further improvement or even the maintenance of current improvements probably will require continued effort. Patients are encouraged to continue to incorporate headache management skills into their daily routine as well as to be on the lookout for the lapses in behavior that can lead to problems in headache control. We reassure patients that the continued practice of headache management skills will require less time and effort than was required when they were learning the skills.

Instruction

Only an introduction to headache management skills is provided during home-based treatment; therefore, we plan what the patient will work on when clinic contacts end, and identify events likely to cause a reoccurrence or worsening of headaches. We help patients identify obstacles to effective self-management and develop plans for coping with these obstacles. We assist patients in identifying behaviors such as increased use of medications, sleep difficulties, and ineffective coping with stress that might suggest they are off track with their headache management program, and discuss how to handle such temporary setbacks. Lastly, we remind patients that life is full of challenges, and explain that they might need an occasional "checkup" or booster session.

ACKNOWLEDGMENTS

Support for this chapter was provided, in part, by a grant from The National Institute of Neurological Disorders and Stroke of the National Institutes of Health (NS32374).

REFERENCES

Bandura A. *Self-Efficacy: The Exercise of Control.* New York: W.H. Freeman, 1997.

Beck AT, Steer RA, Ball R, Ciervo CA, Kabat M. Use of the Beck Anxiety and Depression Inventories for primary care with medical outpatients. *Assessment* 1997; 4:211–219.

Bernstein DA, Borkovec TD. *Progressive Relaxation Training: A Manual for the Helping Professions.* Champaign, IL: Research Press, 1973.

Bernstein DA, Carlson CR. Progressive relaxation: abbreviated methods. In: Lehrer P, Woolfolk RL (Eds). *Principles and Practice of Stress Management.* New York: Guilford Press, 1993, pp 53–85.

Blanchard EB, Andrasik F. *Management of Chronic Headaches: A Psychological Approach.* Elmsford, NY: Pergamon Press, 1985.

Blanchard EB, Kim M, Hermann CU, Steffek BD. Preliminary results of the effects on headache relief of perception of success among tension headache patients receiving relaxation. *Headache Q* 1993; 4:249–253.

Bogaards MC, ter Kuile MM. Treatment of recurrent tension headache: a meta-analytic review. *Clin J Pain* 1994; 10:174–190.

Breslau N, Davis GC. Migraine, physical health and psychiatric disorder: a prospective epidemiologic study in young adults. *J Psychiatr Res* 1993; 27:211–221.

Breslau N, Davis GC, Schultz LR, Peterson EL. Migraine and major depression: a longitudinal study. *Headache* 1994a; 34:387–393.

Breslau N, Merikangas K, Bowden CL. Comorbidity of migraine and major affective disorders. *Neurology* 1994b; 44:S17–S22.

Campbell JK, Penzien DB, Wall EM. Evidence-based guidelines for migraine headache: behavioral and physical treatments. U.S. Headache Consortium, 2000. Available via the Internet: www.aan.com/public/practiceguidelines/headache_gl.htm.

Davidoff RA. *Migraine: Manifestations, Pathogenesis, and Management.* Philadelphia: Davis, 1995.

DeGood DE. *The Headache and Neck Pain Workbook: An Integrated Mind and Body Program.* Oakland, CA: Harbinger, 1997.

Diamond S, Dalessio DJ. *The Practicing Physician's Approach to Headache,* 4th ed. Baltimore: Williams & Wilkins, 1992.

Diener HC. Headache associated with chronic use of substances. In: Olesen J, Tfelt-Hansen P, Welch KMA (Eds). *The Headaches.* Philadelphia: Lippincott, Williams, & Wilkins, 2000, pp 871–877.

French DJ, Holroyd KA, Pinnell C, et al. Perceived self-efficacy and headache-related disability. *Headache* 2000, 40:647–656.

Goncalves JA, Monteiro P. Psychiatric analysis of patients with tension-type headache. In: Olesen J, Schoenen J (Eds). *Tension-Type Headache: Classification, Mechanisms, and Treatment.* New York: Raven Press, 1993, pp 167–172.

Guidetti V, Galli F, Fabrizi P, et al. Headache and psychiatric comorbidity: clinical aspects and outcome in an 8 year follow-up study. *Cephalalgia* 1998; 18:455–462.

Haddock CK, Rowan AB, Andrasik F, et al. Home-based behavioral treatments for chronic benign headache: a meta-analysis of controlled trials. *Cephalalgia* 1997; 17:113–118.

Hermann C, Kim M, Blanchard EB. Behavioral and pharmacological intervention studies of pediatric migraine: an exploratory meta-analysis. *Pain* 1995; 60:239–256.

Holroyd KA. Assessment and psychological treatment of recurrent headache disorders. *J Consult Clin Psychol* 2002; 70:656–677.

Holroyd KA, Penzien DB. Pharmacological vs. nonpharmacological prophylaxis of recurrent migraine headache: a meta-analytic review of clinical trails. *Pain* 1990; 42:1–13.

Holroyd KA, Penzien DB, Hursey K, et al. Change mechanisms in EMG biofeedback training: cognitive changes underlying improvements in tension headache. *J Consult Clin Psychol* 1984; 52:1039–1053.

Holroyd KA, Lipchik GL, Penzien DB. Psychological management of recurrent headache disorders: empirical basis for clinical practice. In: Dobson KS, Craig KD (Eds). *Best Practice: Developing and Promoting Empirically Supported Interventions.* Newbury Park, CA: Sage, 1998, pp 193–212.

Holroyd K, Stensland M, Lipchik G, et al. Psychosocial correlates and impact of chronic tension-type headaches. *Headache* 2000; 40:3–16.

Holroyd KA, Lipchik GL, Penzien DB. Behavioral management of recurrent headache disorders. In: Silberstein SD, Lipton RB, Dalessio DJ (Eds). *Wolff's Headache and Other Headache Pain,* 7th ed. New York: Oxford University Press, 2001a, 562–598.

Holroyd KA, O'Donnell FJ, Stensland M, et al. Management of chronic tension-type headache with tricyclic antidepressant medication, stress-management therapy, and their combination: a randomized controlled trial. *JAMA* 2001b; 285:2208–2215.

Jacobson GP, Ramadan NM, Aggarwal SK, Newman CW. The Henry Ford Hospital Headache Disability Inventory (HDI). *Neurology* 1994; 44:837–842.

Limmroth V, Katsarava Z, Fritsche G, Przywara S, Diener HC. Features of medication overuse headache following overuse of different acute headache drugs. *Neurology* 2002; 59:1011–1014.

Lipchik GL, Holroyd KA, Nash JM. Cognitive-behavioral management of recurrent headache disorders: a minimal therapist contact approach. In: Turk DC, Gatchel RS (Eds). *Psychological Approaches to Pain Management,* 2nd ed. New York: Guilford Publications, 2002, pp 356–389.

Lipton RB, Hamelsky SW, Kolodner K, Steiner M, Stewart W. Migraine, quality of life, and depression: a population based study. *Neurology* 2000; 55:629–635.

Lipton RB, Hamelsky SW, Stewart WF. Epidemiology and impact of headache. In: Silberstein SD, Lipton RB, Dalessio DJ (Eds). *Wolff's Headache and Other Headache Pain,* 7th ed. New York: Oxford University Press, 2001a, pp 85–107.

Lipton RB, Stewart WF, Sawyer J, Edmeads J. Clinical utility of an instrument assessing migraine disability: the Migraine Disability Assessment (MIDAS) questionnaire. *Headache* 2001b; 41:854–861.

Martin N, Holroyd K, Rokiki L. The headache self-efficacy scale: adaptation to recurrent headaches. *Headache* 1993; 33:244–248.

Martin VT, Behbehani MM. Towards a rationale understanding of migraine trigger factors. *Med Clin North Am* 2002.

McCrory D, Penzien D, Hasselblad V, Gray R. *Behavioral and Physical Treatments for Tension-Type and Cervicogenic Headache.* Des Moines: Foundation for Chiropractic Education and Research, 2001.

Merikangas KR, Angst J, Isler H. Migraine and psychopathology: results of the Zurich cohort study of young adults. *Arch Gen Psychiatry* 1990, 47:894–852.

Merikangas KR, Merikangas JR, Angst J. Headache syndromes and psychiatric disorders: association and family transmission. *J Psychiatr Res* 1993; 27:197–210.

Poppen R. *Behavioral Relaxation Training and Assessment.* Elmsford, NY: Pergamon Press, 1988.

Puca F, Genco S, Prudenzano MP. Psychiatric comorbidity and psychosocial stress in patients with tension-type headache from headache centers in Italy. *Cephalalgia* 1999; 19:159–164.

Rasmussen BK. Migraine and tension-type headache in a general population: precipitating factors, female hormones, sleep pattern and relation to lifestyle. *Pain* 1993; 53:65–72.

Rasmussen BK, Jensen R, Schroll M, Olesen J. Epidemiology of headache in a general population—a prevalence study. *J Clin Epidemiol* 1991; 44:1147–1157.

Robbins L. Precipitating factors in migraine: a retrospective review of 494 patients. *Headache* 1994; 34:214–216.

Robbins LD. *Management of Headache and Headache Medications,* 2nd ed. New York: Springer, 2000.

Rowan AB, Andrasik F. Efficacy and cost-effectiveness of minimal therapist contact treatments of chronic headache: a review. *Behav Ther* 1996; 27:207–234.

Sahota PK, Dexter JD. Sleep and headache syndromes: a clinical review. *Headache* 1990; 35:80–84.

Scharff L, Marcus DA. Interdisciplinary outpatient group treatment of intractable headache. *Headache* 1994; 34:73–78.

Schultz J, Luthe W. *Autogenic Training: A Psychophysiologic Approach in Psychotherapy*, Vol. 1. New York: Grune & Stratton, 1959.

Schwartz BS, Stewart WF, Simon MS, Lipton RB. A population-based study of the epidemiology of tension-type headache. *JAMA* 1998; 279:381–383.

Silberstein SD, Dongmei L. Drug overuse and rebound headache. *Curr Pain Headache Rep* 2002; 6:240–247.

Silberstein SD, Merriman G. Sex hormones and headache. In: Goadsby P, Silberstein SD (Eds). *Blue Books of Practical Neurology: Headache*. Boston: Butterworth Heinemann, 1997, pp 143–176.

Silberstein SD, Rosenberg J. Multispecialty consensus on diagnosis and treatment of headache. *Neurology* 2000; 54:1553–1554.

Silberstein SD, Lipton RB, Goadsby PJ. *Headache in Clinical Practice*. Oxford: Isis Medical Media, 1998.

Silberstein SD, Lipton RB, Dalessio DJ (Eds). *Wolff's Headache and Other Headache Pain*. New York: Oxford University Press, 2001.

Spielberger CD, Jacobs G, Crane R, et al. *State-Trait Personality Inventory*. Tampa: University of South Florida Human Resources Institute, 1970.

Spitzer RL, Williams JBW, Kroenke K, et al. Utility of a new procedure for diagnosing mental disorders in primary care: the PRIME MD 1000 study. *JAMA* 1994; 272:1749–1756.

Spitzer RL, Kroenke K, Williams JBW. Validation and utility of a self-report version of the PRIME-MD: the PHQ primary care study. *JAMA* 1999; 282:1737–1744.

Ware JE, Bayliss M, Dahlof C, et al. Developing short, static assessments from the Headache Impact Test (HIT) item pool. *Cephalalgia* 2000; 20:308–309.

Correspondence to: Kenneth A. Holroyd, PhD, Psychology Department, Ohio University, Athens, OH 45701-2979, USA. Tel: 740-593-1085 or 1060; Fax: 740-593-0116; email: holroyd@ohio.edu.

Psychosocial Aspects of Pain: A Handbook for Health Care Providers, Progress in Pain Research and Management, Vol. 27, edited by Robert H. Dworkin and William S. Breitbart, IASP Press, Seattle, © 2004.

18

Temporomandibular Disorders

Richard Ohrbach[a] and Jeffrey Sherman[b]

[a]Department of Oral Diagnostic Sciences, University at Buffalo, Buffalo, New York, USA; [b]Department of Oral Medicine, School of Dentistry, University of Washington, Seattle, Washington, USA

Although management of persistent pain has seen considerable advances in the last two decades and psychological factors are now commonly understood to be important determinants of pain-related disability and treatment seeking, Cartesian dualism remains influential within clinical practice and pain research. Among pain disorders, this dualistic view is profound in the field of temporomandibular disorders (TMD). Consequently, locating the putative (and presumably self-evidential) cause of continuing pain is a frequent goal. Medically minded dentists look toward the muscles of mastication, the temporomandibular joint (TMJ), and dysfunction of the nervous system as causes for TMD pain. Psychologically minded dentists distinguish TMD pain from nociception and link it to central dysregulation, stress, or anxiety-driven muscle tension.

In this chapter, we suggest a model for TMD assessment and treatment that integrates both medical and psychological (which we term biobehavioral, also known as biopsychosocial) factors for its etiology, maintenance, and treatment outcome. We begin with TMD epidemiology and treatment costs, followed by some primary models for TMD etiology and assessment and common biobehavioral treatment approaches. We conclude with a proposal for an empirically based approach that acknowledges medical as well as biobehavioral differences. Our intent is to use the presentation of treatment matching to simultaneously describe stepped care for TMD that could be conceptualized in more than one way and implemented in both medical and dental settings.

TMD comprises a cluster of related musculoskeletal conditions that affect the hard and soft structures of the masticatory system and are primarily characterized by: (1) pain in the pre-auricular area, the ear, the cheeks, and/or the temporal area; (2) limitations in movement of the mandible; and/or (3) joint sounds in the TMJ during functional jaw movements (Dworkin and LeResche 1992). Like other joints, the TMJ is vulnerable to both extrinsic and intrinsic influences as well as age-related degenerative changes. TMD not only influences activities that sustain life such as eating, drinking, and swallowing, but also affects speech and facial expressions. When the disorder is more severe, jaw pain begins to interfere with other functional domains such as work, recreation, and family activities.

TMD is a common condition. In adult population studies, the prevalence of TMD pain that is sufficiently severe to warrant treatment has been estimated to range between 3.7% and 12%, with figures varying for men (0–10%) and women (2–18%) (Von Korff et al. 1988; Goulet et al. 1995; Drangsholt and LeResche 2000). After synthesizing the available cross-sectional and cohort population studies, Drangsholt and LeResche (2000) concluded that TMD is rare in childhood, becomes more prevalent in adolescence, is relatively common during the adult years, seems to decline in older age, and is twice as common in women than in men, affecting 6,670,000 men and 13,350,000 women per year in the United States. Little is yet known about the incidence of new TMD cases; however, it is clear that for many individuals, TMD is either a continuous disorder or a cyclic/recurrent disorder, and the chronicity ranges from several months to multiple decades.

The heterogeneity of TMD affects epidemiological estimates. TMD involving the muscles of mastication (myofascial pain) is much more common in young to middle-aged adults, while TMD involving arthritic changes is more common in the elderly. Clicking in the TMJ is a common finding in approximately 30% of all adults, and clicking alone is no longer considered a valid indicator of a disorder requiring treatment (Truelove 2001).

TMD is not only prevalent, but costly. Approximately five million Americans seek health care for TMD symptoms annually. At a conservative estimate of U.S.$400 per year expense in healthcare visits, over $2 billion is spent each year for TMD treatment in the United States (Drangsholt and LeResche 2000). These direct costs do not take into account indirect costs related to lost work time, reduced productivity, or lost tax revenues.

MODELS TO EXPLAIN TMD

TMDs are deceptively complex. Even though the diagnostic rubric, the clinical tests, the types of diagnoses commonly given, and the treatments that can be effective for most patients are individually and collectively practical and readily understandable, complexity nevertheless emerges quickly.

While many reasons appear to account for this phenomenon, the outcome is that opinions about the etiology and treatment of TMD appear to occupy more of the information bandwidth than do empirical data and sensible theory. Unfounded opinions continue despite significant scientific advances common to all pain disorders, and such discourse continues to sway policy decisions, confuse practitioners and patients alike, and lead to treatments that often cause as many problems as they solve. Nevertheless, general scientific advances in pain have had a profound impact on the area of TMD, and because of many features unique to the masticatory system, TMD in turn provides a special view of chronic pain.

The clinical phenomena of TMD straddle a number of fields, and because the field began within dentistry in the 1930s, the earlier models tended toward structural theories such as how the teeth or the jaws fit together. While strong evidence against them quickly emerged, those earlier theories never disappeared—rather, they were transformed into "new" structural theories (Ohrbach 2003). Consequently, attempts to explain and treat TMD as though it were purely a structural problem have persisted, and the impact of science on clinical practice has been slow. Active structural theories for TMD include the following: missing posterior teeth, malocclusion, disharmony between the occlusion and the TMJ, too much (or too little) vertical growth of the face, and displaced disks of the TMJ (for which there is "real" evidence from magnetic resonance imaging [MRI]). For all of these structural theories, a convincing mechanism responsive to therapeutic intervention has yet to be established.

The structural models have slowly given way to a classic biomedical approach that considers the presenting history and clinical examination findings, coupled with imaging (and other tests) as needed, within the context of traditional medical disorders such as myofascial pain, spasm, dystonias, and arthritis. Mechanisms implicated by this approach include alterations in central pain-regulatory mechanisms and dysregulation of autonomic and neuroendocrine systems. TMD patients have lower pain threshold and tolerance levels when compared to matched, pain-free controls, implying central sensitization (Maixner et al. 1995, 1997). These studies suggest that patients with TMD are more sensitive to noxious stimuli and that this sensitivity is not limited to the face; such patients may have impaired endogenous opioid pain-regulatory mechanisms as well. Bragdon and colleagues (2002) found that compared to pain-free controls, TMD patients show altered endogenous analgesic functioning based on their plasma concentrations of β-endorphins. In other words, TMD patients may have greater central sensitization to pain.

Furthermore, TMD patients also have altered stress responsivity as measured by salivary and plasma cortisol. Cortisol, the principal circulating glucocorticoid, is released by the adrenal gland during acute stress. Typically, cortisol levels increase immediately after wakening and then gradually decrease throughout the day. When compared to pain-free controls, TMD patients had greater salivary cortisol increases to experimental stress than did non-pain controls (Jones et al. 1997). Furthermore, TMD patients were heterogenous with regard to salivary cortisol, comprising a group of cortisol hypersecreters and a group whose salivary cortisol was similar to that of controls. More recently, Korszun and colleagues (2002) found that TMD patients had markedly increased daytime plasma cortisol levels when compared to matched pain-free controls.

Psychological models have also been suggested to explain TMD. Patients often report muscle tension, multiple physical symptoms, and significant stress, anxiety, and depression (Dworkin 1995; Gatchel et al. 1996; Kight et al. 1999; Rollman and Gillespie 2000). The relationship between TMD pain and depression has been repeatedly explored, with much controversy surrounding the causal direction of the relationship. Von Korff and colleagues (1993) prospectively examined rates of first onset of five common pain symptoms and assessed whether premorbid depressive symptoms were associated with risk for pain onset. Participants were interviewed about their history of pain and psychological symptoms at baseline and again 3 years later. Preexisting depressive symptoms were associated with subsequent increased risk of onset for chest pain, headache pain, and possibly TMD pain, but not for back or abdominal pain. The results overall did not indicate a strong causal relationship between depression and risk for subsequent pain onset, however, because severity of depression had no influence.

In contrast, Dohrenwend et al. (1999) examined the familial prevalence of depression within first-degree relatives of patients with TMD-related myofascial pain. Prevalence of affective disorders was elevated in relatives of patients with personal histories of early-onset major depressive disorder, but not in relatives of patients with or without personal histories of early- or late-onset depression. Among the patients with myofascial face pain and depression, the TMD preceded the depression in about 40% and followed it in 44%. Although the authors suggested that living with chronic myofascial face pain contributes to elevated rates of depression, thus supporting the pain as causative, these results indicate that depression may well be a risk factor as often as it is a consequence of pain.

Cartesian duality remains alive in TMD as in other areas of medicine. The research data, however, actively support the validity and utility of transcending dualist views regarding TMD and considering both the biomedical and biobehavioral aspects of TMD simultaneously. The biopsychosocial model of TMD provides an integrated framework for generating specific physical and behavioral interventions for TMD based on both biomedical and psychosocial information (Dworkin et al. 1992). The model presumes some level of physical pathology and considers that psychological and social processes interact with the pathology to result in overt expressions of pain such as functional impairment, disability, and distress. Initial signals of nociception are subjected to higher-order perceptive and appraisal processes that interpret the nociceptive signal as painful or threatening. The result of the appraisal is a behavior, or response, that is expressed in the context of the individual's social role and environment. When these responses include treatment-seeking behaviors and style of symptom presentation in doctors' offices, discerning nociception from pain amidst the overwhelming display of pain behaviors can be very difficult. This complexity highlights the significance of perception and appraisal in understanding suffering. Dworkin and colleagues (1992) have suggested this model as a useful tool in describing the multiple processes that occur simultaneously in TMD patients and all chronic pain patients. This model is the basis for the assessment process that we propose in the next section.

ASSESSMENT OF TMD

Comprehensive assessment of TMD is necessarily based on two simultaneous perspectives: biomedical and biobehavioral. Each is appropriately stepped, depending on the findings at a prior level of evaluation. A stepped approach to assessment is cost-effective, and patients understand and appreciate assessment tailored to the severity of the problem. Moreover, a stepped treatment approach allows better selection of treatment for this complex condition whose cause is often not understandable at the outset. We use the Research Diagnostic Criteria for TMD (RDC/TMD) as the method for organizing the first level of assessment.

The RDC/TMD (Dworkin and LeResche 1992) provide a standardized system for examining and classifying the most commonly appearing subtypes of TMD. The major attributes of the RDC/TMD system that make it especially valuable in clinical research settings are: (1) a carefully documented set of specifications for conducting a systematic clinical examination for TMD; (2) operational definitions stated in measurable terms for major clinical variables (e.g., range of motion, muscle palpation pain); (3) demonstrated reliability for these operational clinical measurement methods; (4) consistent and valid diagnosis (see Table I); and (5) use of a dual-axis system.

Use of the RDC/TMD allows the practitioner to provide a physical assessment based on both objective and subjective criteria, that is, observable

Table I

Research Diagnostic Criteria for Temporomandibular Disorders (RDC/TMD)

Group I: Muscle Disorders

Ia. Myofascial pain (pain in the muscles of mastication)

    1. Pain or ache, at rest or during function, in the jaw, temples, face, preauricular area, inside the ear; plus

    2. Palpation pain in at least 3 of 20 masticatory muscle sites. Palpation pain must be at least present on the side of pain complaint

Ib. Myofascial pain with limited opening

    1. Myofascial pain, as defined above; plus

    2. Pain-free unassisted mandibular opening of less than 40 mm; plus

    3. Maximum assisted opening at least 5 mm greater than pain-free unassisted opening

Group II: Disk Displacements

IIa. Disk displacement with reduction

    1. Reciprocal clicking in the TMJ (click on both opening and closing, or a click on either opening or closing and click during lateral or protrusive excursions)

IIb. Disk displacement without reduction, with limited opening

    1. Report of significant limitation of mandibular opening; plus

    2. Maximum unassisted opening ≤35 mm; plus

    3. Passive stretch increases opening 4 mm or less beyond unassisted opening; plus

    4. Contralateral excursion <7 mm and/or uncorrected deviation to the ipsilateral side on opening; plus

    5. Absence of joint sounds, or presence of joint sounds not meeting criteria for disk displacement with reduction

IIc. Disk displacement without reduction, without limited opening

    1. Report of significant limitation of mandibular opening; plus

    2. Maximal unassisted opening >35 mm; plus

    3. Passive stretch increases opening at least 5 mm; plus

    4. Contralateral excursion ≥7 mm; plus

    5. Presence of joint sounds not meeting criteria for disk displacement with reduction; plus

    6. If joint imaging is requested, it should image the disk in closed and open mouth positions; the imaging modalities of value are arthrography and MRI

Group III: Arthralgia, Arthritis, Arthrosis

IIIa. Arthralgia (pain in the joint)

    1. Pain in one or both joint sites during palpation; plus

    2. One or more self-reports of pain in the region of the joint, pain in joint during maximum unassisted or assisted opening, or lateral excursions; plus

    3. Absence of coarse crepitus

IIIb. Osteoarthritis of the TMJ (inflammatory changes in the joint)

    1. Arthralgia (see above); plus

    2. Coarse crepitus in the joint or joint imaging showing erosions, sclerosis or condylar head or articular eminence, or flattening of the joint surfaces

IIIc. Osteoarthrosis of the TMJ (remodeling of the articulating surfaces)

    1. Absence of arthralgia; plus

    2. Coarse crepitus or joint imaging showing joint changes

Source: Dworkin and LeResche (1992).

measurement of mandibular range of motion, TMJ sounds, radiographic evidence, and subjective reports of pain on palpation of various sites in the head, face, and neck. Examination of the physical axis results in one or more TMD diagnoses within three conceptually sensible and empirically validated groups: (1) muscle disorders; (2) disk displacements; and (3) arthralgia, arthritis, or arthrosis (Table I).

In addition to the physical examination, the biomedical evaluation consists of a standard pain history that includes chief complaint, pain characteristics, modifying factors, lifetime pain and treatment history, medication usage, and comorbid pain conditions. At the time of the biomedical assessment, the patient also completes a standardized self-report questionnaire that assesses (1) symptoms and behaviors of depression, anxiety, and somatization; (2) limitations in using the jaw for mastication, drinking, speech, and emotional expression; (3) characteristic levels of present pain, and worst and average pain over the past 6 months; and (4) jaw-related disability in home, recreation, and vocation areas. This set of variables allows rapid characterization of the patient into functioning well, moderately affected by the pain, or severely affected by the pain. This information, based on reliable and valid measurement of the associated constructs, provides a classification of psychological disturbance (Dworkin and Sherman 2002; Dworkin et al. 2002b) and of the degree of interference the patient has experienced due to pain.

Based on the findings from the first level of evaluation, either the biomedical or biobehavioral assessment, or both, can be expanded. Biomedical evaluation is most commonly expanded to include an MRI of the TMJ to evaluate for the presence of displaced TMJ disks; less commonly other imaging techniques such as computed tomography (CT) will be used to rule out systemic arthritic conditions or other disorders such as tumor. When pain is acute, further evaluations will commonly assess other structures as the nociceptive source, but when pain is chronic, the history and examination as detailed within the RDC/TMD are generally adequate for a biomedical diagnosis (see Table II).

The biobehavioral assessment domain can be expanded to include more comprehensive self-report instruments, psychophysiological assessment, and semi-structured pain psychology interviews (see Table III). We typically do not use other self-report instruments, but common ones include the Minnesota Multiphasic Personality Inventory and the Multidimensional Pain Inventory (MPI). Psychophysiological assessment for TMD is by far most commonly targeted toward electromyographic measurement of the jaw muscles; while this measurement is most commonly taken at "rest," such assessments are less useful than they might seem due to poor operationalization of "rest." A more useful electromyographic assessment focuses on

Table II
Assessment methods

---

1. Biomedical Assessment
  a. Initial
     Chief complaint
     Pain characteristics
     Modifying factors
     Lifetime pain and treatment history
     Medication usage
     Comorbid pain conditions
  b. Stepped
     MRI scan
     CT scan

2. Biobehavioral Assessment
  a. Initial
     Depression, anxiety, and somatization
     Limitations in using the jaw for mastication, drinking, speech, and emotional
       expression
     Characteristic levels of present pain and of worst and average pain over prior 6
       months
     Jaw-related disability in home, recreational, and vocational areas
  b. Stepped
     More comprehensive self-report instruments
     Psychophysiological assessment
     Semi-structured pain psychology interviews

3. Integration
  a. When patients report no impact from the pain: TMD treatment should proceed
     with full attention placed on the biomedical factors
  b. When patients report moderate impact from the pain: treatment includes
     biobehavioral aspects and further assessment
  c. When patients report severe impact from the pain: pain psychology interview
     required

---

jaw postures (e.g., rest as defined by the person's usual pattern, or rest as implemented via behavioral instructions) contrasted with established patterns such as clenching, bracing, and the like, together with a stress challenge to assess muscle response patterning to stress and its cessation.

We rely extensively on the biobehavioral screening instruments listed previously. When patients report no impact from the pain—that is, they are functioning well other than having pain—TMD treatment should proceed with full attention placed on the biomedical factors. When patients report moderate impact from the pain, we recognize that treatment should include attention to the biobehavioral aspects, with the next logical step including further assessment. When patients report severe impact from the pain, we consider a pain psychology interview to be necessary before proceeding with biomedical treatment. This interview consists of the constructs listed in

Table III. However, we also recognize that patients may not be ready for a comprehensive pain psychology interview at the outset, and so the treating dentist ultimately determines the contextualization and timing of the interview (Jensen et al. 2000).

CONTEMPORARY TREATMENTS

TMD, in many respects, can be considered similar to certain aspects of headache and low back pain. Advances in each of those areas are applicable to TMD treatment. Progress in psychological management of headaches and advances in isolating the critical aspects of treatment for acute low back pain are particularly useful. Unique characteristics of TMD warrant specific treatments or modifications of treatments, however.

Medical treatments for TMD consist of the usual medications prescribed for any chronic musculoskeletal pain. These drugs include analgesics such as nonsteroidal anti-inflammatory drugs (NSAIDs), opioids, and acetaminophen; muscle relaxants; and anxiolytic medications. NSAIDs are useful for acute pain, but they rapidly lose their efficacy for chronic pain. Indeed, few randomized clinical trials have been performed using NSAIDs for chronic muscle pain. The other analgesic class often considered for TMD pain is opioid combination drugs; the attraction is better analgesia with fewer gastric complications (from NSAIDs) or liver problems (from acetaminophen). Patients report better pain relief, however, from controlling factors that precipitate pain episodes and from using relaxation as a coping method for pain flare-ups. As such, we find analgesics of little value for chronic TMD of muscular origin, except at the outset of treatment to immediately reduce some nociception while the patient begins to use other treatments.

Relaxants are commonly used for TMD, but their best efficacy may come from bedtime dosing for individuals with nocturnal bruxism. For bruxism, short-term anxiolytic medications are also useful. Tricyclic medications have been advocated as a long-term medication approach to nocturnal bruxism, but the evidence remains weak, consistent with our clinical observations. There are, however, individuals who respond very positively to such agents (e.g., amitriptyline 25 mg at bedtime), with a consistent report of reduced pain and improved sleep. Bruxism is now believed to emerge from multiple causes such as trauma, pain, developmental causes, stress, behavioral causes, and even stroke; several of these causes are perhaps better assessed as part of an overall biobehavioral evaluation, with a goal of integrating biobehavioral treatment with pharmacological treatment to achieve better efficacy than either modality can provide alone.

Table III
Biobehavioral interview questions

Pain Characteristics
1. Where do you experience the pain?
2. When did the pain problem begin?
3. How did the pain problem begin?
4. Describe what your life was like when the pain began.
5. Since the pain began, has it stayed the same, gotten better, or gotten worse?
6. Is there a daily pattern to the pain? Is it better in the morning? Afternoon? Evening?
7. What makes it better?
8. What makes it worse?

Pain Coping
9. What have you tried for the pain, and how effective has each treatment been?
   a. Do you have other ways of coping with the pain?
   b. Have you tried relaxation? What is its effect?
   c. Are there particular thoughts or beliefs associated with your pain or the flare-ups?
   d. How do you communicate pain to your significant other?
   e. Does emotional stress make it worse? Or do you notice a relationship between the pain and stress?
10. How do you manage pain flare-ups?
11. When you're feeling a little better do you try to catch up on things by doing a lot of work? Or when you're having a flare-up do you do less of your usual activities?

Disability and Operant Behaviors
12. What does the pain prevent you from doing?
   a. What are you doing more of since the pain began?
   b. What are you doing less of since the pain began?
   c. How has your overall activity been affected?
13. What would you like to get back to doing if the pain was decreased?

Medical History
14. What medications are you currently using?
   a. How often do you take each medication?
   b. Under what circumstances do you take more than you should?
   c. Are you concerned about using too much medication?
15. How is the rest of your health? Other chronic conditions?
16. Who do you see for these conditions?

Explanatory Model
17. What is your explanation for everything that has been going on?
18. What do you think has to be done to relieve the pain?

Of greater therapeutic utility are physical medicine procedures, including stretching and other muscle exercises, thermal agents, and physical therapy. The basic stretching exercise for TMD pain is elongation of the jaw-closing muscles. Applying thermal agents with stretching improves the stretch and decreases pain. Physical therapy referrals are best oriented toward either

Table III
Continued

Developmental History

19. Where were you born and raised?
20. Were you raised by both parents?
21. How would you describe your home life growing up?
22. How many siblings do you have?
23. What is your relationship now with your parents? Siblings?
24. Is there any history in your family of chronic pain or illness?
25. Is there any history in your family of substance abuse?
26. Is there any history in your family of sexual, verbal, physical abuse or neglect?
27. Is there any history in your family of emotional or mental disorders?

Education and Work History

28. What is your educational background?
29. Please describe your work history.
30. Do you not work due to pain or have you limited your work due to pain?
31. Is there any litigation going on right now or in the past regarding your pain or injury?
32. Are you receiving any workers' compensation or public assistance payments?

Living Status

33. Who do you currently live with?
34. What is your marital status?
35. Any children? Their ages?
36. How would you describe the relationship with your significant other/children?
37. How has the pain affected the relationship with your significant other/children?
38. Is there an impact on sex in the relationship with your significant other?
39. Is there an impact on how you relate to the children?
40. How does/do your significant other/children respond when you are in pain or are having a flare-up?

local treatment for a myofascial condition, or cervical evaluation and treatment due to comorbidity of masticatory myofascial pain and cervical problems, but with a long-term goal of a home-based management program. How patients approach these simple exercises, however, ranges enormously. Common patterns include overstretching and ignoring pain, understretching or avoidance of stretching, insistence on immediate results and abandoning the exercise when results fail to appear, or cyclic use of the exercise. Thus, stretching and toning exercises, while classically considered to be a physical treatment, are often best implemented as a biobehavioral treatment. The results, in addition to improved mobility and decreased pain, include improved self-efficacy and mastery with respect to self-management of pain.

Intraoral appliances are commonly used for treating TMD. While such appliances are often implemented for diurnal wear, we believe that behavioral approaches are far superior. The main application of intraoral appliances is for nocturnal bruxism; their efficacy is generally accepted, although much remains to be better understood. Simple nightguards made from hard acrylic have remained a well-founded treatment; recent studies question whether the appliance needs to be custom made of hard acrylic or can be made from athletic mouth guards; obviously, the latter option is far cheaper. Only one randomized controlled trial (RCT) has successfully shown the equivalent efficacy of both soft and hard nightguards (Truelove et al. 1999), however, and more research is needed before we can make a full recommendation for that type of treatment. Another type of intraoral appliance (the so-called repositioning appliance) is often recommended, but we lack outcomes evidence for this approach, and we believe that such appliances have little use in adults. Moreover, such approaches can cause significant and unnecessary complications.

This short review of accepted medical treatments is intended to highlight the importance of considering the application of biobehavioral treatment concepts in TMD treatment. See Table IV for a listing of standard

Table IV
Standard treatment approaches for TMD

A. *Primarily Medical*
  a. Medications:
     Analgesics (NSAIDs, acetaminophen, opioid combinations)
     Muscle relaxants
     Anxiolytics
     Tricyclic antidepressants
  b. Physical medicine:
     Stretching and other exercises
     Thermal agents
     Physical therapy
     Intraoral appliances for use during sleep

B. *Primarily Biobehavioral*
  a. All of the above
  b. Biofeedback
  c. Relaxation
  d. Structured cognitive-behavioral programs:
     Education
     Practicing self-management activities
     Pacing
     Managing activities
     Monitoring medication usage patterns
     Generalizing relaxation skills to other settings
     Controlling anger
     Managing stress
     Overcoming nonproductive beliefs about pain
     Increasing health-promoting/pleasurable activities
     Preventing relapse

treatment approaches for TMD. All listed medical treatments for TMD are targets for using behavioral methods as well. Although this overlap is also recognized in other chronic pain areas, it is particularly salient for TMD because of the biological primacy of the masticatory system and its significant emotional links.

The primary psychologically oriented approaches include biofeedback, relaxation, and structured cognitive-behavioral treatment. The evidence for biofeedback in the treatment of TMD is as good, if not better than, for any other chronic pain condition. The rationale for using biofeedback in TMD is to help develop competing behaviors as a way to avoid diurnal parafunction. Crider and Glaros (1999) conducted a meta-analysis of treatments using biofeedback for TMD and concluded that a significantly greater proportion of patients treated with biofeedback (69% versus 35%) reported being symptom free or greatly improved when compared to patients treated with a variety of placebo interventions.

The evidence for general relaxation is also excellent. Rather than making the common comparison of biofeedback versus relaxation, we find that each treatment has its place. Biofeedback is often useful as a single session for individuals with TMD pain to learn basic skills in generalizing full relaxation from the experience acquired from a targeted muscle. It is notable how difficult it can be for some individuals to understand the sensations and goals associated with jaw (or bodily) relaxation, and how easy it is for providers to be dismayed due to lack of treatment progress from relaxation training; biofeedback can facilitate this process and at the same time can give important feedback to the provider in terms of patient style. Another method is teaching specific relaxation of the jaw using behavioral means such as teaching a competing response. The other approach to relaxation is general relaxation skills, taught by a variety of methods; the keys to the successful implementation of this method as a pain therapy seem to include whether the patient maintains a daily practice so that he or she can apply the basic learned skills in life situations such as psychophysiological stress responses or pain flare-ups.

Because many individuals have difficulty in applying basic relaxation skills to life situations, cognitive-behavioral treatment helps address problems with pacing, activity management, medication usage patterns, generalizability of relaxation skills to other settings, anger control, stress management, and overcoming nonproductive beliefs about pain. Recently, Mishra and colleagues (2000) and Gardea and colleagues (2001) have examined the efficacy of biofeedback, cognitive-behavioral therapy, and a combined biofeedback and cognitive-behavioral intervention in patients with chronic TMD. Biofeedback alone was found to be the most effective treatment for reducing TMD pain immediately after treatment (Mishra et al. 2000). At 1 year follow-up the combined biofeedback and cognitive-behavioral therapy group showed the most improvement in TMD pain, pain-related disability, and mandibular functioning.

In sum, treatment for chronic TMD pain is more successful when the level of treatment is matched to the severity of the individual's biobehavioral status. The specific physical diagnosis appears to have less influence on outcome, assuming that the standard level of medical care is provided; a core set of standard medical treatments is remarkably consistent for its utility across the different TMD diagnoses.

A NOVEL APPROACH TO TREATMENT OF TMD

We have reviewed numerous medical and psychological approaches to the treatment of TMD and would like to conclude with an evidence-based recommendation for treatment that appreciates individual differences in our patients. This approach combines two treatment modalities established in the chronic pain field, namely minimal-contact interventions (Penzien and Holroyd 1994; Von Korff 1999) and treatment matching based on psychosocial profiles (Rudy et al. 1989).

In an early study, Dworkin and colleagues (1994) compared a minimal-contact cognitive-behavioral intervention in addition to usual care, in comparison to usual care alone. The cognitive-behavioral intervention was presented in a group format of two sessions over the course of 2 weeks and consisted of education about masticatory system functioning and the nature of TMD, followed by education in and practice of relaxation exercises. These sessions were led by a psychologist and a dentist. This treatment was compared to usual dental treatment that consisted of use of a flat-plane occlusal appliance, NSAID medication, passive and active range of jaw motion exercises, modification of parafunctional activity, modification of food texture, and use of thermal agents. Patients receiving the minimal cognitive-behavioral intervention followed by usual care showed greater decreases in pain levels and interference at 1-year follow-up than did patients receiving only usual treatment.

Other minimal interventions have been successful for TMD as well. For the management of myofascial TMD pain, Carlson and colleagues (2001) examined the effectiveness of a two-session, dentist-based skills-training program that involved breathing, postural relaxation, and proprioceptive re-education. This intervention was compared with standard dental care that included a flat-plane intraoral appliance and self-care instructions. Although at 6 weeks pain and interference outcomes were improved for both groups, at 26 weeks the physical self-regulation group reported less pain and greater mobility than did the group receiving standard care, demonstrating the power of implementing biobehavioral concepts taught by the biomedical clinician.

More recently, Townsen and colleagues (2001) utilized an oral habit-reversal treatment in a minimal-therapist-contact intervention delivered by phone and e-mail. Results from 10 females suffering from TMD were compared to a wait-list group, and the results showed that the habit-reversal treatment significantly reduced maladaptive oral habits and led to statistically and clinically significant improvements in mean weekly pain ratings, number of pain-free days per week, and highest weekly pain ratings. Significant reductions in life stress and pain interference were observed following treatment.

While results from minimal-contact interventions in TMD and other chronic pain conditions are compelling, a subsample of the clinic population remains that utilizes considerable health care, has significant psychosocial disability in response to pain, and exhibits elevated levels of depression and somatization. While the results from brief cognitive-behavioral interventions are impressive, Dworkin et al. (1994) and McCreary et al. (1991) noted that those patients who initially reported high levels of pain and interference with daily activities (i.e., dysfunctional chronic pain patients) and those patients initially high in somatization did not benefit from the brief cognitive-behavioral intervention. This led investigators to consider an approach that appreciates the need to match treatment to patients based on psychosocial characteristics as well as medical characteristics (Table V).

The management of TMD depends on the type of biomedical disorder. Guidelines for general biomedical management are available (e.g., Ohrbach and Burgess 1999). However, as with many other chronic conditions, behavioral, psychological, and psychosocial factors are often more predictive of illness outcome than are objective indications and physical pathology (McCreary et al. 1991; Dworkin et al. 1994; Ohrbach and Dworkin 1998). In much the same way that TMD is a heterogeneous group of physical conditions, our patients present with a multitude of psychosocial characteristics. Some patients need minimal education, support, and guidance because they are relatively functional and are coping adaptively; this care is best provided by the biomedical clinician in the context of appropriate biomedical treatments. Other patients, however, may lack coping skills, may be depressed or otherwise disabled, and may need more intensive contact with clinicians skilled in applying biobehavioral treatment concepts to pain disorders.

An appreciation of psychosocial characteristics has guided programmatic research over the last 10 years. In our own laboratory, we have

Table V
Novel treatment approaches for TMD

Minimal Contact Approaches
  1. Psychologist and dentist led
     Group format
     Two sessions at weekly intervals
     Primary focus is TMD education and relaxation training
     Followed by usual physical treatments
  2. Dentist led
     Two sessions
     Primary focus is breathing, postural relaxation, and proprioceptive re-education

Integrated Approach
  Intraoral appliance, biofeedback, stress management

Structured Biobehavioral Program
  1. Dental hygienist-based
     Three treatment sessions and two telephone follow-up calls
     Focus includes:
         Education about TMD
         Guided reading with structured feedback
         General relaxation and stress management training
         Development of a personal care plan to reduce, in a structured manner, stress
             and response patterns to stressors
         Maintenance and relapse prevention
  2. Psychologist-based
     Six-session cognitive-behavioral therapy intervention delivered by a pain
         psychologist in conjunction with usual TMD treatment
     Cognitive-behavioral therapy includes:
         Education about the biopsychosocial model of TMD and the gate control
             theory of chronic pain
         Training in abdominal breathing and progressive muscle relaxation
         Stress management and cognitive restructuring to reduce depressive thoughts
             and behaviors
         Education about pacing and relapse
         Structured homework assignments to assess compliance and reinforce session
             information and practice

---

investigated the validity and clinical utility of the RDC/TMD in identifying subsamples of TMD clinic cases and in treating patients in light of these differences. In previous studies (Dworkin et al. 2002a) we found it useful to characterize TMD patients with Graded Chronic Pain (GCP) scale scores in the Grades I–II range as "psychosocially functional." These patients typically show minimal psychological distress and pain-related interference in the personal, social, and work domains of their lives. In contrast, we have demonstrated that patients classified within Grades III and IV show psychosocial dysfunction that includes high levels of functional disability and depression.

Recognizing the importance of distinguishing levels of psychosocial dysfunction has led to a more targeted approach for TMD treatment. A focus has recently emerged on developing treatments for chronic pain that target specific patient characteristics (Turk et al. 1996; Sherman and Turk 2001). Initial attempts at tailoring TMD treatments were conducted by Turk, Rudy, and colleagues, who found that integrating cognitive-behavioral methods with components of usual TMD care in patient-treatment matching paradigms was more effective than usual treatment alone. Using the MPI to distinguish dysfunctional, interpersonally distressed, and adaptive coping subgroups of TMD patients, Rudy et al. (1989) evaluated differential responses of the subgroups to conservative treatment consisting of an intraoral appliance, biofeedback, and stress management. The results demonstrated that TMD patients significantly improved and maintained the improvements on physical, psychosocial, and behavioral measures. Comparisons across MPI profiles revealed differential patterns of improvement. Notably, the dysfunctional patients showed significantly greater improvements in pain intensity, perceived impact of TMD on their lives, and depression compared with the interpersonally distressed and adaptive coping groups. These findings support the clinical utility of a psychosocial-behavioral classification system that goes beyond medical diagnosis alone, and suggest that individualizing treatments based upon each patient's adaptation to pain may improve treatment efficacy.

Recently, Dworkin and colleagues (2002a,c) completed two RCTs specifically targeted at patients' psychosocial profiles independent of their biomedical diagnosis. In the first study (Dworkin et al. 2002a), subjects with psychosocially functional profiles, that is, GCP scores at II or below, were randomized either into a self-care group where treatment was delivered by a dental hygienist or to a customary treatment group where care was delivered by a dentist. The hygienist sessions included: (1) education about TMD; (2) guided reading with structured feedback; (3) general relaxation and stress management training; (4) development of a personal care plan to reduce, in a structured manner, stress and response patterns to stressors; and (5) maintenance and relapse prevention. These components were delivered over the course of three treatment sessions and two telephone follow-up calls. At the 1-year follow-up evaluation, those participating in the self-care program showed significantly decreased TMD pain, less pain-related interference, and fewer masticatory muscles found to be painful on clinical examination as compared to those randomized to receive the usual TMD treatment.

Concurrent with the prior study, Dworkin and colleagues (2002c) conducted an RCT tailored specifically to TMD patients whose GCP score indicated psychosocially dysfunctional functioning (Grades III and IV). The dysfunctional subgroup of TMD patients was randomized to receive either a six-session cognitive-behavioral intervention delivered by a pain psychologist in conjunction with usual TMD treatment, or to the usual conservative treatment delivered by a dentist specializing in TMD. Cognitive-behavioral therapy included education about the biopsychosocial model of TMD and the gate control theory of chronic pain; training in abdominal breathing and progressive muscle relaxation; stress management and cognitive restructuring to reduce depressive thoughts and behaviors; education about pacing and relapse; and structured homework assignments to assess compliance and reinforce session information and practice. After treatment the comprehensive care group, when compared to the usual treatment group, showed significantly lower levels of pain intensity, significantly higher self-reported ability to control TMD pain, and a strong trend toward lower pain-related activity interference.

Reliable and valid identification of subgroups of TMD patients based on psychosocial axes, together with the results from the cognitive-behavioral interventions and minimal interventions showing significant but different effectiveness in individuals with different psychosocial profiles, suggests a need to tailor treatment to the individual with TMD. It seems reasonable to hypothesize that treatments matched to patient characteristics will be both more clinically effective and more cost effective. The dental setting affords a unique opportunity for delivery of self-care management for psychosocially functional patients. Dental hygienists are often trained as patient educators with respect to oral health behavior change, and with additional training they could provide self-care management education for those with TMD. While the relative costs of providing a dentist-based self-care training program may be prohibitive, a dental hygienist, working under the supervision of a dentist, could provide care that might be more efficacious and cost-effective.

CONCLUSIONS

The practical implications of this chapter can be summarized as follows: (1) Patients with TMD are probably best treated by a specialist dentist rather than a nonspecialist dentist, because the former will be more likely to use a greater range of reversible treatments and to minimize or eliminate the complications that ensue with disturbing frequency following more aggressive treatments. (2) Aggressive treatments for TMD are without evidential support. (3) Patients with TMD receiving treatment from a specialist dentist should simultaneously be monitored for signs of behavioral or psychological dysregulation; if the specialist dentist does not address those issues, the primary physician should consider whether they are important for inclusion in overall management of the patient. (4) Level of behavioral and psychological dysregulation is an important and highly useful assessment variable, and essentially, patients can be classified into three groups: well-functioning, somewhat impacted, and significantly impacted. Many self-report instruments can provide information suitable for this classification; we favor either the GCP or the MPI, supplemented by a general measure of behavior and mood (such as the Beck Depression Inventory or the Symptom Checklist-90 [SCL-90]). (5) Patients with moderate behavioral and psychosocial impact will benefit from basic relaxation skills, education about pain and nociception, and information about managing flare-ups. In the dental setting, these skills can be delivered by a dental hygienist. (6) Patients with significant behavioral and psychosocial impact will benefit from structured treatment with a psychologist or other mental health provider trained in the use of cognitive-behavioral treatment methods applied to pain conditions.

REFERENCES

Bragdon EE, Light KC, Costello NL, et al. Group differences in pain modulation: pain-free women compared to pain-free men and to women with TMD. *Pain* 2002; 96:227–237.

Carlson CR, Bertrand PM, Ehrlich AD, Maxwell AW, Burton RG. Physical self-regulation training for the management of temporomandibular disorders. *J Orofac Pain* 2001; 15:47–55.

Crider AB, Glaros AG. A meta-analysis of the EMG biofeedback treatment of temporomandibular disorders. *J Orofac Pain* 1999; 13(1):29–37.

Dohrenwend BP, Raphael KG, Marbach JJ, Gallagher RM. Why is depression comorbid with chronic myofascial face pain? A family study test of alternative hypotheses. *Pain* 1999; 83:183–192.

Drangsholt M, LeResche L. Temporomandibular disorder pain. In: Crombie IK, Croft PR, Linton SJ, LeResche L, Von Korff M (Eds). *Epidemiology of Pain.* Seattle: IASP Press, 2000, pp 203–233.

Dworkin SF. Behavioral characteristics of chronic temporomandibular disorders: diagnosis and assessment. In: Sessle BJ, Bryant PS, Dionne RA (Eds). *Temporomandibular Disorders and Related Pain Conditions,* Progress in Pain Research and Management, Vol. 4. Seattle: IASP Press, 1995, pp 175–192.

Dworkin SF, LeResche L. Research diagnostic criteria for temporomandibular disorders: review, criteria, examinations and specifications, critique. *J Craniomandib Disord* 1992; 6:301–355.

Dworkin SF, Sherman JJ. Relying on objective and subjective measures of chronic pain: guidelines for use and interpretation. In: Turk DC, Melzack R (Eds). *Handbook of Pain Assessment.* New York: Guilford Press, 2002, pp 619–638.

Dworkin SF, Von Korff M, LeResche L. Epidemiologic studies of chronic pain: a dynamic-ecologic perspective. *Ann Behav Med* 1992; 14:3–11.

Dworkin SF, Turner JA, Wilson L, et al. Brief group cognitive-behavioral intervention for temporomandibular disorders. *Pain* 1994; 59:175–187.

Dworkin SF, Huggins KH, Wilson L, et al. A randomized clinical trial using research diagnostic criteria for temporomandibular disorders axis II to target clinic cases for a tailored self-care TMD treatment program. *J Orofac Pain* 2002a; 16(1):48–63.

Dworkin SF, Sherman J, Mancl L, et al. Reliability, validity, and clinical utility of the research diagnostic criteria for Temporomandibular Disorders Axis II Scales: depression, non-specific physical symptoms, and graded chronic pain. *J Orofac Pain* 2002b; 16(3):207–220.

Dworkin SF, Turner JA, Mancl L, et al. A randomized clinical trial of a tailored comprehensive care treatment program for temporomandibular disorders. *J Orofac Pain* 2002c; 16(4):259–276.

Gardea MA, Gatchel RJ, Mishra KD. Long-term efficacy of biobehavioral treatment of temporomandibular disorders. *J Behav Med* 2001; 24:341–359.

Gatchel RJ, Garafalo JP, Ellis E, Holt C. Major psychological disorders in acute and chronic TMD: an initial examination. *J Am Dent Assoc* 1996; 127:1365–1374.

Goulet JP, Lavigne GJ, Lund JP. Jaw pain prevalence among French speaking Canadians in Quebec and related symptoms of temporomandibular disorders. *J Dent Res* 1995; 74:1738–1744.

Jensen MP, Nielson WR, Romano JM, Hill ML, Turner JA. Further evaluation of the Pain Stages of Change Questionnaire: is the transtheoretical model of change useful for patients with chronic pain? *Pain* 2000; 86:255–264.

Jones DA, Rollman GB, Brook RI. The cortisol response to psychological stress in temporomandibular dysfunction. *Pain* 1997; 72:171–182.

Kight M, Gatchel RJ, Wesley L. Temporomandibular disorders: evidence for significant overlap with psychopathology. *Health Psychol* 1999; 18:177–182.

Korszun A, Young EA, Singer K, et al. Basal circadian cortisol secretion in women with temporomandibular disorders. *J Dent Res* 2002; 81:279–283.

Maixner W, Fillingim R, Booker D, Sigurdsson A. Sensitivity of patients with temporomandibular disorders to experimentally evoked pain. *Pain* 1995; 63:85–102.

Maixner W, Fillingim R, Kincaid S, Sigurdsson A, Harris MB. Relationship between pain sensitivity and resting arterial blood pressure in patients with temporomandibular disorders. *Psychosom Med* 1997; 59:503–511.

McCreary CP, Clark GT, Merril RL, Flack V, Oakley ME. Psychological distress and diagnostic subgroups of temporomandibular disorder patients. *Pain* 1991; 44:29–34.

Mishra KD, Gatchel RJ, Gardea MA. The relative efficacy of three cognitive-behavioral treatment approaches to temporomandibular disorders. *J Behav Med* 2000; 23:293–309.

Ohrbach R. Temporomandibular disorders: conceptualization and diagnostic frameworks. *Alpha Omegan* 2003; 96:15–19.

Ohrbach R, Burgess J. Temporomandibular disorders and orofacial pain. In: Rakel RE (Ed). *Conn's Current Therapy,* 51st ed. Philadelphia: W.B. Saunders, 1999, pp 997–1004.

Ohrbach R, Dworkin SF. Longitudinal changes in TMD: relationship of changes in pain to changes in clinical and psychological variables. *Pain* 1998; 74:315–326.

Penzien DB, Holroyd KA. Psychosocial interventions in the management of recurrent headache disorders: description of treatment techniques. *Behav Med* 1994; 20:64–73.

Rollman GB, Gillespie JM. The role of psychosocial factors in temporomandibular disorders. *Curr Rev Pain* 2000; 4:71–81.

Rudy TE, Turk DC, Zaki HS, Curtin HD. An empirical taxometric alternative to traditional classification of temporomandibular disorders. *Pain* 1989; 36:311–320.

Sherman JJ, Turk DC. Nonpharmacologic approaches to the management of myofascial temporomandibular disorders. *Curr Pain Headache Rep* 2001; 5(5):421–431.

Townsen D, Nicholson RA, Buenaver L, Bush F, Gramling S. Use of a habit reversal treatment for temporomandibular pain in a minimal therapist contact format. *J Behav Ther Exp Psychiatry* 2001; 32:221–239.

Truelove EL. Temporomandibular disorders. In: Eversole LR, Truelove EL (Eds). *Essentials of Oral Medicine*. Hamilton, ON: B.C. Decker, 2001, pp 311–325.

Truelove EL, Huggins KH, Dworkin SF, et al. RCT of splint treatment in TMD: 12-month self report outcomes. *J Dent Res* 1999; 78:292.

Turk DC, Rudy TE, Kubinski JA, Zaki HS, Greco C. Dysfunctional TMD patients: evaluating the efficacy of a tailored treatment protocol. *J Consult Clin Psychol* 1996; 64:139–146.

Von Korff M. Pain management in primary care: an individualized stepped-care approach. In: Gatchel RJ, Turk DC (Eds). *Psychosocial Factors in Pain: Critical Perspectives*. New York: Guilford Press, 1999, pp 360–373.

Von Korff M, Dworkin SF, LeResche L, Kruger A. An epidemiologic comparison of pain complaints. *Pain* 1988; 32:173–183.

Von Korff M, LeResche L, Dworkin SF. First onset of common pain symptoms: a prospective study of depression as a risk factor. *Pain* 1993; 55:251–258.

Correspondence to: Richard Ohrbach, DDS, PhD, Department of Oral Diagnostic Sciences, 355 Squire Hall, University at Buffalo, Buffalo, NY 14214, USA. Tel: 716-829-3590; Fax: 716-829-3554; email: ohrbach@buffalo.edu.

Psychosocial Aspects of Pain: A Handbook for Health Care Providers, Progress in Pain Research and Management, Vol. 27, edited by Robert H. Dworkin and William S. Breitbart, IASP Press, Seattle, © 2004.

19

Psychological and Psychiatric Dimensions of Palliative Care

William S. Breitbart[a,b] and David K. Payne[a,b]

[a]Department of Psychiatry and Behavioral Sciences, Memorial Sloan-Kettering Cancer Center, and [b]Weill Medical College, Cornell University, New York, New York, USA

In the palliative care setting, the management of symptoms becomes the paramount mandate as quality of life becomes the principal goal. Of the most common symptoms, pain represents one of the greatest challenges to the maintenance of quality of life in patients with advanced cancer or acquired immunodeficiency syndrome (AIDS). To provide adequate relief of such pain, a multidisciplinary approach is indicated in which neurologists, neurosurgeons, anesthesiologists, pain management specialists, and physiatrists play a role (Foley 1978, 1985; Breitbart and Holland 1990). With the awareness of the impact of psychological factors in the management of pain, the utilization of psychiatric interventions in the treatment of cancer and AIDS patients with pain and psychological distress has now become an integral part of such a comprehensive approach (Massie and Holland 1987; Breitbart 1989, 1990b).

THE SCOPE OF THE PROBLEM: PREVALENCE OF PAIN IN CANCER AND AIDS

Unfortunately, pain represents one of the most common symptoms in cancer patients, with approximately 70% of patients experiencing severe pain at some time in the course of their illness (Foley 1985), nearly 75% of patients with advanced cancer having pain (Bonica 1990), and 25% of cancer patients dying in severe pain (Twycross and Lack 1983). Variability in the prevalence of pain exists among different types of cancer. Whereas only around 5% of leukemia patients experience pain during the course of their illness, 50–75% of patients with tumors of the lung, gastrointestinal tract, or genitourinary system experience significant pain. The prevalence of pain is highest in patients with cancers of the bone or cervix, with as many as 85% of patients experiencing significant pain during the course of their illness (Foley 1978). Despite its prevalence, pain in patients with cancer and AIDS remains frequently underdiagnosed and inadequately treated (Marks and Sachar 1973; Foley 1985). Although pain represents a significant threat to their quality of life, cancer patients suffer from an average of three additional troubling physical symptoms (Grond et al. 1994). A thorough understanding of a patient's symptom burden allows for a more complete understanding of the impact of pain for each individual.

In patients with AIDS, pain is frequently significant and often neglected, with estimates of its prevalence ranging from 40% to 60%, increasing as the disease progresses (Singer et al. 1993). Studies suggest that over 50% of hospitalized patients with AIDS require treatment for pain and that pain is the presenting complaint in 30%, second only to fever (Lebovits et al. 1989). Pain varies in location and quality, with chest pain occurring in 22%, headache in 13%, oral cavity pain in 11%, abdominal pain in 9%, and peripheral neuropathy in 6%. A retrospective review of pain in an AIDS population reported that 15% of patients had either abdominal pain, peripheral neuropathy, or Kaposi's sarcoma (Newshan et al. 1993). Other reviews report that between 5% and 30% of AIDS patients have painful peripheral neuropathy (Snider et al. 1983; Levy et al. 1985; Cornblath and McArthur 1988). In a descriptive study of pain in advanced AIDS, 53% of patients surveyed had pain, with peripheral neuropathy, abdominal pain, headache, and Kaposi's sarcoma being most common (Schofferman and Brody 1990). Even in ambulatory AIDS patients, 43% of patients reported pain of at least 2 weeks' duration (Breitbart 1996). Painful neuropathy accounted for 50% of pain diagnoses, and lower-extremity pain related to Kaposi's sarcoma was found in 45%. While neuropathic pains are an important clinical problem that has attracted a great deal of attention, the evolving literature on AIDS pain syndromes suggests that pains of somatic and visceral etiologies are more prominent in AIDS. Recent work suggests that of the pains experienced by ambulatory patients with AIDS, approximately 33% are somatic, 35% are visceral, and 33% are neuropathic. In addition, somatic, visceral, and neuropathic pains often occur concurrently, and neuropathic pain is not often the predominant pain (Hewitt et al. 1997).

MULTIDIMENSIONAL CONCEPT OF PAIN
IN TERMINAL ILLNESS

Pain in terminal conditions such as advanced cancer and AIDS, rather than being a purely nociceptive or physical experience, involves complex aspects of human functioning, including personality, affect, cognition, behavior, and social relations (Stiefel 1993). Cicely Saunders coined the term "total pain" to capture the all-encompassing nature of this experience (Saunders 1966). Consequently, analgesic drugs alone do not always lead to pain relief (Hanks 1991), and a more recent study (Syrjala and Chapko 1995) suggests that psychological factors play a modest but important role in pain intensity. The interaction of cognitive, emotional, socioenvironmental, and nociceptive aspects of pain shown in Fig. 1 illustrates the multidimensional nature of pain in terminal illness and suggests the importance of multimodal interventions (Breitbart and Holland 1990). The challenge of untangling and addressing both the physical and psychological issues involved in pain is essential to developing rational and effective management strategies. Psychosocial therapies directed primarily at psychological variables have a profound impact on nociception, while somatic therapies directed at nociception have beneficial effects on the psychological aspects of pain. Ideally, such somatic and psychosocial therapies are used simultaneously in the multidisciplinary approach to pain management in the terminally ill (Breitbart 1989).

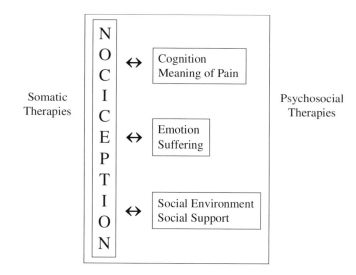

Fig. 1. The multidimensional nature of pain in terminal illness.

PSYCHOLOGICAL FACTORS IN THE PAIN EXPERIENCE

The patient with cancer or AIDS faces many stressors during the course of illness including dependency, disability, and fear of painful death. Such fears are universal; however, the level of psychological distress is variable and depends on medical factors, social supports, coping capacities, and personality. Pain has profound effects on psychological distress in cancer patients, and psychological factors such as anxiety, depression, and the meaning of pain can intensify cancer pain experience. Cancer patients who attribute a new pain to an unrelated benign cause report less interference with activities of daily living and quality of life than do patients who believe that their pain represents progression of disease (Daut and Cleeland 1982). Spiegel and Bloom (1983b) found that women with metastatic breast cancer experience more intense pain if they believe that their pain represents spread of their cancer, and if they are depressed. Beliefs about the meaning of pain and the presence of a mood disturbance are better predictors of level of pain than is the site of metastasis.

Psychosocial variables affect pain in three domains: (1) physical well-being; (2) psychological well-being, consisting of affective factors, cognitive factors, spiritual factors, communication, coping, and the meaning of pain or cancer; and (3) interpersonal well-being, focusing on social support or role functioning (Padilla et al. 1990). In advanced cancer, patients with less anxiety and depression are less likely to report pain (Bond and Pearson 1969; McKegney et al. 1981). A prospective study of cancer patients found that maladaptive coping strategies, lower levels of self-efficacy, and distress specific to the treatment or disease progression were modest but significant predictors of reports of pain intensity (Syrjala and Chapko 1995).

Psychological variables including perceived control over pain, emotional associations with pain, memories of pain, fear of death, depression, anxiety, and hopelessness contribute to the experience of pain in persons with AIDS and can increase suffering (Breitbart et al. 1994). Negative thoughts related to pain are associated with greater pain intensity, psychological distress, and disability in ambulatory patients with AIDS (Payne et al. 1994). Pain appears to have a profound impact on levels of emotional distress and disability. In a pilot study of the impact of pain on ambulatory patients with human immunodeficiency virus (HIV) (Vogl et al. 1999), depression was significantly correlated with the presence of pain. In addition to being significantly more distressed and depressed, 40% of those with pain had suicidal ideation compared to only 20% of those without pain. HIV-infected patients with pain were more functionally impaired, and such functional interference was highly correlated to levels of pain intensity and depression. Those who felt that pain represented a threat to their health reported more intense pain than did those who did not see pain as a threat. Patients with pain were more likely to be unemployed or disabled, and they reported less social support. Singer and colleagues (1993) also reported an association among the frequency of multiple pains, increased disability, and higher levels of depression. A review of the literature examining the relationships between chronic cancer-related pain and psychological distress, social support, and coping strategies suggests that the role of psychological distress in the experience of pain is significant, the role of social support is moderate, and the impact of coping strategies on cancer-related pain is inconclusive (Zaza and Baine 2002).

Not uncommonly, pain that has not responded to somatic therapies is attributed to psychological factors when in fact medical factors have not been adequately appreciated. When the psychiatrist or psychologist is asked to consult on pain management issues in patients with cancer or AIDS, they need to assess whether an accurate pain diagnosis has been made and whether medical analgesic management is adequate. In general, psychological distress in terminally ill patients with pain must initially be assumed to be the consequence of uncontrolled pain. Personality factors may be quite distorted by the presence of pain, and relief of pain often results in the disappearance of a perceived psychiatric disorder (Marks and Sachar 1973; Cleeland and Tearnan 1986).

PSYCHIATRIC DISORDERS AND PAIN IN THE TERMINALLY ILL

An increased frequency of psychiatric disorders is found in cancer patients with pain. The Psychosocial Collaborative Oncology Group Study (Derogatis et al. 1983) examined the prevalence of psychiatric disorders in cancer patients, finding that of the patients who received a psychiatric diagnosis (see Table I), 39% reported significant pain, while only 19% of patients without a psychiatric diagnosis had significant pain. The psychiatric disorders most commonly seen in cancer patients with pain include adjustment disorder with depressed or anxious mood (69%) and major depression (15%). Similar findings of increased frequency of psychiatric disturbance in cancer pain patients has been reported elsewhere (Woodforde and Fielding 1970; Ahles et al. 1983).

A case in point is the diagnosis of epidural spinal cord compression (ESCC), a common neurological complication of systemic cancer that occurs in 5–10% of patients with cancer and can often involve severe pain.

Table I
Rates of psychiatric disorders and prevalence of pain observed
in 215 cancer patients from three cancer centers

Diagnostic Category	Number in Diagnostic Class	Percentage of Psychiatric Diagnoses	Number with Significant Pain*
Adjustment disorders	69	32	68
Major affective disorders	13	6	13
Organic mental disorders	8	4	8
Personality disorders	7	3	7
Anxiety disorders	4	2	4
Total with psychiatric diagnosis	101	47	39 (39%)
Total with no psychiatric diagnosis	114	53	21 (19%)
Total patient population	215	100	60 (28%)

*Score greater than 50 mm on a 100-mm visual analogue scale of pain severity.

These patients are routinely treated with a combination of high-dose dexamethasone (up to 96 mg a day for several weeks and tapering for several weeks) and radiotherapy. A retrospective review noted that 22% of patients with ESCC had been diagnosed with a major depressive syndrome as compared to 4% in the comparison group. Also, delirium was much more common in the dexamethasone-treated patients with ESCC, with 24% being diagnosed with delirium during the course of treatment as compared to only 10% in the comparison group (Stiefel et al. 1989).

In general, cancer patients with advanced disease are a particularly vulnerable group. The incidence of pain, depression, and delirium increases with greater debilitation and advanced stages of illness (Bukberg et al. 1984). Approximately 25% of all cancer patients experience severe depressive symptoms, with the prevalence increasing to 77% in those with advanced illness. The prevalence of organic mental disorders such as delirium among cancer patients requiring psychiatric consultation ranges from 25% to 40%, and may be as high as 85% during the terminal stages of illness (Massie et al. 1983). Narcotic analgesics, such as meperidine, levorphanol, and morphine sulfate, can cause confusional states, particularly in the elderly and terminally ill (Bruera et al. 1989b).

Findings of the psychological impact of pain were similar in an ambulatory AIDS population (Breitbart 1996; Vogl et al. 1999). AIDS patients with pain reported significantly greater depression and functional impairment than did those without pain. Psychiatric disorders, in particular the organic mental disorders such as AIDS dementia complex, can occasionally interfere with adequate pain management. Opioid analgesics, the mainstay of treatment for moderate to severe pain, may worsen dementia or cause sedation, confusion, or hallucinations in patients with neurological complications of AIDS. Psychostimulants to diminish sedation and neuroleptics to clear confusional states can be quite helpful. Other psychiatric disorders that can affect pain management in the AIDS population include substance abuse and personality disorders.

PAIN AND SUICIDE

Suicide and suicidal ideation represent a major complication of uncontrolled pain patients with cancer and AIDS (Breitbart 1987, 1990a; Haller and Miles 2003). The public perceives cancer as an extremely painful disease compared with other medical conditions, and a survey of public opinion revealed that 69% of those polled agreed that cancer pain could cause a person to consider suicide (Levin et al. 1985). Although relatively few cancer patients commit suicide, most suicides observed in this population have severe pain that is inadequately controlled or poorly tolerated (Farberow et al. 1963; Bolund 1985; Levin et al. 1985). Patients with advanced illness are at highest risk and are the most likely to have the complications of pain, depression, or delirium. A review of the psychiatric consultation data at Memorial Sloan-Kettering Cancer Center showed that 33% of cancer patients who were seen for evaluation of suicide risk received a diagnosis of major depression, while approximately 20% met criteria for delirium and more than 50% were diagnosed with an adjustment disorder (Breitbart 1987).

Thoughts of suicide probably occur quite frequently, particularly in the setting of advanced illness (Massie et al. 1994), and seem to act as a steam valve for feelings often expressed by patients as "If it gets too bad, I always have a way out." Once the clinician has developed a trusting and safe relationship with a terminally ill patient, the patient will almost universally reveal that he or she has had occasional thoughts of suicide as a means of escaping the threat of being overwhelmed by pain. Several studies have suggested that suicidal ideation is relatively rare in cancer patients and is probably more accurately understood as an interaction between unmanaged pain and depression (Achte and Vanhkonen 1971; Silberfarb et al. 1980).

A more in-depth evaluation of the role of cancer pain in suicidal ideation was conducted in 185 cancer patients involved in ongoing research protocols of the Memorial Sloan-Kettering Cancer Center Pain and Psychiatry Services. This study revealed that suicidal ideation occurred in 17% of the study population, with the majority reporting suicidal ideation without intent to act (Breitbart 1990a). In accordance with previous observations, in this population of cancer patients who all had significant pain, suicidal ideation was not directly related to pain intensity but was strongly related to degree of depression and mood disturbance. Pain was related to suicidal ideation indirectly in that patients' perception of poor pain relief was associated with thoughts of suicide. Pain has adverse effects on patients' quality of life and sense of control and impairs the family's ability to provide support. Factors other than pain, such as mood disturbance, delirium, loss of control, and hopelessness contribute to the suicide risk among patients with cancer (Bolund 1985).

In patients with AIDS the relative risk of suicide may be 36 times higher than that of males in the general population (Marzuk et al. 1988). Many of the patients in this cohort had advanced AIDS with Kaposi's sarcoma and other potentially painful conditions. In another study of ambulatory AIDS patients, suicidal ideation was highly correlated with the presence of pain, with depressed mood (as measured by the Beck Depression Inventory), and with low T4 lymphocyte counts. While 20% of ambulatory AIDS patients in this study without pain reported suicidal thoughts, over 40% of those with pain reported suicidal ideation and only two (of 110 patients) reported suicidal intent. One of these two men was in the pain group; however, both scored quite highly on measures of depression. No correlations were observed between suicidal ideation and pain intensity or pain relief. The mean visual analogue scale measure of pain intensity for the group overall was 49 mm (range 5–100 mm), thus falling predominantly in the moderate range. As with cancer pain patients, suicidal ideation in AIDS patients with pain is more likely to be related to a concomitant mood disturbance than to the intensity of pain experienced. Although AIDS patients frequently have suicidal ideation, these thoughts are more often context-specific, occurring almost exclusively during exacerbations of the illness that are often accompanied by severe pain or at times of bereavement (Rabkin et al. 1993).

INADEQUATE PAIN MANAGEMENT: ASSESSMENT ISSUES IN THE TREATMENT OF PAIN

Although pain continues to be undertreated in patients with cancer (Cleeland et al. 1994), in AIDS the problem is dramatic (Lebovits et al. 1989; McCormack et al. 1993). These studies suggest that opioid analgesics are underused in the treatment of pain in AIDS. Our group has reported (Breitbart et al. 1994) that, in our cohort of AIDS patients, only 6% of individuals reporting pain in the severe range (8–10 on a 0–10-point numerical rating scale) received an opioid, such as morphine, as recommended in the World Health Organization (WHO) analgesic ladder. This degree of undermedication far exceeds reports published for cancer pain (Cleeland et al. 1994). The factors associated with the undertreatment of pain in cancer and AIDS include gender (women are more often undertreated), education, substance abuse history, and a variety of patient-related barriers (Breitbart et al. 1994). More recently, however, Turk and Okifuji (1999) found no differences between the cancer patients of either sex in terms of past treatments, current analgesic use, pain, or disability. There were differences, however, between psychological subgroups in their pain, mood, and disability regardless of gender, suggesting that gender may be less important than the psychological characteristics of patients in the prescription of analgesic and adjuvant analgesic medications. While opioid analgesics are underused, it is also clear from our work and that of others that adjuvant agents such as the antidepressants are also dramatically underutilized (Lebovits et al. 1989; McCormack et al. 1993; Breitbart et al. 1994). Only 6% of a sample of AIDS patients reporting pain received an adjuvant analgesic drug (none received an antidepressant), despite the fact that this class of analgesic agents is a critical part of the WHO analgesic ladder.

Inadequate management of pain is often due the inability to properly assess pain in all its dimensions (Twycross and Lack 1983; Foley 1985; Breitbart 1989). As mentioned earlier, psychological variables are often proposed to explain continued pain or lack of response to therapy without a full exploration of the role of medical factors. Other causes of inadequate pain management on the part of clinicians include lack of knowledge of current pharmacotherapeutic or psychotherapeutic approaches and a focus on prolonging life rather than alleviating suffering. Pain relief may be hampered by lack of communication between doctor and patient, by limited expectations of patients to achieve pain relief, and by communication problems in patients impaired by organic mental disorders. Other factors include unavailability of narcotics, doctors' fear of causing respiratory depression, and, most importantly, doctors' fear of amplifying addiction and substance abuse. In advanced cancer, factors that predict the undermanagement of pain include a discrepancy between physician and patient in judging the severity of pain, the presence of pain that physicians did not attribute to cancer, better performance status, age of 70 years or over, and female sex (Cleeland et al. 1994).

In addition to difficulty in managing pain in advanced cancer or AIDS, health care providers have consistently demonstrated difficulty in identifying patients' psychological distress and their need for psychiatric intervention. This problem appears to be worse in patients with head and neck cancer or lung cancer and in patients from lower socioeconomic backgrounds. Oncologists' recommendations for psychiatric intervention correlated with progressive disease and with less denial behavior but not with patient distress (Sollner et. al. 2001). However, when oncologists were provided with a simple algorithm for the identification and treatment of depression in cancer patients, patients benefited from even the least complicated psychotropic intervention (Passik et al. 2002).

Patient-related barriers also contribute to the undermanagement of pain. In a study of the barriers to effective cancer pain management that affected patients' responses to pain in hospitalized cancer patients, three factors emerged: poor levels of knowledge about pain, low perceived control over pain, and a deficit in communication about pain. There appears to be a trend for older patients to be more willing to tolerate pain and to perceive less control over their pain (Yates et al. 2002). Although most studies of pain-related barriers to pain have focused on Caucasian patients, minority patients are at risk both for patient-related barriers to pain management and for the undertreatment of their pain. In a study of pain-related concerns in cancer patients, African-American and Hispanic patients reported severe pain and many concerns about pain management. Most patients in both ethnic groups expressed a belief in stoicism and had concerns about possible addiction to opioid medications and the development of tolerance. Although they described their physicians as the most frequent and trusted source of information about cancer pain, they also reported difficulties with communication and a reluctance to complain of pain (Anderson et al. 2002).

Fear of addiction affects both patient compliance and physician management of opioid analgesics, leading to undermedication of pain in cancer and AIDS patients (Charap 1978; Twycross and Lack 1983; Breitbart and Holland 1990). Studies of the patterns of chronic opioid use in patients with cancer have demonstrated that, although tolerance and physical dependence commonly occur, addiction (psychological dependence) is rare and almost never occurs in an individual without a history of drug abuse prior to cancer illness (Kanner and Foley 1981). Escalation of narcotic analgesic use by cancer patients is usually due to progression of cancer or the development of tolerance, where a larger dose is required to maintain the original analgesic effect. Physical dependence is characterized by the onset of signs and symptoms of withdrawal if the opioid is suddenly stopped or an opioid antagonist is administered. Tolerance usually occurs in association with physical dependence, but it does not imply psychological dependence or addiction, which is a behavioral pattern of compulsive drug abuse characterized by a craving for the drug and overwhelming involvement in obtaining and using it for effects other than pain relief. The cancer pain patient with a history of intravenous opioid abuse presents an often unnecessarily difficult management problem. Adequate pain control can ultimately be achieved in such patients by means of appropriate analgesic dosages and intensive staff education.

More problematic however, is the management of pain in the growing segment of the AIDS population that is actively abusing intravenous drugs (Breitbart and Patt 1994). Such active drug use, in particular intravenous opioid abuse, poses several pain treatment difficulties including: (1) high tolerance to opioid analgesics, (2) drug-seeking and manipulative behavior, (3) lack of compliance in taking medications, (4) lack of reliability of patient history, and (5) the risk of spreading HIV while under the influence of substances and consequently disinhibited. Unfortunately, the patient's subjective report is often the best or only indication of the presence and intensity of pain as well as the degree of pain relief achieved by an intervention. Physicians who believe they are being manipulated by drug-seeking individuals are hesitant to use opioid analgesics in appropriate dosages for adequate control of pain, and this reluctance often leads to undermedication. Most clinicians experienced in working with this population of AIDS patients recommend setting clear and direct limits. While that is an important aspect of the care of AIDS patients who use intravenous drugs, it is by no means the whole answer. As much as possible, clinicians should attempt to eliminate the issue of drug abuse as an obstacle to pain management by dealing directly with the problems of opioid withdrawal and drug abuse treatment. Often specialized substance abuse consultation services are available to help manage such patients and initiate drug rehabilitation. Clinicians should avoid making the analgesic drugs the focus of a battle for control with the patient, especially in terminal stages of illness. Clinicians should err on the side of believing patients when they complain of pain, utilizing their knowledge of the specific pain syndrome seen in AIDS patients to corroborate the patient's report if they feel it is unreliable.

The risk of inducing respiratory depression is too often overestimated and can limit appropriate use of opioid analgesics for pain and symptom control. Bruera et al. (1990) demonstrated that, in a population of terminally ill cancer patients with respiratory failure and dyspnea, administration of subcutaneous morphine improved dyspnea without causing a significant deterioration in respiratory function. The adequacy of cancer pain management can be influenced by the lack of concordance between patients' ratings or complaints of their pain and those made by caregivers. Persistent cancer pain is often ascribed to a psychological cause when it does not respond to treatment attempts. In our clinical experience we have noted that patients who report their pain as "severe" are quite likely to be viewed as having a psychological contribution to their complaints. Staff members' ability to empathize with a patient's pain complaint may be limited by the intensity of the complaint. Grossman et al. (1991) found that while there is a high degree of concordance between patient and caregiver ratings of patient pain intensity at the low and moderate levels, this concordance breaks down at high levels. Thus, a clinician's ability to assess a patient's level of pain becomes unreliable once a patient's report of pain intensity rises above 7 on a visual analogue rating scale of 0–10. Physicians must be educated as to the limitations of their ability to objectively assess the severity of a subjective pain experience. Additionally, patient education is often a useful intervention in such cases. Patients are more likely to be believed and adequately treated if they are taught to request pain relief in a nonhysterical, business-like fashion.

PSYCHIATRIC MANAGEMENT OF PAIN IN PALLIATIVE CARE

Optimal treatment of pain associated with advanced disease is multimodal and includes pharmacological, psychotherapeutic, cognitive-behavioral, anesthetic, neurostimulatory, and rehabilitative approaches. In addition to psychotherapeutic interventions, psychoeducational interventions can be helpful. Relatively brief interventions (20 minutes or less) during which patients receive information about pain self-management and misconceptions about pain treatment are addressed can lead to marked decreases in pain among cancer patients (de Wit et al. 2001a; Oliver et al 2001). In general, psychiatric participation in pain management involves the use of psychotherapeutic, cognitive-behavioral, and psychopharmacological interventions, usually in combination, as described below.

PSYCHOTHERAPY AND PAIN

The goals of psychotherapy with medically ill patients with pain are to provide support, knowledge, and skills (Table II). Utilizing short-term supportive psychotherapy focused on the crisis created by the medical illness, the therapist provides emotional support, continuity, information, and assistance in adaptation. The therapist has a role in emphasizing past strengths, supporting previously successful coping strategies, and teaching new coping skills such as relaxation, cognitive coping, skills in managing the use of analgesics including self-observation and documentation of pain levels and medication used, and assertiveness and communication skills. Communication skills are of paramount importance for both patient and family, particularly around pain and analgesic issues. The patient and family are the unit of concern, and need a long-term, supportive relationship within the health care system in addition to specific psychological approaches dealing with pain and dying that a psychiatrist, psychologist, social worker, chaplain, or nurse can provide.

Psychotherapy with the dying patient in pain consists of active listening with supportive verbal interventions and the occasional interpretation (Cassem 1987). Despite the seriousness of the patient's plight, it is not necessary for the psychiatrist or psychologist to appear overly solemn or emotionally restrained. Often, it is only the psychotherapist, of all the patient's caregivers, who is comfortable enough to converse lightheartedly and allow the patient to talk about his or her life and experiences, rather than focus solely on impending death. The dying patient who wishes to talk or ask questions about death and pain and suffering should be allowed to do so freely, with the therapist maintaining an interested, interactive stance. Rather than enforcing death and dying as the therapeutic agenda, the sensitive therapist allows the patient to bring up these issues in his or her own timing. Some patients derive benefit from spiritual guidance, and it is not uncommon for the dying patient to benefit from pastoral counseling if available.

As the dying process progresses, psychotherapy with the individual patient may become limited by cognitive and speech deficits, and at this point the focus of supportive psychotherapeutic interventions shifts primarily to the family. In our experience, a very common concern for family members at this point is the patient's level of alertness. Attempts to control pain are often accompanied by sedation that can limit communication between patient and family. This problem can sometimes become a source of conflict, with some family members disagreeing among themselves or with the

Table II
The goals of psychotherapy with medically ill patients

Goals	Format
Support: provide continuity	*Individuals:* supportive/crisis intervention
Knowledge: provide information	*Family:* patient and family are the unit of
Skills: relaxation, cognitive coping,	concern
use of analgesics, communication	*Group:* share experiences, identify
	successful coping strategies

patient about what constitutes an appropriate balance between comfort and alertness. It can be helpful for the physician to clarify the patient's preferences as they relate to these issues early on so that conflict can be avoided and work related to bereavement can begin.

Group interventions with individual patients (even in advanced stages of disease) and with spouses, couples, and families are a powerful means of sharing experiences and identifying successful coping strategies. The limitations of using group interventions for patients with advanced disease are primarily pragmatic. The patient must be physically comfortable enough to participate and have the cognitive capacity to be aware of group discussion. It is often helpful for family members to attend support groups during the terminal phases of the patient's illness.

Psychotherapeutic interventions that have multiple foci may be most useful. A prospective study of cancer pain showed that cognitive-behavioral and psychoeducational techniques based upon increasing support, self-efficacy, and education may be helpful in assisting patients in dealing with increased pain (Syrjala et al. 1992). Results of this evaluation of patients with cancer pain indicate that psychological and social variables are significant predictors of pain. Distress specific to the illness, self-efficacy, and coping styles were predictors of increased pain.

Utilizing psychotherapy to diminish symptoms of anxiety and depression, factors that can intensify pain, has beneficial effects on the cancer pain experience. In a controlled, randomized prospective study, Spiegel and Bloom (1983a) demonstrated the efficacy of both supportive group therapy for metastatic breast cancer patients and hypnotic pain control exercises. Their support group focused not on interpersonal processes or self-exploration, but rather on a series of themes related to the practical and existential problems of living with cancer. The results showed that patients in the treatment groups reported a decreased level of pain whereas those in the control group reported a large increase in pain.

Although psychotherapy with the cancer patient in pain is primarily non-analytical and is focused on techniques for managing the pain, sessions may shift into a more exploratory mode when patients are in more stable periods. This exploration of reactions to cancer often involves insights into earlier, more pervasive life issues. Some patients choose to continue a more exploratory psychotherapy during extended illness-free periods or survivorship.

COGNITIVE-BEHAVIORAL TECHNIQUES

Cognitive-behavioral techniques can be useful adjuncts to the management of pain in cancer and AIDS patients (Table III). In a meta-analysis of the effect of psychoeducational interventions on pain in adults with cancer, Devine (2003) found relatively strong evidence for the use of relaxation-based cognitive-behavioral interventions, education about analgesic usage, and supportive counseling, although a conclusion about the relative effectiveness of each of these was limited by the relatively small number of studies. Cognitive-behavioral techniques have demonstrated their effectiveness not only in reducing the pain of HIV-related peripheral neuropathy but also in producing improvements in most domains of pain-related functional interference (Evans et. al. 2003a).

Cognitive-behavioral techniques include passive relaxation with mental imagery, cognitive distraction or focusing, progressive muscle relaxation, biofeedback, hypnosis, and music therapy (Cleeland et al. 1986; Cleeland 1987; Fishman and Loscalzo 1987; Loscalzo and Jacobsen 1990). The goal of treatment is to guide the patient toward a sense of control over pain. Some techniques are primarily cognitive in nature, focusing on perceptual and thought processes, and others are directed at modifying patterns of behavior to help patients cope with pain. Behavioral techniques for pain control seek to modify physiological pain reactions, respondent pain behaviors, and operant pain behaviors (see Table IV for definitions).

Primarily cognitive techniques for coping with pain are aimed at reducing the intensity and distress that are part of the pain experience. Techniques include modification of the patient's thoughts about pain or psychological distress, introduction of more adaptive coping strategies, and instruction in relaxation techniques. Cognitive modification or restructuring is an approach derived from cognitive therapy for depression or anxiety and is based on how one interprets events and bodily sensation. It is assumed that patients have dysfunctional automatic thoughts that are consistent with underlying assumptions and beliefs. In both cancer and AIDS pain populations, negative thoughts about pain are significantly related to pain intensity, degree of psychological distress, and level of interference in functional activities (de Wit et al. 2001b; Evans et al. 2003b). By identifying and challenging dysfunctional automatic thoughts and underlying beliefs by restructuring or modifying thought processes, patients can develop a more rational response to pain (Fishman and Loscalzo 1987). Examples of automatic thoughts that worsen the pain experience are: "The intensity of my pain will never diminish" or "Because my pain limits my activities, I am completely helpless." Patients

Table III
Cognitive-behavioral techniques used by pain patients
with advanced disease

Psychoeducation
    Preparatory information
    Self-monitoring

Relaxation
    Passive breathing
    Progressive muscle relaxation

Distraction
    Focusing
    Mental imagery
    Cognitive distraction
    Behavioral distraction.

Combined Techniques (Relaxation and Distraction)
    Passive/progressive relaxation with mental imagery
    Systematic desensitization
    Meditation
    Hypnosis
    Biofeedback
    Music therapy

Cognitive Therapies
    Cognitive distortion
    Cognitive restructuring

Behavioral Therapies
    Modeling
    Graded task management
    Contingency management
    Behavioral rehearsal

---

can be taught to recognize and interrupt such thoughts and proceed to develop a view of the pain experience as time-limited and themselves as functional despite periods in which they are limited.

Although cognitive restructuring may be a useful technique in the earlier stages of cancer and AIDS, the goals change in the palliative care context. In this setting the goal is not necessarily to change the patient's maladaptive thoughts but to utilize techniques designed to diminish the patient's frustration, anxiety, and anger. Helping patients to employ more adaptive coping strategies and to avoid catastrophizing, as well as encouraging an increase in problem-solving skills, may be helpful at this stage (Fishman 1990; Turk and Fernendez 1990; Jensen et al. 1991).

Aside from modifying dysfunctional thoughts and attitudes, the most fundamental behavioral technique is self-monitoring. The development of the ability to monitor one's behaviors allows individuals to notice their dysfunctional reactions to the pain experience and learn to control them. Systematic desensitization (see Table IV) is useful in extinguishing anticipatory anxiety that leads to avoidant behaviors and in remobilizing inactive patients. The hallmark of systematic desensitization is the use of graded task assignments in which the patient takes a series of small behavioral steps toward activities that are anxiety-producing. Contingency management is a method of reinforcing "well" behaviors only, thus modifying dysfunctional operant pain behaviors associated with secondary gain (Cleeland 1987; Loscalzo and Jacobsen 1990).

Cognitive-behavioral interventions that are useful in the setting of advanced illness include techniques ranging from preparatory information and self-monitoring to systematic desensitization and methods of distraction and relaxation (Breitbart and Holland 1988). A review of nonpharmacological interventions in cancer patients suggests that behavioral interventions can effectively control a number of symptoms in cancer patients including anticipatory nausea and vomiting, anxiety related to invasive medical treatments, and treatment-related pain. The most effective pain management techniques appear to be those that utilize methods similar to hypnosis, involving relaxation, suggestion, and distracting imagery (Redd et al. 2001). Most often, techniques such as hypnosis, biofeedback, or systematic desensitization utilize both cognitive and behavioral elements such as muscular relaxation and cognitive distraction.

Patient selection. Many cancer and AIDS patients fear that focusing on their pain will distract their physicians from treating the underlying causes of their disease and consequently are highly motivated to learn and practice cognitive-behavioral techniques. These techniques are often effective not only in pain control, but in restoring a sense of self-control, personal efficacy, and active participation in medical treatment. It is important to note that these techniques must not be used as a substitute for appropriate analgesic management of pain, but rather as part of a comprehensive multimodal approach. The fact that cognitive-behavioral techniques are not associated with side effects makes them attractive in the palliative care setting as a supplement to already complicated medication regimens. The successful use of these techniques should never lead to the erroneous conclusion that the pain was of psychogenic origin and as such not "real." The mechanisms by which these cognitive and behavioral techniques relieve pain are not known; however, they all seem to share the elements of relaxation and distraction. Distraction or redirection of attention helps to reduce awareness of pain, and relaxation lowers both muscle tension and sympathetic arousal (Cleeland 1987).

Table IV
Cognitive-behavioral techniques: definitions and descriptions

Behavioral Therapy
The clinical use of techniques derived from the experimental analysis
of behavior (learning and conditioning) for the evaluation, prevention,
and treatment of physical disease or physiological dysfunction

Cognitive Therapy
A focused intervention targeted at changing maladaptive beliefs and
dysfunctional attitudes; the therapist engages the client in a process of
collaborative empiricism, where these underlying beliefs are
challenged and corrected

Operant Pain
Pain behaviors resulting from operant learning or conditioning; pain
behavior is reinforced and continues because of secondary gain, in the
form of increased attention and caring

Respondent Pain
Pain behaviors resulting from respondent learning or conditioning;
stimuli associated with prior painful experiences can elicit increased
pain and avoidance behavior

Cognitive Restructuring
Redefinition of some or all aspects of the patient's interpretation of the
noxious or threatening experience, resulting in decreased distress,
anxiety, and hopelessness

Self-Monitoring (Pain Diary)
Written or audiotaped chronicle that the patient maintains to describe
specific agreed-upon characteristics associated with pain

Contingency Management
Focusing of patient and family member responses that either reinforce
or inhibit specific behaviors exhibited by the patient; this method
involves reinforcing desired "well" behaviors

Grade Task Assignments
A hierarchy of tasks—physical, cognitive, and behavioral—are
compartmentalized and performed sequentially in manageable steps,
ultimately achieving an identified goal

Systematic Desensitization
Relaxation and distraction exercises are paired with a hierarchy of
anxiety-arousing stimuli presented through mental imagery or in vivo,
resulting in control of fear

Most patients with advanced illness and pain are appropriate candidates
for useful application of these techniques; the clinician, however, should
take into account the intensity of pain and the patient's mental clarity. Ideal
candidates have mild to moderate pain and can expect benefit, whereas
patients with severe pain can expect limited benefit from psychological
interventions unless somatic therapies can lower the level of pain to some

degree. Confusional states interfere dramatically with a patient's ability to focus attention and thus limit the usefulness of these techniques (Loscalzo and Jacobsen 1990). Occasionally these techniques can be modified so as to include mildly cognitive impaired patients; in such cases the therapist often takes a more active role by orienting the patient, creating a safe and secure environment, and evoking a conditioned response to the therapist's voice or presence.

Barriers to engaging patients in cognitive-behavioral therapies can arise either from physicians and nurses or from patients. The health care provider who works with patients with advanced illness may have particular difficulty in becoming comfortable with the use of behavioral therapies. Pharmacotherapy is highly effective in the management of pain and physicians may consider it easier to use than labor-intensive and time-consuming nonpharmacological interventions. Physicians and nurses have typical concerns about the practice of behavioral interventions such as: "What if the patient laughs, and doesn't buy it?" or "It seems too theatrical, unscientific, nonmedical; too New Age!" Overcoming such obstacles will be greatly rewarded. It is imperative that physicians working with patients with advanced illness be aware of the effective nonpharmacological treatments for pain that are available, and be able to make appropriate referrals to practitioners who can provide such interventions.

Patients themselves may be uncertain about the utility of behavioral therapies. Some may ask, "How can breathing take away my pain?" They may be frightened by the word "hypnosis" and its connotations. Hypnosis is often associated with powerful magical properties, and some patients become frightened at the prospect of losing control or being under the influence of someone else. We generally attempt to introduce behavioral interventions only after establishing rapport with a patient. Occasionally, some patients may benefit from a discussion of the theoretical basis of these interventions; however, we stress that it is not important to understand why a technique works, but rather to use the technique that works. Apprehensions must be affirmed and dealt with. Patients must also feel in control of the process at all times and be reassured that they can stop at any time.

General instructions. A general approach to using cognitive-behavioral interventions with patients with advanced illness and pain involves assessing the symptoms, choosing a cognitive-behavioral strategy, and preparing the patient and the setting.

The main purpose of conducting a cognitive-behavioral assessment of pain is to determine what, if any, behavioral interventions are indicated (Loscalzo and Jacobsen 1990). The therapist must initially engage the patient and establish a therapeutic alliance, and then take a history of the pain symptom, review previous efforts to treat the patient's pain, and collect data regarding the nature of the pain and its impact on the patient and his or her family.

The assessment process will lead to a variety of potential behavioral interventions. Choosing the appropriate behavioral strategy involves taking into consideration the patient's medical condition and physical and cognitive limitations, as well as such issues as time constraints and practical matters. For instance, patients with cognitive impairment or delirium will probably be unable to keep a pain diary or use techniques that involve cognitive manipulation.

Relaxation techniques. Several techniques can be used to achieve a mental and physical state of relaxation. Muscular tension, autonomic arousal, and mental distress exacerbate pain (Cleeland 1987; Loscalzo and Jacobsen 1990). Some specific relaxation techniques, described in more detail by Andrasik (this volume), include passive relaxation, focusing attention on sensations of warmth and decreased tension in various parts of the body; progressive muscle relaxation, involving active tensing and relaxing of muscles; and meditation. Other techniques that employ both relaxation and cognitive techniques include hypnosis, biofeedback, and music therapy and are discussed later in this chapter.

Passive relaxation, focused breathing, and passive muscle relaxation exercises involve focusing attention systematically on one's breathing, on sensations of warmth and relaxation, or on release of muscular tension in various body parts. Verbal suggestions and imagery are used to help promote relaxation. Muscle relaxation is an important component of the relaxation response and can augment the benefits of simple focused breathing exercises, leading to a deeper experience of relaxation and self-control.

Progressive or active muscle relaxation involves the active tensing and relaxing of various muscle groups in the body, focusing attention on the sensations of tension and relaxation. In the hospital setting, relaxation is most commonly achieved through a combination of focused breathing and progressive muscle relaxation exercises. Once patients are in a relaxed state, imagery techniques can then be used to induce deeper relaxation and facilitate distraction from or manipulation of a variety of cancer-related symptoms. Passive or active relaxation and focused breathing exercises based upon the work of Erickson (1959), Benson (1975), and others (Loscalzo and Jacobsen 1990) can be helpful.

Imagery and distraction techniques. Clinically, relaxation techniques are most helpful in managing pain when combined with distracting or pleasant imagery. The use of distraction or focusing involves controlling the focus of attention and can be used to make the patient less aware of noxious stimuli (Broome et al. 1992). One can employ imaginative inattention by picturing oneself on a beach. Mental distraction is similar to the practice of counting sheep to aid sleep. Keeping oneself busy is a form of behavioral distraction. Imagery—using one's imagination while in a relaxed state—can be used to transform pain into a warm or cold sensation. One can also imaginatively transform the context of pain, perhaps by imagining oneself in action on the football field instead of the hospital bed. Disassociation is a technique in which patients imagine that a painful body part is no longer part of their body (Fishman and Loscalzo 1987; Breitbart 1989; Breitbart and Holland 1990; Loscalzo and Jacobsen 1990). Not every patient finds these techniques acceptable, and the therapist must try out a number of approaches to determine which are consistent with the patient's style.

Imagery (often referred to as guided imagery) is most effective when the specific image is obtained from the patient. The clinician may ask the patient to close his or her eyes and think of a place, an activity, or an experience where he or she has felt most safe and secure. The clinician may provide suggestions for the patient such as a favorite beach scene, a room in a house, or riding a bicycle in a state park. Once the patient identifies the scene, the clinician may ask the patient to elaborate by providing specific details such as the temperature, season, time of day, and the type of ocean (calm, or with big waves). The clinician then utilizes this information and describes an image for the patient in detail. The skill is for the clinician to be as flexible and as creative as possible, and to elaborate upon the scene, utilizing all aspects of the senses and bodily sensations such as "feel the suns rays touch your skin, allow your skin to feel warm and tingly all over," or " breathe in the fresh, clear air, allow it to fill your lungs with its freshness," or " feel the fresh dew of the grass under your feet." The clinician can focus on "aromas in the garden" or the "sounds of birds singing," always reminding the patient to breath evenly and steadily as he or she feels more and more relaxed and in control. If possible, the clinician should avoid volunteering an image or scene for the patient without being aware of the association or meaning the image may have for the patient. For example, a patient may be afraid of water, and therefore a beach scene may invoke feelings of fear and loss of control.

Hypnosis can be a useful adjunct in the management of cancer pain (Barber and Gitelson 1980; Redd et al. 1983; Spiegel and Bloom 1983a; Spiegel 1985; Levitan 1992). In a controlled trial comparing hypnosis with cognitive-behavioral therapy in relieving mucositis following a bone marrow transplant, patients utilizing hypnosis reported a significant reduction in pain compared to patients who used cognitive-behavioral techniques (Syrjala et al. 1992). The hypnotic trance is essentially a state of heightened and focused concentration, and thus it can be used to manipulate the perception of pain. The depth of the patient's capacity to enter hypnosis will also determine the effectiveness of the technique as well as the strategies employed during each session. One-third of the population is not hypnotizable, and should use other techniques, such as relaxation. Of the two-thirds of patients who are identified as being less, moderately, and highly hypnotizable, three principles underlie the use of hypnosis in controlling pain (Broome et al. 1992): (a) use self-hypnosis; (b) relax, do not fight the pain; and (c) use a mental filter to ease the hurt in pain. Patients who are moderately and highly hypnotizable can often alter sensations in a painful area by changing temperature sensation or experiencing tingling. Less hypnotizable patients can often use an alternative focus by concentrating on a sensation in a nonaffected body part or enjoying a mental image of a pleasant scene. The main disadvantage of hypnosis for cancer patients is that the technique frequently requires more attentional capacity than they generally have.

Biofeedback. Fotopoulos et al. (1978) noted significant pain relief in a group of cancer patients who were taught electromyographic (EMG) and electroencephalographic (EEG) biofeedback-assisted relaxation. Only 2 of 17 patients were able to maintain analgesia after the treatment ended, however. A lack of generalization of effect can be a problem with biofeedback techniques. Although deteriorating physical condition may make a prolonged training period impossible, especially for the terminally ill, most cancer patients can often utilize EMG and temperature biofeedback techniques for learning relaxation-assisted pain control (Cleeland 1987).

Music, aroma, and art therapies. Munro and Mount (1978) have written extensively on the use of music therapy with cancer patients, documenting clinical examples and suggesting mechanisms of action. Music can often capture the focus of attention like no other stimulus. It offers patients a new form of expression and helps them distract themselves from their perception of pain, while expressing themselves in meaningful ways (Schroeder-Sheker 1994).

Aromas have innate relaxing and stimulating qualities. Our colleagues at Memorial Hospital have recently begun to explore the use of aromatherapy to treat procedure-related anxiety related to magnetic resonance imaging scans. Utilizing the scent heliotropin, Manne et al. (1994) reported that two-thirds of the patients found the scent especially pleasant and reported much less anxiety than those who were not exposed to the scent during their scan. As a general relaxation technique, aromatherapy may have an application for pain management, but this possibility remains unstudied.

Art therapy allows children and less verbally skilled adults to express the fears and concerns that they have in a more comfortable fashion. The creative experience can be used both as a important means of providing support and as an avenue for providing patients with psychological insights into their experience (Connell 1992).

PSYCHOTROPIC ADJUVANT ANALGESICS FOR PAIN IN THE PATIENT WITH ADVANCED ILLNESS

The patient with advanced disease and pain has much to gain from the appropriate and maximal utilization of psychotropic drugs. The primary adjuvant analgesics are anticonvulsant and antidepressant medications, but a wide variety of other drugs are also used. To optimize analgesic therapy in patients with neuropathic pain, both opioid and adjuvant analgesics must be used effectively (Farrar and Portenoy 2001). Psychotropic drugs, particularly the tricyclic antidepressants (TCAs), are useful as adjuvant analgesics in the pharmacological management of cancer pain and neuropathic pain. Table V lists the various psychotropic medications with analgesic properties, their routes of administration, and their approximate daily doses. These medications not only are effective in managing symptoms of anxiety, depression, insomnia, or delirium that commonly complicate the course of advanced disease in patients with cancer or AIDS who are in pain, but they also potentiate the analgesic effects of the opioid drugs and have innate analgesic properties of their own (Breitbart 1992).

Antidepressants. A detailed analysis of antidepressant use for psychiatric management of pain is provided by Atkinson et al. (this volume). The current literature supports the use of antidepressants as adjuvant analgesic agents in the management of a wide variety of chronic pain syndromes, including cancer pain (Walsh 1983, 1990; Butler 1984; France 1987; Getto et al. 1987; Magni et al. 1987; Ventafridda et al. 1987; Onghena and Van Houdenhove 1992). While antidepressants are clinically useful as adjuvant analgesics in managing AIDS-related pain (e.g., HIV neuropathies), there are no published controlled clinical trials of their use as analgesics (Lefkowitz and Breitbart 1992). Amitriptyline is the best-studied TCA, and it has been proven effective as an analgesic in a large number of clinical trials addressing a wide variety of chronic pains (Pilowsky et al. 1982; Max et al. 1987, 1988; Sharav et al. 1987; Watson et al. 1992a,b). Other TCAs known to have efficacy as analgesics include imipramine (Kvindesal et al. 1984; Young and Clarke 1985; Sindrup et al. 1989), desipramine (Max et al. 1991; Gordon et al. 1993), nortriptyline (Gomez-Perez et al. 1985), clomipramine (Langohr et al. 1982; Tiengo et al. 1987), and doxepin (Hammeroff et al. 1982).

In general, the TCAs are utilized in cancer pain as adjuvant analgesics, potentiating the effects of opioids, and are rarely used as the primary analgesic

Table V
Psychotropic adjuvant analgesic drugs for pain in patients
with advanced disease

Generic Name	Approximate Daily Dosage Range (mg)	Route
Tricyclic Antidepressants		
Amitriptyline	10–150	p.o., i.m., p.r.
Nortriptyline	10–50	p.o.
Imipramine	12.5–150	p.o., i.m.
Desipramine	12.5–150	p.o.
Clomipramine	10–150	p.o.
Doxepin	12.5–150	p.o., i.m.
Noncyclic Antidepressants		
Trazodone	25–300	p.o.
Fluoxetine	20–60	p.o.
Paroxetine	20–60	p.o.
Monoamide Oxidase Inhibitors		
Phenelzine	45–75	p.o.
Amine Precursors		
L-tryptophan	500–3000	p.o.
Psychostimulants		
Methylphenidate	2.5–20 b.i.d.	p.o.
Dextroamphetamine	2.5–20 b.i.d.	p.o.
Pemoline	18.75–75 b.i.d.	p.o.
Phenothiazines		
Fluphenazine	1–3	p.o., i.m.
Methotrimeprazine	10–20 q6h	p.o., i.m., i.v., s.c.
Butyrophenones		
Haloperidol	1–3	p.o., i.m., i.v., s.c.
Pimozide	2–6 b.i.d.	p.o.
Atypical Neuroleptics		
Olanzapine	2.5–20	p.o.
Antihistamines		
Hydroxyzine	50 q4–6h	p.o., i.m., i.v.
Benzodiazepines		
Alprazolam	0.25–2.0 t.i.d.	p.o.
Clonazepam	0.5–4 b.i.d.	p.o.

Abbreviations: b.i.d. = twice a day; i.m. = intramuscular; i.v. = intravenous; p.o. = oral; p.r. = parenteral; q4–6h = every 4–6 hours; q6h = every 6 hours; s.c. = subcutaneous; t.i.d. = three times a day.

(Botney and Fields 1983; Ventafridda et al. 1987). Ventafridda et al. (1987) reviewed a multicenter clinical trial that used the antidepressants trazodone and amitriptyline to treat chronic cancer pain that had a neuropathic component.

Almost all of these patients were already receiving weak or strong opioids and experienced improved pain control when taking antidepressants. A subsequent randomized, double-blind study found both amitriptyline and trazodone to have similar therapeutic analgesic efficacy (Ventafridda et al. 1987). Magni et al. (1987), reviewing the use of antidepressants in Italian cancer centers, found that a wide range of antidepressants were used for a variety of cancer pain syndromes, with amitriptyline being the most commonly prescribed. In nearly all cases, antidepressants were used in association with opioids. Some evidence indicates that there may be subgroups of patients who respond differentially to tricyclics, and therefore if amitriptyline fails to alleviate pain, another tricyclic should be tried (Watson et al. 1992a). The TCAs are effective as adjuvants in cancer pain through a number of mechanisms that include antidepressant activity (France 1987), potentiation or enhancement of opioid analgesia (Malseed and Goldstein 1979; Botney and Fields 1983; Ventafridda et al. 1990), and direct analgesic effects (Spiegel et al. 1983). Although TCAs have demonstrated their efficacy as an adjuvant analgesic in the management of non-neuropathic pain, recent clinical trials of patients with HIV sensory neuropathy (Kieburtz et al. 1998; Shlay et al. 1998), spinal cord injury pain (Cardenas et al. 2002), and cis-platinum neuropathy (Hammack et al. 2002) have found little benefit of amitriptyline as compared with placebo.

The heterocyclic and noncyclic antidepressant drugs such as trazodone, mianserin, maprotiline, and selective serotonin reuptake inhibitors (SSRIs) including fluoxetine and paroxetine may also be useful as adjuvant analgesics for cancer patients with pain (Costa et al. 1985; Feighner 1985; Hynes et al. 1985; Davidoff et al. 1987; Eberhard et al. 1988). Several case reports suggest that fluoxetine may be a useful adjuvant analgesic in the management of headache (Diamond and Frietag 1989), fibrositis (Geller 1989), and diabetic neuropathy (Theesen and Marsh 1989). In a recent clinical trial, fluoxetine was no better than placebo as an analgesic in painful diabetic neuropathy (Max et al. 1992). Paroxetine is the first SSRI shown to be a highly effective analgesic in the treatment of neuropathic pain (Sindrup et al. 1990), and may be a useful addition to our armamentarium of adjuvant analgesics for cancer pain. Newer antidepressants such as sertraline, venlafaxine, and nefazodone may also eventually prove to be clinically useful as adjuvant analgesics. Nefazodone, for instance, has been demonstrated to potentiate opioid analgesics in an animal model (Pick et al. 1992). More recent evidence suggests that serotonergic-noradrenergic antidepressants may have more consistent antinociceptive effects than serotonergic antidepressants (Fishbain 2000).

In general, it is clear that many antidepressants have analgesic properties. There is no definite indication that any one drug is more effective than the others, although the most experience has been accrued with amitriptyline, which remains the drug of first choice. In terms of appropriate dosage, evidence indicates that the therapeutic analgesic effects of amitriptyline are correlated with serum levels just as the antidepressant effects are, and that analgesic treatment failure is due to low serum levels (Max et al. 1987, 1988; McQuay et al. 1993). A high-dose regimen of up to 150 mg of amitriptyline or higher is suggested (Watson and Evans 1985; Sharav et al. 1987). As to the time course of onset of analgesia or with antidepressants, there appears to be a biphasic process that occurs with immediate or early analgesic effects that occur within hours or days (Botney and Fields 1983; Spiegel et al. 1983; Tiengo et al. 1987) and later, longer analgesic effects that peak over a 4–6-week period (Max et al. 1987, 1988; Pilowsky et al. 1982).

Treatment should be initiated with a small dose of amitriptyline of 10–25 mg at bedtime, especially in debilitated patients, and increased slowly by 10–25 mg every 2–4 days toward 150 mg with frequent assessment of pain and side effects until a beneficial effect is achieved. Maximal effect as an adjuvant analgesic may require continuation of the drug for 2–6 weeks. It may also help to measure serum levels to assure that therapeutic levels are being achieved. Both pain and depression in cancer patients often respond to lower doses (25–100 mg) of antidepressant than are usually required in the physically healthy (100–300 mg), most likely because of impaired metabolism of these drugs. The choice of drug often depends on the side-effect profile, existing medical problems, the nature of depressive symptoms if present, and past response to specific antidepressants. Sedating drugs like amitriptyline are helpful when insomnia complicates the presence of pain and depression on a cancer patient. Anticholinergic properties of some of these drugs should also be kept in mind. Occasionally, in patients who have limited analgesic response to a tricyclic, analgesia can be enhanced with the addition of lithium (Tyler 1974).

Monoamine oxidase (MAO) inhibitors are also less useful in the cancer setting because of dietary restrictions and potentially dangerous interactions with narcotics such as meperidine. Phenelzine is an MAO inhibitor that has adjuvant analgesic properties in patients with atypical facial pain and migraine (Lascelles 1966; Anthony and Lance 1969).

Psychostimulants. Dextroamphetamine and methylphenidate are useful antidepressant agents prescribed selectively for medically ill cancer patients with depression (Kaufmann et al. 1982; Fernandez et al. 1987a). Psychostimulants are also useful in diminishing excessive sedation secondary to opioids, and are potent adjuvant analgesics. Bruera and colleagues (1987,

1989a, 1992) demonstrated that a regimen of 10 mg methylphenidate with breakfast and 5 mg with lunch significantly decreased sedation and potentiated the analgesic effect of opioids in patients with cancer pain. Dextroamphetamine has also been reported to have additive analgesic effects when used with morphine in postoperative pain (Forrest et al. 1977). In relatively low doses, psychostimulants enhance appetite, promote a sense of well-being, and improve feelings of weakness and fatigue in cancer patients. Treatment with dextroamphetamine or methylphenidate usually begins with a dose of 2.5 mg at 8 a.m. and at noon. The dosage is slowly increased over several days until a desired effect is achieved or side effects such as overstimulation, anxiety, insomnia, paranoia, or confusion intervene. Typically a dose greater than 30 mg per day is not necessary, although occasionally patients require up to 60 mg per day. Patients usually are maintained on methylphenidate for 1--2 months, and approximately two-thirds will be able to be withdrawn from methylphenidate without a recurrence of depressive symptoms. Those who do have a recurrence of symptoms can be maintained on a psychostimulant for up to one year without significant abuse problems. Tolerance will develop, and adjustment of dose may be necessary. A strategy we have found useful in treating cancer pain associated with depression is to start a psychostimulant (at a starting dose of 2.5 mg of methylphenidate at 8 a.m. and noon) and then to add a TCA after several days to help prolong and potentiate the short-lasting effect of the stimulant. Pemoline is a unique alternative psychostimulant that is chemically unrelated to amphetamine, but may have similar usefulness as an antidepressant and adjuvant analgesic in cancer patients (Breitbart and Mermelstein 1991). Advantages of pemoline as a psychostimulant in cancer pain patients include the lack of abuse potential, the lack of federal regulation through special triplicate prescriptions, the mild sympathomimetic effects, and the fact that it comes in a chewable tablet form that can be absorbed through the buccal mucosa and thus used by cancer patients who have difficulty swallowing or have intestinal obstruction. In our clinical experience, pemoline is as effective as methylphenidate or dextroamphetamine in treating depressive symptoms and in countering the sedating effects of opioid analgesics. There are no studies of pemoline's capacity to potentiate the analgesic properties of opioids. Pemoline can be started at a dose of 18.75 mg in the morning and at noon, and increased gradually over several days. Typically patients require 75 mg a day or less. Pemoline should be used with caution in patients with liver impairment, and liver function tests should be monitored periodically with longer-term treatment (Nehra et al. 1990).

Neuroleptics. Methotrimeprazine is a phenothiazine that is equianalgesic to morphine, has none of the opioid effects on gut motility, and probably produces analgesia through α-adrenergic blockade (Beaver et al. 1966). In patients who are opioid tolerant, it provides an alternative approach in providing analgesia by a non-opioid mechanism. It is a dopamine blocker and so has antiemetic as well an anxiolytic effects. Methotrimeprazine can produce sedation and hypotension and should be given cautiously by slow intravenous infusion. Other phenothiazines such as chlorpromazine and prochlorperazine are useful as antiemetics in cancer patients, but probably have limited use as analgesics (Maltbie et al. 1979). Fluphenazine in combination with TCAs is helpful in neuropathic pains (Langohr et al. 1982). Haloperidol is the drug of choice in the management of delirium or psychoses in cancer patients, and has clinical usefulness as a coanalgesic for cancer pain (Maltbie et al. 1979). Pimozide, a butyrophenone, is effective as an analgesic in the management of trigeminal neuralgia, at doses of 4–12 mg per day (Lechin et al. 1989). The atypical neuroleptic, olanzapine, reduces both anxiety and opioid usage in cognitively impaired cancer patients with pain; these patients also reported lower pain levels, which suggests that olanzapine may have analgesic properties (Khojainova et al. 2002).

Anxiolytics. Hydroxyzine is a mild anxiolytic with sedating and analgesic properties that are useful in the anxious cancer patient with pain (Beaver and Feise 1976; Rumore and Schlichting 1986). This antihistamine has antiemetic activity as well. One hundred milligrams of parenteral hydroxyzine has analgesic activity approaching 8 mg of morphine, and has additive analgesic effects when combined with morphine. Benzodiazepines are not thought to have direct analgesic properties, although they are potent anxiolytics and anticonvulsants (Coda et al. 1992). Some authors have suggested that their anticonvulsant properties make certain benzodiazepine drugs useful in the management of neuropathic pain. Recently, Fernandez et al. (1987b) showed that alprazolam, a unique benzodiazepine with mild antidepressant properties, was a helpful adjuvant analgesic in cancer patients with phantom limb pain or deafferentation (neuropathic) pain. Clonazepam may also be useful in the management of lancinating neuropathic pains in the cancer setting, and has been reported to be an effective analgesic for patients with trigeminal neuralgia, headache, and post-traumatic neuralgia (Caccia 1975; Swerdlow and Cundhill 1981). Intravenous midazolam in a patient-controlled dosage brought about no reduction in the use of post-operative morphine requirements or in the patient's perception of pain (Egan et al. 1992). Intrathecal midazolam in animal models, however, potentiated morphine analgesia (Liao and Takemori 1990). Diazepam can be useful as an adjuvant analgesic in the management of pain due to skeletal muscle spasms in patients with advanced cancer (Srivastava and Walsh 2003).

Placebo.   A mention of the placebo response is important in order to highlight the misunderstandings and relative harm of this phenomenon (see Fields, this volume, for a detailed discussion). The placebo response is common, and analgesia is mediated through endogenous opioids. The deceptive use of placebo response to distinguish psychogenic pain from "real" pain should be avoided. Placebos are effective in a portion of patients for a short period of time only and are not indicated in the management of cancer pain (Foley 1985).

REFERENCES

Achte KA, Vanhkonen ML. Cancer and the psyche. *Omega* 1971; 2:46–56.

Ahles TA, Blanchard EB, Ruckdeschel JC. The multidimensional nature of cancer related pain. *Pain* 1983; 17:277–288.

Anderson KO, Richman SP, Hurley J, et al. Cancer pain management among underserved minority outpatients: perceived needs and barriers to optimal control. *Cancer* 2002; 94:2295–2304.

Anthony M, Lance JW. MAO inhibition in the treatment of migraine. *Arch Neurol* 1969; 21:263.

Barber J, Gitelson J. Cancer pain: psychological management using hypnosis. *CA Cancer J Clin* 1980; 3:130–136.

Beaver WT, Feise G. Comparison of the analgesic effects of morphine, hydroxyzine and their combination in patients with post-operative pain. In: Bonica JJ, Albe-Fessard (Eds). *Proceedings of the First World Congress on Pain,* Advances in Pain Research and Therapy, Vol. 1. New York: Raven Press, 1976, pp 533–557.

Beaver WT, Wallenstein SL, Houde RW, et al. A comparison of the analgesic effect of methotrimeprazine and morphine in patients with cancer. *Clin Pharmacol Ther* 1966; 7:436–446.

Benson H. *The Relaxation Response.* New York: William Morrow, 1975.

Bolund C. Suicide and cancer: II. Medical and care factors in suicide by cancer patients in Sweden 1973–1976. *J Psychosoc Oncol* 1985; 3:17–30.

Bond MR, Pearson IB. Psychological aspects of pain in women with advanced cancer of the cervix. *J Psychosom Res* 1969; 13:13–19.

Bonica JJ. Cancer pain. In: Bonica JJ (Ed). *The Management of Pain,* 2nd ed, Vol. 1. Philadelphia: Lea and Febiger, 1990, pp 400–460.

Botney M, Fields HC. Amitriptyline potentiates morphine analgesia by direct action on the central nervous system. *Ann Neurol* 1983; 13:160–164.

Breitbart W. Suicide in cancer patients. *Oncology* 1987; 1:49–53.

Breitbart W. Psychiatric management of cancer pain. *Cancer* 1989; 63:2336–2342.

Breitbart W. Cancer pain and suicide. In: Foley KM, Bonica JJ, Ventafridda V (Eds). *Proceedings of the Second International Congress on Cancer Pain,* Advances in Pain Research and Therapy, Vol. 16. New York: Raven Press, 1990a, pp 399–412.

Breitbart W. Psychiatric aspects of pain and HIV disease. *Focus: Guide AIDS Res Counseling* 1990b; 5:1–2.

Breitbart W. Pain management and psychosocial issues in HIV and AIDS. *Am J Hosp Palliat Care* 1996; 13(1):20–29.

Breitbart W. Psychotropic adjuvant analgesics for cancer pain. *Psychooncology* 1998; 7(4):133–145.

Breitbart W, Holland JC. Psychiatric complications of cancer. In: Brain MC, Carbone PP (Eds). *Current Therapy in Hematology Oncology,* Vol. 3. Toronto: B.C. Decker, 1988, pp 268–274.

Breitbart W, Holland J. Psychiatric aspects of cancer pain. In: Foley KM, Bonica JJ, Ventafridda V (Eds). *Proceedings of the Second International Congress on Cancer Pain,* Advances in Pain Research and Therapy, Vol. 16. New York: Raven Press, 1990, pp 73–87.

Breitbart W, Mermelstein H. Pemoline: an alternative psychostimulant in the management of depressive disorders in cancer patients. *Psychosomatics* 1991; 33:352–356.

Breitbart W, Patt R. Pain management in the patient with AIDS. *Hematol Oncol Ann* 1994; 2:391–399.

Broome M, Lillis P, McGahhe T, et al. The use of distraction and imagery with children during painful procedures. *Oncol Nurs Forum* 1992; 19:499–502.

Bruera E, Chadwick S, Brennels C, et al. Methylphenidate associated with narcotics for the treatment of cancer pain. *Cancer Treat Rep* 1987; 71:67–70.

Bruera E, Brenneis C, Paterson AH, et al. Use of methylphenidate as an adjuvant to narcotic analgesics in patients with advanced cancer. *J Pain Sympton Manage* 1989a; 4:3–6.

Bruera E, MacMillan K, Kachin N, et al. The cognitive effects of the administration of narcotics. *Pain* 1989b; 39:13–16.

Bruera E, MacMillan K, Pither J, et al. Effects of morphine on the dyspnea of terminal cancer patients. *J Pain Symptom Manage* 1990; 5:341–344.

Bruera E, Fainsinger R, MacEachern T, et al. The use of methylphenidate in patients with incident cancer pain receiving regular opiates: a preliminary report. *Pain* 1992; 50:75–77.

Bukberg J, Penman D, Holland J. Depression in hospitalized cancer patients. *Psychosom Med* 1984; 43:199–122.

Butler S. Present status of tricyclic antidepressants in chronic pain therapy. In: Benedetti C (Ed). *Recent Advances in the Management of Pain,* Advances in Pain Research and Therapy, Vol. 7. New York: Raven Press, 1984, pp 173–196.

Caccia MR. Clonazepam in facial neuralgia and cluster headache: clinical and electrophysiological study. *Eur Neurol* 1975; 13:560–563.

Cardenas DD, Warms CA, Turner JA, et al. Efficacy of amitriptyline for relief of pain in spinal cord injury: results of a randomized controlled trial. *Pain* 2002; 96:365–373.

Cassem NH. The dying patient. In: Hackett TP, Cassem NH (Eds). *Massachusetts General Hospital Handbook of General Hospital Psychiatry,* 2nd ed. Littleton, MA: PSG, 1987, pp 332–352.

Charap AD. The knowledge, attitudes, and experience of medical personnel treating pain in the terminally ill. *Mt Sinai J Med* 1978; 45:561–501.

Cleeland CS. Nonpharmacologic management of cancer pain. *J Pain Symptom Manage* 1987; 2:523–528.

Cleeland CS, Tearnan BH. Behavioral control of cancer pain. In: Holzman D, Turk D (Eds). *Pain Management.* New York: Pergamon Press, 1986, pp 193–212.

Cleeland C, Gonin R, Hatfield A, et al. Pain and its treatment in outpatients with metastatic cancer. *N Engl J Med* 1994; 330:592–596.

Coda B, Mackie A, Hill H. Influence of alprazolam on opioid analgesia and side effects during steady-stage morphine infusions. *Pain* 1992; 50:309–316.

Connell C. Art therapy as part of a palliative cancer program. *Palliat Med* 1992; 6:18–25.

Cornblath DR, McArthur IC. Predominantly sensory neuropathy in patients with AIDS and AIDS-related complex. *Neurology* 1988; 38:794–796.

Costa D, Mogos I, Toma T. Efficacy and safety of mianserin in the treatment of depression of woman with cancer. *Acta Psychiatr Scand* 1985; 72:85–92.

Daut RL, Cleeland CS. The prevalence and severity of pain in cancer. *Cancer* 1982; 50:1913–1918.

Davidoff G, Guarracini M, Roth E, et al. Trazodone hydrochloride in the treatment of dysesthetic pain in traumatic myelopathy: a randomized, double-blind, placebo-controlled study. *Pain* 1987; 29:151–161.

Derogatis LR, Morrow GR, Fetting J, et al. The prevalence of psychiatric disorders among cancer patients. *JAMA* 1983; 249:751–757.

Devine EC. Meta-analysis of the effect of psychoeducational interventions on pain in adults with cancer. *Oncol Nurs Forum* 2003; 30:75–89.

De Wit R, van Dam F, Loonstra S, et al. Improving the quality of pain treatment by a tailored pain education programme for patients in chronic pain. *Eur J Pain* 2001a; 5:241–256.

De Wit R, van Dam F, Litjens MJ, Abu-Saad HH. Assessment of pain cognitions in cancer patients with chronic pain. *J Pain Sympton Manage* 2001b; 5:911–924.

Diamond S, Frietag FG. The use of fluoxetine in the treatment of headache. *Clin J Pain* 1989; 5:200–201.

Eberhard G, von Knorring L, Nilsson HL, et al. A double-blind randomized study of clomipramine versus maprotiline in patients with idiopathic pain syndromes. *Neuropsychobiology* 1988; 19:25–32.

Egan K, Ready L, Nessly M, et al. Self administration of midazolam for post-operative anxiety: a double blinded study. *Pain* 1992; 49:3–8.

Erickson MH. Hypnosis in painful terminal illness. *Am J Clin Hypnosis* 1959; 1:1117–1121.

Evans S, Fishman B, Spielman L, et al. Randomized trial of cognitive behavior therapy versus supportive psychotherapy for HIV-related peripheral neuropathic pain. *Psychosomatics* 2003a; 44:44–50.

Evans S, Weinberg B, Spielman L, Fishman B. Assessing negative thoughts in response to pain among people with HIV. *Pain* 2003b; 105:239–245.

Farberow NL, Schneidman ES, Leonard CV. Suicide among general medical and surgical hospital patients with malignant neoplasms. *Med Bull Vet Admin* 1963; 9:1–11.

Farrar JT, Portenoy RK. Neuropathic cancer pain: the role of adjuvant analgesics. *Oncology (Hunting)* 2001; 15:1435–1442, 1445; discussion 1445; 1450–1453.

Feighner JP. A comparative trial of fluoxetine and amitriptyline in patients with major depressive disorder. *J Clin Psychiatry* 1985; 46:369–372.

Fernandez F, Adams F, Holmes VF, et al. Methylphenidate for depressive disorders in cancer patients. *Psychosomatics* 1987a; 28:455–461.

Fernandez F, Adams F, Holmes VF. Analgesic effect of alprazolam in patients with chronic, organic pain of malignant origin. *J Clin Psychopharmacol* 1987b; 3:167–169.

Fishbain D. Evidence-based data on pain relief with antidepressants. *Ann Med* 2000; 32:305–316.

Fishman B. The treatment of suffering in patients with cancer pain. In: Foley K, Bonica J, Ventafridda V (Eds). *Proceedings of the Second International Congress on Cancer Pain,* Advances in Pain Research and Therapy, Vol. 16. New York: Raven Press, 1990, pp 301–316.

Fishman B, Loscalzo M. Cognitive-behavioral interventions in the management of cancer pain: principles and applications. *Med Clin North Am* 1987; 71:271–287.

Foley KM. Pain syndromes in patients with cancer. In: Bonica JJ, Ventafridda V, Fink RB, Jones LE, Loeser JD (Eds). *International Symposium on Pain of Advanced Cancer,* Advances in Pain Research and Therapy, Vol. 2. New York: Raven Press, 1978, pp 59–75.

Foley KM. The treatment of cancer pain. *N Engl J Med* 1985; 313:845.

Forrest WH Jr, Brown BW Jr, Brown CR, et al. Dextroamphetamine with morphine for the treatment of post-operative pain. *N Engl J Med* 1977; 296:712–715.

Fotopoulos SS, Graham C, Cook MR. Psychophysiologic control of cancer pain. In: Bonica JJ, Ventafridda V, Fink RB, Jones LE, Loeser JD (Eds). *International Symposium on Pain of Advanced Cancer,* Advances in Pain Research and Therapy, Vol. 2. New York: Raven Press, 1978, pp 231–244.

France RD. The future for antidepressants: treatment of pain. *Psychopathology* 1987; 20:99–113.

Geller SA. Treatment of fibrositis with fluoxetine hydrochloride (Prozac). *Am J Med* 1989; 87:594–595.

Getto CJ, Sorkness CA, Howell T. Antidepressants and chronic nonmalignant pain: a review. *J Pain Symptom Manage* 1987; 2:9–18.

Gomez-Perez FJ, Rull JA, Dies H, et al. Nortriptyline and fluphenazine in the symptomatic treatment of diabetic neuropathy: a double-blind cross-over study. *Pain* 1985; 23:395–400.

Gordon N, Heller P, Gear R, et al. Temporal factors in the enhancement of morphine analgesic by desipramine. *Pain* 1993; 53:273–276.

Grond S, Zech D, Diefenbach C, et al. Prevalence and pattern of symptoms in patients with cancer pain: a prospective evaluation of 1635 cancer patients referred to a pain clinic. *J Pain Symptom Manage* 1994; 9:372–382.

Grossman SA, Sheidler VR, Swedeen K, et al. Correlations of patient and caregiver ratings of cancer pain. *J Pain Symptom Manage* 1991; 6:53–57.

Haller DL, Miles DR. Suicidal ideation among psychiatric patients with HIV: psychiatric morbidity and quality of life. *AIDS Behav* 2003; 7:101–108.

Hammack JE, Michalak JC, Loprinzi CL, et al. Phase III evaluation of nortriptyline for alleviation of symptoms of cis-platinum-induced peripheral neuropathy. *Pain* 2002; 98:195–203

Hammeroff SR, Cork RC, Scherer K, et al. Doxepin effects on chronic pain, depression and plasma opioids. *J Clin Psychiatry* 1982; 2:22–26.

Hanks GW. Opioid responsive and opioid non-responsive pain in cancer. *Br Med Bull* 1991; 47:718–731.

Hewitt D, Breitbart W, Rosenfeld B, et al. Pain syndromes and etiologies in ambulatory AIDS patients. *Pain* 1997; 70:117–123.

Hynes MD, Lochner MA, Bemis K, et al. Fluoxetine, a selective inhibitor of serotonin uptake, potentiates morphine analgesia without altering its discriminative stimulus properties or affinity for opioid receptors. *Life Sci* 1985; 36:2317–2323.

Jensen M, Turner J, Romano J, et al. Coping with chronic pain: a critical review of the literature. *Pain* 1991; 47:249–283.

Kanner RM, Foley KM. Patterns of narcotic use in a cancer pain clinic. *Ann New York Acad Sci* 1981; 362:161–172.

Kaufmann MW, Murray GB, Cassem NH. Use of psychostimulants in medically ill depressive patients. *Psychosomatics* 1982; 23:817–819.

Khojainova N, Santiago-Palma J, Kornick C, et al. Olanzapine in the management of cancer pain. *J Pain Symptom Manage* 2002; 23:346–350.

Kieburtz K, Simpson D, Yiannoutsos C, et al. AIDS Clinical Trial Group 242 Protocol Team. A randomized trial of amitriptyline and mexiletine for painful neuropathy in HIV infection. *Neurology* 1998; 51:1682–1688.

Kvindesal B, Molin J, Froland A, et al. Imipramine treatment of painful diabetic neuropathy. *JAMA* 1984; 251:1727–1730.

Langohr HD, Stohr M, Petruch F. An open and double-blind crossover study on the efficacy of clomipramine (Anafranil) in patients with painful mono- and polyneuropathies. *Eur Neurol* 1982; 21:309–315.

Lascelles RG. Atypical facial pain and depression. *Br J Psychol* 1966; 122:651.

Lebovits AH, Lefkowitz M, McCarthy D, et al. The prevalence and management of pain in patients with AIDS: a review of 134 cases. *Clin J Pain* 1989; 5:245–248.

Lechin F, van der Dijs B, Lechin ME, et al. Pimozide therapy for trigeminal neuralgia. *Arch Neurol* 1989; 9:960–964.

Lefkowitz M, Breitbart W. Chronic pain and AIDS. *Innovat Pain Med* 1992; 36:2–3.

Levin DN, Cleeland CS, Dan R. Public attitudes toward cancer pain. *Cancer* 1985; 56:2337–2339.

Levitan A. The use of hypnosis with cancer patients. *Psychiatry Med* 1992; 10:119–131.

Levy RM, Bredesen DE, Rosenblum ML. Neurological manifestations of the AIDS experience at UCSF and review of the literature. *J Neurosurg* 1985; 62:475–495.

Liao J, Takemori A. Quantitative assessment of antinociceptive effects of midazolam, amitriptyline, and carbamazepine alone and in combination with morphine in mice. *Anesthesiology* 1990; 73:A753.

Loscalzo M, Jacobsen PB. Practical behavioral approaches to the effective management of pain and distress. *J Psychosoc Oncol* 1990; 8:139–169.

Magni G, Arsie D, DeLeo D. Antidepressants in the treatment of cancer pain: a survey in Italy. *Pain* 1987; 29:347–353.

Malseed RT, Goldstein FJ. Enhancement of morphine analgesics by tricyclic antidepressants. *Neuropharmacology* 1979; 18:827–829.

Maltbie AA, Cavenar JO, Sullivan JL, et al. Analgesia and haloperidol: a hypothesis. *J Clin Psychiatry* 1979; 40:323–326.

Manne S, Redd W, Jacobsen P, et al. Fragrance administration to reduce anxiety during MR imaging. *J Magn Reson Imaging* 1994; 4:623–626.

Marks RM, Sachar EJ. Undertreatment of medical inpatients with narcotic analgesics. *Ann Intern Med* 1973; 78:173–181.

Marzuk P, Tierney H, Tardiff K, et al. Increased risk of suicide in persons with AIDS. *JAMA* 1988; 259:1333–1337.

Massie MJ, Holland JC. The cancer patient with pain: psychiatric complications and their management. *Med Clin North Am* 1987; 71:243–258.

Massie JM, Holland JC, Glass E. Delirium in terminally ill cancer patients. *Am J Psychiatry* 1983; 140:1048–1050.

Massie M, Gagnon P, Holland J. Depression and suicide in patients with cancer. *J Pain Symptom Manage* 1994; 9:325–331.

Max MB, Culnane M, Schafer SC, et al. Amitriptyline relieves diabetic-neuropathy pain in patients with normal and depressed mood. *Neurology* 1987; 37:589–596.

Max MB, Schafer SC, Culnane M, et al. Amitriptyline, but not lorazepam, relieves postherpetic neuralgia. *Neurology* 1988; 38:427–432.

Max MB, Kishore-Kumar R, Schafer SC, et al. Efficacy of desipramine in painful diabetic neuropathy: a placebo-controlled trial. *Pain* 1991; 45:3–10.

Max MB, Lynch SA, Muir J, et al. Effects of desipramine, amitriptyline, and fluoxetine on pain in diabetic neuropathy. *N Engl J Med* 1992; 326:1250–1256.

McCormack JP, Li R, Zarowny D, et al. Inadequate treatment of pain in ambulatory HIV patients. *Clin J Pain* 1993; 9:279–283.

McKegney FP, Bailey CR, Yates JW. Prediction and management of pain in patients with advanced cancer. *Gen Hosp Psychiatry* 1981; 3:95–101.

McQuay H, Carroll D, Glynn C. Dose-response for analgesic effect of amitriptyline in chronic pain. *Anesthesia* 1993; 48:281–285.

Munro SM, Mount B. Music therapy in palliative care. *CMAJ* 1978; 119:1029–1034.

Nehra A, Mullick F, Ishak KG, Zimmerman HJ. Pemoline-associated hepatic injury. *Gastroenterology* 1990; 99:1517–1519.

Newshan G, Wainapel S, Schmitz D. Pain characteristics and their management in persons with AIDS. *J Assoc Nurses AIDS Care* 1993; 4:53–59.

Oliver JW, Kravitz RL, Kaplan SH, et al. Individualized patient education and coaching to improve pain control among cancer outpatients. *J Clin Oncol* 2001; 19:2206–2212.

Onghena P, Van Houdenhove B. Antidepressant-induced analgesia in chronic non-malignant pain: a meta-analysis of 39 placebo-controlled studies. *Pain* 1992; 49:205–219.

Padilla G, Ferrell B, Grant M, et al. Defining the content domain of quality of life for cancer patients with pain. *Cancer Nurs* 1990; 13:108–115.

Passik S, Kirsh KL, Theobald D, et al. Use of a depression screening tool and a fluoxetine-based algorithm to improve the recognition and treatment of depression in cancer patients: a demonstration project. *J Pain Symptom Manage* 2002; 24:318–327.

Pick CG, Paul D, Eison MS, et al. Potentiation of opioid analgesia by the antidepressant nefazodone. *Eur J Pharmacol* 1992; 211:375–381.

Pilowsky I, Hallett EC, Bassett DL, et al. A controlled study of amitriptyline in the treatment of chronic pain. *Pain* 1982; 14:169–179.

Rabkin J, Remien R, Katoff L, et al. Suicidality in AIDS long-term survivors: what is the evidence? *AIDS Care* 1993; 5:401–411.

Redd WB, Reeves JL, Storm FK, et al. Hypnosis in the control of pain during hyperthermia treatment of cancer. In: Bonica JJ, Lindblom U, Iggo A (Eds). Proceedings of the Third World Congress on Pain, Advances in Pain Research and Theory, Vol. 5. New York: Raven Press, 1983, pp 857–861.

Redd WH, Montgomery GH, DuHamel KN. Behavioral intervention for cancer treatment side effects. *J Natl Cancer Inst* 2001; 93:810–823.

Rumore M, Schlichting D. Clinical efficacy of antihistamines as analgesics. *Pain* 1986; 25:7–22.

Saunders CM. Terminal patient care. *Geriatrics* 1966; 12:70–74.

Schofferman J, Brody R. Pain in far advanced AIDS. In: Foley KM, Bonica JJ, Ventafridda V (Eds). Proceedings of the Second International Congress on Cancer Pain, Advances in Pain Research and Therapy, Vol. 16. New York: Raven Press, 1990, pp 379–386.

Schroeder-Sheker T. Music for the dying: a personal account of the new field of music thanatology—history, theories, and clinical narratives. *J Holist Nurs* 1994; 12:83–99.

Shlay JC, Chaloner K, Max MB, et al. Community programs for clinical research on AIDS. Acupuncture and amitriptyline for pain due to HIV-related peripheral neuropathy: a randomized controlled trial. *JAMA* 1998; 280:1590–1595

Sharav Y, Singer E, Schmidt E, et al. The analgesic effect of amitriptyline on chronic facial pain. *Pain* 1987; 31:199–209.

Silberfarb PM, Manrer LH, Cronthamel CS. Psychological aspects of neoplastic disease. I: Functional status of breast cancer patients during different treatment regimens. *Am J Psychiatry* 1980; 137:450–455.

Sindrup SH, Ejlertsen B, Froland A, et al. Imipramine treatment in diabetic neuropathy: relief of subjective symptoms without changes in peripheral and autonomic nerve function. *Eur J Clin Pharmacol* 1989; 37:151–153.

Sindrup SH, Gram LF, Brosen K, et al. The selective serotonin reuptake inhibitor paroxetine is effective in the treatment of diabetic neuropathy symptoms. *Pain* 1990; 42:135–144.

Singer EJ, Zorilla C, Fahy-Chandon B, et al. Painful symptoms reported for ambulatory HIV-infected men in a longitudinal study. *Pain* 1993; 54:15–19.

Snider WD, Simpson DM, Nielsen S, et al. Neurological complications of AIDS; analysis of 50 patients. *Ann Neurol* 1983; 14:403–418.

Sollner W, DeVries A, Steixner E, et al. How successful are oncologists in identifying patient distress, perceived social support, and need for psychosocial counseling? *Br J Cancer* 2001; 84:179–185.

Spiegel D. The use of hypnosis in controlling cancer pain. *CA Cancer J Clin* 1985; 4:221–231.

Spiegel D, Bloom JR. Group therapy and hypnosis reduce metastatic breast carcinoma pain. *Psychosom Med* 1983a; 4:333–339.

Spiegel D, Bloom JR. Pain in metastatic breast cancer. *Cancer* 1983b; 52:341–345.

Spiegel K, Kalb R, Pasternak GW. Analgesic activity of tricyclic antidepressants. *Ann Neurol* 1983; 13:462–465.

Srivastava M, Walsh D. Diazepam as an adjuvant analgesic to morphine for pain due to skeletal muscle spasm. *Support Care Cancer* 2003;11:66–69.

Stiefel F. Psychosocial aspects of cancer pain. *Support Care Cancer* 1993; 1:130–134.

Stiefel FC, Breitbart W, Holland JC. Corticosteroids in cancer: neuropsychiatric complications. *Cancer Invest* 1989; 7:479–491.

Swerdlow M, Cundill JG. Anticonvulsant drugs used in the treatment of lancinating pains: a comparison. *Anesthesia* 1981; 36:1129–1134.

Syrjala K, Chapko M. Evidence for a biopsychosocial model of cancer treatment-related pain. *Pain* 1995; 61:69–79.

Syrjala K, Cummings C, Donaldson G. Hypnosis or cognitive behavioral training for the reduction of pain and nausea during cancer treatment: a controlled trial. *Pain* 1992; 48:137–146.

Theesen KA, Marsh WR. Relief of diabetic neuropathy with fluoxetine. *DICP* 1989; 23:572–574.

Tiengo M, Pagnoni B, Calmi A, et al. Clomipramine compared to pentazocine as a unique treatment in postoperative pain. *Int J Clin Pharmacol Res* 1987; 7:141–143.

Turk D, Fernendez E. On the putative uniqueness of cancer pain: do psychological principles apply? *Behav Res Ther* 1990; 28:1–13.

Turk D, Okifuji A. Does sex make a difference in the prescription of treatments and the adaptation to chronic pain by cancer and non-cancer patients? *Pain* 1999; 82:139–148.

Twycross RG, Lack SA. Symptom control in far advanced cancer: pain relief. London: Pitman Brooks, 1983.

Tyler MA. Treatment of the painful shoulder syndrome with amitriptyline and lithium carbonate. *CMAJ* 1974; 111:137–140.

Ventafridda V, Bonezzi C, Caraceni A, et al. Antidepressants for cancer pain and other painful syndromes with deafferentation component: comparison of amitriptyline and trazodone. *Ital J Neurol Sci* 1987; 8:579–587.

Ventafridda V, Bianchi M, Ripamonti C, et al. Studies on the effects of antidepressant drugs on the antinociceptive action of morphine and on plasma morphine in rat and man. *Pain* 1990; 43:155–162.

Vogl D, Rosenfeld B, Breitbart W, et al. Symptom prevalence, characteristics, and distress in AIDS outpatients. *J Pain Symptom Manage* 1999; 18(4):253–262.

Walsh TD. Antidepressants and chronic pain. *Clin Neuropharmacol* 1983; 6:271–295.

Walsh TD. Adjuvant analgesic therapy in cancer pain. In: Foley KM, Bonica JJ, Ventafridda V (Eds). *Proceedings of the Second International Congress on Cancer Pain,* Advances in Pain Research and Therapy, Vol. 16. New York: Raven Press, 1990, pp 155–165.

Watson CP, Evans RJ. A comparative trial of amitriptyline and zimelidine in post-herpetic neuralgia. *Pain* 1985; 23:387–394.

Watson CP, Evans RJ, Reed K, et al. Amitriptyline versus placebo in post herpetic neuralgia. *Neurology* 1992a; 32:671–673.

Watson C, Chipan M, Reed K, et al. Amitriptyline versus maprotiline in postherpetic neuralgia: a randomized double-blind crossover trial. *Pain* 1992b; 48:29–36.

Woodforde JM, Fielding JR. Pain and cancer. *J Psychosom Res* 1970; 14:365–370.

Yates PM, Edwards HE, Nash RE, et al. Barriers to effective cancer pain management: a survey of hospitalized cancer patients in Australia. *J Pain Symptom Manage* 2002; 23:393–405.

Young RJ, Clarke BF. Pain relief in diabetic neuropathy: the effectiveness of imipramine and related drugs. *Diabet Med* 1985; 2:363–366.

Zaza C, Baine N. Cancer pain and psychosocial factors: a critical review of the literature. *J Pain Symptom Manage* 2002; 24:526–542.

Correspondence to: William S. Breitbart, MD, Department of Psychiatry and Behavioral Sciences, Memorial Sloan-Kettering Cancer Center, 1242 Second Avenue, Box 421, New York, NY 10021, USA. Email: breitbaw@mskcc.org.

Part V

Specific Populations

Psychosocial Aspects of Pain: A Handbook for Health Care Providers, Progress in Pain Research and Management, Vol. 27, edited by Robert H. Dworkin and William S. Breitbart, IASP Press, Seattle, © 2004.

20

Identifying and Treating Patients with Drug Abuse Problems

Steven D. Passik and Kenneth L. Kirsh

Symptom Management and Palliative Care Program, Markey Cancer Center, University of Kentucky, Lexington, Kentucky, USA

Nearly one-third of the U.S. population has experimented with illicit drugs, and substance use disorders are estimated to have a base rate of 6–15% (Regier et al. 1984; Collier and Kopstein 1991; Groerer and Brodsky 1992). In addition, more than four million Americans used prescription drugs in 2000 for nonmedical purposes. This high prevalence of nonmedical drug use, along with concerns of drug abuse and addiction, often has negatively influenced the manner in which pain is treated. Patients who have current or previous histories of drug abuse along with progressive life-threatening diseases present numerous physical and psychosocial issues that may affect medical treatment and pain and symptom management. Many physicians do not specialize in addiction issues and may encounter difficulty in their efforts to treat these patients efficiently. Moreover, there is a lack of clarity in defining abuse or addiction in the chronic pain setting. Even when patients do not have bona fide histories of addiction, problematic behavior can become manifest at times during pain therapy. The meaning of these behaviors is often complex.

Another issue that has detrimental effects on pain management is opiophobia, or the fear of prescribing opioid analgesics, which may result in the undertreatment of chronic pain (Cohen 1980; Shine and Demas 1984; Morgan 1986). Opiophobia may stem from multiple concerns, including fear of opening the door to abuse, fear of creating full-blown addiction in patients, fear of regulatory and legal sanction, and fear of inducing respiratory depression. While it is estimated that approximately 3–16% of chronic pain patients are addicted to opioids, this estimate may not reflect the true rate of addiction in this population due to diversity in patient samples and discrepancies in defining addiction (Haller and Butler 1991; Fishbain 1996; Miotto et al. 1996). Empirical data also indicate that substance use disorders are more prevalent in the chronic pain population than in the general population (Katon et al. 1985; Fishbain et al. 1986; Atkinson et al. 1991; Gatchel et al. 1994).

Due to these issues and despite national guidelines for the treatment of cancer pain, undertreatment of both malignant and nonmalignant pain continues. It is estimated that 40–50% of patients with metastatic disease and 90% of patients with terminal cancer experience unrelieved pain (Ward et al. 1993; Glajchen et al. 1995; Ramer et al. 1999). Furthermore, there is a greater potential for inadequate treatment of pain if the patient has a history of substance abuse (Joranson and Gibson 1994). This chapter will examine relevant conceptual and clinical aspects of aberrant behavior that can improve the identification and treatment of patients who manifest noncompliance behaviors ranging from the innocuous to the illegal.

CHALLENGES IN DEFINING ABUSE AND ADDICTION IN THE MEDICALLY ILL

Chronic opioid therapy has been gaining acceptance as an appropriate and effective method of pain management not only in cancer patients, but also in patients experiencing chronic nonmalignant pain (Portenoy and Foley 1986; Urban et al. 1986; Portenoy 1990, 1994; Zenz et al. 1992). Despite this growing acceptance, chronic opioid therapy continues to be controversial due to the possibility that some patients may be at increased risk for developing opioid addiction or for increasing premorbid addiction behaviors (Miotto et al. 1996). Therefore, clinicians must pay particular attention to the assessment of outcomes while patients are receiving chronic opioid therapy. These outcomes include pain relief, psychosocial functioning, side effects, and possible aberrant drug-taking behaviors (Compton et al. 1998; Passik and Weinreb 2000).

Challenges are also encountered in attempting to identify a substance use disorder in medical patients because the definition of both abuse and addiction has been elicited from addicted populations without medical illness. This situation may ultimately lead to confusion in the medical setting. Clarification of this terminology is therefore crucial for improving the diagnosis and management of substance abuse in the oncology setting (Passik and Portenoy 1998a,b).

UNDERTREATMENT OF PAIN

Various compelling studies provide evidence that pain is undertreated in the medically ill (Ward et al. 1993; Glajchen et al. 1995; Ramer et al. 1999). In addition, clinical experience suggests that inadequate management of symptoms and related pain may be the motivation for aberrant drug-taking behaviors. *Pseudoaddiction* is the term utilized to delineate the distress and drug-seeking behaviors, sometimes similar to those of addicts, that can occur in the context of unrelieved pain (Weissman and Haddox 1989). The most important element of this syndrome is that adequate pain relief eliminates aberrant behaviors (Passik et al. 1998; Passik and Portenoy 1998a).

The possibility of pseudoaddiction presents numerous challenges regarding the assessment of known substance abusers who develop illness. Clinical evidence indicates that aberrant behaviors evoked by unrelieved pain can become so dramatic that some patients appear to return to illicit drug use as a means of self-medication, while others utilize less blatant patterns of behavior that may also raise concerns regarding the possibility of true addiction. While it may be apparent that drug-related behaviors are aberrant, the intent of these behaviors may be difficult to discern in the context of unrelieved symptoms (Passik et al. 1998; Passik and Portenoy 1998a).

DIFFERENTIATING ABERRANT DRUG-TAKING BEHAVIORS

The continuum of drug-related behaviors ranges from less aberrant behaviors such as aggressive requests for medication to more aberrant ones such as frequent unsanctioned dose escalation. The ability to classify these questionable behaviors as outside the social or cultural norm presupposes that there is certainty regarding the parameters of normative behavior. However, in the area of prescription drug utilization we lack empirical data defining these parameters. A specific behavior in which a large proportion of patients engage may be normative, and judgments concerning aberrancy should be influenced accordingly (Passik et al. 1998; Passik and Portenoy 1998a).

This issue was the focus of a pilot study performed at Memorial Sloan-Kettering Cancer Center, which revealed that 26% of cancer patients admitted borrowing anxiolytics from a family member at some time. The high incidence of this behavior among cancer patients raises concerns regarding its predictive validity as an indicator of a diagnosis related to substance abuse. Clearly, we need empirical data that clarify the prevalence of drug-taking behaviors and attitudes in different populations of medically ill patients to help guide clinical thinking concerning behaviors that manifest during treatment (Passik et al. 1998; Passik and Portenoy 1998a).

DISEASE-RELATED VARIABLES

Alterations in physical and psychosocial functioning caused by medical illness and its treatment, which may be difficult to differentiate from the morbidity associated with drug abuse, also challenge the main concepts utilized to define addiction. This difficulty may particularly complicate the ability to assess a concept that is crucial to the diagnosis of addiction: "use despite harm." For example, it can be difficult to discern problematic behaviors in the patient who develops social withdrawal or cognitive changes after brain irradiation for metastases. Even if impaired cognition is clearly related to medication used in treatment, this effect might only represent a narrow therapeutic window rather than the patient's utilization of analgesics to attain these psychic effects (Passik et al. 1998; Passik and Portenoy 1998a). Additionally, in situations where disease and pain have severely limited psychological, social, and vocational functioning, it can be difficult to ascribe harm to particular drug-taking behaviors in the context of so much dysfunction.

Accurate assessment of drug-related behaviors in medical patients usually requires detailed information concerning the role of the drug in the patient's life. Therefore, mild mental clouding or the amount of time spent in bed may be insignificant when compared to other outcomes such as noncompliance with primary therapy related to drug use as well as behaviors that compromise relationships with physicians, other health care professionals, and family members (Passik et al. 1998; Passik and Portenoy 1998a).

NEW DEFINITIONS OF ABUSE AND ADDICTION
FOR THE MEDICALLY ILL

Various definitions of abuse that include the phenomena related to physical dependence or tolerance are not applicable to patients who receive potentially abusable drugs for legitimate medical purposes (see Table I). A differential diagnosis should be explored if questionable behaviors occur during pain treatment. A true addiction is only one of several possible explanations, but is more likely when the patient engages in behaviors such as multiple unsanctioned dose escalations and attempts to obtain opioids from

Table I
Terms to consider when evaluating a chronic pain patient
for possible substance use disorders

Term	Definition	Utility
Physical dependence	The development of substance-specific symptoms of withdrawal after the abrupt stopping of a medication; these symptoms can be physiological only (i.e., absence of psychological or behavioral maladaptive patterns)	Not useful for determining substance use disorders because all patients may express dependence
Tolerance	The development of a need to take increasing doses of a medication to obtain the same effect; tachyphylaxis is the term used when this process happens quickly	Not useful for determining substance use disorders because all patients may express tolerance
Addiction	The development of a maladaptive pattern of medication use that leads to clinically significant impairment or distress in personal or occupational roles. This syndrome also includes a great deal of time used to obtain and use the medication or to recover from its effects, loss of control over medication use, and continuation of medication use after medical or psychological adverse effects have occurred	Very useful; clearcut addiction is heralded by the tenet of "use despite harm." Management will involve clear planning and extensive follow-up of the patient
Pseudoaddiction	Pattern of drug-seeking behavior of pain patients receiving inadequate pain management that can be mistaken for addiction	Potentially useful; best diagnosed retrospectively, after effective opioid therapy is achieved
Abuse/impulsive drug use	The intentional misuse of a medication, either overuse or use for a purpose not prescribed (i.e., mood alteration); physical dependence is not present	Potentially useful; abuse may be experimentation or related to diversion and criminal activity; monitor carefully
Aberrant drug takers	Those with personality disorders who exhibit aberrant drug-taking behaviors by utilizing prescription medications to express fear and anger or to improve chronic boredom	Potentially useful; patients need psychiatric referral and follow-up concomitant with their pain management

multiple prescribers. The diagnosis of pseudoaddiction must also be considered if the patient is reporting distress related to unrelieved symptoms. Behaviors such as aggressively complaining about the need for higher doses or occasional unilateral drug escalations may be indications that the patient's pain is undermedicated. Impulsive drug use may also indicate another psychiatric disorder, diagnosis of which may have therapeutic implications. For example, patients with borderline personality disorders may be categorized as exhibiting aberrant drug-taking behaviors if they use prescription medications to express fear and anger or to improve chronic boredom. Similarly, patients who use opioids to self-medicate for symptoms of anxiety or depression, insomnia, or problems of adjustment may be classified as aberrant drug takers. Occasionally, aberrant drug-related behaviors appear to be causally related to mild encephalopathy, with confusion regarding the appropriate therapeutic regimen. Problematic behaviors rarely imply criminal intent such as when patients report pain but intend to sell or divert medications. These diagnoses are not mutually exclusive, and a thorough psychiatric assessment is vitally important in an effort to categorize questionable behaviors properly in both the population without a prior history of substance abuse and that of known substance abusers who have a higher incidence of psychiatric comorbidity (Passik et al. 1998; Passik and Portenoy 1998).

CLINICAL MANAGEMENT

Out-of-control aberrant drug-taking among medically ill patients (with or without a prior history of substance abuse) represents a serious and complex clinical occurrence. Perhaps the more difficult situations involve the patient who is actively abusing illicit or prescription drugs or alcohol concomitantly with medical therapies. The following guidelines can be useful whether the patient is an active drug abuser, has a history of substance abuse, or is not complying with the therapeutic regimen. The principles outlined help clinicians to establish structure and control and monitor drug consumption so that they can prescribe freely and without prejudice.

MULTIDISCIPLINARY APPROACH

A multidisciplinary team approach is recommended for the management of substance abuse in the palliative care setting. Mental health professionals with specialization in the addictions can be instrumental in helping palliative care team members develop strategies for management and patient treatment compliance, although often such professionals are not readily available. Providing care to these patients can lead to feelings of anger and frustration among staff. Such feelings can unintentionally compromise the level of patient care surrounding the patient's pain management and may contribute to feelings of isolation and alienation by the patient. A structured multidisciplinary approach can be effective in helping the staff better understand the patient's needs and develop effective strategies for controlling pain and aberrant drug use simultaneously. Staff meetings can be helpful in establishing treatment goals, facilitating compliance, and coordinating the multidisciplinary team.

ASSESSMENT

The first member of the medical team, frequently a nurse, to suspect problematic drug taking or a history of drug abuse should alert the patient's palliative care team, thus beginning the multidisciplinary assessment and management process (Lundberg and Passik 1997). A physician should assess the potential of withdrawal or other pressing concerns and begin involving staff trained in social work or psychiatry to begin planning management strategies. It is crucial to obtain as detailed as possible a history of duration, frequency, and desired effect of drug use. Frequently, clinicians avoid asking patients about substance abuse out of fear that they will anger the patient or that they are incorrect in their suspicion of abuse. However, such approaches will most likely contribute to continued problems with treatment compliance and frustration among staff. Empathic and truthful communication is always the best approach. The use of a careful, graduated interview approach can be instrumental in slowly introducing the assessment of drug use. This approach entails starting the assessment interview with broad questions about the role of drugs such as nicotine and caffeine in the patient's life and gradually becoming more specific in focus to include illicit drugs. Such an approach is helpful in reducing the denial and resistance that the patient may express. This interviewing style also assists in the detection of coexisting psychiatric disorders, which can significantly contribute to aberrant drug-taking behavior. Studies suggest that 37–62% of alcoholics have one or more coexisting psychiatric disorders. Anxiety, personality disorders, and mood disorders are the most commonly encountered (Penick et al. 1994). The assessment and treatment of comorbid psychiatric disorders can greatly enhance management strategies and reduce the risk of relapse. The patient's desired effects from illicit drugs can often be a clue to comorbid psychiatric disorders—for example, drinking alcohol to quell panic symptoms.

DEVELOPMENT OF A MULTIDISCIPLINARY TREATMENT PLAN

Drug abuse is often a chronic, progressive disorder. Therefore, the development of clear treatment goals is essential. Team members should not expect a complete remission of the patient's substance use problems. The distress of coping with a life-threatening illness and the availability of prescription drugs for symptom control can make complete abstinence an unrealistic goal (Passik and Portenoy 1998b). Rather, a harm reduction approach should be employed that aims to enhance social support, maximize treatment compliance, and contain the harm caused by episodic relapse (see Table II). The following guidelines are recommended for the management of patients with a substance disorder. The clinician should first establish a relationship based on empathic listening and accept the patient's report of distress. Second, it is important to utilize non-opioid and behavioral interventions when possible, but not as substitutes for appropriate pain management. Third, the team should consider tolerance, route of administration, and duration of action when prescribing medications for pain and symptom management. Pre-existing tolerance should be taken into account for patients who are actively abusing drugs or are being maintained on methadone maintenance programs.

Table II
Managing chronic pain patients with substance use problems:
a harm reduction approach

Step 1: Establish the Relationship
Focus on developing rapport with the patient
Use empathy, active listening, and nonjudgmental language

Step 2: Use Non-Opioid Therapies and Behavioral Interventions
Consider anticonvulsants for neuropathic components of pain
  disorder
NSAIDs for swelling and muscle tension
Relaxation training, including biofeedback, progressive muscle
  relaxation, imagery, and distraction

Step 3: Evaluate Opioid History
Consider pre-existing tolerance
Avoid undermedication of opioids, which will lead to greater abuse
  and aberrancy of behaviors

Step 4: Opioid Choice
Consider results of step 3
Choose long-acting versus short-acting whenever possible
Limit rescue medications

Step 5: Reassess Frequently
Document behaviors and revisit issues on a timely basis
Reassess effectiveness of treatment regimen, being aware of need to
  avoid undertreatment
Evaluate whether patient is engaging in other parts of therapy
  (psychosocial interventions, physical therapy, taking NSAIDs, etc.)
  and not focusing solely on opioids

Abbreviation: NSAIDs = nonsteroidal anti-inflammatory drugs.

Failure to recognize existing tolerance can result in undermedication and may contribute to the patient's attempts to self-medicate. Fourth, the team should consider using longer-acting drugs such as the fentanyl patch and sustained-release opioids. Their longer duration and slow onset may help to reduce aberrant drug-taking behaviors when compared to the rapid onset and increased frequency of dosage associated with short-acting drugs. Finally, the team should make plans to frequently reassess the adequacy of pain and symptom control.

OUTPATIENT MANAGEMENT PLAN

A number of strategies can promote treatment compliance in an outpatient setting. A written contract between the team and patient helps to provide structure to the treatment plan, establishes clear expectations of the roles played by both parties, and outlines the consequences of aberrant drug taking. The inclusion of spot urine toxicology screens in the contract can be useful in maximizing treatment compliance. Expectations regarding attendance of clinic visits and the management of one's supply of medications should also be stated. For example, the clinician may wish to limit the amount of drug dispensed per prescription and make refills contingent upon clinic attendance. When prescribing pain medications and other drugs used in symptom control, the physician must provide the patient with clear instructions about the parameters of responsible drug taking. This practice can help to reduce hesitation to prescribe drugs for pain and symptom management if the patient manages his or her medication responsibly. The clinician should consider requiring the patient to attend 12-step programs, perhaps asking the patient document his or her attendance as a condition for ongoing prescribing. With the patient's consent, the clinician may wish to contact the patient's sponsor and make him or her aware that the patient is being treated for chronic illness that requires medications such as opioids. This action will reduce the potential for the patient to be stigmatized as being noncompliant with the ideals of the 12-step program. Finally, the team should involve family members and friends in the treatment to help bolster social support and functioning. Becoming familiar with the family may help the team identify family members who are themselves drug abusers and who may potentially divert the patient's medications and contribute to the patient's noncompliance. Mental health professionals can help family members with referrals to drug treatment and codependency groups, as a way to help the patient receive optimal medical care.

INPATIENT MANAGEMENT PLAN

The guidelines discussed above for outpatient settings can be expanded to address the management of a patient with substance abuse problems who has been admitted to the hospital for treatment of a life-threatening illness. The aims are to promote the safety of patient and staff, contain manipulative behaviors by patients, enhance the use of medication appropriately used for pain and symptom management, and communicate an understanding of pain and substance abuse management. The first point of order is to discuss the patient's drug use in an open manner. In addition, it is necessary to reassure the patient that steps will be taken to avoid adverse events such as drug withdrawal symptoms. For certain specific situations, such as for preoperative patients, patients should be admitted several days in advance when possible for stabilization of the drug regimen. Also, it is important to provide the patient with a private room near the nurses' station to help nurses monitor the patient and discourage attempts to leave the hospital to purchase illicit drugs. Further, the team should require visitors to check in with nursing staff prior to visitation. In some cases, it may be necessary to search visitors' packages in order to stem the patient's access to drugs. As a final point, the team should collect daily urine specimens for random toxicology analysis and frequently reassess pain and symptom management.

As with pain regimens, management approaches should be tailored to reflect the clinician's assessment of the severity of drug abuse. Open and honest communication between the clinician and the patient reassures the patient that these guidelines were established in his or her best interest. In some cases, these guidelines may fail to curtail aberrant drug use despite repeated interventions by staff. At that point, the patient should be considered for discharge, but our experience suggests that this is only necessary in the most recalcitrant of cases. The clinician should involve members of the staff and administration for discussion about the ethical and legal implications of such a decision.

URINE TOXICOLOGY SCREENING

Clinicians must control and monitor drug use in all patients, a daunting task in some active abusers. In some cases, a major issue is compliance with treatments for the underlying disease, which may be so poor that the substance abuse shortens life expectancy by preventing the effective administration of primary therapy. Prognosis may also be altered by the use of drugs in a manner that negatively interacts with therapy or predisposes to other serious morbidity. The goals of care can be very difficult to define when poor compliance and risky behavior appear to contradict a reported desire for disease-modifying therapies.

Urine toxicology screening has the potential to be a very useful tool to the practicing clinician, both for diagnosing potential abuse problems and for monitoring patients with an established history of abuse. However, recent work suggests that urine toxicology screens are employed infrequently in tertiary care centers (Passik et al. 2000). In addition, when such screens are ordered, documentation tends to be inconsistent regarding the reasons for ordering as well as any follow-up recommendations based on the results. Indeed, the survey found that nearly 40% of the charts surveyed listed no reason for obtaining the urine toxicology screen, and the ordering physician could not be identified nearly 30% of the time. Staff education efforts can help to address this problem and may ultimately make urine toxicology screens a vital part of treating pain in oncology patients.

METHADONE

Oral methadone is a potent opioid that can be successfully used to replace oral morphine in cancer patients, although continuous assessment is necessary for proper use in order to avoid toxic effects (Mercadante et al. 1996; Ripamonti et al. 1998). Practitioners should consider using methadone with cancer patients due to several of its outstanding properties. First, it is well absorbed enterally and thus retains much of its analgesic efficacy. Second, it readily crosses the blood-brain barrier and has a relatively long half-life of approximately 25 hours, with analgesia effects of approximately 6–8 hours. Third, tolerance develops rather slowly, leading to more persistent effects. Finally, less irritability is associated with it compared to shorter-acting, euphoria-producing opioids (Carrol et al. 1994; Lawlor et al. 1998).

It must be stressed that patients who have addiction concerns with opioids such as heroin cannot be given methadone both as an analgesic and as part of a maintenance recovery program. Practitioners sometimes assume that patients receiving methadone from a maintenance program do not need further pain medication, but this is simply not true (Parrino 1991). Methadone-maintained patients in a recovery program are fully tolerant of the maintenance dose and experience no analgesic effect from the methadone (Zweben and Payte 1990). Therefore, other routes of pain control must be explored.

PATIENTS IN RECOVERY

Pain management with patients in recovery presents a unique challenge. Depending on the structure of the recovery program (e.g., Alcoholics Anonymous or methadone maintenance programs), a patient may fear ostracism from the program's members or may have an increased fear regarding susceptibility to re-addiction. The first choice should be to explore non-opioid therapies with these patients, who may require referral to a pain center (Parrino 1991). Alternate therapies may include the use of nonsteroidal anti-inflammatory drugs, anticonvulsants (for neuropathic components), biofeedback, electrical stimulation, neuroablative techniques, acupuncture, or behavioral management. If the pain condition is so severe that opioids are required, care must be taken to structure their use with opioid management contracts, random urine toxicology screens, and occasional pill counts. If possible, attempts should be made to include the patient's recovery program sponsor in order to garner his or her cooperation and aid in successful monitoring of the condition.

CONCLUSION

While even the most prudent actions on their part cannot obviate the risk of all aberrant drug-related behavior, clinicians must recognize that virtually any drug that acts on the central nervous system, and any route of drug administration, can be abused. The problem does not lie in the drugs themselves. The effective management of patients with pain who engage in aberrant drug-related behavior necessitates a comprehensive approach that recognizes the biological, chemical, social, and psychiatric aspects of substance abuse and addiction and provides practical means to manage risk, treat pain effectively, and assure patient safety.

Treating medically ill patients who are experiencing chronic pain and have a substance use disorder is clearly both complex and challenging, because each issue can significantly complicate the other. However, to treat these patients optimally, clinicians must identify and effectively manage substance abuse issues. While previous studies have shed light on the particular diagnostic meanings of various behaviors and have afforded clinicians the opportunity to recognize those behaviors that are truly aberrant in a given population, far too often clinicians are prejudiced in their perceptions of these behaviors due to anecdotal accounts. Certain behaviors are universally judged as aberrant regardless of limited data, while other behaviors found common in non-addicts that may seem aberrant based on face value may have little predictive value for true addiction.

The future holds several challenges regarding the state of pain management in medically ill patients with past or present histories of substance abuse. Empirical data are needed to understand what aberrant drug-related behaviors are normative in the medically ill. A survey will probably need to be done based on specific illnesses to maximize our understanding. For instance, common aberrant behaviors that we have uncovered in cancer patients (such as increasing medication dose once or twice) may or may not be similar to behaviors found in patients with other disorders such as sickle cell anemia or chronic low back pain. In essence, what is needed is a formal study of the epidemiology of pain behaviors in multiple illnesses.

REFERENCES

Atkinson JH, Slater MA, Patterson TL, et al. Prevalence, onset and risk of psychiatric disorders in men with chronic lower back pain: a controlled study. *Pain* 1991; 45:111–121.

Carrol E, Fine E, Ruff R, et al. A four-drug pain regimen for head and neck cancers. *Laryngoscope* 1994; 104:694–700.

Cohen F. Postsurgical pain relief: patient's status and nurses' medication choices. *Pain* 1980; 9:265–274.

Collier JD, Kopstein AN. Trends in cocaine abuse reflected in emergency room episodes reported to DAWN. *Public Health Rep* 1991; 106:59–68.

Compton P, Darakjian MA, Miotto K. Screening for addiction in patients with problematic substance use: evaluation of a pilot assessment tool. *J Pain Symptom Manage* 1998; 16:355–363.

Fishbain DA. Report on the prevalence of drug/alcohol abuse and dependence in chronic pain patients. *Subst Use Misuse* 1996; 31(8):945–946.

Fishbain DA, Goldberg M, Meagher BR, et al. Male and female chronic pain patients categorized by DSM-III diagnostic criteria. *Pain* 1986; 26:181–197.

Gatchel RJ, Polatin PB, Mayer TG, et al. Psychopathology and the rehabilitation of patients with chronic low back pain disability. *Arch Phys Med Rehabil* 1994; 75:666–670.

Glajchen M, Fitzmartin RD, Blum D, et al. Psychosocial barriers to cancer pain relief. *Cancer Pract* 1995; 3(2):76–82.

Groerer J, Brodsky M. The incidence of illicit drug use in the United States 1962–1989. *Br J Addict* 1992; 87:1345.

Haller DL, Butler S. Use and abuse of prescription and recreation drugs by chronic pain patients. In: Hariss LS (Ed). *Problems in Drug Dependence*. Washington, DC: Government Printing Office, 1991, pp 456–457.

Joranson DE, Gibson AM. Policy issues and imperatives in the use of opioids to treat pain in substance abusers. *J Law Med Ethics* 1994; 22(3):215–223.

Katon W, Eyon K, Miller D. Chronic pain: lifetime psychiatric diagnosis and family history. *Am J Psychiatry* 1985; 142:1156–1160.

Lawlor P, Turner K, Hanson J, et al. Dose ratio between morphine and methadone in patients with cancer pain: a retrospective study. *Cancer* 1998; 82:1167–1173.

Lundberg JC, Passik SD. Alcohol and cancer: a review for psycho-oncologists. *Psychooncology* 1997; 6:253–266.

Marks RM, Sacher EJ. Undertreatment of medical inpatients with narcotic analgesics. *Ann Intern Med* 1973; 78:173–181.

Mercadante S, Sapio R, Serretta M, et al. Patient-controlled analgesia with oral methadone in cancer pain: preliminary report. *Ann Oncol* 1996; 7:613–617.

Miotto MD, Compton P, Ling W, et al. Diagnostic addictive disease in chronic pain patients. *Psychosomatics* 1996; 3(37):223–235.

Morgan JP. *American Opiophobia: Customary Underutilization of Opioid Analgesia.* New York: Hawthorne, 1986, pp 163–173.

Parrino M. *State Methadone Treatment Guidelines.* TIPS 1 DHHS Publication No. (SMA) 93. Washington, DC: Department of Health and Human Services, 1991.

Passik SD, Portenoy RK. Substance abuse issues in palliative care. In: Berger A, Portenoy R, Weissman D (Eds). *Principles and Practice of Supportive Oncology.* Philadelphia: Lippincott-Raven, 1998a, pp 513–524.

Passik SD, Portenoy RK. Substance abuse disorders. In: Holland JC (Ed). *Psychooncology.* New York: Oxford University Press, 1998b, pp 576–586.

Passik SD, Weinreb HJ. Managing chronic nonmalignant pain and overcoming obstacles to the use of opioids. *Adv Ther* 2000; 17:70–80.

Passik SD, Portenoy RK, Ricketts PL. Substance abuse issues in cancer patients part 1: prevalence and diagnosis. *Oncology* 1998; 12(4):517–521.

Passik S, Schreiber J, Kirsh et al. A chart review of the ordering and documentation of urine toxicology screens in a cancer center: do they influence patient management? *J Pain Symptom Manage* 2000; 19:40–44.

Penick E, Powell B, Nickel E, et al. Comorbidity of lifetime psychiatric disorders among male alcoholics. *Alcohol Clin Exp Res* 1994; 18:1289–1293.

Portenoy RK. Chronic opioid therapy in nonmalignant pain. *J Pain Symptom Manage* 1990; S(Suppl):S46–S62.

Portenoy RK. Opioid therapy for chronic nonmalignant pain and current status. In: Fields HL, Liebeskind JC (Eds). *Pharmacological Approaches to the Treatment of Chronic Pain: New Concepts and Critical Issues,* Progress in Pain Research and Management, Vol. 1. Seattle: IASP Press, 1994, pp 247–287.

Portenoy RK, Foley KM. Chronic use of opiate analgesics in nonmalignant pain: report of 38 cases. *Pain* 1986; 25:171–186.

Ramer L, Richardson JL, Cohen MZ, et al. Multimeasure pain assessment in an ethnically diverse group of patients with cancer. *J Transcult Nurs* 1999; 10(2):94–101.

Regier DA, Myers JK, Dramer M, et al. The HIMH epidemiology catchment area program. *Arch Gen Psychiatry* 1984; 41:934.

Ripamonti C, Groff L, Brunelli D, et al. Switching from morphine to oral methadone in treating cancer pain: what is the equianalgesic dose ratio? *J Clin Oncol* 1998; 16:3216–3221.

Shine D, Demas P. Knowledge of medical students, residents and attending physicians about opioid abuse. *J Med Educ* 1984; 59:501–507.

Urban BJ, France RD, Steinberger EK, et al. Long-term use of narcotic/antidepressant medication in the management of phantom limb pain. *Pain* 1986; 24:191–196.

Ward SE, Goldberg N, Miller-McCoulry V, et al. Patient-related barriers to management of cancer pain. *Pain* 1993; 52:319–324.

Weissman DE, Haddox JD. Opioid pseudoaddiction—an iatrogenic syndrome. *Pain* 1989; 36:363–366.

Zenz M, Strumpf M, Tryba M. Long-term opiate therapy in patients with chronic nonmalignant pain. *J Pain Symptom Manage* 1992; 7:69–77.

Zweben JE, Payte JT. Methadone maintenance in the treatment of opioid dependence: a current perspective. *West J Med* 1990; 152:588–599.

Correspondence to: Steven D. Passik, PhD, Symptom Management and Palliative Care Program, Markey Cancer Center, University of Kentucky, 800 Rose Street, CC449, Lexington, KY 40536-0093, USA. Tel: 859-323-5163; Fax: 859-257-7715; email: spassik@uky.edu.

Psychosocial Aspects of Pain: A Handbook for Health Care Providers, Progress in Pain Research and Management, Vol. 27, edited by Robert H. Dworkin and William S. Breitbart, IASP Press, Seattle, © 2004.

21

Psychosocial and Psychiatric Aspects of Pain in Children

Patrick J. McGrath

Departments of Psychology, Pediatrics, and Psychiatry, Dalhousie University; Pediatric Pain Service, IWK Health Centre, Halifax, Nova Scotia, Canada

Historically, children's pain has been poorly managed (Eland and Anderson 1977). Although the last 20 years have seen a great deal of research and much progress in clinical practice (Asprey 1994), the translation of research into practice has lagged. This chapter will try to help bridge this gap by taking an evidence-based approach to the psychosocial and psychiatric aspects of pain in children. However, any short chapter can only scratch the surface. More detailed information is available in specialized textbooks such as that by Schechter et al. (2002), in the series I have coedited (Finley and McGrath 1998, 2000; McGrath and Finley 1999, 2003), in an edited volume on pain in neonates (Anand et al. 2000), and in the *Pediatric Pain Letter* (www.dal.ca/~pedpain/pplet/pplet.html).

Psychosocial and psychiatric aspects of pain cannot be considered outside of the context of biological aspects of pain. However, psychosocial factors cannot simply be reduced to biology. We will never be able to completely understand the 3-year-old who falls while playing in day care and starts to cry simply in terms of peripheral neurons firing and brain areas responding. We will always need to understand the history of the child's experience with pain, the modeling and reinforcement she has received in day care and in her home, the "culture" of the day care and of the child, and the social context in which she fell. Craig (2002) has developed a model for understanding pain from this perspective (Fig. 1). Failure to consider the social context limits our ability to understand and help our patients. Effective psychosocial intervention for pain may occur at any point in the model. For example, an intervention that increases the accuracy of the decoding of pain signals or fosters appropriate action on the part of the caregiver should be considered a pain intervention.

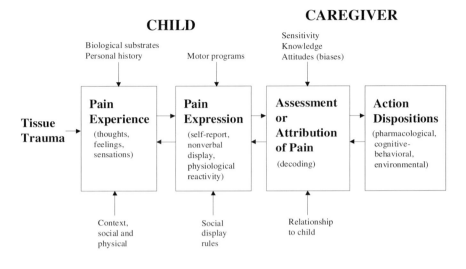

Fig. 1. The world of a child in pain: a sociocommunications model. Reprinted from Craig (2002), with permission.

Recognizing the biological substrate underlying psychological and social phenomena is important in understanding the nature of the pain and in providing both pharmacological and psychosocial treatments. For example, central sensitization may help explain some seemingly inexplicable aspects of chronic and recurrent pain such as hypersensitivity to stimulation and spread of pain, which are often assumed to be of psychiatric or psychological origin. Similarly, relaxation may alleviate headache by means of changes in the biological substrate, perhaps in terms of changes in muscles or in responses to stress. However, relaxation is best delivered as a psychosocial treatment rather than a drug. Drugs that relax muscles are not effective or indicated in the management of headaches (Larsson et al. 1990), while relaxation training has proven effective in many well-designed trials (Hermann et al. 1995; Holden et al. 1999).

Unfortunately, when pain is disabling and presents in a way that cannot be readily explained by health professionals, there has been a tendency to assume that the cause is psychological: "It's all in your head." Patients usually perceive the tendency to label pain as psychogenic without any positive evidence for psychogenicity as doctors blaming patients for their pain. Of course, all pain, no matter if it is caused by a tumor in the brain or by anxiety, is profoundly influenced by psychological processes. Many of us are familiar with the stomach pain that we may experience when we have to give an important presentation, or will recall having exaggerated pain when we were children to avoid a test at school. These common experiences represent psychogenic pain because they are primarily created by psychological processes. Psychogenic pain is usually detected and the situation is corrected by the child and the family long before they seek professional help. The vast majority of children whose families seek help for pain are not suffering from psychogenic pain. Often the cause of their pain is unknown and puzzling, and psychological factors may play a role, but it is not good science or good clinical practice to assume psychogenic causation. Of course, psychosocial treatments may be very helpful, even if the cause is not psychological.

Understanding the complex matrix of psychological and biological factors will help us comprehend how children understand pain and learn how to help them. Simplistic psychological or biological models, in which pain is thought to be either biological ("real") or psychological ("in your head"), do a disservice to our patients.

Children and adolescents with recurrent pain differ in the amount of interference pain causes in their lives. Some are able to carry on their normal activities and successfully fulfill their roles as members of their families, as students, and as peers. Others may have significant interference with activities (disability) and considerable disruption of their social roles (handicap). Disability and handicap are often major targets of psychosocial interventions for chronic pain. When a child is missing school, successful return to school is often the first goal of a pain treatment program.

Although research and practice on pain in children borrow heavily from adult work, developmental factors are more important in children than in adults (Table I). First of all, children tend to have some different types of pain than do adults. For example, only a small number of children have neuropathic pain, but many infants have colic. Second, measurement of pain in children requires developmentally appropriate methods. Behavioral or observational tools and self-report measures are the most useful. These measures have been generated and validated using social science methods. Third, some treatments have different effects depending on the age of the patient. For example, neuropathic pains such as complex regional pain syndrome type I appear to be more amenable to a combination of physical therapy, psychological interventions, and medical treatment in children than the same disorder in adults (Lee et al. 2002). Fourth, children are dependent on adults in terms of the environment in which they find themselves. Adults must voice their children's concerns and advocate for them for pain relief.

In this chapter we have arbitrarily divided the pediatric age range into three categories: infants and neonates, children between 1 year and 12 years,

Table I
Developmental issues related to psychosocial issues in pediatric pain

Approx. Age	Developmental Stage	Pain Issue
6 months		Colic resolves
12 months	Ambulation	Children begin to injure themselves and experience frequent pain from minor accidents
18 months	Use of speech to describe pain	Children become increasingly able to describe pain
5 years	Learning of less and more and the ability to put things in order (seriation)	Children begin to be able to use pain self-report rating scales
9 years		Peak prevalence of recurrent abdominal pain
10 years	Thinking about thinking (metacognition)	Children can begin to change their thinking and use stress management techniques without immediate supervision
11–12 years	Puberty	1. Bias to females having more frequent and severe pain begins 2. Menstrual pain begins 3. Prevalence of most recurrent pains increases for both sexes
14 years	Independence from parents	Average age for children to begin to self-medicate using over-the-counter medications

and adolescents. However, age and the developmental progression that comes with age form a continuum rather than distinct categories. For example, the differences between an infant of 11 months and a child of 1 year obviously are not as great as those between a child of 1 year and a child of 6 years. Similarly, some 16-year-olds are more mature than some 19-year-olds.

PAIN IN NEONATES AND INFANTS

SOURCES OF PAIN

Neonates and infants can suffer from medically related pain (pain from medical conditions, surgical pain, or pain from invasive procedures other than surgery) and from recurrent pain, usually of unknown origin. Healthy, full-term neonates and infants usually experience only a few instances of medical pain.

The most common acute pain is that from medical procedures such as heel sticks. Johnston et al. (1997a) determined that 239 patients in the neonatal intensive care unit (NICU) had a total of 2,134 invasive procedures over a week-long study period. Medication was given for less than 1% of the procedures. In contrast to the situation 15 years ago, most operative procedures on babies in the NICU are now covered by anesthesia and analgesia (Johnston et al. 1997a).

The most common surgical procedure that healthy infants have in North America is male circumcision. The rate of circumcision in the United States and Canada appears to be around 50%, but data are weak (American Academy of Pediatrics 1999). The rate in most other areas of the world is generally quite low, except where circumcision is done for religious reasons. Circumcision is very painful, and analgesia, such as ring blocks, can be very effective, but the rate of use of sufficient analgesia appears to be low.

Colic, which is excessive crying without apparent reason, is the most common recurrent pain in infants. Prevalence varies from 1.5% to 11.9% depending on the definition used (Reijneveld et al. 2001). The underlying cause for colic is unknown. Colic is not life-threatening but may have a serious impact on the family's quality of life.

PSYCHOSOCIAL INTERVENTIONS

Psychosocial interventions for pain are widely used with neonates, often in combination with pharmacological interventions. Two types of psychosocial interventions are important in this age group. The first type of intervention is focused on the organization or environment of the NICU following policies and procedures designed to promote the optimum development of the infant. The second type of intervention consists of specific behavioral interventions.

The best known and most widely used organizational (or environmental) strategies are based on the synactive theory of development proposed by Als (1982). The Newborn Individualized Developmental Care and Assessment Program (NIDCAP) combines naturalistic observation with structured observations to develop an assessment that guides interventions. This approach includes both environmental and behavioral strategies. Although not focused exclusively on pain, this approach has had a major impact on pain management (Franck and Lawhon 2000).

Many environmental strategies are designed to reduce noxious stimuli. These include: (1) decreasing overall lighting and establishing a day/night cycle; (2) decreasing noise from equipment and staff; (3) decreasing handling and clustering caregiving; and (4) limiting painful procedures to those that will make a specific contribution to the infant's outcome (Franck and Lawhon 2000).

Another type of environmental strategy involves the implementation of policies in the unit that support the infant's development. These include policies on use of developmental care, policies on family-centered care, and policies on implementation of individual assessment and care. Research is lacking on how policies and procedures such as these come to be implemented, but it appears that leadership by influential local individuals and education of staff may be important.

Behavioral interventions are another form of psychosocial intervention. These can be divided into several different types and include: (1) those designed to increase containment of the infant, (2) sensory stimulation that is not painful, (3) non-nutritive sucking, (4) sweet taste, and (5) procedural interventions.

Containment or positioning of the infant by nesting, swaddling, maintaining a flexed position, or providing postural supports promotes self-regulation and calms the reaction to pain. The effects are complex and may depend on the age of the infant (Fearon et al. 1997), but these strategies are clearly effective. Sensory, nonpainful stimulation, including rocking, has proven effective in modulating behavioral state (Campos 1994). However, the evidence for reducing pain from procedures such as heel sticks (Johnston et al. 1997b) is equivocal.

Non-nutritive sucking on a pacifier has proven effective in reducing pain from procedures. The mechanism is thought to involve non-opioid pathways activated by stimulation of orotactile and mechanoreceptor mechanisms (Gibbins and Stevens 2001). Sweet taste has been studied mostly using sucrose solutions. Sucrose, which has been effective in numerous trials, probably acts by means of an opioid mechanism that is age dependent (Stevens et al. 2001; Anseloni et al. 2002; Carbajal et al. 2002). Studies on its long-term effectiveness are now underway. There have been criticisms that use of pacifiers and pacifiers with sucrose for painful procedures may discourage breastfeeding, but there is no evidence that the very brief use of a pacifier changes the course of breastfeeding. Procedural interventions that reduce pain include the use of mechanized lancets (Harpin and Rutter 1983), the use of venipuncture rather than heel sticks (Shah et al. 1997), and the adequate training of the staff (Franck and Lawhon 2000).

As mentioned, the most common recurrent pain of infancy is colic or excessive crying. Although there is some debate whether colic is a pain-based disorder, it appears to most parents as if their child is in pain. With colic, psychosocial interventions are helpful. A recent meta-analysis (Garrison and Christakis 2000) found that reducing stimulation was highly effective and that on average one would have to treat only two infants to have a significant improvement (number needed to treat = 2). Given the prevalence of colic and the lack of medical interventions that are safe and effective, behavioral interventions should be more widely used.

PSYCHIATRIC AND PSYCHOSOCIAL FACTORS

Psychiatric issues have not been extensively investigated in regard to pain in neonates and infants. However, recent work by Oberlander and his colleagues (2002) has shown that prolonged use of selective serotonin reuptake inhibitors by mothers during pregnancy has an effect of dampening the pain response in the infant. The implications of this finding are unclear.

Little work has focused on psychosocial influences on pain in neonates and infants. Although considerable discussion has centered on how parents' attention to their child may increase or decrease pain expression, there are few data on the topic. Sweet et al. (1999) found that greater maternal responsiveness (not just at the time of injection but also a week earlier) increased an infant's pain response to injection.

SUMMARY

Our understanding of pain in neonates and infants has dramatically changed in the last decade. Psychosocial interventions for pain have been shown to be effective and are now common in many NICUs. Little is known about psychosocial influences on pain and the role of psychiatric factors.

PAIN IN CHILDREN AGED 1–12 YEARS

SOURCES OF PAIN

Development is a continuous process that does not always correspond exactly to chronological age. As children grow from infancy to 12 years, there are significant changes in pain, but also significant continuities. The types of pain that children have and their response to pain change over time. Children between 1 and 12 years of age are subject to everyday pain, routine medical procedure pain, and the beginnings of recurrent pains. Recurrent headaches increase with age, becoming most prominent in early adolescents.

Everyday pain refers to pain from normal bumps and falls. The vast majority of these do not and should not receive any home or medical treatment. Two studies (Fearon et al. 1996; von Baeyer et al. 1998) have shown that young children have frequent incidents in day care, that girls are more expressive of pain than boys, and that the vast majority of pain in a day care center is ignored. Through these everyday pains, children learn about the reaction of their caregivers to pain.

For most children, medical pain consists primarily of routine immunizations. Although the pain is short-lived, many children experience needles as painful. Younger children report and seem to experience more pain from the same procedures than do older children (Fradet et al. 1990). Children in hospital frequently receive no treatment for postoperative pain that they think should be treated (Demyttenaere et al. 2001).

Headache (McGrath and Larsson 1997), abdominal pain (Faull and Nicol 1986), back pain (Taimela et al. 1997), and limb pain can occur in children before the age of 12 years. The prevalence of headache is lower than in older children, but abdominal pain seems to peak between 9 and 10 years of age (Apley and Naish 1957).

PSYCHOSOCIAL INTERVENTIONS

Cohen has developed brief, cost-effective coaching and distraction procedures that can be implemented by nurses in busy practices (Cohen et al. 1997, 1999; Cohen 2002). These procedures have a very significant impact on children's pain and distress from routine immunization. They appear to prevent negative views of needle procedures such as immunization (Cohen et al. 2001). In Cohen's intervention, nurses prompt children to select a video, and then ask the child questions during the procedure and prompt the child to watch the video that he or she has chosen.

Few studies have focused on headache treatment at this age. However, two excellent studies by Sanders et al. (1989, 1994) demonstrated that recurrent abdominal pain can be effectively treated with a combination of child and parent training in six sessions. Children learned how to manage their stress with self-management training. Parents learned how to promote healthy behavior and discourage sick role behavior in their children. This intervention was superior to a control condition in which a parent took the child to see a gastroenterologist. The cognitive-behavioral treatment continued to be effective at a 6-month follow-up.

PSYCHOSOCIAL AND PSYCHIATRIC FACTORS

We are beginning to understand the role that psychosocial factors play in pain in children. Although there is good evidence of psychological causes (psychogenic pain) in only a small percentage of pain problems, psychological factors are important influences in children's pain. For example, a population-based study by Aromaa et al. (2000) in Finland found that children with headache were more likely than pain-free children to have fathers who were extremely sensitive to pain, were less likely to have their parents talk to comfort them when in pain, and had parents who were more often anxious, frightened, excited, and nervous in reaction to their child's pain and who tried less often to hold the child or divert his or her attention during a temper tantrum.

There is also clear evidence that pain and the disability that can accompany painful conditions aggregate in families (Goodman et al. 1997; Kristjansdottir 2000). Other studies have shown the importance of modeling of pain behavior by parents (Mikail and von Baeyer 1990; Walker et al. 1994).

Research on the role of individual personality factors in child pain has not been well developed. Temperament is correlated with pain response (Lee and White-Traut 1996), but the relationship is not always very strong (Bournaki 1997). Chen et al. (2000) found that pain-sensitive temperament (the child's typical reaction to painful situations) predicted a child's reaction to lumbar punctures. Children with recurrent abdominal pain have more daily stressors than do pain-free children, and these stressors are related to their abdominal pain (Walker et al. 2001).

The literature is sparse on psychiatric aspects of pain in this age group. Children with psychiatric disorders may have a different risk for pain or may react differently to pain. An important feature of separation anxiety is the report of pain, usually headaches or stomachaches, in response to the threat of separation from parents. Pain from separation anxiety typically begins when the child perceives the risk of separation and ends when the risk is over. Treatment should focus on the underlying separation anxiety using cognitive-behavioral methods that focus on successful separation. Successful treatment of the separation anxiety will help resolve this psychogenic pain. Children may have a specific phobia to medical and or dental procedures. Needle phobia is not uncommon and has been related to avoidance and lack of cooperation in health care. Parental fear of needles and children's negative experiences appear to be major causes of needle phobia in children (Townend et al. 2000; Arnrup et al. 2002). Children with depression may often complain of pain, and children with recurrent pain are at slightly increased risk of depressive feelings (Larsson 1991). Simultaneous treatment of the headache and the depression is appropriate. Autistic children may react in a less coherent and consistent way to pain, and thus their pain may not be recognized by caregivers. There is no evidence of pain insensitivity in autism. Although there is a well-known but rare syndrome of congenital insensitivity to pain with anhidrosis (CIPA), most mentally retarded children do not appear to have impaired perception of pain. Children with mental retardation appear to be at higher risk for pain because of their comorbid condition, the procedures that they undergo, and the undervaluing of children with mental retardation (Breau et al. 2000; Stallard et al. 2001). One study has found that children with aggressive behavior disorders were less sensitive to experimental pain than were other children (Seguin et al. 1996).

SUMMARY

Children frequently experience pain in their everyday life. Almost all children have pain from minor procedures. Pain from needles can be efficiently managed using psychosocial interventions by nurses. Recurrent abdominal pain is common in children and is well managed by psychosocial interventions. The role of family and individual differences in pain in children is beginning to be understood. Some psychiatric disorders predispose to pain while others may decrease pain.

PAIN IN ADOLESCENTS

By adolescence, even though some behavior is immature and knowledge may be limited, cognitive abilities are quite mature. Most adolescents have metacognitive abilities (i.e., they can think about thinking). They understand causal relationships and are aware of the consequences of their actions.

SOURCES OF PAIN

Adolescents report less pain with needle procedures than do children, perhaps because they can use self-control strategies, or because they can understand the reason needles are required and can fully understand that the pain will be very brief. However, because adolescents have more influence on whether or not they receive health care, they may be more able than younger children to avoid procedures if they are afraid of pain. This may be especially true of dental care, which they may avoid because of fear of needles and pain (Peretz and Efrat 2000).

Headaches and back pain (Goodman and McGrath 1991; Goodman et al. 1997; Kristjansdottir 1997; Taimela et al. 1997) increase sharply in adolescence, with females more likely to be affected (Unruh and Campbell 1999). Few adolescents with these pain problems are depressed, but there is a considerable burden on quality of life (Nodari et al. 2002). Chronic daily headache may be the most burdensome (Winner and Gladstein 2002).

PSYCHOSOCIAL INTERVENTIONS

Psychosocial treatments for headaches have been developed and widely evaluated. Treatments include relaxation training and cognitive interventions and consist of a series of sessions during which the adolescent is taught to identify stressful situations and stress responses. Adolescents then learn methods to control stress. These methods are most commonly a combination of relaxation training using tension-relaxation exercises, suggestion, and breathing exercises. These skills may be supplemented by training in cognitive methods that teach the adolescent how to think about situations differently. Typically, these treatments are delivered by a psychologist in 8–10 face-to-face sessions. Excellent evidence testifies to the effectiveness of these approaches (Hermann et al. 1995; Holden et al. 1999). However, there is good evidence that similar results can be obtained using telephone-based (McGrath et al. 1992) or Web-based interventions (Hicks et al. 2002) at less cost to the health care system. No reports have documented similar psychosocial treatment trials for back pain.

CHRONIC ILLNESSES

Several types of chronic illness are accompanied by pain, but surprisingly little is know about the prevalence or psychosocial treatment of these problems. Few treatment trials using psychosocial interventions have been undertaken. The little evidence there is suggests that cognitive-behavioral treatment may have promising results (Walco et al. 1999).

We lack satisfactory epidemiological studies of pain in arthritis in the pediatric age range. However, a recent study of a single clinic found that pain upon referral as documented in the clinical record was not a good predictor of the diagnosis of juvenile rheumatoid arthritis (McGhee et al. 2002). Earlier studies have shown mixed results (Beales et al. 1983).

Inflammatory bowel disease is characterized by pain, but again, few studies have documented the frequency, severity, and duration of pain in this population. Although stress may play a role in exacerbations and may even help trigger the initial incident, most children and adolescents with inflammatory bowel disease are not psychologically disturbed (Gold et al. 2000). Many may have reduced quality of life (Griffiths et al. 1999). Although no clinical trials have tested psychosocial interventions with children or adolescents with inflammatory bowel disease, clinical experience suggests that this approach may help some children.

Adolescents with cystic fibrosis are at risk for pain, especially in the last 6 months of life (Ravilly et al. 1996); treatment is usually pharmacological.

Cerebral palsy is a nonprogressive disorder of varying severity and type. Pain is a frequent complaint, but very little work has examined pain in this population of children and adolescents. Pain is also common in spina bifida, occurring weekly or more often in 56% of patients (C. Clancy et al., unpublished manuscript). Pain studies are lacking, and no studies have examined psychosocial factors or treatments in pain in this population of children and adolescents.

Sickle cell disease, in which pain is a major symptom, is a group of genetic blood disorders that occur when the sickle hemoglobin gene is inherited from both parents. Pain occurs from occlusive crises in small blood vessels, and chronic pain also arises from repeated crises. Anie and Green (2002) recently conducted a systematic review in which they identified five randomized or quasi-randomized trials involving 158 patients. Focusing on psychological interventions, the authors found that family education and cognitive-behavioral therapy can help patients cope with sickle cell disease, but that better trials are needed.

Cancer pain has been well documented (e.g., Ljungman et al. 2000); it occurs frequently from disease prior to diagnosis and from procedures during treatment. Although awareness and treatment have increased, much remains to be done. The psychosocial factors in cancer pain in children and adolescents are not well understood. Psychosocial interventions have been widely used and evaluated for procedure pain. The most useful strategy may be to combine pharmacological and psychosocial interventions.

Specialists in chronic illness frequently do not ask their patients about pain. Unless they are asked, patients will not report their pain and will come to believe that their doctor is not interested or that nothing can be done. Research is needed on prevalence, psychosocial interventions, and psychosocial factors.

SUMMARY

Recurrent pain becomes much more common in adolescents. Psychogenic pain is clinically rare, but psychological influences on pain and on disability and handicap are common in adolescence. Few studies have examined pain in adolescents with psychiatric disorders. Studies have shown that psychosocial interventions are effective in management of recurrent headache pain. Few studies have examined psychosocial factors in chronic illness, but this is an important area for research and clinical awareness. Although little research has been done, psychosocial interventions in chronic illness show promise.

CONCLUSIONS

Psychosocial issues are critically important in pain in infants, children, and adolescents. The most important aspects are the effectiveness of psychosocial interventions and the need to consider psychosocial factors. Psychogenic pain is not an important clinical phenomenon. Psychiatric disorders may increase or decrease pain perception. Chronic illness is an area that needs much more attention from a pain perspective.

REFERENCES

Als H. Toward a synactive theory of development: a promise for the assessment and support of infant individuality. *Infant Mental Health J* 1982; 3:229–243.

American Academy of Pediatrics. Task Force on Circumcision. Circumcision policy statement. *Pediatrics* 1999; 103(3):686–693.

Anand KJS, Stevens B, McGrath PJ (Eds). *Pain in Neonates,* 2nd ed. Amsterdam: Elsevier, 2000.

Anie KA, Green J. Psychological therapies for sickle cell disease and pain. *Cochrane Database Syst Rev* 2002; (2):CD001916.

Anseloni VC, Weng HR, Terayama R, et al. Age-dependency of analgesia elicited by intraoral sucrose in acute and persistent pain models. *Pain* 2002; 97:93–103.

Apley J, Naish N. Recurrent abdominal pains: a field survey of 1,000 school children. *Arch Dis Child* 1957; 165–170.

Arnrup K, Berggren U, Broberg AG, Lundin SA, Hakeberg M. Attitudes to dental care among parents of uncooperative vs. cooperative child dental patients. *Eur J Oral Sci* 2002; 110(2):75–82.

Aromaa M, Sillanpaa M, Rautava P, Helenius H. Pain experience of children with headache and their families: a controlled study. *Pediatrics* 2000; 106:207–275.

Asprey JR. Postoperative analgesic prescription and administration in a pediatric population. *J Pediatr Nurs* 1994; 9:150–157.

Beales JG, Keen JH, Holt PJ. The child's perception of the disease and the experience of pain in juvenile chronic arthritis. *J Rheumatol* 1983; 10:61–65.

Bournaki MC. Correlates of pain-related responses to venipunctures in school-age children. *Nurs Res* 1997; 46(3):147–154.

Breau LM, McGrath PJ, Camfield C, Rosmus C, Finley GA. Preliminary validation of an observational pain checklist for persons with cognitive impairments and inability to communicate verbally. *Dev Med Child Neurol* 2000; 42:609–616.

Campos RG. Rocking and pacifiers: two comforting interventions for heelstick pain. *Res Nurs Health* 1994; 17(5):321–331.

Carbajal R, Lenclen R, Gajdos V, Jugie M, Paupe A. Crossover trial of analgesic efficacy of glucose and pacifier in very preterm neonates during subcutaneous injections. *Pediatrics* 2002; 110(2 Pt 1):389–393.

Chen E, Craske MG, Katz ER, Schwartz E, Zeltzer LK. Pain-sensitive temperament: does it predict procedural distress and response to psychological treatment among children with cancer? *J Pediatr Psychol* 2000; 25(4):269–278

Cohen LL. Reducing infant immunization distress through distraction. *Health Psychol* 2002; 21(2):207–211.

Cohen LL, Blount RL, Panopoulos G. Nurse coaching and cartoon distraction: an effective and practical intervention to reduce child, parent, and nurse distress during immunizations. *J Pediatr Psychol* 1997; 22:355–370.

Cohen LL, Blount RL, Cohen RJ, Schaen ER, Zaff JF. Comparative study of distraction versus topical anesthesia for pediatric pain management during immunizations. *Health Psychol* 1999; 18(6):591–598.

Cohen LL, Blount RL, Cohen RJ, et al. Children's expectations and memories of acute distress: short- and long-term efficacy of pain management interventions. *J Pediatr Psychol* 2001; 26(6):367–374.

Craig KD. Pain in infants and children: sociodevelopmental variations on the theme. In: Maria Adele Giamberardino (Ed). *Pain 2002—An Updated Review: Refresher Course Syllabus.* Seattle: IASP Press, 2002.

Demyttenaere S, Finley GA, Johnston CC, McGrath PJ. Pain treatment thresholds in children after major surgery. *Clin J Pain* 2001; 17(2):173–177.

Eland JM, Anderson JE. The experience of pain in children. In: Jacox A (Ed). *Pain: A Source Book for Nurses and Other Health Professionals,* 1st ed. Boston: Little Brown, 1977, pp 453–478.

Faull C, Nicol AR. Abdominal pain in six-year-olds: an epidemiological study in a new town. *J Child Psychol Psychiatry* 1986; 27:251–260.

Fearon I, Kisilevsky BS, Hains SM, Muir DW, Tranmer J. Swaddling after heel lance: age-specific effects on behavioral recovery in preterm infants. *J Dev Behav Pediatr* 1997; 18(4):222–232.

Fearon I, McGrath PJ, Achat H. "Booboos": the study of everyday pain among young children. *Pain* 1996; 68:55–62.

Finley GA, McGrath PJ (Eds). *Measurement of Pain in Infants and Children,* Progress in Pain Research and Management, Vol. 10. Seattle: IASP Press, 1998.

Finley GA, McGrath PJ. (Eds) *Acute and Procedure Pain in Infants and Children,* Progress in Pain Research and Management, Vol. 20. Seattle: IASP Press, 2001.

Fradet C, McGrath PJ, Kay J, Adams S. A prospective survey of reactions to blood tests by children and adolescents. *Pain* 1990; 40:53–60.

Franck LS, Lawhon G. Environmental and behavioural strategies to prevent and manage neonatal pain. In: Anand KJS, Stevens B, McGrath PJ (Eds). *Pain in Neonates,* 2nd ed. Elsevier, Amsterdam, 2000.

Garrison MM, Christakis DA. A systematic review of treatments for infant colic. *Pediatrics* 2000; 106:184–190.

Gibbins S, Stevens B. Mechanisms of sucrose and non-nutritive sucking in procedural pain management in infants. *Pain Res Manage* 2001; 6(1):21–28.

Gold N, Issenman R, Roberts J, Watt S. Well-adjusted children: an alternate view of children with inflammatory bowel disease and functional gastrointestinal complaints. *Inflamm Bowel Dis* 2000; 6(1):1–7.

Goodman JE, McGrath PJ. The epidemiology of pain in children and adolescents: a review. *Pain* 1991; 46:247–264.

Goodman JE, McGrath PJ, Forward SP. Aggregation of pain complaints and pain-related disability and handicap in a community sample of families. In: Jensen TS, Turner JA, Wiesenfeld-Hallin Z (Eds). *Proceedings of the 8th World Congress on Pain,* Progress in Pain Research and Management, Vol. 8. Seattle: IASP Press, 1997, pp 673–682.

Griffiths AM, Nicholas D, Smith C. et al. Development of a Quality-Of-Life Index for pediatric inflammatory bowel disease: dealing with differences related to age and IBD type. *J Pediatr Gastroenterol Nutr* 1999; 28:S46–S52.

Harpin VA, Rutter N. Making heel pricks less painful. *Arch Dis Child* 1983; 58(3):226–228.

Hermann C, Kim M, Blanchard EB. Behavioral and prophylactic pharmacological intervention studies of pediatric migraine: an exploratory meta-analysis. *Pain* 1995; 60:239–256.

Hicks CL, von Baeyer CL, McGrath PJ. Online psychological treatment for pediatric recurrent pain: a randomized evaluation. *Pain Res Manage* 2002; 7(Suppl A):30A.

Holden EW, Deichmann MM, Levy JD. Empirically supported treatments in pediatric psychology: recurrent pediatric headache. *J Pediatr Psychol* 1999; 24:91–109.

Johnston CC, Collinge JM, Henderson SJ, Anand KJS. A cross-sectional survey of pain and pharmacological analgesia in Canadian neonatal intensive care units. *Clin J Pain* 1997a; 13:308–312.

Johnston CC, Stremler RL, Stevens BJ, Horton LJ. Effectiveness of oral sucrose and simulated rocking on pain response in preterm neonates. *Pain* 1997b; 72(1–2):193–199.

Kristjansdottir G. Familial aggregation and pain theory relating to recurrent pain experiences in children. *Acta Paediatr* 2000; 89:1403–1405.

Larsson BS. Somatic complaints and their relationship to depressive symptoms in Swedish adolescents. *J Child Psychol Psychiatry* 1991; 32:821–832.

Larsson BS, Melin L, Doberl A. Recurrent tension headache in adolescents treated with self-help relaxation training and a muscle relaxant drug. *Headache* 1990; 30:665–671.

Lee LW, White-Traut RC. The role of temperament in pediatric pain response. *Issues Compr Pediatr Nurs* 1996; 19(1):49–63.

Lee BH, Scharff L, Sethna NF, et al. Physical therapy and cognitive-behavioral treatment for complex regional pain syndromes. *J Pediatr* 2002; 141(1):135–140.

Ljungman G, Gordh T, Sorensen S, Kreuger A. Pain variations during cancer treatment in children: a descriptive survey. *Pediatr Hematol Oncol* 2000; 17(3):211–221.

McGhee JL, Burks FN, Sheckels JL, Jarvis JN. Identifying children with chronic arthritis based on chief complaints: absence of predictive value for musculoskeletal pain as an indicator of rheumatic disease in children. *Pediatrics* 2002; 110(2 Pt 1):354–359.

McGrath PJ, Finley GA (Eds). *Chronic and Recurrent Pain in Children and Adolescents.* Seattle: IASP Press, 1999.

McGrath PJ, Finley GA (Eds). *Pediatric Pain: Biological and Social Context,* Progress in Pain Research and Management, Vol. 26. Seattle: IASP Press, 2003.

McGrath PJ, Larsson B. Headache in children and adolescents. *Psychiatr Clin North Am* 1997; 6:843–861.

McGrath PJ, Humphreys P, Keene D, et al. The efficacy and efficiency of a self-administered treatment for adolescent migraine. *Pain* 1992; 49:321–324.

Mikail SF, von Baeyer CL. Pain, somatic focus, and emotional adjustment in children of chronic headache sufferers and controls. *Soc Sci Med* 1990; 31(1):51–59.

Nodari E, Battistella PA, Naccarella C, Vidi M. Quality of life in young Italian patients with primary headache. *Headache* 2002; 42(4):268–274.

Oberlander TF, Eckstein Grunau R, Fitzgerald C, et al. Prolonged prenatal psychotropic medication exposure alters neonatal acute pain response. *Pediatr Res* 2002; 51(4):443–453.

Peretz B, Efrat J. Dental anxiety among young adolescent patients in Israel. *Int J Paediatr Dent* 2000; 10(2):126–132

Ravilly S, Robinson W, Suresh S, Wohl ME, Berde CB. Chronic pain in cystic fibrosis. *Pediatrics* 1996; 98(4 Pt 1):741–747.

Reijneveld SA, Brugman E, Hirasing RA. Excessive infant crying: the impact of varying definitions. *Pediatrics* 2001; 108(4):893–897.

Sanders MR, Rebgetz M, Morrison M, Bor W. Cognitive-behavioral treatment of recurrent nonspecific abdominal pain in children: an analysis of generalization, maintenance, and side effects. *J Consult Clin Psychol* 1989; 57:294–300,

Sanders MR, Shepherd RW, Cleghorn G, Woolford H. The treatment of recurrent abdominal pain in children: a controlled comparison of cognitive-behavioral family intervention and standard pediatric care. *J Consult Clin Psychol* 1994; 62:306–314.

Schechter NL, Berde CB, Yaster M (Eds). *Pain in Infants, Children, and Adolescents,* 2nd ed. Philadelphia: Lippincott, Williams, and Wilkins, 2002.

Seguin JR, Pihl RO, Boulerice B, Tremblay RE, Harden PW. Pain sensitivity and stability of physical aggression in boys. *J Child Psychol Psychiatry* 1996; 37:823–834.

Shah VS, Taddio A, Bennett S, Speidel BD. Neonatal pain response to heel stick vs venepuncture for routine blood sampling. *Arch Dis Child Fetal Neonatal Ed* 1997; 77(2):F143–144.

Stallard P, Williams L, Lenton S, Velleman R. Pain in cognitively impaired, non-communicating children. *Arch Dis Child* 2001; 85:460–462.

Stevens B, Yamada J, Ohlsson A. Sucrose for analgesia in newborn infants undergoing painful procedures. *Cochrane Database Syst Rev* 2001; (4):CD001069.

Sweet SD, McGrath PJ, Symons D. The roles of child reactivity and parenting context in infant pain response. *Pain* 1999; 80:655–661.

Taimela S, Kujala UM, Salminen JJ, Viljanen T. The prevalence of low back pain among children and adolescents: a nationwide, cohort-based questionnaire survey in Finland. *Spine* 1997; 22:1132–1136.

Townend E, Dimigen G, Fung D. A clinical study of child dental anxiety. *Behav Res Ther* 2000; 38(1):31–46.

Unruh AM, Campbell MA. Gender variation in children's pain. In: McGrath PJ, Finley GA (Eds). *Chronic and Recurrent Pain in Children and Adolescents,* Progress in Pain Research and Management, Vol. 13. Seattle: IASP Press, 1999.

von Baeyer CL, Baskerville S, McGrath PJ. Everyday pain in three- to five-year-old children in day care. *Pain Res Manage* 1998; 3:111–116.

Walco GA, Sterling CM, Conte PM, Engel RG. Empirically supported treatments in pediatric psychology: disease-related pain. *J Pediatr Psychol* 1999; 24(2):155–167.

Walker LS, Garber J, Greene JW. Somatic complaints in pediatric patients: a prospective study of the role of negative life events, child social and academic competence, and parental somatic symptoms. *J Consult Clin Psychol* 1994; 62(6):1213–1221.

Walker LS, Garber J, Smith CA, Van Slyke DA, Claar RL. The relation of daily stressors to somatic and emotional symptoms in children with and without recurrent abdominal pain. *J Consult Clin Psychol* 2001; 69(1):85–91.

Winner P, Gladstein J. Chronic daily headache in pediatric practice. *Curr Opin Neurol* 2002; 15(3):297–301.

Correspondence to: Patrick J. McGrath, OC, PhD, FRCS, Department of Psychology, Dalhousie University, Halifax, Nova Scotia, Canada B3H 4J1. Email: patrick.mcgrath@dal.ca.

Psychosocial Aspects of Pain: A Handbook for Health Care Providers, Progress in Pain Research and Management, Vol. 27, edited by Robert H. Dworkin and William S. Breitbart, IASP Press, Seattle, © 2004.

22

Psychosocial Aspects of Pain in Older People

Michael J. Farrell and Stephen J. Gibson

National Ageing Research Institute, Parkville, Victoria, Australia

Pain is at once a universal and individual experience. A complaint of pain is instantly recognizable. We can all draw upon our personal history to recollect the aversive nature of a painful sensation along with the emotional responses that accompanied the experience. Yet while the experience is unmistakable, pain is subject to profound plasticity. A myriad of factors can shape the experience of pain, operating both within and among individuals to produce diverse presentations of a common denomination. The literature of pain is replete with physiological, psychological, social, and cultural factors that demonstrate associations with the experience and expression of pain. Of growing interest to pain researchers and clinicians alike is the influence of aging on the pain experience.

Aging is a prime candidate as a pain-modulating factor. Increasing age has the potential to influence pain through changes in the neural substrates of nociception, modification of emotional responses, and developmental and cohort-related effects on cognition. Advanced age is also associated with increased risk for many diseases that are accompanied by complaints of pain, and with increased risk for disorders that impede attempts to adequately assess and manage pain in older people. The impetus to examine the effects of aging on pain is driven by an urgent demographic imperative. The post-World War II generation constitutes a substantial proportion of the population in Western societies, and is growing older during a period characterized by dwindling fertility rates. By mid-century, the over-65-year-old age group will represent 20–35% of populations in many developed countries (United Nations 1995). Responding to the needs of a growing number of older people will become a major challenge for pain practitioners. This chapter will draw upon the gerontology and pain literatures to describe the impact of aging on pain from a psychosocial perspective. It will also examine issues related to the assessment and management of older people with persistent pain.

EPIDEMIOLOGY

Age has a differential effect on the likelihood of acute and chronic pain. The point prevalence of acute pain is stable across the adult life span at a level of approximately 5% (Crook et al. 1984; Kendig et al. 1996). Chronic pain increases in prevalence up to the seventh decade, reaching a plateau thereafter, and may decline in age groups termed the "old old" (75–85 years) and "oldest old" (85+ years; Helme and Gibson 1999, 2001). Although the pattern of chronic pain prevalence is relatively consistent across studies, it is not possible to be definitive in respect to absolute levels of pain prevalence due to marked variations among epidemiological reports. Discrepancies among studies in chronic pain prevalence reflect differences in the time sample under consideration, the method of survey, and the type and sites of pain nominated. Studies that have incorporated samples with a wide age range have reported the prevalence of chronic pain as 10–40% in early adulthood, 20–80% in late middle age, and 15–70% in the oldest members of the community (Brattberg et al. 1989, 1997; Andersson et al. 1993; Magni et al. 1993; Mobily et al. 1994; Kendig et al. 1996; Kind et al. 1998; Bassols et al. 1999; Blyth et al. 2001). The plateau and possible decline in pain prevalence among the oldest cohorts are surprising in light of the age-related epidemiology of many disorders that usually give rise to pain. The factors contributing to the prevalence of pain in persons over the age of 75 years have yet to be elucidated, although limited longitudinal data would argue against selective mortality among older people complaining of pain (Bagge et al. 1992). It is also interesting to note that studies of pain prevalence from samples restricted to older people report rates of chronic pain that tend to exceed the highest levels identified in the population studies (Helme and Gibson 1999). The discrepancy among results from different sampling approaches may arise due to the inclusion of frail older people in samples that target this age group.

The age-related prevalence of chronic pain is due to an amalgam of disorders affecting diverse pain regions that do not invariably share the same pattern across the life span. The epidemiology of osteoarthritis is most compatible with the age-related increase of chronic pain (Felson et al. 1987; Hochberg et al. 1991), and probably drives the prevalence of pain in older cohorts by sheer weight of numbers. It is interesting to note that while the prevalence of radiological osteoarthritis increases with age, the presence of pain does not demonstrate differential age-related risk after accounting for disease severity (Hochberg et al. 1989; Davis et al. 1992; Carman et al. 1994). Furthermore, data from samples including sequestered populations, such as residents of aged care facilities, support a gradual increase in osteoarthritis in the oldest old (Felson et al. 1995).

In distinction to articular pain, evidence indicates that headache (Sternbach 1986; D'Alessandro et al. 1988; Kay et al. 1992; Andersson et al. 1993), abdominal pain (Lavsky-Shulan et al. 1985; Kay et al. 1992), and chest pain (Sternbach 1986; Von Korff et al. 1988; Tibblin et al. 1990; Andersson et al. 1993) peak in later middle age (45–55 years) and decline in prevalence in older age groups. The epidemiology of visceral pain may be a consequence of increasingly frequent instances of atypical disease presentations with advancing age. Visceral disorders usually associated with pain, including myocardial infarct, peritonitis, peptic ulcer, intestinal obstruction, and pneumonia are more likely to be painless in older people (Albano et al. 1975; Konu 1977; MacDonald et al. 1983; Wroblewski and Mikulowski 1991). The interaction of age and the absence of pain in visceral disorders has important implications for the clinical management of older people and also constitutes an interesting phenomenon from the perspective of the pain researcher. The underlying reasons for an age-related increase in atypical pain presentations have yet to be elucidated but certainly warrant attention.

PAIN APPRAISAL

The experience of pain is laden with biological significance. The sudden onset of pain engages reflex behaviors, demands attention, and prompts complex behaviors that diminish the risk of exacerbation of injury. During recovery, pain associated with increased sensitivity (hyperalgesia) heightens awareness of the vulnerability of tissues undergoing repair processes. Persistent pain can accompany disorders with a chronic course, accurately reflecting tissue integrity. On the other hand, pain persisting after the resolution of tissue damage serves a dubious biological function. Acute and chronic pains are intrinsically unpleasant, and this attribute of the experience is intimately related to the capacity of pain to arouse (Price 2000). However, not all emotional and behavioral responses to pain are automatic. The integration of pain is dependent on cognitive appraisal of the meaning of the experience and interaction with behavioral outcomes. A growing body of evidence indicates that aging is associated with substantive differences in the appraisal of pain.

Older people may consider some pain to be a normal companion of aging (Hofland 1992). Empirical studies examining pain appraisals and aging support the contention that older people expect to experience pain as they age (Harkins 1988; Liddell and Locker 1997; Ruzicka 1998; Weiner and Rudy 2000), although this finding has not been universal (Gagliese and Melzack 1997b). Unlike in younger people, the presence of mild symptoms does not affect self-rated health in older people (Ebrahim et al. 1991; Mangione et al. 1993). This style of attribution has important implications for the probable response to mild pain in older people. It seems likely that older people are less threatened by mild pain, less likely to experience emotional disturbance, and less prone to seek treatment. However, the propensity of older people to ascribe pain to the process of aging is confined to mild symptoms. When pain becomes severe, older people are more likely to interpret the experience as a sign of serious illness and seek medical assistance more rapidly than younger people (Leventhal et al. 1993; Stoller 1993). It is important that clinicians dealing with older people are aware of this age-related interaction between pain intensity and pain appraisal. Mild pain, which could be eminently treatable, may go unnoticed in older people and so diligence is required to identify cases. Experiences of severe pain in old and young alike are appraised as a sign of serious illness and need to be acknowledged accordingly.

When pain is of sufficient severity to come to clinical attention, patients acknowledge to varying degrees the role of organic and psychological factors in the modulation of pain. The influence of age on beliefs about pain operates differentially. The conviction that organic issues are important in determining the pain experience (i.e., that pain is a result of tissue damage) is apparent to a similar degree in old and young people (Gagliese and Melzack 1997b). While both old and young people concede that psychological factors can influence pain (Gagliese and Melzack 1997b), older people are less inclined to acknowledge that pain leads to mood disturbance (Cook et al. 1999). The de-emphasis of emotional responses to pain among older people is a recurring anecdote in the pain literature and has recently been assessed psychometrically with an instrument designed to capture pain attitudes with salience for all age groups (Yong et al. 2001). A "stoic-reticence" to communicate pain is most pronounced in older people, who are also more hesitant to label mildly noxious events as painful. The contemporary view of stoicism as a lack of emotional involvement, a lack of emotional expression, and enhanced emotional control (Wagstaff and Rowledge 1995) resonates with the propensity of older people to report lesser degrees of negative affect (Gibson 1997). It appears that the stoic attitudinal style of older people may also operate in their appraisal of pain.

Taken together, the various pain appraisals and beliefs of older people appear paradoxical. On the one hand, older people are inclined to interpret pain as a sign of organic disease, are threatened by the implications of severe pain, and seek medical assistance accordingly. Conversely, older people are reluctant to communicate the true nature of their pain, preferring to preserve a stoic demeanor, and are less likely to acknowledge the emotional consequences of their predicament.

COPING AND SELF-EFFICACY

A common objective of the patient with pain is to find a cure. Unfortunately, the abolition of pain is not always an option, particularly in older people with chronic conditions. When pain persists, patients adopt strategies of variable efficacy to cope with their situation. The perception of patients with chronic pain regarding the success of their efforts to cope does not appear to differ across the adult age spectrum (Harkins 1988; Keefe and Williams 1990; Keefe et al. 1991; Corran et al. 1994; Gagliese et al. 2000). The acknowledgment that personal resources and strategies are important for the experience of pain, as articulated by the internal scale of the Locus of Control questionnaire, also remains constant across the life span (Gibson and Helme 2000). However, older people, notably the oldest old, are more likely to subscribe to the view that chance events are important determinants of the pain experience (Gibson and Helme 2000). It is possible to argue that the endorsement of a chance locus of control could be a reasonable appraisal of symptoms arising from many of the chronic, progressive disorders that afflict the older population. The differential effect of age on loci of control argues for the orthogonal nature of the constructs and alerts the clinician to the nuances of patients' appraisals of the factors influencing their pain. An older person endorsing chance as an important determinant of pain may be equally likely to embrace the more adaptive view that personal efforts will bring about change.

The coping strategies employed by older people to ameliorate the experience and consequences of pain have been subject to empirical investigation, with mixed results. In essence, smaller studies have suggested trends that coalesce into significant effects in larger samples (Keefe and Williams 1990; Sorkin et al. 1990; Keefe et al. 1991; McCracken 1993; Corran et al. 1994). The most consistent finding is the greater use of praying and hoping among older people. In all likelihood, the increased use of praying and hoping reported among older people is a stable attribute of the current cohort. The alternative hypothesis, of a developmental change in religiosity as a pain-coping strategy, must await longitudinal studies to be supported or refuted. Old and young pain patients may also differ in the degree to which they employ ignoring as a coping strategy. Ignoring appears to be more in favor with younger people (Corran et al. 1994). The modest effects of age on the use of coping strategies may also be modulated by pain intensity. In a report on rheumatoid arthritis patients, age differences in coping strategies were only in evidence under circumstances of mild pain (Watkins et al. 1999). The implications of the interaction between pain intensity and age on the use of coping strategies in rheumatoid arthritis patients may not extend beyond this clinical group given that the aforementioned differences in praying and hoping and ignoring pain were identified in samples of pain clinic patients, where complaints of mild pain are unlikely.

It would appear that older people with persistent pain are likely to adopt slightly different coping styles compared to their younger counterparts. The clinical significance of aging effects on coping strategies is dependent on the outcomes associated with the strategies. Praying and hoping, more common in the current cohort of older people, do not appear to explain a significant degree of variance in pain report, mood state, or functional impact in the old or the young (Corran et al. 1994). Greater use of ignoring pain, an attribute more frequent among younger people, is associated with less mood disturbance in this age group (Corran et al. 1994). It is not immediately apparent why older people do not engage in, and benefit from, "ignoring" as a pain reduction strategy. Although similar across age groups in frequency of use, self-coping statements appears to be more efficacious for older people, being associated with less mood disturbance and less functional impact (Corran et al. 1994). The tenure of self-coping statements is compatible with the stoic appraisal of pain that seems to be a feature of the older pain patient. Consequently, it may be judicious for the clinician dealing with older people to reinforce the propensity of this age group to maintain a "stiff upper lip."

COMORBIDITY

Epidemiologists have studied the relative risk of pain with reference to the differential likelihood of painful disorders. The burden of disease in older people also includes disorders that are not primarily painful. Indeed, the weight of pathology, painful or otherwise, in older people is a major distinguishing factor for this age group. Comorbidity is possibly the single most important factor in the heterogeneity of clinical presentations in older people and is a major influence on assessment and treatment options.

Comorbidity may also influence the experience and expression of pain through two major effects: disease-specific effects and the accumulative effects of disease burden.

DISEASE BURDEN

Physiological functions are affected by aging to various degrees. Primary age-related decline in physiological performance may not result in substantive impairments but is characterized by reduced functional reserve. The older person may consequently be vulnerable to the perturbation of physiological systems that have diminished tolerance (Hayflick 2000). Reduced reserves consequently increase the likelihood of disease onset. The plight of older people with illness is frequently compounded by the concurrence and interaction of multiple disease states. Chronic disease states can place further stress on physiological processes. The stress of disease burden is more likely to manifest in functions that are most compromised by primary age-related change.

The experience of pain is dependent on a highly integrated system, the components of which are unlikely to exhibit uniform levels of age-related change. Comorbidity is most likely to accentuate those aspects of the pain experience that are subject to age-related change. Psychophysical approaches have suggested that the acuity of pain perception is diminished in older people (Gibson and Farrell, in press). The exact mechanisms contributing to the increase in pain threshold with advancing age are yet to be established. The accumulative effect of disease burden may further accentuate the decreased sensitivity of older people at the lower end of the response curve, possibly making older people more vulnerable to minor injury due to lack of adequate protective responses. However, it is the potential interaction of age and comorbidity on the experience of pain at levels in excess of the pain threshold that has the most relevance for the clinician dealing with older people. Recent evidence suggests that aging is associated with impairment of the endogenous analgesic system (Washington et al. 2000). Consistent reports of decreased tolerance to prolonged noxious stimuli in older people (Collins and Stone 1966; Woodrow et al. 1972; Walsh et al. 1989; Edwards et al. 2001) may be a manifestation of failing downregulation of the nociceptive system. Deterioration in the waning efficacy of endogenous analgesic systems due to stress associated with intercurrent disease could make older people particularly vulnerable to intensely noxious stimuli. A recent abstract at the World Congress on Pain presented evidence compatible with increased levels of clinical pain among older people with a greater weight of pathology (Neufeld et al. 2002). Older pain clinic patients with four or more systems affected by disease had scores on the McGill Pain Questionnaire that were 31.3% greater than those of older patients with no more than three systems affected by disease. The magnitude of this effect further highlights the need to direct clinical attention to the pain management of the oldest and frailest members of our communities.

SPECIFIC DISEASE EFFECTS

The interaction of disease and the experience of pain may vary as a function of the type of illness. Specific conditions rather than disease load could explain some of the potential effects of comorbidity on pain perception. Painless conditions that increase in prevalence with advancing age have the capacity to modulate painful symptoms arising from intercurrent disorders. A salient example is hypertension, which has both an age-related increase in prevalence and a demonstrable association with reduced pain sensitivity (Bots et al. 1991; France 1999). However, the aging disorder that has attracted most attention as a potential modifier of the pain experience is dementia.

Dementia rarely occurs in younger people. The prevalence of dementia in those aged 65–69 years is 1.5%, increasing exponentially up to the end of the ninth decade to a level of 22.2% in those aged 85–89 years (Ritchie and Kildea 1995). Dementia prevalence after the age of 90 years continues to increase but does not accelerate to the same degree, reaching a peak of 44.8% at age 95–99 years. The dementia syndrome can be caused by a myriad of disorders, the most common of which is Alzheimer's disease. Cerebrovascular disease is the second most frequent cause of dementia, and a significant proportion of cases present with features compatible with a mixed diagnosis of vascular disease and Alzheimer's disease (Zekry et al. 2002). The dementia syndrome is characterized by progressive cognitive dysfunction, of which memory impairment is a defining attribute (American Psychiatric Association 1994).

The interface between dementia and the experience and expression of pain is difficult to posit, given the variable manifestations of the syndrome and the multiple disorders that contribute to the onset of cognitive impairment (Farrell et al. 1996). In Alzheimer's disease the sensory-discriminative aspects of pain perception appear to be preserved (Benedetti et al. 1999; Gibson et al. 2001), a finding that is compatible with current understanding of the pathology of Alzheimer's disease (Hof 1997) and of the supraspinal processing of pain (Coghill et al. 1999). The most likely interface between pain and dementia, irrespective of etiology, is the potential for distorted cognition to fundamentally change the meaning and emotional ramifications of the pain experience. The current evidence would suggest that older people with cognitive impairment are less likely to report pain (Parmelee et al. 1993; Werner et al. 1998; Krulewitch et al. 2000), although the implications of this effect should be tempered by the possibility that some pathologies may be less prevalent among groups with dementia. Of particular note is the finding that regular use of nonsteroidal anti-inflammatory drugs for the management of arthritis offers some protection against the development of Alzheimer's disease (in 't Veld et al. 2001). It would also appear that cognitive impairment is associated with decreased clinical pain intensity and affective ratings (Parmelee 1996; Werner et al. 1998; Scherder et al. 1999; Cohen-Mansfield and Lipson 2002). A report of increased pain tolerance under experimental conditions in subjects with cognitive impairment further supports a significant interaction between dementia and pain at suprathreshold intensities (Benedetti et al. 1999). The contribution of pain beliefs and appraisals to the experience of pain in older people with dementia has yet to be tested but remains a priority for pain and aging research.

As cases with dementia progress, communication becomes increasingly disturbed, and ultimately patients may lose the ability to communicate altogether. The impairment or inability of patients with dementia to verbally communicate their distress has major implications for the identification and treatment of pain in this vulnerable group of older people. The consistent finding that older people with dementia are less likely than their cognitively intact counterparts to receive analgesia despite comparable levels of morbidity is cause for concern (Morrison and Siu 2000; Scherder and Bouma 2000). It seems very likely that impaired communication contributes significantly to the undertreatment of pain in older people with dementia, and clinicians must be especially vigilant when managing patients with cognitive impairment.

PSYCHOPATHOLOGY AND PSYCHIATRIC SYNDROMES IN OLDER PEOPLE WITH CHRONIC PAIN

DEPRESSION

The strong association of chronic pain and depression is a well-established phenomenon, and age does not appear to influence this relationship. Despite some exceptions (Corran et al. 1997; Riley et al. 2000), the weight of evidence from clinical pain samples supports consistent rates of depression (Herr and Mobily 1993; Corran et al. 1994; Benbow et al. 1996; Wijeratne et al. 2001) and a consistent number of depressive symptoms across the age spectrum (Middaugh et al. 1988; Sorkin et al. 1990; Herr and Mobily 1993;

McCracken 1993; Turk et al. 1995; Gagliese and Melzack 1997b; Cossins et al. 1999). Presumably, emotional distress greatly increases the likelihood of admission to a pain service, and we should exercise caution before extrapolating findings from highly selected pain clinic samples to other settings. However, epidemiological data from a community-dwelling sample also support a consistent pain-related risk for depression across the age spectrum (Magni et al. 1993). Depression among subjects with chronic pain was 16.4% compared to a prevalence of 5.7% in the sample without pain and did not vary significantly as a function of age.

The absence of an aging effect on the nexus of pain and depression needs to be assessed with reference to the general prevalence of depression. Both the likelihood of a depression diagnosis and the level of depressive symptomatology peak in late middle age and decline thereafter (Gibson 1997; Henderson et al. 1998; Jorm 2000). The lack of synchrony in age-associated rates of depression among persons with and without chronic pain suggests that the interaction between the aging process and the experience of pain has a significant impact on the manifestation of mood disturbance. Examining the literature of depression and aging may reveal potential explanations for the interplay of pain, age, and mood.

Reasons for the general age-related decrease in depression are probably multifactorial and incorporate methodological issues including survivorship (Wulsin et al. 1999) and sequestration of the frailest members of the older population in residential facilities (Ames 1993; Katz et al. 1995). Primary aging explanations for decreased mood disturbance in older people include decreased emotional responsiveness, increased emotional control, and psychological immunization associated with repeated exposure to adverse life events (Jorm 2000). Two further explanations for the age-related decrease of depression are particularly important in the context of chronic pain. The first involves the differential effects of age on associated risk factors for depression, and the second relates to age-related changes in the phenomenology and reporting of depressive symptoms.

Empirical studies have identified a wide range of psychological and social factors that are associated with increased risk of depression. When examining the effect of aging it is judicious to control for risk factors that may covary with age. In most instances, controlling for differential rates of marital status, level of education, income, employment, and gender distribution leads to the unmasking or an accentuating of age-related decreases of depression (Comstock and Helsing 1976; Eaton and Kessler 1981; Frerichs et al. 1981; Mirowsky and Ross 1992; Regier et al. 1993; Henderson et al. 1998). However, comorbidity is an important risk factor primarily associated with older people that warrants specific attention. Comorbidity greatly increases the likelihood of depression in older people. Rates of major depression from 11% to 30% have been reported in elderly clinical populations (Rapp et al. 1991; Lyness et al. 1999). Suicide rates are much higher for older people with health problems (Gurland et al. 1988). Reports have suggested that more than 85% of older people committing suicide have an active disease, in addition to depression, immediately preceding their death (Ouslander 1982). The unique place of comorbidity in older people means that it is rarely examined across the age spectrum because there is a relative absence of active disease in younger, healthier people. Chronic pain can be construed as a type of morbidity that allows meaningful comparisons across age groups. The consistent rate of depression among chronic pain sufferers of disparate age suggests that any protection against the onset of depression afforded by increased age is obviated by the concurrence of pain. It could be that the propensity among older people to experience less emotional response is not sufficient to counteract the mood-altering effects of persistent pain. This path of reasoning highlights the clinical importance of chronic pain as a major factor in the emotional well-being of many older people.

The aging effect on rates of depression, independent of pain, has been examined from the perspective of the phenomenology and measurement of the clinical condition. Instruments for assessing depression vary in the extent to which they identify aging effects, suggesting an age bias in some psychometric measures (Lyness et al. 1995; Newmann et al. 1996). If a psychometric instrument is employed to flag potential cases of depression then it is advisable to select a measure with demonstrable validity in older people. Item bias can also occur in the questions that constitute depression inventories. It is possible for old and young groups to achieve comparable mean scores on depression scales but differ significantly in the frequency of endorsement of particular items (Gallo et al. 1994). This issue certainly has implications for measurement, but also has ramifications for the probable presentation of depression in older people. While older people with depression are more likely to report sleep problems, to complain of fatigue, and to contemplate death, they are less likely to report depressed mood and anhedonia (an inability to experience pleasure) (Gallo et al. 1994; Newmann et al. 1996; Christensen et al. 1999). Older people are also more inclined to ascribe somatic depressive symptoms to physical causes, an effect that operates independently of competing explanations from physical comorbidities (Knauper and Wittchen 1994; Heithoff 1995). The clinician who is confronted with an older person complaining of persistent pain should be mindful that the manifestation of a concurrent depressive condition may differ significantly from the clinical presentation of younger patients.

ANXIETY

The level of anxiety among older people with chronic pain is not well established. Existing evidence would suggest that older chronic pain patients are less likely to be anxious than their younger counterparts (McCracken 1993; Corran et al. 1994; Benbow et al. 1995; Cossins et al. 1999; Riley et al. 2000; Cook and Chastain 2001). This evidence is consistent with most reports of anxiety disorders from diverse samples of older people (Henderson et al. 1998). The reason for the decreased levels of anxiety in older people have not been established, but may be related to a general decrease in the reporting of negative emotional features with advancing age (Gibson 1997).

Although consistently reported in studies of mood, the decrease in anxiety among older people is of modest proportions. The prevalence of anxiety among community-dwelling young to middle-aged people is on the order of 8.3%, compared to 5.5% in people over the age of 65 (Flint 1994). The decrease in symptoms of anxiety among older people with chronic pain has been reported as approximately 25% less than in their younger counterparts (McCracken 1993; Corran et al. 1994; Benbow et al. 1995; Cossins et al. 1999; Riley et al. 2000; Cook and Chastain 2001). This substantial decrease is more noteworthy because it underscores the divergence between anxiety and depression in their respective relationships with chronic pain and aging.

Anxiety and depression frequently occur in unison in the broader population of older people (Lenze et al. 2001). Generalized anxiety, as opposed to specific phobic disorders, is less frequently diagnosed in the absence of depressive features in older people. It is important to recognize psychiatric comorbidity because cases with concurrent depression and anxiety tend to present with more severe pathology and are less responsive to treatment (Lenze et al. 2001). Casten and colleagues (1995) tested the unique contributions of anxiety and depression as predictors of pain report in a sample of older people. The results of the path model used in this study were consistent with a greater role for anxiety as a predictor of pain report. The greater weight of research devoted to pain and depression has tended to de-emphasize the role of anxiety in the presentation of chronic pain patients. It may be judicious to focus clinical attention on the identification and management of anxiety in older people with chronic pain despite the relative decrease in the prevalence of anxiety with advancing age.

SOMATOFORM DISORDERS

It has been postulated that somatoform disorders are less likely to be diagnosed in older people (Portenoy and Farkash 1988). It is possible that the weight of pathology in older pain patients may militate against a psychogenic disorder (Wijeratne and Hickie 2001). An isolated report (Helme et al. 1996b) from a pain clinic for older people identified 8.7% of patients who were diagnosed with a somatoform pain disorder according to the criteria defined in the DSM-IV (American Psychiatric Association 1994). A study examining psychiatric conditions among pain clinic patients identified no cases of pain disorder in young or older groups, leaving unanswered the question of age-related risk of somatoform disorder (Wijeratne et al. 2001).

AGING AND SOCIAL ISSUES RELATED TO PAIN

During old age, individuals typically enjoy greater freedom to pursue personal life interests and pastimes as well as a reduced level of societal and vocational responsibility. Advanced age may also be associated with impaired mobility, economic constraints, and death of one's friends or spouse, leading to social isolation. These changes in social functioning might be expected to influence pain and its expression. Fordyce (1978) suggested that older persons may be more likely to complain of pain in order to receive social contact from friends and family that would otherwise be unavailable. One empirical study has shown that social factors such as income, residential status, and frequency of social support were similar in older adults with and without chronic pain (Roy and Thomas 1987). However, within a sample of older patients at a pain clinic, increased levels of social support appeared to be associated with increased levels of pain (Helme et al. 1996a). Conversely, the loss of a partner and bereavement might affect mood state and thereby pain. Widowhood is associated with an increased risk for pain in community-dwelling older people. Widows with mood disturbance are also more likely to experience pain that is moderate to severe (Bradbeer et al. 2003). There is a clear and urgent need for further research into social factors that have a moderating influence on the expression of pain in older people. For example, type and level of social support, widowhood, and economic prosperity all deserve further study that will ultimately contribute to a more comprehensive understanding of age differences in the pain experience.

ASSESSMENT AND TREATMENT

PAIN ASSESSMENT IN OLDER PEOPLE

Evidence from a variety of sources would suggest that any measurement approach found to be useful in young adult populations has the potential for use with many older persons (Parmelee 1994; Helme and Gibson 1998).

However, the heterogeneity of cognitive and communication abilities among older people dictates that assessment must be tailored according to capacity. Three broad classes of pain assessment have been applied in older populations: self-report scales, behavioral-observation measures, and third-party proxy ratings.

Single-item scales of self-reported pain intensity, such as verbal descriptor scales, numeric rating scales, colored analogue scales, and the pictorial pain faces scale, all possess some attributes of validity and reliability when used in healthy older adults and even in those with mild cognitive impairment (see Herr and Garand 2001 for review). Some evidence supports the validity of visual analogue scales (VAS) (Scherder and Bouma 2000), although concerns have been raised about the suitability of this measure for use with older patients (Herr and Mobily 1993; Ferrell 1995; Benesch et al. 1997; Tiplady et al. 1998). In particular, it has been suggested that older persons may have difficulties with the more abstract nature of the scaling properties of the VAS (Kremer et al. 1981; Herr and Mobily 1993). Multidimensional word descriptor inventories such as the McGill Pain Questionnaire have also been questioned due to their complexity and the need for advanced language skills (Herr and Mobily 1991). However, most data would support the use of pain inventories in older adults with and without cognitive impairment (Helme et al. 1989; Corran et al. 1991; Ferrell 1995; Gagliese and Melzack 1997a; Weiner et al. 1998), although completion rates may not be as favorable as for single-item scales (Parmelee 1994; Ferrell 1995; Hadjistavropoulos et al. 1997).

Comorbid medical illnesses, physical impairments in vision or hearing, severe cognitive impairment, and difficulties with verbal communication skills can complicate routine psychometric pain assessment. Behavioral-observation measures of pain that can bypass many of these difficulties have been examined for use in frail older populations such as nursing home residents and the demented elderly. Standardized protocols have been developed (e.g., Keefe and Block 1982) to monitor the frequency of pain-related behaviors including guarding, bracing, rubbing, grimacing, and sighing. Inter-rater reliability and concurrent validity appear to be adequate in older nursing home residents, including those with mild to moderate cognitive impairment (Simons and Malabar 1995; Weiner et al. 1996, 1998, 1999; Kovach et al. 1999). However, the level of agreement between resident and staff perceptions of pain as indexed by behavioral markers was relatively poor (Weiner et al. 1999).

Behavioral-observation measures incorporate an approach that involves coding of discrete facial expressions as nonverbal indicators of pain (Craig et al. 2001). A characteristic pain face has been noted (including lowered eyebrows, raised cheeks, closed eyes, and parting or tightening of lips), and despite some individual differences, this expression is instantly recognizable by third-party observers. The complexity and speed of facial gestures can lead to errors of judgment, but recently a facial action coding system has been developed with the aid of videotaped recordings. When this technique was used in frail older adults, inter-rater reliability was excellent, and there was good evidence of discriminate and concurrent validity when compared to patient self-report (Hadjistavropoulos et al. 1997, 1998, 2002). In fact, in older adults with dementia, facial expressions of pain during needle injections correlated very closely with patients' self-report (Hadjistavropoulos et al. 1997). No such correlation was found when considering the acute exacerbation of musculoskeletal pain upon movement (Hadjistavropoulos et al. 2000), and there may be some age differences in the correspondence between pain self-report and the intensity of facial reactions (Matheson 1997). Nonetheless, these findings are encouraging and may offer another method of pain measurement that is sensitive to differences in functional capacity and can capitalize on the available communication repertoire of persons at the end stage of the life span.

The final class of measures involves third-party proxy ratings of pain by medical staff, caregivers, or others who know the individual well. Given that pain is a latent and subjective experience that is really only accessible to the individual who is suffering, this method cannot be recommended for routine pain assessment. However, such measures may be of value when no other method is available. For instance, some studies with older demented patients have shown a reasonable level of agreement (70%) between nursing staff and patient ratings in identifying the presence of pain (Krulewitch et al. 2000; Weiner et al. 1998; Werner et al. 1998). On the other hand, staff often underestimate the presence of pain, there is often poor inter-rater reliability, and estimates of pain intensity may vary widely between patient and proxy ratings (Weiner et al. 1998; Krulewitch et al. 2000). It is likely that a lifetime partner or long-term caregiver might be better able to identify times of pain, but studies to verify this possibility have yet to be undertaken.

In summary, asking older patients to describe their pain with a self-rating scale is the first assessment option when verbal communication is possible. The choice of self-rating scale is dependent on cognitive abilities, in that simple scales are more likely to be completed than multidimensional scales. The failure of a cognitively impaired patient to complete one type of self-rating scale does not preclude the possibility that an alternative instrument may prompt a salient response (Ferrell et al. 1995), and consequently the clinician should have a range of scales available when assessing older people. Behavioral-observation measures can augment verbal reports or provide information about pain when verbal communication is impaired. Established behavioral-observation methods are preferable to third-party judgments by virtue of the relative quality of information, but detailed observational strategies are resource-intensive and of less utility in many settings populated by the frailest members of the older community.

TREATMENT CONSIDERATIONS IN OLDER PEOPLE

A wide range of pharmacological, surgical, psychological, behavioral, and physical therapies have demonstrated effects in people with chronic pain. The focus of this review is on treatments with a psychosocial emphasis (for details on other treatment approaches see the guidelines of the American Geriatrics Society [2002]). The vast majority of treatments for chronic pain have been developed in younger people, and there have been few investigations of age differences in the treatment response over the life span. Pain clinicians have no option but to extrapolate treatment guidelines from younger patients, tempering their judgments according to the frailties of their older patients (Portenoy and Farkash 1988). It is not entirely clear why there has been limited interest in pursuing age differences, although recent evidence indicates a substantial age bias against patient referral and prognosis as well as bias against the perceived effectiveness of many treatment approaches (Kee et al. 1998).

Considerable evidence supports the use of psychological approaches for the management of pain in younger people (see Gatchel and Turk 1999 for review). Uncontrolled, essentially descriptive studies have also shown that older people benefit from relaxation training (Arena et al. 1988, 1991), biofeedback (Nicholson and Blanchard 1993), behavior therapy (Miller and LeLieuvre 1982), and cognitive-behavioral programs (Puder 1988). One recent randomized, controlled trial examined cognitive-behavioral therapy in nursing home residents (Cook 1998). Cognitive-behavioral therapy involving 10 weekly sessions of education, reconceptualization of pain and belief structures, training in coping skills, relaxation, and goal setting greatly improved self-rated pain and functional disability, but not depressed mood. These effects were maintained at 4-month follow-up. In combination, these findings discourage the attitude that older people are less accepting of psychological approaches to pain management (Kee et al. 1996), but without formal age-comparative data, it is impossible to evaluate relative treatment efficacy across different age groups. Other psychological approaches such as hypnosis, psychotherapy, and stress reduction have not received systematic investigation across the age spectrum and have limited support for efficacy in the management of chronic pain.

Multidisciplinary pain management facilities offer state-of-the-art treatment for more complex chronic pain problems, particularly when conventional strategies have failed (Flor et al. 1992; Guzman et al. 2002). Several authors have noted the importance of modifying standard treatment protocols in order to accommodate the special needs of older patients (Arena et al. 1988; Portenoy and Farkash 1988; Gibson et al. 1996). Modifications include setting age-relevant treatment goals, recognizing comorbid disease and its influence on treatment decisions, allowing more time for assessment and treatment instructions, and ensuring that the older person takes an active role in the treatment process and has good self-efficacy skills for the recommended treatment approach (Gibson et al. 1996). It may also be important to ensure that the social milieu of the clinic is appropriate for older persons, because group therapy is more effective if participants share similar life experience, have similar aspirations, and face similar problems. The available literature on treatment outcome for older adults provides strong support for multidisciplinary treatment (see Gibson et al. 1996 for review). With few exceptions (Painter et al. 1980; Aronoff and Evans 1982; Guck et al. 1986), it appears that older adults can show substantial post-treatment benefits (Hallett and Pilowsky 1982; Ysla et al. 1986; Middaugh et al. 1988; Helme et al. 1989, 1996b; Farrell and Gibson 1993; Hodgson et al. 1993; Kolter-Cope and Gerber 1993; Cutler et al. 1994; Groves et al. 2002). The studies favoring the response of older people to multidisciplinary treatment have not been of sufficient methodological rigor to allow uncritical acceptance of the effect, and a randomized, controlled trial has yet to be reported. Despite this caveat, clinicians should actively consider multidisciplinary approaches for older people with chronic pain.

CONCLUSION

Advanced age is associated with changes in the likelihood, manifestation, and consequences of pain. The magnitude of age-related change in pain presentations is not always substantial, although comorbidity can accentuate differences and complicate management. The interplay of pain and comorbidity generally and that of pain and dementia specifically are critical issues that remain unresolved. However, our understanding of the effects of age on pain has become increasingly sophisticated, thanks to a growing body of literature that continues to inform clinical practice.

ACKNOWLEDGMENTS

M.J. Farrell was in receipt of a Neil Hamilton Fairley Fellowship from the National Health and Medical Research Council during preparation of this manuscript.

REFERENCES

Albano WA, Zielinski CM, Organ CH. Is appendicitis in the aged really different? *Geriatrics* 1975; 30:81–88.

American Geriatrics Society. The management of persistent pain in older persons. *J Am Geriatr Soc* 2002; 50:S205–S224.

American Psychiatric Association. *Diagnostic and Statistical Manual of Mental Disorders,* 4th ed. Washington, DC: American Psychiatric Association, 1994.

Ames D. Depressive disorders among elderly people in long-term institutional care. *Aust NZ J Psychiatry* 1993; 27:379–391.

Andersson HI, Ejlertsson G, Leden I, Rosenberg C. Chronic pain in a geographically defined general population: studies of differences in age, gender, social class, and pain localization. *Clin J Pain* 1993; 9:174–182.

Arena JG, Hightower NE, Chong GC. Relaxation therapy for tension headache in the elderly: a prospective study. *Psychol Aging* 1988; 3:96–98.

Arena JG, Hannah SL, Bruno GM, Meador KJ. Electromyographic biofeedback training for tension headache in the elderly: a prospective study. *Biofeedback Self Regul* 1991; 16:379–390.

Aronoff GM, Evans WO. The prediction of treatment outcome at a multidisciplinary pain center. *Pain* 1982; 14:67–73.

Bagge E, Bjelle A, Eden S, Svanborg A. A longitudinal study of the occurrence of joint complaints in elderly people. *Age Ageing* 1992; 21:160–167.

Bassols A, Bosch F, Campillo M, Canellas M, Banos JE. An epidemiological comparison of pain complaints in the general population of Catalonia (Spain). *Pain* 1999; 83:9–16.

Benbow SJ, Cossins L, Bowsher D. A comparison of young and elderly patients attending a regional pain centre. *Pain Clinic* 1995; 8:323–332.

Benbow S, Cossins L, Wiles JR. A comparative study of disability, depression and pain severity in young and elderly chronic pain patients. *Abstracts: 8th World Congress on Pain*. Seattle: IASP Press, 1996, pp 289.

Benedetti F, Vighetti S, Ricco C, et al. Pain threshold and tolerance in Alzheimer's disease. *Pain* 1999; 80:377–382.

Benesch LS, Szigeti E, Ferraro FR. Tools for assessing chronic pain in rural elderly women. *Home Health Care Nurse* 1997; 15:207–212.

Blyth FM, March LM, Brnabic AJ, et al. Chronic pain in Australia: a prevalence study. *Pain* 2001; 89:127–134.

Bots ML, Grobbee DE, Hofman A. High blood pressure in the elderly. *Epidemiol Rev* 1991; 13:294–314.

Bradbeer M, Helme RD, Yong HH, Kendig HL, Gibson SJ. Widowhood and other demographic associations of pain in independent older people. *Clin J Pain* 2003;19(4):247–254.

Brattberg G, Thorslund M, Wikman A. The prevalence of pain in a general population: the results of a postal survey in a county of Sweden. *Pain* 1989; 37:215–222.

Brattberg G, Parker MG, Thorslund M. A longitudinal study of pain: reported pain from middle age to old age. *Clin J Pain* 1997; 13:144–149.

Carman WJ, Sowers M, Hawthorne VM, Weissfeld LA. Obesity as a risk factor for osteoarthritis of the hand and wrist: a prospective study. *Am J Epidemiol* 1994; 139:119–129.

Casten RJ, Parmelee PA, Kleban MH, Lawton MP, Katz IR. The relationships among anxiety, depression, and pain in a geriatric institutionalized sample. *Pain* 1995; 61:271–276.

Christensen H, Jorm AF, Mackinnon AJ, et al. Age differences in depression and anxiety symptoms: a structural equation modelling analysis of data from a general population sample. *Psychol Med* 1999; 29:325–339.

Coghill RC, Sang CN, Maisog JM, Iadarola MJ. Pain intensity processing within the human brain: a bilateral, distributed mechanism. *J Neurophysiol* 1999; 82:1934–1943.

Cohen-Mansfield J, Lipson S. Pain in cognitively impaired nursing home residents: how well are physicians diagnosing it? *J Am Geriatr Soc* 2002; 50:1039–1044.

Collins LG, Stone LA. Pain sensitivity, age and activity level in chronic schizophrenics and in normals. *Br J Psychiatry* 1966; 112:33–35.

Comstock GW, Helsing KJ. Symptoms of depression in two communities. *Psychol Med* 1976; 6:551–563.

Cook AJ. Cognitive-behavioral pain management for elderly nursing home residents. *J Gerontol B Psychol Sci Soc Sci* 1998; 53:51–59.

Cook AJ, Chastain DC. The classification of patients with chronic pain: age and sex differences. *Pain Res Manage* 2001; 6:142–151.

Cook AJ, DeGood DE, Chastain DC. Age differences in pain beliefs. *Abstracts: 9th World Congress on Pain.* Seattle: IASP Press, 1999, pp 557–558.

Corran TM, Helme RD, Gibson SJ. An assessment of psychometric instruments used in a geriatric outpatient clinic. *Aust Psychol* 1991; 26:128–131.

Corran TM, Gibson SJ, Farrell MJ, Helme RD. Comparison of chronic pain experience between young and elderly patients. In: Gebhart GF, Hammond DL, Jensen TS (Eds). *Proceedings of the 7th World Congress on Pain,* Progress in Pain Research and Management, Vol. 2. Seattle: IASP Press, 1994, pp 895–906.

Corran TM, Farrell, MJ, Helme RD, Gibson SJ. The classification of patients with chronic pain: age as a contributing factor. *Clin J Pain* 1997; 13:207–214.

Cossins L, Benbow S, Wiles JR. A comparison of outcome in young and elderly patients attending a pain clinic. *Abstracts: 9th World Congress on Pain.* Seattle: IASP Press, 1999, p 90.

Craig KD, Prkachin KM, Grunau RVE. The facial expression of pain. In: Turk D, Melzack R (Eds). *Handbook of Pain Assessment.* New York: Guilford Press, 2001, pp 153–169.

Crook J, Rideout E, Browne G. The prevalence of pain complaints in a general population. *Pain* 1984; 18:299–314.

Cutler RB, Fishbain DA, Rosomoff RS, Rosomoff HL. Outcomes in treatment of pain in geriatric and younger age groups. *Arch Phys Med Rehabil* 1994; 75:457–464.

D'Alessandro R, Benassi G, Lenzi PL, et al. Epidemiology of headache in the Republic of San Marino. *J Neurol Neurosurg Psychiatry* 1988; 51:21–27.

Davis MA, Ettinger WH, Neuhaus JM, Barclay JD, Segal MR. Correlates of knee pain among US adults with and without radiographic knee osteoarthritis. *J Rheumatol* 1992; 19:1943–1949.

Eaton WW, Kessler LG. Rates of symptoms of depression in a national sample. *Am J Epidemiol* 1981; 114:528–538.

Ebrahim S, Brittis S, Wu A. The valuation of states of ill-health: the impact of age and disability. *Age Ageing* 1991; 20:37–40.

Edwards RR, Doleys DM, Fillingim RB, Lowery D. Ethnic differences in pain tolerance: clinical implications in a chronic pain population. *Psychosom Med* 2001; 63:316–323.

Farrell MJ, Gibson SJ. Outcomes for geriatric pain clinic patients. *Proceedings of the 14th Scientific Meeting of the Australian Pain Society.* Sydney: APS Press, 1993, pp 48.

Farrell MJ, Katz B, Helme RD. The impact of dementia on the pain experience. *Pain* 1996; 67:7–15.

Felson DT, Naimark A, Anderson J, et al. The prevalence of knee osteoarthritis in the elderly: the Framingham Osteoarthritis Study. *Arthritis Rheum* 1987; 30:914–918.

Felson DT, Zhang Y, Hannan MT, et al. The incidence and natural history of knee osteoarthritis in the elderly: the Framingham Osteoarthritis Study. *Arthritis Rheum* 1995; 38:1500–1505.

Ferrell BA. Pain evaluation and management in the nursing home. *Ann Intern Med* 1995; 123:681–687.

Ferrell BA, Ferrell BR, Rivera L. Pain in cognitively impaired nursing home patients. *J Pain Symptom Manage* 1995; 10:591–598.

Flint AJ. Epidemiology and comorbidity of anxiety disorders in the elderly. *Am J Psychiatry* 1994; 151:640–649.

Flor H, Fydrich T, Turk DC. Efficacy of multidisciplinary pain treatment centers: a meta-analytic review. *Pain* 1992; 49:221–230.

Fordyce WE. Evaluating and managing chronic pain. *Geriatrics* 1978; 33:59–62.

France CR. Decreased pain perception and risk for hypertension: considering a common physiological mechanism. *Psychophysiology* 1999; 36:683–692.

Frerichs RR, Aneshensel CS, Clark VA. Prevalence of depression in Los Angeles County. *Am J Epidemiol* 1981; 113:691–619.

Gagliese L, Melzack R. Age differences in the quality of chronic pain: a preliminary study. *Pain Res Manage* 1997a; 2:157–162.

Gagliese L, Melzack R. Lack of evidence for age differences in pain beliefs. *Pain Res Manage* 1997b; 2:19–28.

Gagliese L, Jackson M, Ritvo P, Wowk A, Katz J. Age is not an impediment to effective use of patient-controlled analgesia by surgical patients. *Anesthesiology* 2000; 93:601–610.

Gallo JJ, Anthony JC, Muthen BO. Age differences in the symptoms of depression: a latent trait analysis. *J Gerontol* 1994; 49:251–264.

Gatchel RJ, Turk DC. *Psychosocial Factors in Pain: Critical Perspectives*. New York: Guilford Press, 1999.

Gibson SJ. The measurement of mood states in older adults. *J Gerontol B Psychol Sci Soc Sci* 1997; 52:19–28.

Gibson SJ, Farrell MJ. A review of age differences in the neurophysiology of nociception and the perceptual experience of pain. *Clin J Pain;* in press.

Gibson SJ, Helme RD. Cognitive factors and the experience of pain and suffering in older persons. *Pain* 2000; 85:375–383.

Gibson SJ, Farrell MJ, Katz B, Helme RD. Multidisciplinary management of chronic non-malignant pain. In: Ferrell BR, Ferrell BA (Eds). *Pain in the Elderly*. Seattle: IASP Press, 1996, pp 91–99.

Gibson SJ, Voukelatos X, Ames D, Flicker L, Helme RD. An examination of pain perception and cerebral event-related potentials following carbon dioxide laser stimulation in patients with Alzheimer's disease and age-matched control volunteers. *Pain Res Manage* 2001; 6:126–132.

Groves F, Garland K, Mendelson G, Gibson SJ. Multidisciplinary pain treatment outcome differs as a function of age. *Abstracts: 10th World Congress on Pain*. Seattle: IASP Press, 2002, p 70.

Guck TP, Meilman PW, Skultety FM, Dowd ET. Prediction of long-term outcome of multidisciplinary pain treatment. *Arch Phys Med Rehabil* 1986; 67:293–296.

Gurland BJ, Wilder DE, Berkman C. Depression and disability in the elderly: reciprocal relations and changes with age. *Int J Geriatr Psychiatry* 1988; 3:163–179.

Guzman J, Esmail R, Karjalainen K. et al. Multidisciplinary bio-psycho-social rehabilitation for chronic low back pain. *Cochrane Database Syst Rev* 2002; 1:CD000963.

Hadjistavropoulos T, Craig KD, Martin N, Hadjistavropoulos H, McMurtry B. Toward a research outcome measure of pain in frail elderly in chronic care. *Pain Clinic* 1997; 10:71–79.

Hadjistavropoulos T, La Chapele D, MacLeod F, et al. Cognitive functioning and pain reactions in hospitalized elders. *Pain Res Manage* 1998; 3:145–151.

Hadjistavropoulos T, LaChapelle DL, MacLeod FK, Snider B, Craig KD. Measuring movement-exacerbated pain in cognitively impaired frail elders. *Clin J Pain* 2000; 16:54–63.

Hadjistavropoulos T, LaChapelle DL, Hadjistavropoulos HD, Green S, Asmundson GJ. Using facial expressions to assess musculoskeletal pain in older persons. *Eur J Pain* 2002; 6:179–187.

Hallett EC, Pilowsky I. The response to treatment in a multidisciplinary pain clinic. *Pain* 1982; 12:365–374.

Harkins SW. Pain in the elderly. In: Dubner R, Gebhart GF, Bond MR (Eds). *Proceedings of the Vth World Congress on Pain.* Amsterdam: Elsevier Science, 1988, pp 355–367.

Hayflick L. The future of ageing. *Nature* 2000; 408:267–269.

Heithoff K. Does the ECA underestimate the prevalence of late-life depression? *J Am Geriatr Soc* 1995; 43:2–6.

Helme RD, Gibson SJ. Measurement and management of pain in older people. *Aust J Ageing* 1998; 17:5–9.

Helme RD, Gibson SJ. Pain in older people. In: Crombie IK, Croft PR, Linton SJ, LeResche L, Von Korff M (Eds). *Epidemiology of Pain.* Seattle: IASP Press, 1999, pp 103–112.

Helme RD, Gibson SJ. The epidemiology of pain in elderly people. *Clin Geriatr Med* 2001; 17:417–431.

Helme RD, Katz B, Neufeld M, et al. The establishment of a geriatric pain clinic for older people. *Aust J Ageing* 1989; 8:27–30.

Helme RD, Gibson SJ, Farrell MJ. The influence of social factors on the chronic pain experience in older people. *Abstracts: 8th World Congress on Pain.* Seattle: IASP Press, 1996a, p 519.

Helme RD, Katz B, Gibson SJ, et al. Multidisciplinary pain clinics for older people: do they have a role? *Clin Geriatr Med* 1996b; 12:563–582.

Henderson AS, Jorm AF, Korten AE, et al. Symptoms of depression and anxiety during adult life: evidence for a decline in prevalence with age. *Psychol Med* 1998; 28:1321–1328.

Herr KA, Garand L. Assessment and measurement of pain in older adults. *Clin Geriatr Med* 2001; 17:457–478.

Herr KA, Mobily PR. Pain assessment in the elderly: clinical considerations. *J Gerontol Nurs* 1991; 17:12–19.

Herr KA, Mobily PR. Comparison of selected pain assessment tools for use with the elderly. *Appl Nurs Res* 1993; 6:39–46.

Hochberg MC, Lawrence RC, Everett DF, Cornoni-Huntley J. Epidemiologic associations of pain in osteoarthritis of the knee: data from the National Health and Nutrition Examination Survey and the National Health and Nutrition Examination-I Epidemiologic Follow-up Survey. *Semin Arthritis Rheum* 1989; 18:4–9.

Hochberg MC, Lethbridge-Cejku M, Plato CC, Wigley FM, Tobin JD. Factors associated with osteoarthritis of the hand in males: data from the Baltimore Longitudinal Study of Aging. *Am J Epidemiol* 1991; 134:1121–1127.

Hodgson JE, Suda KT, Bruce BK, Rome JD. Depression in the elderly chronic pain patient. *Abstracts: 7th World Congress on Pain.* Seattle: IASP Press, 1993, p 582.

Hof PR. Morphology and neurochemical characteristics of the vulnerable neurons in brain aging and Alzheimer's disease. *Eur Neurol* 1997; 37:71–81.

Hofland SL. Elder beliefs: blocks to pain management. *J Gerontol Nurs* 1992; 18:19–23.

in 't Veld BA, Ruitenberg A, Hofman A, et al. Nonsteroidal antiinflammatory drugs and the risk of Alzheimer's disease. *N Engl J Med* 2001; 345:1515–1521.

Jorm AF. Does old age reduce the risk of anxiety and depression? A review of epidemiological studies across the adult life span. *Psychol Med* 2000; 30:11–22.

Katz IR, Parmalee PA, Streim J. Depression in older patients in residential care: significance of dysphoria. *Am J Geriatr Psychiatry* 1995; 3:161–169.

Kay L, Jorgensen T, Schultz-Larsen K. Abdominal pain in a 70-year-old Danish population: an epidemiological study of the prevalence and importance of abdominal pain. *J Clin Epidemiol* 1992; 45:1377–1382.

Kee WG, Middaugh SJ, Pawlick KL. Persistent pain in older people: evaluation and treatment. In: Gatchel RJ, Turk DC (Eds). *Psychosocial Factors in Pain: Critical Perspectives.* New York: Guilford Press, 1996, pp 371–402.

Kee WG, Middaugh SJ, Redpath S, Hargadon R. Age as a factor in admission to chronic pain rehabilitation. *Clin J Pain* 1998; 14:121–128.

Keefe FJ, Block AR. Development of an observational method for assessing pain behavior in chronic low back pain patients. *Behav Ther* 1982; 13:363–375.

Keefe FJ, Williams DA. A comparison of coping strategies in chronic pain patients in different age groups. *J Gerontol* 1990; 45:161–165.

Keefe FJ, Caldwell DS, Martinez S, et al. Analyzing pain in rheumatoid arthritis patients: pain coping strategies in patients who have had knee replacement surgery. *Pain* 1991; 46:153–160.

Kendig H, Helme RD, Teshuva K. *Health Status of Older People Project: Data from a Survey of the Health and Lifestyles of Older Australians.* Report to the Victorian Health Promotion Foundation, 1996.

Kind P, Dolan P, Gudex C, Williams A. Variations in population health status: results from a United Kingdom national questionnaire survey. *BMJ* 1998; 316:736–741.

Knauper B, Wittchen HU. Diagnosing major depression in the elderly: evidence for response bias in standardized diagnostic interviews? *J Psychiatr Res* 1994; 28:147–164.

Kolter-Cope S, Gerber KE. Is age related to response to treatment for chronic pain. *Abstracts: 7th World Congress on Pain.* Seattle: IASP Press, 1993, p 582.

Konu V. Myocardial infarction in the elderly: a clinical and epidemiological study with a one-year follow-up. *Acta Med Scand Suppl* 1977; 604:3–68.

Kovach CR, Weissman DE, Griffie J, Matson S, Muchka S. Assessment and treatment of discomfort for people with late-stage dementia. *J Pain Symptom Manage* 1999; 18:412–419.

Kremer E, Atkinson JH, Ignelzi RJ. Measurement of pain: patient preference does not confound pain measurement. *Pain* 1981; 10:241–248.

Krulewitch H, London MR, Skakel VJ, et al. Assessment of pain in cognitively impaired older adults: a comparison of pain assessment tools and their use by nonprofessional caregivers. *J Am Geriatr Soc* 2000; 48:1607–1611.

Lavsky-Shulan M, Wallace RB, Kohout FJ. et al. Prevalence and functional correlates of low back pain in the elderly: the Iowa 65+ Rural Health Study. *J Am Geriatr Soc* 1985; 33:23–28.

Lenze EJ, Mulsant BH, Shear MK, et al. Comorbidity of depression and anxiety disorders in later life. *Depress Anxiety* 2001; 14:86–93.

Leventhal EA, Leventhal H, Schaefer P, Easterling D. Conservation of energy, uncertainty reduction, and swift utilization of medical care among the elderly. *J Gerontol* 1993; 48:78–86.

Liddell A, Locker D. Gender and age differences in attitudes to dental pain and dental control. *Community Dent Oral Epidemiol* 1997; 25:314–318.

Lyness JM, Cox C, Curry J, et al. Older age and the underreporting of depressive symptoms. *J Am Geriatr Soc* 1995; 43:216–221.

Lyness JM, Caine ED, King DA, et al. Psychiatric disorders in older primary care patients. *J Gen Intern Med* 1999; 14:249–254.

MacDonald JB, Baillie J, Williams BO, Ballantyne D. Coronary care in the elderly. *Age Ageing* 1983; 12:17–20.

Magni G, Marchetti M, Moreschi C, Merskey H, Luchini SR. Chronic musculoskeletal pain and depressive symptoms in the National Health and Nutrition Examination. I. Epidemiologic Follow-up Study. *Pain* 1993; 53:163–168.

Mangione CM, Marcantonio ER, Goldman L, et al. Influence of age on measurement of health status in patients undergoing elective surgery. *J Am Geriatr Soc* 1993; 41:377–383.

Matheson DH. The painful truth: interpretation of facial expression of pain in older adults. *J Nonverbal Behav* 1997; 21:223–238.

McCracken LM. Age, pain and impairment: results from two clinical samples. *Abstracts: 7th World Congress on Pain.* Seattle: IASP Press, 1993, p 99.

Middaugh SJ, Levin RB, Kee WG, Barchiesi FD, Roberts JM. Chronic pain: its treatment in geriatric and younger patients. *Arch Phys Med Rehabil* 1988; 69:1021–1026.

Miller C, LeLieuvre RB. A method to reduce chronic pain in elderly nursing home residents. *Gerontologist* 1982; 22:314–317.

Mirowsky J, Ross CE. Age and depression. *J Health Soc Behav* 1992; 33:187–205; 206–212.

Mobily PA, Herr KA, Clark MK, Wallace RB. An epidemiologic analysis of pain in the elderly: the Iowa 65+ Rural Health Study. *J Aging Health* 1994; 6:139–154.

Morrison RS, Siu AL. A comparison of pain and its treatment in advanced dementia and cognitively intact patients with hip fracture. *J Pain Symptom Manage* 2000; 19:240–248.

Neufeld M, Katz B, Farrell MJ, Gibson SJ. The influence of comorbid disease on clinical presentation of older chronic pain patients. *Abstracts: 10th World Congress on Pain*. Seattle: IASP Press, 2002, p 303.

Newmann JP, Klein MH, Jensen JE, Essex MJ. Depressive symptom experiences among older women: a comparison of alternative measurement approaches. *Psychol Aging* 1996; 11:112–126.

Nicholson NL, Blanchard EB. A controlled evaluation of behavioral treatment of chronic headache in older people. *Behav Ther* 1993; 24:395–408.

Ouslander JG. Physical illness and depression in the elderly. *J Am Geriatr Soc* 1982; 30:593–599.

Painter JR, Seres JL, Newman RI. Assessing benefits of the pain center: why some patients regress. *Pain* 1980; 8:101–113.

Parmelee PA. Assessment of pain in the elderly. In: Lawton MP, Tevesi JA (Eds). *Annual Review of Gerontology and Geriatrics,* Vol. 14. New York: Springer, 1994, pp 281–301.

Parmelee PA. Pain in cognitively impaired older persons. *Clin Geriatr Med* 1996; 12:473–487.

Parmelee PA, Smith B, Katz IR. Pain complaints and cognitive status among elderly institution residents. *J Am Geriatr Soc* 1993; 41:517–522.

Portenoy RK, Farkash A. Practical management of non-malignant pain in the elderly. *Geriatrics* 1988; 43:29–40, 44–47.

Price DD. Psychological and neural mechanisms of the affective dimension of pain. *Science* 2000; 288:1769–1772.

Puder RS. Age analysis of cognitive-behavioral group therapy for chronic pain outpatients. *Psychol Aging* 1988; 3:204–207.

Rapp SR, Parisi SA, Wallace CE. Comorbid psychiatric disorders in elderly medical patients: a 1-year prospective study. *J Am Geriatr Soc* 1991; 39:124–131.

Regier DA, Farmer ME, Rae DS, et al. One-month prevalence of mental disorders in the United States and sociodemographic characteristics: the Epidemiologic Catchment Area study. *Acta Psychiatr Scand* 1993; 88:35–47.

Riley JL III, Wade JB, Robinson ME, Price DD. The stages of pain processing across the lifespan. *J Pain* 2000; 1:162–170.

Ritchie K, Kildea D. Is senile dementia "age-related" or "ageing-related"? Evidence from meta-analysis of dementia prevalence in the oldest old. *Lancet* 1995; 346:931–934.

Roy R, Thomas M. Elderly persons with and without pain: a comparative study. *Clin J Pain* 1987; 3:102–106.

Ruzicka SA. Pain beliefs: what do elders believe? *J Holist Nurs* 1998; 16:369–382.

Scherder EJ, Bouma A. Visual analogue scales for pain assessment in Alzheimer's disease. *Gerontology* 2000; 46:47–53.

Scherder E, Bouma A, Borkent M, Rahman O. Alzheimer patients report less pain intensity and pain affect than non-demented elderly. *Psychiatry* 1999; 62:265–272.

Simons W, Malabar R. Assessing pain in elderly patients who cannot respond verbally. *J Adv Nurs* 1995; 22:663–669.

Sorkin BA, Rudy TE, Hanlon RB, Turk DC, Stieg RL. Chronic pain in old and young patients: differences appear less important than similarities. *J Gerontol* 1990; 45:64–68.

Sternbach RA. Survey of pain in the United States: the Nuprin Pain Report. *Clin J Pain* 1986; 2:49–53.

Stoller EP. Interpretations of symptoms by older people. *J Aging Health* 1993; 5:58–81.

Tibblin G, Bengtsson C, Furness B, Lapidus L. Symptoms by age and sex. *Scand J Prim Health Care* 1990; 8:9–17.

Tiplady B, Jackson SH, Maskrey VM, Swift CG. Validity and sensitivity of visual analogue scales in young and older healthy subjects. *Age Ageing* 1998; 27:63–66.

Turk DC, Okifuji A, Scharff L. Chronic pain and depression: role of perceived impact and perceived control in different age cohorts. *Pain* 1995; 61:93–101.

United Nations. *World Population Prospects.* New York: United Nations, 1995.

Von Korff M, Dworkin SF, Le Resche L, Kruger A. An epidemiologic comparison of pain complaints. *Pain* 1988; 32:173–183.

Wagstaff GF, Rowledge AM. Stoicism: its relation to gender, attitudes toward poverty, and reactions to emotive material. *J Soc Psychol* 1995; 135:181–184.

Walsh NE, Schoenfeld L, Ramamurthy S, Hoffman J. Normative model for cold pressor test. *Am J Phys Med Rehabil* 1989; 68:6–11.

Washington LL, Gibson SJ, Helme RD. Age-related differences in the endogenous analgesic response to repeated cold water immersion in human volunteers. *Pain* 2000; 89:89–96.

Watkins KW, Shifren K, Park DC, Morrell RW. Age, pain, and coping with rheumatoid arthritis. *Pain* 1999; 82:217–228.

Weiner DK, Rudy TE. Attitudinal barriers to effective pain management in the nursing home. In: Devor M, Rowbotham MC, Wiesenfeld-Hallin Z (Eds). *Proceedings of the 9th World Congress on Pain,* Progress in Pain Research and Management, Vol. 16. Seattle: IASP Press, 2000, pp 1097–2003.

Weiner D, Pieper C, McConnell E, Martinez S, Keefe F. Pain measurement in elders with chronic low back pain: traditional and alternative approaches. *Pain* 1996; 67:461–467.

Weiner D, Peterson B, Keefe F. Evaluating persistent pain in long term care residents: what role for pain maps? *Pain* 1998; 76:249–257.

Weiner D, Peterson B, Keefe F. Chronic pain-associated behaviors in the nursing home: resident versus caregiver perceptions. *Pain* 1999; 80:577–588.

Werner P, Cohen-Mansfield J, Watson V, Pasis S. Pain in participants of adult day care centers: assessment by different raters. *J Pain Symptom Manage* 1998; 15:8–17.

Wijeratne C, Hickie I. Somatic distress syndromes in later life: the need for paradigm change. *Psychol Med* 2001; 31:571–576.

Wijeratne C, Shome S, Hickie I, Koschera A. An age-based comparison of chronic pain clinic patients. *Int J Geriatr Psychiatry* 2001; 16:477–483.

Woodrow KM, Friedman GD, Siegelaub AB, Collen MF. Pain tolerance: differences according to age, sex and race. *Psychosom Med* 1972; 34:548–556.

Wroblewski M, Mikulowski P. Peritonitis in geriatric inpatients. *Age Ageing* 1991; 20:90–94.

Wulsin LR, Vaillant GE, Wells VE. A systematic review of the mortality of depression. *Psychosom Med* 1999; 61:6–17.

Yong HH, Gibson SJ, Horne DJ, Helme RD. Development of a pain attitudes questionnaire to assess stoicism and cautiousness for possible age differences. *J Gerontol B Psychol Sci Soc Sci* 2001; 56:279–284.

Ysla R, Rosomoff RS, Rosomoff HL. Functional improvement in geriatric pain patients. *Arch Phys Med Rehabil* 1986; 67:685.

Zekry D, Hauw JJ, Gold G. Mixed dementia: epidemiology, diagnosis, and treatment. *J Am Geriatr Soc* 2002; 50:1431–1438.

Correspondence to: Michael J. Farrell, PhD, Howard Florey Institute, National Neuroscience Facility, University of Melbourne, Level 2, 161 Barry Street, Parkville, Victoria 3010, Australia. Email: m.farrell@pcomm.hfi.unimelb.edu.au.

Part VI

Special Issues

Psychosocial Aspects of Pain: A Handbook for Health Care Providers, Progress in Pain Research and Management, Vol. 27, edited by Robert H. Dworkin and William S. Breitbart, IASP Press, Seattle, © 2004.

23

The Influence of Coping Styles and Personality Traits on Pain

Michael E. Geisser

The Spine Program, Department of Physical Medicine and Rehabilitation, University of Michigan Medical Center, Ann Arbor, Michigan, USA

Individual responses to pain are recognized as important determinants of the pain experience. First, cognitive and emotional factors are believed to directly influence the sensory transmission of pain, through cortical influences on "pain gates" that modulate afferent pain transmission (Melzack and Wall 1965). Second, persons with pain (particularly chronic pain) demonstrate widely different emotional and behavioral responses to similar levels of pain intensity and physical impairment, and research has consistently demonstrated that clinical pain intensity has little or no relation to functional impairment (Flor and Turk 1988; Millard et al. 1991; Vlaeyen et al. 1995; Geisser and Roth 1998; Geisser et al. 2000). Third, there is little relationship in some chronic pain patients between physical pathology and pain, leading researchers to suggest that certain types of chronic pain are primarily psychological in nature (Fordyce 1979; White and Gordon 1982; Sanders 1985; Weintraub 1988; Owen-Salters et al. 1996). While this proposal may be attributable in part to lack of knowledge regarding the pathophysiology of certain pain condtions, the above findings highlight the importance of psychosocial factors in the experience of pain, particularly chronic pain. Even prospectively, psychosocial factors have been found to be significant predictors of chronicity. For example, in a study of factory workers, Bigos and colleagues (1992) found that work satisfaction and personality factors were significantly related to the later development of a chronic pain problem, while physical findings were not. Such investigations have expanded our knowledge of the factors that contribute to the onset and maintenance of pain, and may lead to interventions designed to reduce the likelihood of developing a chronic pain condition.

This chapter will focus on personality and coping in relation to the experience of pain. Various attitudes and beliefs about pain will also be discussed, as these factors are believed to directly influence the experience of pain, as well as attempts to cope with it. The reader should be advised that some divergent findings appear in relation to studies of acute and chronic pain. These differences will highlighted.

MODELS OF COPING

Personality traits are characterized as "patterns of perceiving, relating to, and thinking about the environment and oneself that are exhibited in a wide range of social and personal contexts" (American Psychiatric Association 1994). *Beliefs* are defined as the cognitions (beliefs, appraisals, or expectancies) that one has about one's pain (Jensen et al. 1991). Finally, *coping* is defined as purposeful efforts to manage or modify the negative impact of stress (Lazarus and Folkman 1984).

Coping responses are often categorized in different ways. Although the best method of categorization is debatable, coping strategies are typically divided into one of two categories: active or problem-focused strategies, which are directed at solving or relieving the source of stress; and passive or emotion-focused strategies, which are efforts designed to manage the emotional impact of stress. More recently, Jensen and colleagues (1995) proposed the dimensions of illness-focused versus wellness-focused coping behaviors, whereby the former strategies concentrate on avoiding pain and illness, while the latter behaviors are aimed at promoting health. Examples of the former include medication taking and guarding, while the latter include strategies such as exercise, relaxation, and the use of coping self-statements.

The most popular model of coping with illness, including pain, has been proposed by Lazarus and Folkman (1984). These authors characterize coping as a dynamic process that is influenced by the person as well as the environment, and is constantly changing. The authors propose that coping is influenced by dispositions, which they indicate are stable biological, personality, and social role characteristics that influence how a person responds to stress. Coping is also influenced by appraisals or beliefs, because perceptions regarding the threat value of a particular event are hypothesized to affect emotional responses and coping. Finally, coping responses are viewed as the cognitive and behavioral efforts to manage specific external and internal demands that are appraised as taxing or exceeding an individual's resources. The authors propose that coping must be examined over time within the context of a specific stressor so that change can be observed in thoughts, feelings, and behavior as the requirements of the situation change.

As outlined in this model, personality, pain beliefs, and coping attempts are all relevant to the process of coping with pain.

PERSONALITY

NORMAL CONSTRUCTS

Research on pain and personality has focused on variables representing "normal" personality dimensions, as well as dimensions of personality that are viewed as being reflective of psychopathology or a personality disorder as defined by the American Psychiatric Association (1994) in the *Diagnostic and Statistical Manual of Mental Disorders,* 4th edition (DSM-IV). Studies examining normal personality traits will be presented first.

One construct that has been studied extensively in relation to pain is the

roversion. Based predominantly on), it is hypothesized that introverts are l stimulation because persons high in of cortical arousal, making them more pain. Several studies utilizing various and different pain-induction techniques nd to report lower pain thresholds and of equal intensity as being more pain- nd Gatchel 2000). Introverts also tend painful procedures, and require greater nic pain, Phillips and Gatchel (2000) plain less about pain and have higher to introverts. However, these authors ng studies examining relationships be- experience of pain in clinical popula-

he influence of social desirability on ttings, this personality dimension may of appearing to be "a good patient or more pain tolerant. Kohn et al. (1989) ial desirability and introversion-extro- task. The authors hypothesized that influence of introversion-extroversion e the influence of arousal on pain by decreasing the desire to stop enduring pain. They determined that social desirability had no influence on pressure pain ratings or tolerance, while greater psychological arousal was associated with decreased pain tolerance and higher pain ratings. Geisser et al. (1992) also reported no relationship between social desirability and cold-pressor pain threshold and tolerance.

Internal locus of control, or the belief that one has personal control over an event, has been proposed to influence pain through increasing the likelihood that one will employ active attempts to cope with one's pain problem, leading to better adjustment. Studies examining the relationship between locus of control and chronic pain have found that persons with high internal locus of control report lower levels of disability (Spinhoven et al. 1989), less pain (Toomey et al. 1991), and lower levels of affective distress (Rudy et al. 1988). In addition, high internal locus of control is associated with improved immediate and long-term treatment outcomes (Harkapaa et al. 1991, 1996). Change from external to higher internal locus of control is also associated with greater reductions in pain following treatment (Lipchik et al. 1993).

Neuroticism is a personality trait that consists of a constant preoccupation with things that might go wrong, and a strong emotional reaction of anxiety to these thoughts (Eysenck 1960). Neuroticism is believed to influence illness and adjustment by leaving an individual prone to the effects of stress, and persons high in this trait may cope poorly with medical problems because they tend to experience chronic negative emotions that lead to fearfulness, low self-esteem, and distress (Wade and Price 2000). In addition, these persons typically display a cognitive style that leaves them prone to thinking about events in a catastrophic fashion, magnifying the negative aspects of a situation.

Neuroticism was found to be associated with greater psychological distress among persons with rheumatoid arthritis independent of pain intensity and degree of depressive symptoms (Affleck et al. 1992). Neuroticism is also associated with pain behavior among older persons (Lauver and Johnson 1997), and is predictive of psychological distress among persons with chronic low back pain (BenDebba et al. 1997). In prospective studies, Breslau et al. (1996) have found neuroticism to be predictive of migraine headache, and Pietri-Taleb et al. (1994) found it to predictive of later development of neck pain among machine operators.

Anxiety sensitivity is a relatively new construct in the pain literature. It is defined as the fear of anxiety-related bodily sensations that stems from the belief that these sensations are a signal of harm or damage to the body. Anxiety sensitivity is thought to be related to a trait predisposition to fear pain, and is significantly associated with avoidance of potentially painful activity (Asmundson and Norton 1995). Plehn et al. (1998) found that anxiety sensitivity was significantly associated with poorer social functioning, vitality, and psychological functioning among a heterogeneous sample of persons with chronic pain. Among normal, healthy persons undergoing an experimental pain task, Keogh and Cochrane (2002) found that those who were high in anxiety sensitivity demonstrated a greater interpretive bias and reported more negative pain experiences. In addition, the authors indicated that greater affective pain experience was associated with a tendency to misinterpret innocuous bodily sensations among persons high in anxiety sensitivity.

Few studies have examined the impact of more adaptive personality traits on pain. One such trait that has received attention in the general medical literature is optimism, defined as a tendency to hold positive expectations regarding the future (Garafolo 2000). Unfortunately, little research has examined the relationship between optimism and pain (Garafolo 2000).

ABNORMAL CONSTRUCTS

Some models of chronic pain suggest that personality traits play a significant role in the development and maintenance of the disorder. For example, Engel (1959) proposed that chronic pain arises from developmental experiences that enhance the prominence of pain in childhood, which in turn gives rise to the use of pain as a defense mechanism in adulthood. Studies attempting to examine and empirically validate the model (Turk and Flor 1984; Roy 1985; Gamsa 1994) have all concluded that there is no consistent empirical evidence to support the model's applicability for the majority of chronic pain patients.

Most recent studies have failed to find a relationship between specific personality traits or disorders and chronic pain (Weisberg 2000). Rather, most studies find high rates of all DSM-IV Axis II (personality) disorders in chronic pain populations (Gatchel et al. 1996; Monti et al. 1998).

A more contemporary model of the relationship between abnormal personality and pain is based on stress-diathesis principles (Weisberg and Keefe 1997). It has been proposed that pain serves as a stressor that exacerbates the severity of preexisting pathological personality traits. This exacerbation in pathological traits leads to a higher prevalence of personality disorders, which inhibit the ability to effectively cope with pain and contribute to the maintenance of both pain and psychopathology.

DIRECTIONS FOR RESEARCH

Personality traits, as reviewed above, have been found to be significantly related to pain and adjustment, as well as treatment outcome. Among "normal" personality traits, Wade and Price (2000) indicate that neuroticism has demonstrated consistent and significant relationships to the experience of pain. Few studies have examined the impact of positive personality dimensions on pain, such as optimism, and these types of personality dimensions may warrant study in the future. Research examining the influence of pathological personality characteristics on pain has been unsuccessful in identifying particular personality dimensions that are specific to pain. A stress-diathesis model of personality and pain therefore appears consistent with existing data.

Few systematic studies have been conducted to examine the impact of various interventions on personality disorders. Data on potential interventions for "normal" personality dimensions are even more scant. In general, most personality disorders are viewed to be relatively refractory to treatment. Thus, we lack data that may be applicable to modify personality in relation to pain. In addition, while some persons have personality dimensions such as neuroticism that may increase the likelihood of seeking psychological treatment, persons with other personality traits may not be easy to engage in therapy.

Alternatively, it may be beneficial to attempt to tailor interventions to improve pain coping based on the personality style of the individual. Some studies suggest that the effectiveness of specific coping styles varies depending on the personality characteristics of the individual. This issue will be discussed further in the summary at the end of this chapter.

PAIN BELIEFS

Beliefs about pain have important influences on behavioral and emotional responses to pain. Several pain belief measures have been validated in pain populations, including the Survey of Pain Attitudes (SOPA; Jensen et al. 1994b) and the Pain Beliefs and Perceptions Inventory (Williams et al. 1994). Beliefs assessed by the SOPA include: (1) perceived control over one's pain (control); (2) the belief that one is unable to function because of pain (disability); (3) the belief that pain is a signal of damage and that exercise and activity therefore should be limited (harm); (4) the belief that pain is influenced by one's emotional state (emotions); (5) the belief that taking medications is appropriate for treating chronic pain (medication); (6) the belief that aid should be received from family members when one is in pain (solicitude); and (7) the belief that a medical cure exists for one's pain (cure). In a study examining the relationship of the SOPA to measures of pain, disability, health care utilization, and demographics, Jensen et al.

(1994b) found that beliefs that emotions affect pain, that others should be solicitous in response to pain, and that one is disabled by pain were positively associated with psychosocial dysfunction. The harm and disability subscales were associated with greater self-report of physical disability. The only subscale that was significantly associated with health care utilization was the belief that medication is appropriate for treating pain, which was associated with a higher number of emergency room visits.

Williams and colleagues (1994) examined the relationship between four dimensions of beliefs, assessed by the Pain Beliefs and Perceptions Inventory, and various aspects of the pain experience. The authors found that greater endorsement of beliefs that pain is constant were significantly associated with greater pain intensity. They also reported that beliefs that pain is permanent were associated with greater anxiety, that beliefs that pain is mysterious were associated with greater overall psychological distress, and that attitudes associated with blaming oneself for pain were associated with greater self-report of depressive symptoms. For a comprehensive review of these and other measures, please refer to the recent, excellent review by DeGood and Tait (2001).

PAIN-RELATED FEAR

Pain-related fear (the belief that pain is a sign of damage or harm to the body, and that activities that might cause pain should be avoided) is increasingly being recognized as an important contributor to disability and adjustment among persons with chronic pain. Pain-related fear is believed to contribute to pain and disability in several ways. One factor is that persons high in pain-related fear begin to avoid situations they believe may cause pain (Hill et al. 1955; Lethem et al. 1983; Philips 1987; Kori et al. 1990). Research also suggests that these persons tend to overestimate the amount of pain experienced during functional activity (Flor and Turk 1988; McCracken et al. 1993; Crombez et al. 1996), leading to greater activity avoidance. In this fashion, pain-related fear and associated avoidance of activity are believed to contribute to disability independently of pain itself. Pain-related fear and avoidance also lead to greater physical deconditioning, which in turn heightens disability (Crombez et al. 1999). In addition, pain-related fear is related to musculoskeletal abnormalities such as muscle guarding while bending, which in turn may directly contribute to the pain experience (Watson et al. 1997).

Several studies provide strong support to the notion that pain-related fear is significantly related to greater perceived disability, even when controlling for biomedical factors, demographic variables, and self-reported pain

(Waddell et al. 1993; Jensen et al. 1994b; Vlaeyen et al. 1995). Two studies (Asmundson et al. 1997; McCracken et al. 1999) have demonstrated that pain-related fear is associated with a profile of high psychological distress, high interference due to pain, low perceived control over pain, and low activity levels on the Multidimensional Pain Inventory (Kerns et al. 1985). Studies have also reported that decreases in pain-related fear during treatment are associated with improved physical functioning, decreased depression and pain severity, and lower interference due to pain (Jensen et al. 1994a; McCracken and Gross 1998).

These findings extend to the observation of functional activity among persons with chronic back pain. Vlaeyen et al. (1999) determined that pain-related fear was inversely related to the ability to hold a heavy bag until pain or physical discomfort made it impossible to continue. Crombez et al. (1999) reported that higher peak torque on a task of isokinetic trunk extension and flexion was associated with lower pain-related fear. Similar findings were obtained on measures of knee extension and flexion, as well as trunk rotation. Geisser et al. (2000) found that beliefs that activities that cause pain should be avoided were significantly related to poorer performance on a lifting task even when controlling for factors such as clinical pain, physiological and perceived effort, and body mass index.

Interventions to reduce pain-related fear such as exposure to feared activities are potentially powerful interventions for chronic pain. Using a repeated-measures design, Vlaeyen et al. (2002) examined six subjects with chronic low back pain who underwent baseline observation and then received either in vivo exposure to feared light-normal activity followed by exposure to graded activity (exercise), or graded activity followed by in vivo exposure. Examples of light-normal activities utilized include lifting a child, riding a bicycle, mopping the floor, and lifting a crate from the trunk of a car. Among subjects who received in vivo exposure first, significant decreases in fear were observed following this exposure and were maintained over time. Subjects who received graded activity demonstrated declines in fear only when in vivo exposure was introduced. In addition, in vivo exposure also reduced negative thoughts about pain, fear of pain, and self-reported disability. These treatment gains were maintained at a 1-year follow-up. Interestingly, decreases in self-reported pain were also observed, even though pain was not a target of the intervention, and one might expect pain to increase with greater function. The authors proposed that declines in pain-related fear may reduce pain vigilance, resulting in declines in reported pain intensity.

SELF-EFFICACY

Perceived self-efficacy has consistently been shown to be related to both acute and chronic pain, as well as to pain treatment outcome. Self-efficacy is the confidence one has that a particular behavior or other action can be performed and will produce a desired outcome. For example, Litt (1988) found that perceived self-efficacy to manage pain was a significant predictor of pain tolerance during a cold-pressor task, and that changes in self-efficacy predicted changes in cold-pressor performance. Bandura et al. (1987) examined cold-pressor tolerance among normal, healthy subjects who received naloxone or placebo, in addition to various instructional sets to cope with pain. The authors found evidence to support the hypothesis that self-efficacy influences pain through influencing endogenous opioid production and increasing attempts to cope with pain. In a study of patients who had undergone orthopedic surgery, Pellino and Ward (1998) found that perceived control over pain partially mediated the relationship between pain severity and patient satisfaction. The authors found that while individuals who reported severe pain were less satisfied with pain relief compared to persons with less pain, perceived control over pain had the greatest impact on satisfaction with pain relief.

Self-efficacy is highly associated with the experience of pain in chronic pain populations as well. For example, Buckelew (1994) found that self-efficacy for function was significantly related to pain behavior among persons with fibromyalgia, while depression was unrelated. Lackner et al. (1996) reported that functional self-efficacy was significantly related to function among persons with chronic low back pain, independent of expectancies of pain and reinjury. Asghari and Nickolas (2001) found that self-efficacy beliefs for managing pain significantly predicted pain behavior and activity avoidance 9 months later in a heterogeneous sample of persons with chronic pain.

OTHER BELIEFS ABOUT PAIN

The development of feelings of victimization (the belief that one is wrongfully suffering because of someone else's mistake or carelessness) and entitlement (the belief that one is "owed" or should be compensated) may be important factors in the experience of chronic pain, particularly among persons with accident-related pain. DeGood and Kiernan (1996) found that chronic pain patients who blamed their injury on their employer or another source tended to have significantly higher levels of affective distress compared to patients who indicated that no one was at fault for their pain. These persons also tended to be more refractory to past treatment, were more likely to indicate that their pain would limit their activity, and had higher levels of anticipated pain. Patients who blamed their employer for their pain were also more likely to be unemployed at follow-up.

Perceptions or beliefs about the cause or etiology of pain appear to have a significant impact on adjustment. Several studies highlight the importance a patient places on understanding the cause of illness-related symptoms (Leventhal and Nerenz 1983; Weiner 1985; Rimer 1990), and this is true for chronic pain as well (Reading 1982; Skevington 1983). For example, Packard (1979) surveyed headache sufferers and physicians to ask "what the head-ache patient wants" from medical consultation. While physicians ranked pain relief and medication as most important, patients indicated that an explanation for the cause of their headache was their primary concern. Deyo and Diehl (1986) observed that the greatest source of patient dissatisfaction following treatment for low back pain was the failure to obtain an adequate explanation for the cause. Cherkin et al. (1989) examined patients in a health maintenance organization who were receiving treatment for low back pain by either their primary care physician or a chiropractor. Patients re-ported a threefold increase in being "very satisfied" with chiropractic care compared to the family physician, and this difference appeared to be related to the amount of information obtained regarding the cause and treatment of pain. Lacroix et al. (1990) found that accuracy of patients' understanding for the basis of their pain significantly predicted return to work while orthope-dic evaluation of the severity of the condition, number of "nonorganic" examination signs, and scales 1 and 3 of the Minnesota Multiphasic Person-ality Inventory (MMPI) did not.

Geisser and Roth (1998) examined patients' agreement with their pain diagnosis and several dimensions of the experience of chronic pain. Patients who disagreed with their clinical diagnosis were more likely to be diagnosed with musculoskeletal pain and reported the highest levels of pain, as well as the greatest levels of affective distress. Patients who were unsure of or disagreed with their diagnosis tended to report a greater belief in pain being a signal of harm, described themselves as more disabled, reported lower perceived control over their pain, and had a greater tendency to use mal-adaptive coping skills. Roth et al. (1998) examined the characteristics of patients with myofascial pain and patients with rheumatological or neuro-logical pain conditions. The authors found that persons with myofascial pain were less accurate in identifying their diagnosis, less satisfied with their care, and more likely to indicate that they had a physiological cause to their pain that was "more serious and different" than that identified by their doctors. These studies suggest that addressing a person's beliefs about the etiology of his or her pain, and challenging erroneous beliefs about the cause, may be beneficial in facilitating adjustment.

Recently, Kerns et al. (1997) applied the transtheoretical model of change (Prochaska and DiClemente 1984) to persons with pain to examine how willingness to accept rehabilitative approaches to treating chronic pain related to conservative pain treatment outcome. The authors indicated that chronic pain patients can be placed into one of four stages in relation to accepting self-management approaches for their pain: precontemplation, in which persons express little interest in changing; contemplation, in which persons think about changing but appear to be far from a decision; preparation, in which persons are likely to consider specific active steps to changing; and action, in which action is finally taken. A fifth stage, maintenance, has further been proposed that includes working to maintain changes in health behavior. These authors developed an instrument, the Pain Stages of Change Questionnaire (PSOCQ), to assess the stage of change of chronic pain patients in relation to their readiness to accept pain self-management approaches. The authors hypothesized that persons in the latter stages of change would benefit most from cognitive-behavioral therapy, an intervention that focuses on teaching cognitive and behavioral coping strategies to manage pain. Two subsequent studies, however, have questioned the validity and utility of the measure. Jensen et al. (2000) indicated that the measure was not particularly useful for classifying persons with chronic pain into one of the four specific stages. Strong et al. (2002) indicated that the factor structure of the scale seemed to only reflect two stages, and that a measure of pain self-efficacy was a better predictor of treatment outcome than the PSOCQ.

APPLICATIONS FOR PAIN MANAGEMENT

Both pain self-efficacy and pain-related fear have consistently been shown to be related to chronic pain adjustment. Other pain beliefs such as blame regarding injury, entitlement, and knowledge of pain etiology appear to merit further study. While readiness to adopt a rehabilitation approach to managing pain is viewed as a clinically important factor in relation to conservative treatment outcome, recent studies examining the utility of the PSOCQ have not been supportive. Perhaps the measure needs to be refined or reexamined. Other pain beliefs, such as beliefs regarding the utility of medication use for pain, may be beneficial in predicting certain aspects of the chronic pain experience such as the likelihood to seek out interventional treatments for pain.

Given that self-efficacy appears to significantly contribute to the experience of pain, it would be beneficial to examine factors that may modify this trait. In acute pain situations, this change may be achieved through introducing methods of pain management that are controlled by the patient. In chronic pain populations, changing self-efficacy may be more difficult. According to social learning theory (Bandura 1977), mastery experiences are believed to have the greatest impact on increasing self-efficacy. Thus, interventions that teach various pain management strategies might be improved by giving the patient opportunities to practice and master the skills. In addition, in chronic pain populations, it might be beneficial to distinguish whether measures of self-efficacy are reflective of perceived control over pain, or whether low scores on such measures are reflective of hopelessness or helplessness (Geisser et al. 1999). It has been observed that chronic pain patients use problem-focused coping infrequently (Turner et al. 1987) and perceive themselves as having little control over their pain (Rosenstiel and Keefe 1983; Turner and Clancy 1986). Also, one might predict that greater self-efficacy would be associated with more frequent use of problem-focused or active coping in chronic pain populations. Instead, factor analytic studies using the Coping Strategies Questionnaire (CSQ; Rosenstiel and Keefe 1983) suggest that perceived control over pain and ability to decrease pain are inversely associated with a factor that includes a positive contribution from catastrophizing, or responses to pain that characterize it as being awful, horrible, and unbearable. This factor is generally labeled as a construct representing helplessness or hopelessness (Rosenstiel and Keefe 1983; Keefe et al. 1987; Turner et al. 1987; Jensen et al. 1992; Dozois et al. 1996). These findings suggest that low scores on measures of perceived control over pain in chronic pain populations may reflect hopelessness or helplessness more than high scores on these scales measure the degree of perceived control over pain.

Exposure to feared pain situations may prove to be powerful interventions for chronic pain. In fact, reduction of pain-related fear may be responsible in part for the success of interventions that emphasize functional restoration (e.g., Mayer et al. 1987), because the physiological benefits of activity and exercise that are part of these programs are not likely to be apparent over the short time course of the treatment program. It would be beneficial to examine whether the functional gains in these types of programs are clinically relevant and generalizable to activities such as return to work and resumption of leisure activities. In addition, we must question how much we should attempt to increase a person's function before increases in pain begin to emerge. For some persons, given their pain condition and functional demands, fear of movement and reinjury may be adaptive. In addition, it is unclear as to whether exposure is beneficial for persons who are low in pain-related fear and who have a good sense of the relationship between particular activities and pain.

COPING WITH PAIN

Many pain-coping strategies have been empirically examined, and the types of strategies studied tend to be driven by the assessment measures utilized. The Coping Strategies Questionnaire (CSQ; Rosenstiel and Keefe 1983) is one of the most frequently employed measures in the literature, and consists mainly of cognitive coping strategies, with the exception of one behavioral strategy (increasing activity). The cognitive strategies typically used by persons with pain include diverting attention away from pain, reinterpreting pain sensations, ignoring pain sensations, making positive coping self-statements, praying and hoping that pain will go away, and catastrophizing. The scale also has two additional items where persons rate how much control they have over pain, and how much they are able to decrease their pain. More recently, Jensen et al. (1995) introduced the Chronic Pain Coping Inventory (CPCI). This measure includes behavioral coping strategies that are often targeted in pain management treatment, such as exercise, stretching, and relaxation. Other coping strategies assessed by this instrument include guarding; resting; asking for assistance; using opioid, nonsteroidal, and sedative-hypnotic medications; persisting at tasks, making coping self-statements, and seeking social support. The authors indicate that guarding, resting, and asking for assistance were associated with increased disability and decreased activity levels among persons with chronic pain, while task persistence was associated with decreased disability when rated by a significant other (Jensen et al. 1995).

Tan et al. (2001) compared the CSQ and CPCI in a large sample of predominantly male persons with chronic pain. The authors reported that the CSQ catastrophizing scale was the most powerful predictor of depression. The authors indicated that the CPCI was somewhat more strongly predictive of disability, and that guarding was the strongest single predictor of this variable. Catastrophizing also was the best predictor of pain intensity.

Recent reviews on coping with pain have been written by Boothby et al. (1999) and DeGood (2000). In addition, a comprehensive review of pain coping measures is provided in the chapter mentioned earlier by DeGood and Tait (2001).

In a review of studies primarily on acute pain, Fernandez and Turk (1989) reported that imagery methods were the most effective coping methods of controlling pain, whereas strategies involving the repetition of cognitions or acknowledgment of the sensations were the least effective. In addition, cognitive coping strategies were found to be superior in alleviating pain compared to no-treatment or expectancy controls. Examining acute pain perception in normal, healthy subjects, Geisser et al. (1992) assessed the coping strategies used during a cold-pressor test using a modified version of the CSQ. The results indicated that subjects who were classified as pain tolerant reported less pain catastrophizing, greater use of coping self-statements, and a greater tendency to ignore pain sensations. Studies teaching various pain management strategies to normal, healthy persons have found that strategies such as distraction (Hodes et al. 1990) and goal specification (Thorn and Williams 1989) increase pain tolerance.

Among persons with acute painful burn injuries, Ulmer (1997) noted that catastrophizing was positively associated with pain intensity. Haythornthwaite et al. (2001) indicated that burn patients taught to focus on their sensations during burn dressing changes experienced less pain as compared to patients who were encouraged to distract themselves with music and to others who received usual care. Although this finding is somewhat counterintuitive given the research presented above on distraction, the authors suggest that sensory focus decreases overall perception of pain through inhibiting emotional responses to the stimuli. Logan et al. (1995) also found that sensory focus decreased pain among persons undergoing root canal therapy, but only among persons who also had a high desire for control together with low perceived control.

Few studies have concluded that coping strategies help a person to better adapt to chronic pain. This point is illustrated in a study by Snow-Turek et al. (1996), in which the authors noted that both the active and passive coping dimensions of the CSQ and Vanderbilt Pain Management Inventory (Brown and Nicassio 1987) were significantly related to chronic pain adjustment. However, they concluded that the passive coping dimensions of both measures tended to be more highly related to poorer pain adjustment, compared to the influence of the active coping dimensions on better adjustment to pain. One study by Keefe et al. (1987) found that osteoarthritis patients scoring high on a factor of self-control and rational thinking of the CSQ had lower pain ratings, less reported psychological disability and physical disability, and lower levels of global psychological distress.

More commonly, studies among persons with chronic pain find a relationship between maladjustment and specific coping styles, particularly catastrophizing. For example, Spinhoven et al. (1989) found that chronic low back pain patients who reported high levels of pain, functional impairment, anxiety, depression, and neuroticism scored higher on the CSQ factor of helplessness (high catastrophizing and low ability to control or decrease pain). Geisser et al. (1994a) reported that the pain avoidance factor on the CSQ (diverting attention and praying and hoping) was significantly associated with higher pain. Also, catastrophizing was positively related to negative affect and to a dysfunctional profile of pain coping, even when the investigators controlled for level of depression. Martin et al. (1996) examined responses to the CSQ among 80 persons with fibromyalgia. The authors found that coping attempts (a composite scale combining reinterpreting pain, ignoring pain, diverting attention, making coping self-statements, and increasing activity) was associated with higher levels of physical and total disability, but with less psychosocial disability. Catastrophizing was associated with greater total disability. More recently, Jensen et al. (2002) reported that catastrophizing measured 1 month after limb amputation was significantly associated with greater pain severity, pain interference, and depression at a 5-month follow-up.

Differences in coping responses have also been reported as a function of age and gender. Watkins et al. (1999) reported that older adults with rheumatoid arthritis were more likely than younger adults to employ maladaptive strategies when faced with mild pain. Overall, the authors found that subjects engaged in more active coping strategies when confronted with mild pain, and more maladaptive strategies when faced with severe pain. Keefe et al. (2000) indicated that women with chronic pain tended to report more pain, disability, and pain behavior. Using multiple regression analyses, the authors reported that this effect was mediated by catastrophizing.

While catastrophizing clearly has a significant impact on the experience of pain, several conceptual concerns have been raised about the construct. Early studies on catastrophizing suggested that maladaptive responses to pain mirrored responses typically seen in persons with depression, suggesting that catastrophizing is merely a symptom of depression rather than a separate entity (Sullivan and D'Eon 1990). However, later studies found catastrophizing to be significantly related to pain and pain-related disability independent of the influence of depression and negative affect (Keefe et al. 1989, 1990b; Geisser et al. 1994b; Geisser and Roth 1998; Sullivan et al. 1998). Also, there has been considerable debate as to whether catastrophizing is best conceptualized as a coping strategy or as a belief or appraisal (Jensen et al. 1991; Geisser et al. 1999; Sullivan et al. 2001). Sullivan et al. (2001) outline several conceptual models of catastrophizing, and review the evidence for each. These authors indicate that there is evidence to support both notions, and suggest that catastrophizing can be conceptualized as a coping response because overt expressions of catastrophizing may reflect attempts to elicit support and sympathy from others. Further research is needed to determine which model of catastrophizing is most appropriate.

The method of examining coping strategies may have a significant impact on the findings and conclusions reached. Previous reviews on coping with pain (Jensen et al. 1991; Boothby et al. 1999; DeGood 2000) have noted that most research has been cross-sectional, and that future research should employ experimental designs allowing for the examination of cause-and-effect relationships. A good illustration of how results may differ depending on how one looks at the data is apparent in a study by Keefe et al. (1997). These authors utilized a daily diary method of assessing coping and outcome variables such as pain and mood over a 30-day period among persons with rheumatoid arthritis. When analyzing the data across subjects, daily coping efficacy (a rating of the effectiveness of coping) was not associated with pain coping or with pain intensity, and more frequent use of coping strategies was associated with greater pain. However, when examining within-person trends in the data, high levels of coping self-efficacy were significantly associated with decreased pain levels the following day. In addition, coping attempts and relaxation contributed to improvements in next-day pain and in positive mood. The authors point out that the across-subject analyses might reflect the fact that subjects make greater coping attempts when faced with higher levels of pain. However, the benefits of these efforts may be delayed and not observable in a cross-sectional slice of time.

APPLICATIONS FOR PAIN MANAGEMENT

When examining coping with acute pain, a number of active or problem focused coping strategies appear to be beneficial in reducing pain such as distraction, sensory focus, goal setting, and coping self-statements. In contrast, when looking at coping with chronic pain, few active or problem-focused strategies appear to be related to better adaptation. It is possible that these findings may be a function of the populations studied, and how we study them. For example, as noted above, longitudinal studies may be needed to examine the positive benefits of coping. In addition, most chronic pain and coping studies have been conducted on persons presenting for treatment. Very little research has focused on persons from community samples who do not seek care for their pain, presumably because they are coping more effectively with it. Although more severe chronic pain may be less manageable, as noted above, evidence suggests that interventions such as coping skills training and cognitive-behavioral therapy are beneficial in improving adaptation among persons with chronic pain (Keefe et al. 1990a; Morley et al. 1999). Given the above findings, it would also be beneficial to examine the impact of strategies designed to modify beliefs or coping strategies that are believed to be related to poorer adaptation to pain. For example,

Thorn et al. (2002) outlined a treatment program to reduce catastrophizing among persons with chronic pain. Interventions designed to improve coping with chronic pain may benefit from the addition of specific interventions for reducing the use of pain-coping strategies typically associated with poorer pain adjustment.

As noted by DeGood (2000), studies examining coping with pain have been limited because they typically only measure the coping strategies included in standardized measures that are deemed to be important. It might be beneficial for future studies to examine coping in a qualitative way to examine whether persons with chronic pain use strategies that are not captured by the assessment tools commonly employed. For example, few studies have examined the impact of religious coping on pain, despite the fact that many people view this type of coping as extremely beneficial to their adjustment.

SUMMARY

Psychological factors such as personality, pain beliefs, and coping are thought to be extremely important in the development and maintenance of pain, particularly chronic pain. While certain personality styles such as neuroticism have consistently been found to be related to pain, research has yet to established whether specific interventions designed to modify personality traits are effective in improving adaptation to pain. What may prove to be more efficacious and less costly is the strategy of tailoring interventions to fit particular personality styles. A study by Efran et al. (1989) is illustrative. These authors found that "blunters," or persons who prefer to cope with stressors by not seeking out details or information about a situation, performed best on an acute pain task when given a coping style that encouraged distraction. Subjects who were identified as "monitors," persons who prefer to cope with stress by seeking out as much information as possible, showed a trend toward better pain tolerance when given instructions to concentrate on the sensations they experienced. In addition, as mentioned above, it would be beneficial to examine the impact of personality styles that may enhance pain coping, such as optimism, on the experience of pain.

Previous reviews on coping with pain have emphasized the need to examine factors that moderate or mediate the relationship between pain and coping (Jensen et al. 1991; Boothby et al. 1999; DeGood 2000). One factor that has emerged in the literature as a moderator variable is pain intensity. Jensen et al. (1992) found that coping self-statements were related to poorer adjustment, but only among persons with high levels of pain. Peters et al.

(2000) found that persons with a greater duration of pain displayed higher levels of pain catastrophizing, and also received a greater number of solicitous responses from their spouses. It has been suggested in the general literature on coping with illness that emotion-focused pain strategies such as catastrophizing might be beneficial in situations where the person has little control or the situation is ambiguous, whereas problem-focused strategies might be beneficial in situations where personal control is greater, and there is less uncertainty about the medical problem (Auerbach 1989; Hilton 1989). Thus, one may need to consider what type of coping strategies might be effective given the circumstances faced by the individual. For example, encouraging a person with high, uncontrollable pain to increase their activity and to try to employ various strategies to manage their pain may only serve to increase their pain and their frustration over their inability to manage it. In some pain populations, we may need to encourage people to try and adapt to a certain level of disability rather than overcome their pain.

An example of this latter point is outlined in a study by Schmitz et al. (1996). The authors propose that accommodative pain coping (which they define as a downgrading of aspirations, positive reappraisal, and goal and preference adjustment) might facilitate adaptation to a greater degree than what they refer to as "assimilative coping." They define the latter as engaging in instrumental activities aimed at changing the problem, performing self-corrective strategies to increase competence, and engaging in self-corrective strategies to reduce the problem. The authors found that accommodative coping was associated with better adjustment to pain, and that ability to adjust goals reduced the impact of pain on psychological well-being. In addition, problem-focused coping was associated with better adjustment, but only among persons with a high degree of flexible goal adjustment. This study illustrates that teaching adaptive coping strategies to chronic pain patients may not necessarily be beneficial unless one can reduce barriers to more optimal functioning (e.g., by modifying a patient's unrealistic beliefs or providing more realistic expectations regarding the effects of different coping strategies).

Given the complexity of coping styles, it may be necessary to try to tailor coping interventions to the individual, taking into consideration factors other than just personality. Of course, from a research perspective, this approach would make it difficult to study standardized interventions. However, it may be possible to tailor interventions to groups of persons based on psychological and pain profiling. For example, Riley and Robinson (1998) reported that cognitive coping strategies as measured by the CSQ were only related to better adjustment among chronic pain patients with MMPI-2 profiles that tended to have scores within normal limits on each scale. Thus, it may be beneficial to try to teach problem-focused coping skills to persons with less pain and psychopathology, and accommodative skills to persons with higher levels of psychopathology and pain. In addition, it might be helpful to try to focus on reduction of factors such as catastrophizing in this latter population so as to facilitate adjustment.

It would be beneficial to examine whether modifications in a few key factors can produce change in a number of different areas of the pain experience. Some factors might be important only in certain areas of adjustment. For example, Turner et al. (2000) found that catastrophizing was independently associated with emotional responses to pain, while pain beliefs displayed an independent association with disability. Catastrophizing was unrelated when the investigators controlled for pain beliefs. Thus, when emotional adjustment is a key presenting complaint in a person with pain, interventions such as those aimed at modifying catastrophizing might be most beneficial. For persons who are highly disabled, it may be beneficial to modify factors such as pain-related fear.

Targeting a few key components in the coping process, however, may facilitate adaptation in a number of different areas. The study by Vlaeyen et al. (2002) presented earlier is illustrative of this notion, because modifying pain-related fear not only reduced disability but also affected subjects' emotional status, catastrophizing, and level of pain, even though the latter was not a target of the intervention. It would be beneficial to examine whether these findings can be replicated, and to determine what types of pain patients might benefit from such an intervention.

Lastly, several studies have indicated that a number of psychological variables can predict pain chronicity with a high degree of accuracy (e.g., Pulliam et al. 2001; Hazard et al. 1996). It would be of interest to examine whether interventions aimed at modifying these risk factors in high risk persons shortly after the onset of pain are beneficial in reducing chronicity.

In summary, several psychological factors are important in terms of coping with pain. However, further research is needed to determine what types of strategies are optimal in what types of persons, and under what circumstances. Such research may be crucial because emphasizing certain strategies as part of an intervention may be detrimental in some situations based on the person's current psychological status and pain condition. While some interventions such as exposure to feared activities hold a great deal of promise in pain treatment, we need to examine under what circumstances we should try to increase function in patients with pain, and when we should teach them to accommodate to their pain problem.

REFERENCES

Affleck G, Tennen H, Urrows S, Higgins P. Neuroticism and the pain-mood relation in rheumatoid arthritis: insights from a prospective daily study. *J Consult Clin Psychol* 1992; 60:119–126.

American Psychiatric Association. *Diagnostic and Statistical Manual of Mental Disorders,* 4th ed. Washington, DC: American Psychiatric Association, 1994.

Asmundson GJG, Norton GR. Anxiety sensitivity in patients with physically unexplained chronic back pain: a preliminary report. *Behav Res Ther* 1995; 33:771–777.

Asmundson GJG, Norton GR, Allerdings MD. Fear and avoidance in dysfunctional chronic back pain patients. *Pain* 1997; 69:321–236.

Asghari A, Nickolas MK. Pain self-efficacy and pain behaviour: a prospective study. *Pain* 2001; 94:85–100.

Auerbach SM. Stress management and coping research in the health care setting: an overview and methodological commentary. *J Consult Clin Psychol* 1989; 57:388–395.

Bandura A. *Social Learning Theory.* Englewood Cliffs, NJ: Prentice Hall, 1977.

Bandura A, O'Leary A, Taylor B, Gauthier J, Gossard D. Perceived self-efficacy and pain control: opioid and nonopioid mechanisms. *J Pers Soc Psychol* 1987; 53:563–571.

BenDebba M, Torgerson WS, Long DM. Personality traits, pain duration and severity, functional impairment, and psychological distress in patients with persistent low back pain. *Pain* 1997; 72:115–125.

Bigos SJ, Battie, MC Spengler DM, et al. A longitudinal, prospective study of industrial back injury reporting. *Clin Orthop* 1992; 279:21–34.

Boothby JL, Thorn BE, Stroud MW, Jensen MP. Coping with pain. In: Gatchel RJ, Turk DC (Eds). *Psychosocial Factors in Pain.* New York: Guilford Press, 1999, pp 343–359.

Breslau N, Chilcoat HD, Andreski P. Further evidence on the link between migraine and neuroticism. *Neurology* 1996; 47:663–667.

Brown GK, Nicassio PM. Development of a questionnaire for the assessment of active and passive coping strategies in chronic pain patients. *Pain* 1987; 31:53–64.

Buckelew SP, Parker JC, Keefe FJ, et al. Self-efficacy and pain behavior among subjects with fibromyalgia. *Pain* 1994; 59:377–384.

Cherkin DC, MacCornack FA, Berg AO. Managing low back pain: a comparison of the beliefs and behaviors of family physicians and chiropractors. *West J Med* 1989; 149:475–480.

Crombez G, Vervaet L, Baeyens F, Lysens R, Eelen P. Do pain expectancies cause pain in chronic low back patients? A clinical investigation. *Behav Res Ther* 1996; 34:919–925.

Crombez G, Vlaeyen JWS, Heuts PHTG, Lysens R. Pain-related fear is more disabling than pain itself: evidence on the role of pain-related fear in chronic back pain disability. *Pain* 1999; 80:329–339.

DeGood DE. Relationship of pain-coping strategies to adjustment and functioning. In: Gatchel RJ, Weisberg JN (Eds). *Personality Characteristics of Patients with Chronic Pain.* Washington DC: American Psychological Association Press, 2000, pp 129–164.

DeGood DE, Kiernan B. Perception of fault in patients with chronic pain. *Pain* 1996; 64:153–159.

DeGood DE, Tait RC. Assessment of pain beliefs and coping. In: Turk DC, Melzack R (Eds). *Handbook of Pain Assessment,* 2nd ed. New York: Guilford Press, 2001, pp 320–345.

Deyo RA, Diehl AK. Patient satisfaction with medical care for low-back pain. *Spine* 1986; 11:28–30.

Dozois DJA, Dobson KS, Wong M, Hughes D, Long A. Predictive utility of the CSQ in low back pain: individual vs. composite measures. *Pain* 1996; 66:171–180.

Efran JS, Chorney RL, Ascher LM, Lukens MD. Coping styles, paradox, and the cold pressor test. *J Behav Med* 1989; 12:91–103.

Engel GL. 'Psychogenic' pain and the pain-prone patient. *Am J Med* 1959; 26:899–918.

Eysenck HJ. *Structure of Human Personality.* New York: Wiley, 1960.

Fernandez E, Turk DC. The utility of cognitive coping strategies for altering pain perception: a meta-analysis. *Pain* 1989; 38:123–135.

Flor H, Turk DC. Chronic back pain and rheumatoid arthritis: predicting pain and disability from cognitive variables. *J Behav Med* 1988; 11:251–265.

Fordyce WE. Environmental factors in the genesis of low back pain. In: Bonica JJ, Liebeskind JC, Albé-Fessard DG (Eds). *Proceedings of the Second World Congress on Pain,* Advances in Pain Research and Therapy, Vol. 3. New York: Raven Press, 1979, pp 659–666.

Gamsa A. The role of psychological factors in chronic pain: I. A half century of study. *Pain* 1994; 57:5–15.

Garafolo JP. Perceived optimism and chronic pain. In: Gatchel RJ, Weisberg JN (Eds). *Personality Characteristics of Patients with Chronic Pain.* Washington, DC: American Psychological Association Press, 2000, pp 203–217.

Gatchel RJ, Garafolo JP, Ellis E, Holt C. Major psychological disorders in acute and chronic TMD: an initial examination. *J Am Dent Assoc* 1996; 127:1365–1374.

Geisser ME, Roth RS. Knowledge of and agreement with pain diagnosis: relation to pain beliefs, pain severity, disability, and psychological distress. *J Occup Rehabil* 1998; 8:73–88.

Geisser ME, Robinson ME, Pickren W. Coping styles among pain sensitive and pain tolerant individuals on the cold-pressor test. *Behav Ther* 1992; 23:31–41.

Geisser ME, Robinson ME, Henson CD. The Coping Strategies Questionnaire and chronic pain adjustment: a conceptual and empirical reanalysis. *Clin J Pain* 1994a; 10:98–106.

Geisser ME, Robinson ME, Keefe FJ, Weiner ML. Catastrophizing, depression and the sensory, affective and evaluative aspects of chronic pain. *Pain* 1994b; 59:79–84.

Geisser ME, Robinson ME, Riley JL. Pain beliefs, coping, and adjustment to chronic pain: let's focus more on the negative. *Pain Forum* 1999; 8:161–168.

Geisser ME, Haig AJ, Theisen ME. Activity avoidance and function in persons with chronic back pain. *J Occup Rehabil* 2000; 10:215–227.

Harkapaa K, Jarikoski A, Mellin G, Hurri H, Luoma J. Health locus of control beliefs and psychological distress as predictors for treatment outcome in low back pain patients: results of a 3-month follow-up of a controlled intervention study. *Pain* 1991; 46:35–41.

Harkapaa K, Jarikoski A, Estlander A. Health optimism and control beliefs as predictors for treatment outcome of a multimodal back treatment program. *Psychol Health* 1996; 12:123–134.

Haythornthwaite JA, Lawrence JW, Fauerbach JA. Brief cognitive interventions for burn pain. *Ann Behav Med* 2001; 23:42–49.

Hazard RG, Haugh LD, Reid S, Preble JB, MacDonald L. Early prediction of chronic disability after occupational low back injury. *Spine* 1996; 21:945–951.

Hill HE, Belleville RE, Wikler A. Studies on anxiety associated with anticipation of pain. *Arch Neurol Psychiatry* 1955; 73:602–608.

Hilton BA. The relationship of uncertainty, control, commitment, and threat of recurrence to coping strategies used by women diagnosed with breast cancer. *J Behav Med* 1989; 12:39–54.

Hodes RL, Howland EW, Lightfoot N, Cleeland CS. The effects of distraction on responses to cold-pressor pain. *Pain* 1990; 41:109–114.

Jensen MP, Turner JA, Romano, JM, Karoly P. Coping with chronic pain: a review of the literature. *Pain* 1991; 47:249–283.

Jensen MP, Romano JM, Turner JA. Chronic pain coping measures: individual vs. composite scores. *Pain* 1992; 51:273–280.

Jensen MP, Turner JA, Romano JM. Correlates of improvement in multidisciplinary treatment of chronic pain. *J Consult Clin Psychol* 1994a; 62:172–179.

Jensen MP, Turner JA, Romano JM, Lawler BK. Relationship of pain-specific beliefs to chronic pain adjustment. *Pain* 1994b; 57:301–309.

Jensen MP, Turner JA, Romano JM, Strom SE. The Chronic Pain Coping Inventory: development and preliminary validation. *Pain* 1995; 60:203–216.

Jensen MP, Nielson WR, Romano JM, Hill ML, Tuner JA. Further evaluation of the pain stages of change questionnaire: is the transtheoretical model of change useful for patients with chronic pain? *Pain* 2000; 86:255–264.

Jensen MP, Ehde DM, Hoffman AJ, et al. Cognitions, coping and social environment predict adjustment to phantom limb pain. *Pain* 2002; 95:133–142.

Keefe FJ, Caldwell DS, Queen KT, et al. Pain coping strategies in osteoarthritis patients. *J Consult Clin Psychol* 1987; 55:208–212.

Keefe FJ, Brown GK, Wallston KA, Caldwell DS. Coping with rheumatoid arthritis pain: catastrophizing as a maladaptive strategy. *Pain* 1989; 37:51–56.

Keefe FJ, Affleck G, Lefebvre JC, et al. Pain coping strategies and coping efficacy in rheumatoid arthritis: a daily process analysis. *Pain* 1997; 69:35–42.

Keefe FJ, Caldwell DS, Williams DA, et al. Pain coping skills training in the management of osteoarthritic knee pain: a comparative study. *Behav Ther* 1990a; 21:49–62.

Keefe FJ, Caldwell DS, Williams DA, et al. Pain coping skills training in the management of osteoarthritic knee pain. II: Follow-up results. *Behav Ther* 1990b; 21:435–447.

Keefe FJ, Lefebvre JC, Egert JR, et al. The relationship of gender to pain, pain behavior, and disability in osteoarthritis patients: the role of catastrophizing. *Pain* 2000; 87:325–334.

Kerns RD, Turk DC, Rudy TE. The West Haven-Yale Multidimensional Pain Inventory (WHYMPI). *Pain* 1985; 23:345–356.

Kerns RD, Rosenberg R, Jamison RN, Caudill MA, Haythornthwaite J. Readiness to adopt a self-management approach to chronic pain: the Pain Stages of Change Questionnaire. *Pain* 1997; 72:227–234.

Keogh E, Cochrane M. Anxiety sensitivity, cognitive biases, and the experience of pain. *J Pain* 2002; 3:320–329.

Kohn PM, Cowles MP, Dzinas K. Arousability, need for approval, and situational context as factors in pain tolerance. *J Res Pers* 1989; 23:214–224.

Kori SH, Miller RP, Todd DD. Kinesiophobia: a new view of chronic pain behavior. *Pain Manage* 1990; 3:35–43.

Lackner JM, Carosella AM, Feuerstein M. Pain expectancies, pain, and functional self-efficacy expectancies as determinants of disability in patients with chronic low-back disorders. *J Consult Clin Psychol* 1996; 64:212–220.

Lacroix JM, Powell J, Lloyd GJ, et al. Low-back pain: factors of value in predicting outcome. *Spine* 1990; 15:495–499.

Lauver SC, Johnson JL. The role of neuroticism and social support in older adults with chronic pain behavior. *Pers Indiv Differences* 1997; 23:165–176.

Lazarus RS, Folkman S. *Stress, Appraisal, and Coping*. New York: Springer, 1984.

Lethem J, Slade PD, Troup JDG, Bentley G. Outline of a fear-avoidance model of exaggerated pain perceptions. *Behav Res Ther* 1983; 21:401–408.

Leventhal H, Nerenz DR. A model for stress research with some implications for the control of stress disorders. In: Meichenbaum D, Jarenko M (Eds). *Stress Reduction and Prevention*. New York: Plenum Press, 1983, pp 5–38.

Lipchik G, Miles K, Covington E. Effects of multidisciplinary pain management treatment on locus of control and pain beliefs in chronic non-terminal pain. *Clin J Pain* 1993; 9:49–57.

Litt MD. Self-efficacy and perceived control: cognitive mediators of pain tolerance. *J Pers Soc Psychol* 1988, 54:149–160.

Logan HL, Baron RS, Kohout F. Sensory focus as therapeutic treatments for acute pain. *Psychosom Med* 1995; 57:475–484.

Martin MY, Bradley LA, Alexander RW, et al. Coping strategies predict disability in patients with primary fibromyalgia. *Pain* 1996; 68:45–53.

Mayer TG, Gatchel RJ, Mayer H. A prospective two year study of functional restoration in industrial low back injury: an objective assessment procedure. *JAMA* 1987; 258:1763–1767.

McCracken LM, Gross RT. The role of pain-related anxiety reduction in the outcome of multidisciplinary treatment for chronic low back pain: preliminary results. *J Occup Rehabil* 1998; 8:179–189.

McCracken LM, Gross RT, Sorg PJ, Edmands TA. Prediction of pain in patients with chronic low back pain: effects of inaccurate prediction and pain-related anxiety. *Behav Res Ther* 1993; 31:647–652.

McCracken LM, Spertus IL, Janeck AS, Sinclair D, Wetzel FT. Behavioral dimensions of adjustment in persons with chronic pain: pain-related anxiety and acceptance. *Pain* 1999; 80:283–289.

Melzack R, Wall PD. Pain mechanisms: a new theory. *Science* 1965; 150:971–979.

Millard RW, Wells N, Thebarge RW. A comparison of models describing reports of disability associated with chronic pain. *Clin J Pain* 1991; 7:283–291.

Monti D, Herring C, Schwartzman R, Marchese M. Personality assessment of patients with complex regional pain syndrome Type I. *Clin J Pain* 1998; 14:295–302.

Morley S, Eccleston C, Williams A. Systematic review and meta-analysis of randomized, controlled trials of cognitive behavior therapy for chronic pain in adults, excluding headache. *Pain* 1999; 80:1–13.

Owen-Salters E, Gatchel RJ, Polatin PB, Mayer TG. Changes in psychopathology following functional restoration of chronic low back pain patients: a prospective study. *J Occup Rehabil* 1996; 6:215–223.

Packard RC. What does the headache patient want? *Headache* 1979; 19:370–374.

Pellino TA, Ward SE. Perceived control mediates the relationship between pain severity and patient satisfaction. *J Pain Symptom Manage* 1998; 15:110–116.

Peters ML, Sorbi MJ, Kruise DA, et al. Electronic diary assessment of pain, disability, and psychological adaptation in patients differing in duration of pain. *Pain* 2000; 84:181–192.

Pietri-Taleb F, Riihimaki H, Viikari-Juntura E, Lindstrom K. Longitudinal study on the role of personality characteristics and psychological distress in neck trouble among working men. *Pain* 1994; 58:261–167.

Philips HC. Avoidance behavior and its role in sustaining chronic pain. *Behav Res Ther* 1987; 25:273–279.

Phillips JM, Gatchel RJ. Extroversion-introversion and chronic pain. In: Gatchel RJ, Weisberg JN (Eds). *Personality Characteristics of Patients with Chronic Pain*. Washington, DC: American Psychological Association Press, 2000, pp 181–202.

Plehn K, Peterson RA, Williams DA. Anxiety sensitivity: its relationship to functional status in patients with chronic pain. *J Occup Rehabil* 1998; 8:213–222.

Prochaska JO, DiClemente CC. *The Transtheoretical Approach: Towards a Systematic Eclectic Framework*. Homewood, IL: Dow Jones Irwin, 1984.

Pulliam CB, Gatchel RJ, Gardea MA. Psychosocial differences in high risk versus low risk acute low-back pain patients. *J Occup Rehabil* 2001; 11:43–52.

Reading AE. Attribution and the management of the pain patient. In: Antaki C, Brewin C (Eds). *Attributions and Psychological Change*. New York: Academic Press, 1982, pp 157–174.

Riley JL, Robinson ME. Validity of MMPI-2 profiles in chronic pain patients: differences in path models of coping and somatization. *Clin J Pain* 1998; 14:215–227.

Rimer BK. Perspectives on interpersonal theories in health education and health behavior. In: Glanz K, Lewis FM, Rimer BK (Eds). *Health Behavior and Health Education*. San Francisco: Jossey-Bass, 1990, pp 140–157.

Rosenstiel AK, Keefe FJ. The use of coping strategies in chronic low back pain patients: relationship to patient characteristics and current adjustment. *Pain* 1983; 17:33–44.

Roth RS, Horowitz K, Bachman JE. Chronic myofascial pain: knowledge of diagnosis and satisfaction with treatment. *Arch Phys Med Rehabil* 1998; 79:966–970.

Roy R. Engel's pain-prone disorder patient: 25 years after. *Psychother Psychosom* 1985; 43:126–135.

Rudy TE, Kerns RD, Turk DC. Chronic pain and depression: toward a cognitive-behavioral mediation model. *Pain* 1988; 35:129–140.

Sanders SH. Cross-validation of the Back Pain Classification Scale with chronic, intractable pain patients. *Pain* 1985; 22:271–277.

Schmitz U, Saile H, Nilges P. Coping with chronic pain: flexible goal adjustment as an interactive buffer against pain-related distress. *Pain* 1996; 67:41–51.

Skevington SM. Social cognitions, personality and chronic pain. *J Psychosom Res* 1983; 27:421–428.

Snow-Turek AL, Norris M, Tan G. Active and passive coping strategies in chronic pain patients. *Pain* 1996; 64:455–462.

Spinhoven P, Ter Kuile MM, Linssen CG, Gazendam B. Pain coping strategies in a Dutch population of chronic low back pain patients. *Pain* 1989; 37:77–83.

Strong J, Westbury K, Smith G, McKenzie I, Ryan W. Treatment outcome in individuals with chronic pain: is the Pain Stages of Change Questionnaire (PSOCQ) a useful tool? *Pain* 2002; 97:65–73.

Sullivan MJL, D'Eon JL. Relation between catastrophizing and depression in chronic pain patients. *J Abnorm Psychol* 1990; 99:260–263.

Sullivan MJL, Standish W, Waite H, Sullivan M, Tripp DA. Catastrophizing, pain and disability in patients with soft-tissue injuries. *Pain* 1998; 77:253–260.

Sullivan MJL, Thorn B, Haythornthwaite JA, et al. Theoretical perspectives on the relation between catastrophizing and pain. *Clin J Pain* 2001; 17:52–64.

Tan G, Jensen MP, Robinson-Whelen S, Thornby JI, Monga TN. Coping with chronic pain: a comparison of two measures. *Pain* 2001; 90:127–133.

Thorn BE, Williams GA. Goal specification alters perceived pain intensity and tolerance latency. *Cognit Ther Res* 1989; 13:171–183.

Thorn BE, Boothby JL, Sullivan MJL. Targeted treatment of catastrophizing for the management of chronic pain. *Cognit Behav Pract* 2002; 9:127–138.

Toomey TC, Mann JD, Abashian S, Thompson-Pope S. Relationship between perceived self-control of pain, pain description, and functioning. *Pain* 1991; 45:129–133.

Turk DC, Flor H. Etiological theories and treatment for chronic back pain: II. psychological models and interventions. *Pain* 1984; 19:209–233.

Turner JA, Clancy S. Strategies for coping with chronic low back pain: relationship to pain and disability. *Pain* 1986; 24:355–364.

Turner JA, Clancy S, Vitaliano PP. Relationships of stress, appraisals of coping, to chronic low back pain. *Behav Res Ther* 1987; 25:281–288.

Turner JA, Jensen MP, Romano JM. Do beliefs, coping and catastrophizing independently predict functioning in patients with chronic pain? *Pain* 2000; 85:115–125.

Ulmer JF. An exploratory study of pain, coping and depressed mood following burn injury. *J Pain Symptom Manage* 1997; 13:148–157.

Vlaeyen JWS, Kole-Snijders AMJ, Rotteveel AM, Rvesink R, Heuts PHTG. The role of fear of movement/(re)injury in pain disability. *J Occup Rehabil* 1995; 5:235–252.

Vlaeyen JWS, Seelen HAM, Peters M, et al. Fear of movement/(re)injury and muscular reactivity in chronic low back pain patients: an experimental investigation. *Pain* 1999; 82:297–304.

Vlaeyen JWS, de Jong J, Geilen M, Heuts PHTG, van Breulelen G. The treatment of fear of movement/(re)injury in chronic low back pain: further evidence on the effectiveness of exposure in vivo. *Clin J Pain* 2002; 18:251–261.

Waddell G, Newton M, Henderson I, Somerville D, Main C. A Fear-Avoidance Beliefs Questionnaire (FABQ) and the role of fear-avoidance beliefs in chronic low back pain and disability. *Pain* 1993; 52:157–168.

Wade JB, Price DD. Nonpathological factors and chronic pain: implications for assessment and treatment. In: Gatchel RJ, Weisberg JN (Eds). *Personality Characteristics of Patients with Chronic Pain.* Washington, DC: American Psychological Association Press, 2000, pp 89–107.

Watkins KW, Shifren K, Park DC, Morrell RW. Age, pain and coping with rheumatoid arthritis. *Pain* 1999; 82:217–228.

Watson PJ, Booker CK, Main CJ. Evidence for the role of psychological factors in abnormal paraspinal activity in patients with chronic low back pain. *J Musculoskeletal Pain* 1997; 5:41–56.

Weiner B. An attributional theory of achievement motivation and emotion. *Psychol Rev* 1985; 93:548–575.

Weintraub MI. Regional pain is usually hysterical. *Arch Neurol* 1988; 45:914–915.

Weisberg JN. Studies investigating the prevalence of personality disorders in patients with chronic pain. In: Gatchel RJ, Weisberg JN (Eds). *Personality Characteristics of Patients with Chronic Pain.* Washington, DC: American Psychological Association Press, 2000, pp 181–202, 221–239.

Weisberg JN, Keefe FJ. Personality disorders in the chronic pain population: basic concepts, empirical findings, and clinical implications. *Pain Forum* 1997; 6:1–9.

White AA, Gordon SC. Synopsis: workshop on idiopathic low back pain. *Spine* 1982; 7:141–149.

Williams DA, Robinson ME, Geisser ME. Pain beliefs: assessment and utility. *Pain* 1994; 59:71–78.

Correspondence to: Michael Geisser, PhD, The Spine Program, Department of Physical Medicine and Rehabilitation, University of Michigan Medical Center, 325 E. Eisenhower Parkway, Ann Arbor, MI 48108, USA. Tel: 734-998-7805; Fax: 734-998-7914; email: mgeisser@umich.edu.

Psychosocial Aspects of Pain: A Handbook for Health Care Providers, Progress in Pain Research and Management, Vol. 27, edited by Robert H. Dworkin and William S. Breitbart, IASP Press, Seattle, © 2004.

24

Compensation Claims for Chronic Pain: Effects on Evaluation and Treatment

Raymond C. Tait

Department of Psychiatry, Saint Louis University School of Medicine, St. Louis, Missouri, USA

Few areas in the chronic pain literature generate as many disparate findings and opinions as those elicited by patients involved in litigation such as compensation proceedings for potentially compensable injuries. Depending upon the source, psychosocial factors associated with compensable injuries either augment symptoms (Jamison et al. 1988; Chapman and Brena 1989; Fishbain et al. 1991, 1995; Hayes et al. 1993; Rohling et al. 1995; Rainville et al. 1997; Iverson et al. 2001) or cause no increase in symptoms (Melzack et al. 1985; Jamison et al. 1988; Hendler and Kozikowski 1993; McGuigan 1995; Thimineur et al. 2000). Similarly, psychosocial factors related to compensation either interfere with treatment response (Chapman and Brena 1989; Greenough and Fraser 1989; Aronoff 1991; Rohling et al. 1995; Atlas et al. 1996; Bellamy 1997; Fordyce 1997; Butterfield et al. 1998; Feuerstein et al. 1999; Cassidy et al. 2000) or have no such effect (Trabin et al. 1987; Mayer et al. 1998; Atlas et al. 2000).

Whatever the empirical evidence, opinions about pain and compensation are strongly held. Evidence of the emotions provoked by the topic is found in the classic definition of "compensation neurosis": "a state of mind, borne of fear, kept alive by avarice, stimulated by lawyers, and cured by a verdict" (Kennedy 1946). In addition to the latter term, a variety of other disparaging terms also have been coined: "American disease" (although the Swiss might take issue with this nomenclature; Nachemson 1994), "barristogenic illness," "functional overlay," "malingering," "post-accident syndrome," "psychogenic invalidism," "railway spine," "secondary gain," and "symptom magnification" (Bellamy 1997). These and other terms reflect widely held negative stereotypes of pain patients who are involved in compensation proceedings.

Such stereotypes derive partly from the scope of problems associated with compensation-related pain, partly from disparities between expressed symptoms and levels of perceived disability, and partly from treatment outcomes that fall short of expectations (Deyo et al. 1995; May et al. 1999). Work-related musculoskeletal injuries involving the lumbar spine, while only a small portion of all compensation-related injuries, are the leading cause of work disability in the United States (U.S. Department of Labor 2000). While the incidence of these injuries may have declined somewhat in recent years (Frank et al. 1996; Pope and Andersson 1997; Silverstein et al. 1997), annual costs associated with workers' compensation approached $20 billion in 1996 (AFL-CIO 1997). If expenses associated with lost work time and other sources of compensation are considered, the costs are much higher (Webster and Snook 1994; Frymoyer 1997). Further, efforts to minimize disability associated with such injuries have often been unsuccessful (Garofalo and Polatin 1999) and may even have exacerbated the problem in some respects (Hadler 1997).

This chapter discusses psychosocial factors associated with symptom presentation and response to treatment among patients reporting pain associated with compensable injuries. Patients with compensable injuries include those who have retained legal representation for a painful injury (either at work or in another setting), those involved in workers' compensation proceedings without legal representation, and those covered under Social Security disability and other disability programs (Durbin 1997). This chapter addresses issues relevant to each of these situations.

The first section below describes several models that have been applied to compensable injuries associated with pain. The second section addresses associations between compensation status and symptom presentation. Outcome studies are the focus of the third section. The fourth section discusses systemic factors that may influence evaluation and treatment of chronic pain claimants. The chapter concludes with comments aimed at integrating research efforts and with suggestions for future studies.

CONCEPTUAL ISSUES

While a variety of models of diagnosis and rehabilitation have informed thinking on pain-related disability (Schultz et al. 2000), two primary models represent much of the literature regarding claimants with intractable pain: a biomedical model and a biopsychosocial model (Hadjistavropoulos 1999). The former model uses physical examination findings and diagnostic testing to identify lesions and assess impairment. This model underlies most medical ratings of impairment, even though such ratings often are difficult to make reliably (Greenwood 1985; Clark and Haldeman 1993; Michel et al. 1997; Hinderer et al. 2000). In the absence of identifiable lesions or clear medical impairment, patients frequently are diagnosed with either somatization (Katz and Tait 2000) or a pain disorder (American Psychiatric Association 1994). The latter diagnosis requires four elements: (1) persistent pain that interferes with social, emotional, or occupational function; (2) pain that is not intentionally produced; (3) pain that is maintained or exacerbated by psychological factors; (4) symptoms that are not better accounted for by another diagnosis. Functionally, the biomedical model, requiring a psychiatric diagnosis in the absence of bona fide physical findings, reflects a dualistic view of pain (if it is not physical, it must be mental).

Biopsychosocial models, developed after the introduction of the gate control theory (Melzack and Wall 1965), also have been applied to compensation-related pain. Unlike the biomedical model, biopsychosocial models accommodate both medical and psychosocial factors. One variant of the biopsychosocial model emphasizes operant factors that condition patient pain behaviors (Fordyce et al. 1973, 1985). Basic to the operant model is the concept that behaviors are shaped by external contingencies. Hence, reinforcing contingencies that may be associated with the exhibition of pain behaviors, such as sympathy, money, and exoneration from burdensome responsibilities, are likely to increase the frequency of those behaviors. When such reinforcers are absent, the frequency of pain behaviors is likely to decline. The model has obvious implications for situations that involve potential social and financial rewards such as those associated with disability systems. These implications were spelled out in a report released through the International Association for the Study of Pain (Fordyce 1995), which identified social factors likely to play a role in maintaining pain-related disability and provided suggestions for minimizing the effects of those factors. It is worth noting, however, that many of the recommendations have spawned controversy (e.g., Merskey 1996).

An alternative biopsychosocial model views adjustment to persistent pain as a multifactorial phenomenon with biological, psychological, medicolegal, and social components (Schultz et al. 2000). The Glasgow Illness Model (Waddell et al. 1993) exemplifies this view (see Fig. 1). While nociception is at the core of this model, it includes a host of additional elements. One element that contributes to adjustment involves such cognitive phenomena as fear-avoidance beliefs (McCracken and Gross 1993; Vlaeyen et al. 1995; Asmundson and Taylor 1996), attitudes (Jensen et al. 1994), and coping skills (Keefe et al. 1997; Boothby et al. 1999). Another factor involves affective distress and psychiatric disorders (Robinson and

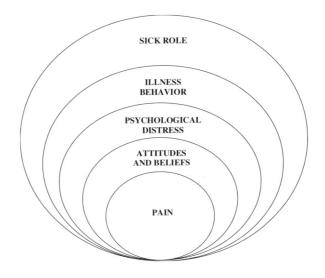

Fig. 1. The Glasgow Illness Model (adapted with permission from Waddell et al. 1993).

Riley 1999; Sullivan 2001). Additionally, pain behaviors (Keefe et al. 2001), functional limitations (King et al. 1998), and social and cultural influences (Carron et al. 1985; Jacob and Kerns 2001) are important contributors to adjustment. Because it includes social influences, the biopsychosocial model can accommodate operant factors associated with pain behavior. Many biopsychosocial factors will be evident in the literature reviewed in the following sections.

SYMPTOM PRESENTATION

MALINGERING

Malingering, "the intentional production of false or grossly exaggerated physical or psychological symptoms, motivated by external incentives" (American Psychiatric Association 1994), accounts for little variance in symptom reporting associated with compensation because of its infrequency (Wallis and Bogduk 1996). Physician estimates of this phenomenon may differ (Leavitt and Sweet 1986), but fewer than 5% of low back patients are generally believed to be malingerers (Fordyce 1995; Hadjistavropoulos 1999).

In fact, the evidence suggests that under-reporting of work-related injuries is more common. Biddle et al. (1998) compared a database of 30,000 known or suspected cases of occupational illness or injury in Michigan, USA, against a workers' compensation claims database. Because of deficiencies in the database, the investigators could only classify claims as "certainly" or "possibly" related to a specific work injury. For musculoskeletal injuries, approximately 12% of injuries were categorized as "certain," while another 35% of injuries were labeled as "possible." Thus, even if all "possible" and "certain" claims became actual claims, over 50% of workers with work-related injuries or illnesses chose not to pursue a claim.

Similarly, researchers have examined relations between economic cycles and applications for compensation benefits. Early work suggested that pain-related claims for work-related disability may increase in recessionary times, presumably as a way to cope with threats to job stability (Volinn et al. 1988; Clemmer and Mohr 1991). A larger and more recent study, however, tracked economic cycles in Ontario between 1975 and 1993. This study showed that both acute and chronic back pain claims increased during economic booms and decreased during slumps (Brooker et al. 1997). In contrast to the former studies, the latter pattern was seen as evidence of a straightforward association between increased workload and increased likelihood of injury, a pattern consistent with biomechanical rather than psychosocial moderators of disability claims.

COMPENSATION STATUS

Numerous studies have compared patients involved in workers' compensation claims or personal injury litigation against patients not involved in such proceedings. As noted earlier, some studies have found either lower symptom reports associated with compensation status (e.g., Melzack et al. 1985) or no association between symptom levels and compensation status (Mendelson 1984; Trabin et al. 1987; Tait et al. 1990). Most research, however, has found higher symptom levels in patients involved in compensation claims (Mendelson 1986; Tait et al. 1988; Lee et al. 1993; Harness and Chase 1994; Fishbain et al. 1995; Vlaeyen et al. 1995; Atlas et al. 1996; Turk and Okifuji 1996; Rainville et al. 1997; Iverson et al. 2001). While the preponderance of evidence suggests that compensation claimants report more severe symptoms (Rohling et al. 1995), other variables may moderate these findings. Of particular interest are studies examining interactions of compensation status with employment status and claim type.

EMPLOYMENT STATUS

McGuigan (1995) examined the effects of compensation and employment status on attribution style, depression, and perceived pain control in 112 male patients. Results showed no effects of compensation status, but significant effects of work status on depression. Using a similar study design, Sanderson et al. (1995) examined several measures of disability in 269 consecutive patients. While they found main effects for work and compensation status, the compensation patients who were unemployed accounted for most of the variance. Compensation patients who were employed did not differ in disability status from patients not involved in compensation.

Grossi et al. (1999) examined length of work absence as a factor associated with pain intensity, disability, emotional distress, and burnout. Using a sample of 586 consecutive patients, they found that patients on sick leave generally reported higher symptom levels than did patients who continued to work. Moreover, patients on extended sick leave reported the highest levels of both burnout and psychiatric symptoms.

While the results of these studies suggest that work status contributes to the distress and dysfunction often attributed to compensation status, interpretation of the results is complicated by the correlational nature of the studies. In particular, it is impossible to assess whether patients with more severe symptoms are more likely to be unemployed or, instead, whether the unemployed develop more severe symptoms. Similarly, it is impossible to evaluate the potential influences of premorbid adjustment. While causality is impossible to infer in light of these considerations, the studies do serve to underscore the importance of assessing both employment and compensation status.

CLAIM STATUS

Several studies have shown that the status of a compensation claim may moderate the general compensation effects described earlier. Guest and Drummond (1992) found that patients awaiting case settlement were more distressed and less functional than were patients who recently had settled their cases. A similar pattern emerged in a study that compared patients anticipating financial compensation with those not expecting compensation (Hayes et al. 1993); those anticipating compensation reported more intense pain, more widespread pain, more nonorganic signs, and more distress than did patients not anticipating financial gain. Similarly, evidence indicates that patients awaiting resolution of a claim obtain higher levels of health care services than patients whose claims have been resolved (Hojsted et al. 1999).

While the studies described above were correlational, a naturalistic study conducted in Canada involved a more rigorous design (Cassidy et al. 2000). In anticipation of a statutory change from tort to no-fault compensation for motor vehicle accidents in the province of Saskatchewan on January 1,

1995, the investigators collected data on accidents occurring 6 months before the change to 12 months after. Individuals involved in motor vehicle accidents before the change in statute were more likely to retain legal representation and reported more intense and widespread pain than did those injured after the change. Further, the change to a no-fault system was associated with a 54% decrease in time to case closure. Interestingly, despite these differences, no changes in work absenteeism were associated with the change in statute.

While the above research suggests that claim status is associated in a straightforward manner with increased symptoms, other research is inconsistent with this pattern. Jamison et al. (1988) studied pain behavior, emotional distress, levels of activity, and prescription drug use in patients with no compensation involvement, with time-limited involvement (workers' compensation), or with unlimited compensation (Social Security Disability Insurance; SSDI). SSDI claimants were the most symptomatic of the groups, exhibiting more pain behavior, more drug use, and more symptom dramatization, while patients involved with workers' compensation did not differ significantly from noncompensation patients. Similarly, Tait et al. (1990) found an interaction between compensation and legal representation. Patients involved in workers' compensation proceedings who had retained attorneys were less depressed and anxious than were compensation patients who had not done so. Patients not involved in such proceedings, however, demonstrated a different pattern. Noncompensation patients who had retained lawyers were more depressed and anxious than were noncompensation patients who had not done so. These results suggest that the decision to retain legal representation was adaptive for compensation patients, perhaps because they were likely to be involved in adversarial proceedings. For noncompensation patients, however, the decision was not adaptive, perhaps because those patients faced different stressors.

While there is some inconsistency in symptom presentation associated with types of compensation and litigation status, the studies provide both correlational and more rigorous evidence suggesting that symptom reports generally are higher among patients involved in pain-related claims. This pattern, consistent with other research involving chronic pain patients (Marbach et al. 1990; Deshields et al. 1995), is also compatible with social psychological research that has shown that efforts to influence how others perceive us are ubiquitous (Mechanic 1972; Arkin and Sheppard 1989). Hence, the above pattern of results is probably less surprising than would be a pattern in which data showed impression management not to be a factor.

OUTCOMES

Conventional wisdom holds that treatment outcomes are poor for chronic pain patients involved in compensation proceedings across a range of treatments, including behavioral interventions (Block et al. 1980; Turk et al. 1983), rehabilitative treatment (Rainville et al. 1997), customary medical care (Greenough and Fraser 1989; Hadler et al. 1995), and surgery (Walsh and Dumitru 1988; Epker and Block 2001). A recent meta-analysis of studies conducted between 1966 and 1991 provided further support for this view (Rohling et al. 1995). Because of the weight of this evidence, some pain treatment programs have gone so far as to bar patients involved in ongoing litigation from entry into treatment (Aronoff 1991).

Not so clear, however, are the factors that may account for the negative outcomes. As has already been indicated, malingering cannot account for the pattern. This section reviews two broad categories of research relevant to factors that influence compensation-related outcomes: (1) outcomes associated with treatment (medical, rehabilitative, and multidisciplinary); and (2) outcomes following the settlement of personal injury claims.

OUTCOMES FOLLOWING TREATMENT

One of the early studies of potential moderators of treatment response among compensation patients attempted to separate the effects of compensation and work status (Dworkin et al. 1985). A retrospective chart review was used to identify predictors of short- and long-term outcomes. While univariate analyses showed that both compensation and employment status predicted short-term outcomes, multiple regression analyses showed that employment status accounted for most of the variance. A similar pattern emerged for long-term outcomes, leading the authors to recommend that further research target the role of employment status in the treatment of compensation patients. Consistent with the results of this study, subsequent research has shown that both employment status (Spitzer 1987; Frank et al. 1996) and time off work (Lancourt and Kettelhut 1992; Waddell 1996) predict response to treatment in compensation patients.

Another variable that has been investigated involves the status of the compensation claim. Becker et al. (1998) looked at differences in response to multidisciplinary treatment among patients who were receiving disability benefits, those who were not receiving benefits, and those who were applying for benefits. Results showed that patients receiving benefits and those not receiving benefits made comparable improvements on measures of pain, distress, and disability. Patients applying for disability benefits, however, showed little change, a pattern that suggested that socioeconomic problems interfered with their response to treatment. Others also have reported results showing that unresolved financial disputes negatively affect outcomes (Wright et al. 1999) and inflate health care utilization (Hojsted et al. 1999).

Expectancies regarding treatment also have been studied. A retrospective study examined relations between short-term outcomes and prior surgical history, reported pain intensity, and expectations regarding return to work among compensation and noncompensation patients (Burns et al. 1995). Compensation patients generally demonstrated poor outcomes relative to noncompensation patients. When return-to-work expectations were considered, however, a different picture emerged. Compensation patients with positive expectations fared as well as noncompensation patients, so that the compensation effect was largely a function of patients with poor expectations.

While not, strictly speaking, a study of compensation (81% of patients in the study were on workers' compensation and the remainder feared job loss), a recent investigation of response to functional restoration treatment is relevant (Pfingsten et al. 1997). This study showed that self-perceived disability prior to treatment was highly predictive of return to work following treatment, a pattern also identified in other work (Feuerstein and Thebarge 1991; Lancourt and Kettelhut 1992; Gatchel et al. 1995b; Szpalski et al. 1995). Similarly, an Australian study examined the impact of an educational media campaign on a large cohort of physicians and patients (Buchbinder et al. 2001). The study measured beliefs regarding low back pain, as well as compensation claims and costs. Results indicated that both physicians and patients modified their beliefs regarding the management of back pain. Further, a 2-year follow-up showed a 15% reduction in low back claims and a 20% reduction in costs. Taken together, these studies point to the importance of beliefs and expectations in shaping a good treatment response for patients, including those involved in compensation, while also underscoring that maladaptive beliefs and negative expectations can undermine response to treatment.

Other psychosocial risk factors associated with poor response to treatment have been identified. For example, several studies have shown that patients reporting higher levels of pain are less likely to demonstrate good outcomes, especially return to work (Lancourt and Kettelhut 1992; Gatchel et al. 1995b; Klenerman et al. 1995). Similarly, Gatchel et al. (1995a) found that somatic preoccupation was associated with poor return to work among patients with chronic low back pain. Depression (Hasenbring et al. 1994) and fear-avoidance beliefs (Hasenbring et al. 1994; Klenerman et al. 1995) also have been identified as predictors of poor outcomes. In these and other studies, psychological factors have been more predictive of outcomes than medical factors (Gatchel and Gardea 1999).

In light of the above findings, it is not surprising that the most effective treatments for intractable pain following work-related and other compensable injuries have aimed at both functional and psychological factors. The model for this kind of program, a combination of aggressive, goal-oriented rehabilitation and psycho-educational treatment, has achieved high rates of return to work for patients with chronic low back pain (Mayer et al. 1986, 1987; Cutler et al. 1994), postsurgical low back pain (Mayer et al. 1998), and cervical spine disorders (Wright et al. 1999). Numerous other studies report successful outcomes for patients with chronic pain conditions (Alaranta et al. 1994; Hazard et al. 1994; Hazard 1995; Corey et al. 1996; Rainville et al. 1996; Kishino et al. 2000). Interestingly, behavioral treatments specifically targeting fear-avoidance beliefs and behavior also have reported good success, even for patients who have failed multidisciplinary treatment (Vlaeyen et al. 1995, 2001; Vlaeyen and Linton 2000). The success of such interventions among compensation patients suggests that unaddressed but modifiable behavioral and psychosocial factors, rather than compensation status itself, account for a significant percentage of problematic outcomes.

OUTCOMES FOLLOWING CLAIM SETTLEMENT

While the literature concerning outcomes of treatment reflects both problems and promise, such inconsistencies cannot be ascribed to research associated with post-settlement outcomes. An early, archival study of 50 cases presenting with "gross neurotic symptoms" reported that symptoms of "accident neurosis" largely resolved following resolution of a claim (Miller 1961). A similar conclusion was reached in another study based largely on personal observations (Parker 1970).

Subsequent empirical studies, however, have consistently failed to support the latter conclusion (Mendelson 1992; Kolbinson et al. 1996). For example, Mendelson (1995) interviewed 760 litigants following settlement of their claims. Of the 264 individuals not working at the time of settlement, 198 (75%) still were not working an average of 23 months after settlement. Kelly and Smith (1981) followed a smaller cohort of patients after claim settlement, finding that 90% of those not working at the time of settlement were not working 2 years later. Greenough and Fraser (1989) interviewed 150 compensation and 150 noncompensation patients from 1 to 5 years after their initial injuries, finding that the settlement had no effect on adjustment for either group. Norris and Watt (1983) followed 61 patients with whiplash symptoms, two-thirds of whom were litigating. The investigators categorized patients according to degree of medical findings (no physical abnormality versus reduced range of motion versus objective neurological loss). No differences were found in post-settlement symptoms associated with compensation status: 50–66% reported no change in their symptoms, and approximately 25% reported symptoms worsening after settlement. In short, contrary to initial claims, the data on long-term outcomes following case settlement indicate that these patients are not "cured by a verdict." It is testimony to the power of stereotyping that perceptions persist in the health care professions that run counter to this evidence.

SYSTEMIC FACTORS INVOLVED IN COMPENSATION

Although the discussion to this point has focused on patient factors associated with symptom presentation and treatment, it is important to recognize systemic factors that also may influence these matters. Hadler (1987) has noted that injured workers who consult physicians encounter a dynamic quite different from that faced by patients who seek medical advice for a noncompensable injury. In the latter case, patients consult physicians with symptoms that secondarily interfere with function. Physicians diagnose and treat the presenting symptoms, expecting that symptomatic improvement will ameliorate function. In the occupational medicine context, however, patients who present to physicians do so with a primary symptom of work incapacity. Because physicians are charged primarily with minimizing work incapacity, other symptoms can be of secondary importance. This situation may cause physicians to downplay the significance of symptoms, leading patients to lose confidence in their diagnosis (Tait et al. 1988). At the same time, patients may promote their symptoms either in response to distress or in an effort to convince physicians of their work incapacity (MacLeod et al. 2001), leading physicians either to discount symptom reports (e.g., Clayer et al. 1986; Tarasuk and Eakin 1995; Merskey and Teasell 2000) or to develop pessimistic expectations regarding treatment outcomes (Simmonds and Kumar 1996). This dynamic can undermine effective working relationships between patients and physicians, relationships that probably are more important when dealing with chronic rather than acute problems. In turn, problematic physician-patient interactions may contribute to iatrogenic disability (Sullivan and Loeser 1992; Loeser and Sullivan 1995).

A recent study demonstrates the pernicious nature of the compensation dynamic (Hadler et al. 1995). The investigators followed patients who had low back injuries of comparable severity and whose treatment was covered through either workers' compensation or standard insurance. At 12 weeks, rates of return to work were similar for both groups. However, patients in the compensation group rated their functional well-being as significantly worse than did those who received treatment under the noncompensation format. The results suggest problems endemic to the compensation system itself.

Several studies have addressed elements of compensation systems that may contribute to iatrogenesis. Gallagher and colleagues (1995) have found evidence that patients involved in compensation proceedings are referred too late for multidisciplinary treatment. While empirical research suggests that multidisciplinary treatment should be considered for patients who have not demonstrated substantial improvement within 3 months (Frank et al. 1996, 1998), much longer delays are common in chronic pain patients (Gallagher and Myers 1996). Because the likelihood of return to work diminishes with each passing month of disability (Crook and Moldofsky 1994; Waddell 1996), delays in referral may contribute meaningfully to failure to return to work (Matheson and Brophy 1997). Among other factors, these delays may reflect negative attitudes toward treatment at pain centers that may be held by referring physicians, case managers, insurers, and others involved in compensation-related claims (Simmonds and Kumar 1996; Robinson et al. 1998).

Referral delays are not the only aspect of treatment of compensable injuries that may prejudice outcomes. Evidence indicates that negative stereotypes, such as those described earlier by Miller (1961), continue to influence medical thinking (Gallagher et al. 1995). When asked to rate the severity of symptoms presented by patients involved in compensation claims, both the lay public (Tait and Chibnall 1994; Chibnall and Tait 1995) and health care providers (Quintner 1995; Tarasuk and Eakin 1995; Merskey and Teasell 2000) tend to discount symptoms presented by patients involved in such proceedings. Moreover, as noted earlier, the negative stereotypes are not one-sided. Patients involved in compensation claims related to intractable pain seem to place less confidence in physician diagnoses than do patients not so involved (Tait et al. 1988).

Because of the dynamics described above, coping with compensation systems can be stressful. It appears that one way in which patients cope with such stress is to seek legal representation, a tactic that may reduce levels of depression and anxiety (Tait et al. 1990). Furthermore, patients who retain legal representation may receive higher impairment and disability ratings than those who do not (Chibnall and Tait 2000). On the other hand, while the decision to seek legal representation may have adaptive elements, it may be a mixed blessing. Evidence indicates that legal representation is associated with longer claim durations and perhaps with higher levels of post-settlement disability (Waddell 1996; Hadler 1997; Chibnall and Tait 2000).

Aside from ethical issues and emotional stressors associated with negative stereotypes, there is reason to believe that such stereotypes can create self-fulfilling prophecies (Tarasuk and Eakin 1995; May et al. 1999; Merskey and Teasell 2000). A long-term study of a large cohort of consecutive patients referred for orthopedic evaluation and treatment exemplifies the issue. In this study, Atlas et al. (2000) reported that compensation patients exhibited rates of return to work that were comparable to those achieved by patients not involved in compensation, although the compensation group rated pain severity as higher. Patients who underwent surgery, however, reported lower symptom levels than did nonsurgical patients, and patients in the compensation group underwent significantly less surgery than did noncompensation patients. While the conclusions that may be drawn are speculative, the pattern of findings suggests that surgical decision-making may have been influenced by compensation status, a pattern noted by others (Merskey and Teasell 2000). In turn, this situation could leave compensation patients with higher levels of residual symptoms.

Stereotypes also appear to influence other forms of medical decision-making. Chibnall and Tait (2000) found considerable variability among occupational medicine physicians in the management of workers who sustained low back injuries that required impairment ratings. Aside from the high levels of variability in diagnostic testing and treatment, the results suggested that workers belonging to a racial minority incurred lower expenditures for treatment. In a re-analysis of the data, Tait and Chibnall (2001) found that both race and legal representation were associated with differences in disability management. Costs associated with temporary total disability (TTD) payments disbursed to claimants for excused work absences were comparable for African Americans and Caucasians when both had legal representation. Without legal representation, however, TTD costs for African Americans were 10% of those for Caucasians. A similar pattern applied for impairment ratings, where African Americans without legal representation received ratings that were only approximately 20% of those given to Caucasians.

CONCLUDING COMMENTS

If nothing else, the studies reviewed above suggest that the effects of compensation or litigation status on symptom presentation and treatment response are inadequately explained by reference to a "greenback poultice" (a term used in the United States to explain remission of pain following settlement of litigation). This is not to say that patients with potentially compensable injuries present and respond to treatment similarly to patients not involved in compensation proceedings. In fact, the data generally show that compensation patients present more severe and disabling symptoms and respond more poorly to treatment (unless the treatment explicitly targets functional and psychosocial factors). Instead, there appear to be factors that interact with compensation status to influence symptom presentation and treatment response.

For example, patients with compensable injuries report more severe symptoms under certain conditions. One involves employment: employed patients involved in compensation claims report symptom levels comparable to those of noncompensation patients, while unemployed patients involved in compensation report symptom levels that are significantly higher. Similarly, emotionally distressed patients report more severe symptoms related to pain and disability than do nondistressed patients, whose symptom reports are generally comparable to those of noncompensation patients. Other factors, such as return-to-work expectations, also appear to influence symptom report.

Response to treatment also appears to be associated with moderating variables. Compensation patients who are employed respond to treatment as well as do patients not involved in compensation proceedings, while those who are unemployed respond more poorly. Similarly, patients with compensable injuries who expect to return to work demonstrate a good response to treatment relative to patients not involved in compensation, while compensation patients without such expectations fare less well. Contrariwise, patients who anticipate financial compensation and face economic uncertainty do not respond well to treatment, while those with more secure financial arrangements do better.

A diathesis-stress model (Monroe and Simons 1991; Dworkin and Banks 1999) may represent a way to integrate the findings described above. According to this model, patient vulnerabilities (diatheses) are activated in response to stressors that they confront, such that the interaction of stressors and diatheses occasions psychological and functional pathology. For patients who are hardy (Younkin and Betz 1996; Abramson 2000), diatheses are relatively few and the likelihood of pathology relatively low, while less hardy patients exhibit greater pathology in response to similar levels of stress. Regardless of the level of hardiness that patients exhibit, however, the model postulates that pathology is increasingly likely with higher levels of stress (either additive stressors or stressors with which patients cope poorly). Hence, even the hardiest patients exhibit diatheses under high stress conditions.

Fig. 2 depicts a diathesis-stress model for the development of pain-related disability that might apply to patients who incur potentially compensable injuries. A partial list of diatheses includes five variables, each of which has been linked to outcomes in pain research: low levels of education (Frymoyer and Cats-Baril 1987; Hasenbring et al. 1994), coping skill deficits (Boothby et al. 1999), maladaptive beliefs and/or low expectancies regarding functional recovery (Burns et al. 1995; Klenerman et al. 1995), premorbid emotional status (Gatchel et al. 1995b), and ethnicity (Gatchel et al. 1995a). While all five items represent subject variables, ethnicity is likely to represent a diathesis because of societal factors, including potential disparities in treatment provided to African Americans (Tait and Chibnall 2001).

These vulnerabilities interact with two sets of stressors associated with painful occupational injuries. One set involves stressors relevant to any chronic pain experience. These include, at a minimum, the prospect of coping not only with pain, but also the distress, disability, and role changes

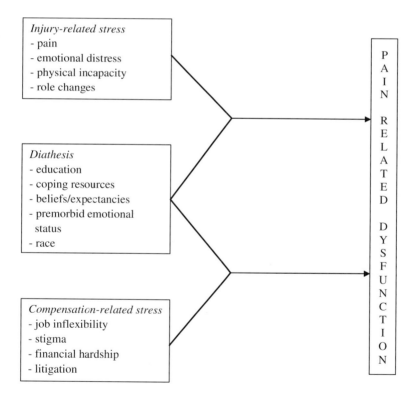

Injury-related stress
- pain
- emotional distress
- physical incapacity
- role changes

Diathesis
- education
- coping resources
- beliefs/expectancies
- premorbid emotional
  status
- race

Compensation-related stress
- job inflexibility
- stigma
- financial hardship
- litigation

PAIN RELATED DYSFUNCTION

Fig. 2. The diathesis-stress model for pain-related disability with compensable injury (see text for details).

often associated with refractory pain (Tait et al. 1989). While a percentage of patients facing this set of stressors possess diatheses likely to hamper a productive adjustment, many manage these stressors reasonably well with standard medical care (Chapman et al. 1979; Frymoyer 1992).

The second set of stressors associated with the compensation process not only adds to those associated with pain, but may represent hardships with which patients are poorly equipped to cope (e.g., job inflexibility, financial hardship, litigation, stigma). The diathesis-stress model predicts that a significant percentage of patients who cope satisfactorily with injury-related stressors will prove incapable of coping with compensation-related stress (Monroe and Simons 1991). Not only would this group be expected to exhibit higher levels of disability, but, as the literature indicates, it also would be expected to respond less well to standard treatment than patients exposed only to the first set of stressors.

Recent treatment paradigms have addressed the vulnerabilities and stresses of the group coping both with chronic pain and compensation. Many of these programs target each element of the diathesis-stress model: vulnerabilities (e.g., deficient coping skills, maladaptive beliefs), injury-related stresses (e.g., physical incapacity), and compensation-related stresses (e.g., job inflexibility). Data from these treatment programs suggest that good outcomes can be obtained in a substantial number of patients with attention to these areas. Unfortunately, such integrated treatment continues to represent the exception rather than the rule (Frank et al. 1998).

Of course, treatment programs cannot address all of the stressors associated with compensation systems, such as stigmatization, disparities in treatment, and inflexible work settings. These and other stressors appear endemic to the current system of workers' compensation (Hadler 1997). Further research should target these issues. Similarly, further studies are needed that examine long-term outcomes, including those for patients who have "graduated" from compensation proceedings, to assess long-term adaptation when stresses associated with compensation systems have moderated. Models such as the diathesis-stress model may be of use in guiding this research, especially if they can identify patient and system variables associated with long-term outcomes.

ACKNOWLEDGMENT

This work was supported in part by grant no. RO1-HS 13087-01 from the Agency for Healthcare Research and Quality.

REFERENCES

Abramson LY. Optimistic cognitive styles and invulnerability to depression. In: Gilham JE (Ed). *The Science of Optimism and Hope: Research Essays in Honor of Martin E.P. Seligman*. Philadelphia: Templeton Foundation Press, 2000, pp 75–98.

AFL-CIO. *Stop the Pain*. Washington, DC: American Federation of Labor and Congress of Industrial Organizations, 1997.

Alaranta H, Rytokoski U, Rissanen A, et al. Intensive physical and psychosocial training program for patients with chronic low back pain: a controlled clinical trial. *Spine* 1994; 19:1339–1449.

American Psychiatric Association. *Diagnostic and Statistical Manual of Mental Disorders*, 4th ed. Washington, DC: American Psychiatric Association, 1994.

Aronoff GM. Chronic pain and the disability epidemic. *Clin J Pain* 1991; 7:330–338.

Arkin RM, Sheppard JA. Strategic self-presentation: an overview. In: Cody M, McLaughlin M (Eds). *Psychology of Tactical Communication*. Clevedon: Multilingual Matters, 1989, pp 175–193.

Asmundson GJG, Taylor S. Role of anxiety sensitivity in pain-related fear and avoidance. *J Behav Med* 1996; 19:577–586.

Atlas SJ, Deyo RA, Keller RB, et al. The Maine lumbar spine study, part II: 1-year outcomes of surgical and nonsurgical management of sciatica. *Spine* 1996; 21:1777–1786.

Atlas SJ, Chang Y, Kammann E, et al. Long-term disability and return to work among patients who have a herniated lumbar disc: the effect of disability compensation. *J Bone Joint Surg Am* 2000; 82-A:4–15.

Becker N, Hojsted J, Sjogren P, Eriksen J. Sociodemographic predictors of treatment outcome in chronic non-malignant pain patients. Do patients receiving or applying for disability pension benefit from multidisciplinary pain treatment? *Pain* 1998; 77:279–287.

Bellamy R. Compensation neurosis: financial reward for illness as nocebo. *Clin Orthop* 1997; 336:94–106.

Biddle J, Roberts K, Rosenman KD, Welch EM. What percentage of workers with work-related illnesses receive workers' compensation benefits? *J Occup Environ Med* 1998; 40:325–331.

Block AR, Kremer E, Gaylor M. Behavioral treatment of chronic pain: variables affecting treatment efficacy. *Pain* 1980; 8:367–375.

Boothby JL, Thorn BE, Stroud MW, Jensen MP. Coping with pain. In: Gatchel RJ, Turk DC (Eds). *Psychosocial Factors in Pain: Critical Perspectives*. New York: Guilford Press, 1999, pp 343–359.

Brooker A-S, Frank JW, Tarasuk VS. Back pain claim rates and the business cycle. *Soc Sci Med* 1997; 45:429–439.

Buchbinder R, Jolley D, Wyatt M. Population based intervention to change back pain beliefs and disability: three part evaluation. *Bone Muscle Joint* 2001; 322:1516–1520.

Burns JW, Sherman ML, Devine J, Mahoney N, Pawl R. Association between workers' compensation and outcome following multidisciplinary treatment for chronic pain: roles of mediators and moderators. *Clin J Pain* 1995; 11:94–102.

Butterfield PG, Spencer PS, Redmond N, Feldstein A, Perrin N. Low back pain: predictors of absenteeism, residual symptoms, functional impairment, and medical costs in Oregon workers' compensation recipients. *Am J Ind Med* 1998; 34:559–567.

Carron H, DeGood DE, Tait R. A comparison of low back pain patients in the United States and New Zealand: psychosocial and economic factors affecting severity of disability. *Pain* 1985; 21:77–89.

Cassidy JD, Carroll LJ, Cote P, et al. Effect of eliminating compensation for pain and suffering on the outcome of insurance claims for whiplash injury. *N Engl J Med* 2000; 342:1179–1186.

Chapman CR, Sola AE, Bonica JJ. Illness behavior and depression compared in pain center and private practice patients. *Pain* 1979; 6:1–7.

Chapman SL, Brena SF. Pain and litigation. In: Melzack R, Wall P (Eds). *The Textbook of Pain*. New York: Churchill Livingstone, 1989, pp 1032–1041.

Chibnall JT, Tait RC. Observer perceptions of low back pain: effects of pain report and other contextual factors. *J Appl Soc Psychol* 1995; 25:418–439.

Chibnall JT, Tait RC. Disability management of low back injuries by employer-retained physicians: ratings and costs. *Am J Ind Med* 2000; 38:529–538.

Clark W, Haldeman S. The development of guideline factors for the evaluation of disability in neck and back injuries. *Spine* 1993; 18:1736–1745.

Clayer JR, Bookless-Pratz CL, Ross MW. The evaluation of illness behaviour and exaggeration of disability. *Br J Psychiatry* 1986; 148:296–299.

Clemmer DI, Mohr DL. Low-back injuries in a heavy industry. II. Labor market forces. *Spine* 1991; 16:831–834.

Corey DT, Koepfler LE, Etlin D, Day HI. A limited functional restoration program for injured workers: a randomized trial. *J Occup Rehabil* 1996; 6:239–249.

Crook J, Moldofsky H. The probability of recovery and return to work from work disability as a function of time. *Qual Life Res* 1994; 3:S97–S109.

Cutler RB, Fishbain DA, Rosomoff HL, et al. Does nonsurgical pain center treatment of chronic pain return patients to work? A review and meta-analysis of the literature. *Spine* 1994; 19:643–652.

Deshields TL, Tait RC, Gfeller JD, Chibnall JT. Relationship between social desirability and self-report in chronic pain patients. *Clin J Pain* 1995; 11:189–193.

Deyo RA, Cherkin D, Conrad D, Volinn E. Cost, controversy, crisis: low back pain and the health of the public. *Annu Rev Public Health* 1995; 12:141–156.

Durbin D. Workplace injuries and the role of insurance: claims costs, outcomes, and incentives. *Clin Orthop* 1997; 336:18–32.

Dworkin RH, Banks SM. A vulnerability-diathesis-stress model of chronic pain: herpes zoster and the development of postherpetic neuralgia. In: Gatchel RJ, Turk DC (Eds). *Psychosocial Factors in Pain: Critical Perspectives*. New York: Guilford Press, 1999, pp 247–269.

Dworkin RH, Handlin DS, Richlin DM, Brand L, Vannucci C. Unraveling the effects of compensation, litigation, and employment on treatment response in chronic pain. *Pain* 1985; 23:49–59.

Epker J, Block AR. Presurgical psychological screening in back pain patients: a review. *Clin J Pain* 2001; 17:200–205.

Feuerstein M, Thebarge RW. Perceptions of disability and occupational stress as discriminators of work disability in patients with chronic pain. *J Occup Rehabil* 1991; 1:185–195.

Feuerstein M, Burrell, LM, Miller VI, et al. Clinical management of carpal tunnel syndrome: a 12-year review of outcomes. *Am J Ind Med* 1999; 35:232–245.

Fishbain DA, Goldberg M, Steele-Rosomoff R, Rosomoff H. Chronic pain patients and the nonorganic physical sign of nondermatomal sensory abnormalities (NDSA). *Psychosomatics* 1991; 32:294–303.

Fishbain DA, Rosomoff HL, Cutler RB, Steele-Rosomoff R. Secondary gain concept: a review of the scientific evidence. *Clin J Pain* 1995; 11:6–21.

Fordyce WE. *Back Pain in the Workplace*. Seattle: IASP Press, 1995.

Fordyce WE. On the nature of illness and disability: an editorial. *Clin Orthop* 1997; 336:47–51.

Fordyce WE, Fowler RS, Lehmann JF, et al. Operant conditioning in the treatment of chronic pain. *Arch Phys Med Rehabil* 1973; 54:399–408.

Fordyce WE, Roberts AH, Sternbach RA. The behavioural management of chronic pain: a response to critics. *Pain* 1985; 22:113–125.

Frank JW, Brooker A-S, DeMaio SE, et al. Disability resulting from occupational low back pain. Part II: What do we know about secondary prevention? A review of the scientific evidence on prevention after disability begins. *Spine* 1996; 21:2918–2929.

Frank J, Sinclair S, Hogg-Johnson S, et al. Preventing disability from work-related low-back pain. *CMAJ* 1998; 158:1625–1631.

Frymoyer JW. Predicting disability from low back pain. *Clin Orthop* 1992; 279:101–109.

Frymoyer JD. Cost and control of industrial musculoskeletal injuries. In: Nordin M, Andersson GBJ, Pope MH (Eds). *Musculoskeletal Disorders in the Workplace: Principles and Practice*. St. Louis: Mosby-Year Book, 1997, pp 62–71.

Frymoyer JW, Cats-Baril W. Predictors of low back pain disability. *Clin Orthop* 1987; 221:89–98.

Gallagher RM, Myers P. Referral delay in back pain patients on worker's compensation: costs and policy implications. *Psychosomatics* 1996; 37:270–284.

Gallagher RM, Williams B, Skelly J, et al. Worker's compensation and return-to-work in low back pain. *Pain* 1995; 61:299–307.

Garofalo JP, Polatin P. Low back pain: an epidemic in industrialized countries. In: Gatchel RJ, Turk DC (Eds). *Psychosocial Factors in Pain*. New York: Guilford Press, 1999; pp 164–174.

Gatchel RJ, Gardea MA. Psychosocial issues: their importance in predicting disability, response to treatment, and search for compensation. *Neurol Clin* 1999; 17:149–166.

Gatchel RJ, Polatin PB, Kinney RK. Predicting outcome of chronic back pain using clinical predictors of psychopathology: a prospective analysis. *Health Psychol* 1995a; 14:415–420.

Gatchel RJ, Polatin PB, Mayer TG. The dominant role of psychosocial risk factors in the development of chronic low back pain disability. *Spine* 1995b; 20:2702–2709.

Greenough CG, Fraser RD. The effects of compensation on recovery from low-back injury. *Spine* 1989; 14:947–955.

Greenwood JG. Low-back impairment-rating practices of orthopaedic surgeons and neurosurgeons in West Virginia. *Spine* 1985; 10:773–776.

Grossi G, Soares JJF, Angesleva J, Perski A. Psychosocial correlates of long-term sick-leave among patients with musculoskeletal pain. *Pain* 1999; 80:607–619.

Guest GH, Drummond PD. Effect of compensation on emotional state and disability in chronic back pain. *Pain* 1992; 48:125–130.

Hadjistavropoulos T. Chronic pain on trial: the influence of litigation and compensation on chronic pain syndromes. In: Block AR, Kremer EF, Fernandez E (Eds). *Handbook of Pain Syndromes*. Mahwah, NJ: Lawrence Erlbaum, 1999, pp 59–76.

Hadler NM. Regional musculoskeletal diseases of the low back: cumulative trauma versus single incident. *Clin Orthop* 1987; 221:33–41.

Hadler NM. Work incapacity from low back pain: the international quest for redress. *Clin Orthop* 1997; 336:79–93.

Hadler NM, Carey TS, Garrett J, et al. The influence of indemnification by workers' compensation insurance on recovery from acute backache. *Spine* 1995; 20:2710–2715.

Harness DM, Chase PF. Litigation and chronic facila pain. *J Orofac Pain* 1994; 8:289–292.

Hasenbring M, Marienfeld G, Kuhlendahl D, Soyka D. Risk factors of chronicity in lumbar disc patients. *Spine* 1994; 19:2759–2765.

Hayes B, Solyom CAE, Wing PC, Berkowitz J. Use of psychometric measures and nonorganic signs testing in detecting nomogenic disorders in low back pain patients. *Spine* 1993; 18:1254–1262.

Hazard RG. Spine update: functional restoration. *Spine* 1995; 20:2345–2348.

Hazard RG, Haugh LD, Green PA, Jones PL. Chronic low back pain: the relationship between patient satisfaction and pain, impairment, and disability outcomes. *Spine* 1994; 19:881–887.

Hendler NH, Kozikowski JG. Overlooked physical diagnoses in chronic pain patients involved in litigation. *Psychosomatics* 1993; 34:494–501.

Hinderer SR, Rondinelli RD, Katz RT. Measurement issues in impairment rating and disability evaluation. In: Rondinelli RD, Katz RT (Eds). *Impairment Rating and Disability Evaluation*. Philadelphia: W.B. Saunders, 2000, pp 35–52.

Hojsted J, Alban A, Hagild K, Eriksen J. Utilisation of health care system by chronic pain patients who applied for disability pensions. *Pain* 1999; 82:275–282.

Iverson GL, King RJ, Scott JG, Adams RL. Cognitive complaints in litigating patients with head injuries or chronic pain. *J Forensic Neuropsychol* 2001; 2:19–30.

Jacob MC, Kerns RD. Assessment of the psychosocial context of the experience of chronic pain. In: Turk DC, Melzack R (Eds). *The Handbook of Pain Assessment,* 2nd ed. New York: Guilford Press, 2001; 362–379.

Jamison RN, Matt DA, Parris WCV. Effects of time-limited vs. unlimited compensation on pain behavior and treatment outcome in low back pain patients. *J Psychosom Res* 1988; 32:277–283.

Jensen MP, Turner JA, Romano JM. Correlates of improvement in multidisciplinary treatment of chronic pain. *J Consult Clin Psychol* 1994; 62:172–179.

Katz RT, Tait RC. Disability evaluation and unexplained pain. In: Rondinelli RD, Katz RT (Eds). *Impairment Rating and Disability Evaluation.* Philadelphia: W.B. Saunders, 2000, pp 257–274.

Keefe FJ, Affleck G, Lefebvre JC, et al. Pain coping strategies and coping efficacy in rheumatoid arthritis: a daily process analysis. *Pain* 1997; 69:35–42.

Keefe FS, Williams DA, Smith S. Assessment of pain behaviors. In: Turk DC, Melzack R (Eds). *Handbook of Pain Assessment,* 2nd ed. New York: Guilford Press, 2001, pp 170–187.

Kelly R, Smith BN. Post-traumatic syndrome: another myth discredited. *J R Soc Med* 1981; 74:275–277.

Kennedy F. The mind of the injured worker: its effect on disability periods. *Comp Med* 1946:1:19–24.

King PM, Tuckwell N, Barrett TE. A critical review of functional capacity evaluations. *Phys Ther* 1998; 78:852–866.

Kishino ND, Polatin PB, Brewer S, Hoffman K. Long-term effectiveness of combined spine surgery and functional restoration: a prospective study. *J Occup Ther* 2000; 10:235–239.

Klenerman L, Slade PD, Stanley IM, et al. The prediction of chronicity in patients with an acute attack of low back pain in a general practice setting. *Spine* 1995; 20:478–484.

Kolbinson DA, Epstein JB, Burgess JA. Temporomandibular disorders, headaches, and neck pain following motor vehicle accidents and the effect of litigation: review of the literature. *J Orofac Pain* 1996; 10:101–125.

Lancourt J, Kettelhut M. Predicting return to work for lower back pain patients receiving worker's compensation. *Spine* 1992; 17:629–640.

Leavitt F, Sweet JJ. Characteristics and frequency of malingering among patients with low back pain. *Pain* 1986; 25:357–364.

Lee J, Giles K, Drummond PD. Psychological disturbances and an exaggerated response to pain in patients with whiplash injury. *J Psychosom Res* 1993; 37:105–110.

Loeser JD, Sullivan M. Disability in the chronic low back pain patient may be iatrogenic. *Pain Forum* 1995; 4:114–121.

MacLeod FK, LaChapelle DL, Hadjistavropoulos T, Pfeifer JE. The effect of disability claimants' coping styles on judgments of pain, disability, and compensation: a vignette study. *Rehabil Psychol* 2001; 46:417–435.

Marbach JJ, Lennon MC, Link BG, Dohrenwend BP. Losing face: sources of stigma as perceived by chronic facial pain patients. *J Behav Med* 1990; 13:583–604.

Matheson LN, Brophy RG. Aggressive early intervention after occupational back injury: some preliminary observations. *J Occup Rehabil* 1997; 7:107–117.

May C, Doyle H, Chew-Graham C. Medical knowledge and the intractable patient: the case of chronic low back pain. *Soc Sci Med* 1999; 48:523–534.

Mayer TG, Gatchel RJ, Kishino N, et al. A prospective short-term study of chronic low back pain patients utilizing novel objective functional measurement. *Pain* 1986; 25:53–68.

Mayer TG, Gatchel RJ, Mayer H, et al. A prospective two-year study of functional restoration in industrial low back injury: an objective assessment procedure. *JAMA* 1987; 258:1763–1767.

Mayer T, McMahon MJ, Gatchel RF, et al. Socioeconomic outcomes of combined spine surgery and functional restoration in workers' compensation spinal disorders with matched controls. *Spine* 1998; 23:598–606.

McCracken LM, Gross RT. Does anxiety affect coping with pain? *Clin J Pain* 1993; 9:253–259.

McGuigan JB. Attributional style and depression in men receiving treatment for chronic pain. *J Appl Rehabil Coun* 1995; 26:21–25.

Mechanic D. Social psychologic factors affecting the presentation of bodily complaints. *N Engl J Med* 1972; 286:1132–1139.

Melzack R, Wall PD. Pain mechanisms: a new theory. *Science* 1965; 150:971–979.

Melzack R, Katz J, Jeans ME. The role of compensation in chronic pain: analysis using a new method of scoring the McGill Pain Questionnaire. *Pain* 1985; 23:101–112.

Mendelson G. Compensation, pain complaints, and psychological disturbance. *Pain* 1984; 20:169–177.

Mendelson G. Chronic pain and compensation: a review. *J Pain Symptom Manage* 1986; 1:135–144.

Mendelson G. Compensation and chronic pain. *Pain* 1992; 48:121–123.

Mendelson G. 'Compensation neurosis' revisited: outcome studies of the effects of litigation. *J Psychosom Res* 1995; 39:695–706.

Merskey H. Re: Back pain in the workplace. *Pain* 1996; 65:111–114.

Merskey H, Teasell RW. The disparagement of pain: social influences on medical thinking. *Pain Res Manage* 2000; 5:259–270.

Michel A, Kohlmann T, Raspe H. The association between clinical findings on physical examination and self-reported severity in back pain. *Spine* 1997; 22:296–304.

Miller H. Accident neurosis. *BMJ* 1961; 1:919–925, 992–998.

Monroe SM, Simons AD. Diathesis-stress theories in the context of life stress research: implications for the depressive disorders. *Psychol Bull* 1991; 110:406–425.

Nachemson A. Chronic pain—the end of the welfare state? *Qual Life Res* 1994; 3:S11–S17.

Norris SH, Watt I. The prognosis of neck injuries resulting from rear-end vehicle collisions. *J Bone Joint Surg Br* 1983; 65:608–611.

Parker N. Accident neurosis. *Med J Aust* 1970; 2:362–265.

Pfingsten M, Hildebrandt J, Leibing E, Franz C, Saur P. Effectiveness of a multimodal treatment program for chronic low-back pain. *Pain* 1997; 73:77–85.

Pope MH, Andersson GBH. Prevention. In: Nordin M, Andersson GBJ, Pope MH (Eds). *Musculoskeletal Disorders in the Workplace: Principles and Practice.* St. Louis, MO: Mosby-Year Book, 1997, pp 244–249.

Quintner JL. The Australian RSI debate: stereotyping and medicine. *Disabil Rehabil* 1995; 17:256–262.

Rainville J, Sobel J, Banco R, Levine H, Childs L. Low back and cervical spine disorders. *Orthop Clin North Am* 1996; 27:729–746.

Rainville J, Sobel JB, Hartigan C, Wright A. The effect of compensation involvement on the reporting of pain and disability by patients referred for rehabilitation of chronic low back pain. *Spine* 1997; 22:2016–2024.

Robinson ME, Riley JL. The role of emotion in pain. In: Gatchel RJ, Turk DC (Eds). *Psychosocial Factors in Pain: Critical Perspectives.* New York: Guilford Press, 1999, pp 74–88.

Robinson JP, Allen T, Fulton LD, Martin DC. Perceived efficacy of pain clinics in the rehabilitation of injured workers. *Clin J Pain* 1998; 14:202–208.

Rohling ML, Binder LM, Langhinrichsen-Rohling J. Money matters: a meta-analytic review of the association between financial compensation and the experience and treatment of chronic pain. *Health Psychol* 1995; 14:537–547.

Sanderson PL, Todd BD, Holt GR, Getty CJM. Compensation, work status, and disability in low back pain patients. *Spine* 1995; 20:554–556.

Schultz IZ, Crook J, Fraser K, Joy PW. Models of diagnosis and rehabilitation in musculoskeletal pain-related occupational disability. *J Occup Rehabil* 2000; 10:271–293.

Silverstein BA, Stetson DS, Keyserling WM, Fine LF. Work-related musculoskeletal disorders: comparison of data sources for surveillance. *Am J Ind Med* 1997; 31:600–608.

Simmonds M, Kumar S. Does knowledge of a patient's workers' compensation status influence clinical judgments? *J Occup Rehabil* 1996; 6:93–107.

Spitzer WO. Diagnosis of the problem (the problem of diagnosis). *Spine* 1987; 12 (7S):S16–S22.

Sullivan MD. Assessment of psychiatric disorders. In: Turk DC, Melzack R (Eds). *Handbook of Pain Assessment,* 2nd ed. New York: Guilford Press, 2001, 275–291.

Sullivan MD, Loeser JD. The diagnosis of disability: treating and rating disability in a pain clinic. *Arch Intern Med* 1992; 152:1829–1835.

Szpalski M, Nordin M, Skovron ML, Melot C, Cukier D. Health care utilization for low back pain in Belgium. *Spine* 1995; 20:431–442.

Tait RC, Chibnall JT. Observer perceptions of chronic low back pain. *J Appl Soc Psychol* 1994; 24:415–431.

Tait RC, Chibnall JT. Work injury management of refractory low back pain: relations with ethnicity, legal representation and diagnosis. *Pain* 2001; 91:47–56.

Tait RC, Margolis RB, Krause SJ, Liebowitz E. Compensation status and symptoms reported by patients with chronic pain. *Arch Phys Med Rehabil* 1988; 69:1027–1029.

Tait RC, Chibnall JT, Duckro PN, Deshields TL. Stable factors in chronic pain. *Clin J Pain* 1989; 5:323–328.

Tait RC, Chibnall JT, Richardson WD. Litigation and employment status: effects on patients with chronic pain. *Pain* 1990; 43:37–46.

Tarasuk VS, Eakin JM. The problem of legitimacy in the experience of work-related back injury. *Qualitative Health Res* 1995; 5:204–221.

Thimineur M, Kaliszewski T, Sood P. Malingering and symptom magnification: a case report illustrating the limitations of clinical judgment. *Conn Med* 2000; 64:399–401.

Trabin T, Rader C, Cummings C. A comparison of pain management outcomes for disability compensation and non-compensation patients. *Psychol Health* 1987; 1:341–351.

Turk DC, Okifuji A. Perception of traumatic onset, compensation status, and physical findings: impact on pain severity, emotional distress, and disability in chronic pain patients. *J Behav Med* 1996; 19:435–453.

Turk DC, Meichenbaum DH, Genest M. *Pain and Behavioural Medicine: A Cognitive-Behavioral Perspective*. New York: Guilford Press, 1983.

U.S. Department of Labor. *Lost-Worktime Injuries and Illnesses: Characteristics and Resulting Time Away from Work,* Publication USDL 00-115. Washington, DC: U.S. Department of Labor, 2000.

Vlaeyen JW, Linton SJ. Fear-avoidance and its consequences in chronic musculoskeletal pain : a state of the art. *Pain* 2000; 85:317–332.

Vlaeyen JWS, Kole-Snijders AMJ, Boeren RGB, van Eek H. Fear of movement/(re)injury in chronic low back pain and its relation to behavioral performance. *Pain* 1995; 62:363–372.

Vlaeyen JW, de Jong J, Geilen M, Heuts PH, van Breukelen G. Graded exposure in vivo in the treatment of pain-related fear: a replicated single-case experimental design in four patients with chronic low back pain. *Behav Res Ther* 2001; 39:151–166.

Volinn E, Lai D, McKinney S, Loeser JD. When back pain becomes disabling: a regional analysis. *Pain* 1988; 33:33–39.

Waddell G. Low back pain: a twentieth century health care enigma. *Spine* 1996; 21:2820–2825.

Waddell G, Newton M, Henderson I, Somerville D, Main CJ. A fear-avoidance beliefs questionnaire (FABQ) and the role of fear-avoidance beliefs in chronic low back pain and disability. *Pain* 1993; 52:157–168.

Wallis BJ, Bogduk N. Faking a profile: can naïve subjects simulate whiplash responses? *Pain* 1996; 66:223–227.

Walsh NE, Dumitru D. The influence of compensation on recovery from low back pain. *Occup Med: State Art Rev* 1988; 3:109–120.

Webster BS, Snook SH. The cost of 1989 Workers' Compensation low back pain claims. *Spine* 1994; 19:1111–1116.

Wright A, Mayer TG, Gatchel RJ. Outcomes of disabling cervical spine disorders in compensation injuries. *Spine* 1999; 24:178–183.

Younkin SL, Betz NE. Psychological hardiness: a reconceptualization and measurement. In: Miller TW (Ed). *Theory and Assessment of Stressful Life Events*. Madison, CT: International Universities Press, 1996, pp 161–178.

Correspondence to: Raymond C. Tait, PhD, Department of Psychiatry, Saint Louis University School of Medicine, 1221 S. Grand Boulevard, St. Louis, MO 63104, USA. Tel: 314-268-5589; Fax: 314-268-5736; email: taitrc@slu.edu.

Psychosocial Aspects of Pain: A Handbook for Health Care Providers, Progress in Pain Research and Management, Vol. 27, edited by Robert H. Dworkin and William S. Breitbart, IASP Press, Seattle, © 2004.

25

What Impact Does Childhood Experience Have on the Development of Chronic Pain?

Stephen Morley

Academic Unit of Psychiatry and Behavioural Sciences, School of Medicine, University of Leeds, Leeds, United Kingdom

The idea that childhood experiences influence the adult is well established in human cultures and is represented in common aphorisms and proverbs such as, "the child is the father of the man." The idea is underpinned by more than a century of clinical observation and research that has moved technical theories and findings, especially those relating to early adversity, into the everyday world.

In translating technical information into everyday knowledge, some studies become emblematic representations of facts. Within the field of pain, Melzack and Scott's (1957) paper on the impact of an early, pain-free, restricted environment on dogs' later pain avoidance behavior has perhaps served this function. Contemporary publications that may similarly come to represent key findings and thus acquire iconic status are Taddio et al.'s (1997) report that circumcised infants showed a stronger pain response to subsequent routine vaccination than uncircumcised infants, and Drossman et al.'s (1990) report that women with functional gastrointestinal disorders were more likely than those with an organic diagnosis to report a history of forced sexual intercourse. These examples encapsulate the notions that less-than-optimal environments and particular adverse events may influence later experience and behavior.

Both of these ideas are represented in current psychosocial models that use a general diathesis-stress framework to formulate the development of chronic pain and to explain differences in individuals' response to the experience of chronic pain. This framework hypothesizes that individuals vary with respect to their propensity (predisposing factors and pre-existing vulnerabilities) to develop chronic pain in response to the onset of acute pain. For the most part these models are formulated at a meta-level; they do not offer specific hypotheses about necessary and sufficient conditions for the emergence of chronic pain, nor do they make precise predictions for testing specific relationships (Dworkin and Banks 1999). Dworkin and Banks have proposed a specific model for postherpetic neuralgia that separates vulnerability and diathesis. In this model the *diathesis* is the illness or injury that instigates acute pain; it is necessary but not sufficient for the development of chronic pain. Two other constructs are needed to complete the explanation: *stress* refers to the psychosocial influences just prior to and at the time of the diathesis, and *vulnerability* refers to the neurobiological and psychosocial factors that predispose individuals to develop chronic pain. Ingram et al. (1998) report that few precise definitions of vulnerability are available in the scientific literature. Their review of the literature led them to propose a definition of vulnerability as an "internal and stable feature of the person that predisposes him or her to the development of psychopathology under specified conditions such as the occurrence of stressful events." They also note that individuals who are resistant to the deleterious effects of such events can be considered to possess stable features that render them resilient to the influence of events, but they explain that resilience does not imply absolute immunity.

A major issue is whether basic relationships between classes of childhood events and chronic pain can be established and what sort of impact they might have on the development of chronic pain. At least three functional relationships are distinguishable. First, some aspect of childhood experience may change the individual in such a way that his or her later adult behavior will lead to increased risk for injury and chronic pain. For example, a child's psychosocial environment might encourage increased risk taking that results in behavior that will lead to injury and pain. This behavior would result in an increased incidence of chronic pain in groups where this vulnerability is established. Melzack and Scott's (1957) study in dogs provides an example of this mechanism.

In the second model, particular childhood experiences may alter the individual's sensitivity to pain. In these circumstances the risk for exposure to events that can lead to injury and chronic pain is the same as in the general population, but the individual's greater sensitivity means that he or she has a lowered threshold to the occurrence of the event and to developing chronic pain. With respect to acute pain it would appear that Taddio et al.'s (1997) observation on increased behavioral responsiveness to injections subsequent to circumcision in male infants is an example of this mechanism. However, it remains to be determined whether such mechanisms can persist into adulthood and result in an increased incidence of chronic pain (Fitzgerald and Walker 2003). It is also possible that many other, and perhaps more extreme, events with more complex psychological and social meanings, such as sexual and physical abuse, confer an increased vulnerability to chronic pain.

In the third functional relationship, a childhood experience may affect systems that determine variation in the expression, course, and resolution of chronic pain rather than its incidence and prevalence. The essential issue here is that chronic pain is not a single entity but involves a complex and dynamic affective, cognitive, and behavioral experience. For example, it is possible that childhood experience may alter the affective system so that vulnerable individuals are no more likely to develop chronic pain but are more liable to show extreme, potentially maladaptive, affective responses if they do experience it.

These three idealized models are simplified, and it is possible that adverse childhood experiences and environments may both increase the incidence and influence the course of chronic pain. In all three models, functional relationships result in increased incidence of chronic pain. Simple epidemiological methods that report the association between chronic pain and childhood events will need greater elaboration. At present it appears that the literature on childhood experiences has not explicitly separated these possible functional relationships. Most studies on adverse childhood experiences, for example sexual and physical abuse, have been concerned predominantly with questions of prevalence as a first step in determining the presence of an association.

The question arises as to what sort of psychosocial events and environments in childhood could bestow vulnerability to the later development of chronic pain. In order to illustrate some of the complexities involved in attempting to answer the question, this chapter will consider two broad classes of the many possible events and environments to which children may be exposed: first, severe adverse events, especially abuse; and second, modeling and the family environment.

ADVERSE EVENTS IN CHILDHOOD

Determining the relationship between childhood experiences and chronic pain hinges on the use of two fundamental study designs shown in Fig. 1. This simple diagram cross-tabulates the presence and absence of chronic pain and the presence and absence of any specified childhood experience. The association can be investigated with two methods. The case-control

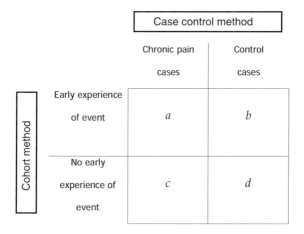

Fig. 1. Case-control and cohort designs.

method compares the frequency of a childhood experience in cases with and
without chronic pain by comparing the ratios $a/(a + c)$ and $b(b + d)$, whereas
the cohort method identifies groups with and without the specified childhood event and compares the rates of chronic pain in the groups, $a/(a + b)$
and $c/(c + d)$. For practical reasons it is relatively easier to run case-control
studies because the sample sizes can be constrained and the sample matched
on putative relevant variables. Case-control studies are always retrospective;
data on the early experience must be derived either from archival sources or
from the memory of the participants. Cohort methods may be prospective,
but because prospective studies are difficult to set up, many cohort studies
are retrospective. For example, investigators may ask subjects about their
exposure to early events so that they can compare the prevalence of the
target symptom, syndrome, or diagnosis in subgroups of individuals exposed
or not exposed to certain events during childhood. Most studies of childhood
experience and chronic pain have used a case-control method.

Numerous published case-control studies have reported an increased
incidence of early adverse experiences, predominantly child sexual abuse, in
various chronic pain conditions including pelvic pain (Walker et al. 1988;
Lampe et al. 1997, 2000; Collett et al. 1998), fibromyalgia (Walker et al.
1988; Boisset-Pioro et al. 1995; Taylor et al. 1995; Imbierowicz and Egle
2003), low back pain (Schofferman et al. 1993; Nickel et al. 2002), breast
pain (Colegrave et al. 2001), gastrointestinal pain (Drossman et al. 1990;
Walker et al. 1995), and unspecified chronic pain (Goldberg et al. 1999;
Goldberg and Goldstein 2000). These studies, representing different investigators across several different countries with varying health care regimes

(and therefore differing patterns of referral to clinics), have all observed an association between early adverse experience (e.g., sexual abuse) and chronic pain, albeit in studies with relatively small samples of fewer than 100 subjects.

Nevertheless, these studies share problems common to all case-control studies. First, the selection of the cases and their controls is likely to be influenced by many characteristics. Cases drawn from clinics will be the product of multiple, often unknown, selection influences operating in the process of referral to the clinic. Investigators can often control for these influences by concurrently assessing variables hypothesized to be important, such as demographic and social class and psychological and medical status. A crucial aspect of the case-control design is the selection of the comparative control group. As far as possible, investigators must control for confounding factors when selecting control subjects. Given the multiplicity of possible confounding factors, the choice of control subjects is often a difficult decision between theoretically desirable characteristics and pragmatic concerns of recruitment. Taken individually, all of the above studies might be judged to be deficient on these grounds, but one might argue that the accumulated weight of the findings across different control groups and diagnoses must count in favor of the hypothesis that early adverse experience is associated with an increase in the later prevalence of chronic pain. Alternatively, a skeptic could rightly question the reasonableness of accumulating "bad" evidence. The second inherent feature of case-control designs is the retrospective nature of the assessment of the key variable. On occasions it may be possible to examine documented evidence of the putative causal variable collected at the time of its occurrence, but by its nature childhood sexual, physical, and emotional abuse is often hidden at the time and researchers must frequently rely on the memory of the participants. The fallible and reconstructive nature of memory is extensively documented, and participants in studies in this field are likely to be influenced by several possible mechanisms such as the "search after meaning," repression of emotionally charged memories, and their current state. Memory of early childhood experience may not inevitably be unreliable, but steps should be taken to assess and control the problem (Brewin et al. 1993).

Despite the apparently persuasive narrative of these reports, data based on larger samples from more representative populations with better documentary evidence of the early childhood event would be more compelling. A number of studies meet some of these desiderata. Linton (1997, 2002) reported data on back pain and childhood abuse collected from a general population in Sweden. Unlike the authors of many population-based studies, Linton also included a clinical sample to enable a direct comparison of rates of adverse experience. He observed no substantial differences in the rates of sexual abuse between the clinic group and persons in the population with "pronounced pain." In the first study, Linton (1997) found evidence of an association between both childhood sexual abuse and physical abuse and pronounced pain, but only for females. In the second report, Linton (2002) followed the same cohort for 12 months and observed that among those who reported no back pain at baseline, individuals who had been physically abused in childhood had a higher inception rate for reporting back pain at follow-up.

Although Linton's study was based on a large community sample, it did rely on the participants' recall to assess childhood adversity. McBeth and colleagues (1999, 2001) partly overcame this problem in a study of a community sample in the United Kingdom. They selected a sample with psychological distress as assessed by a validated screening instrument and determined their current status with a standardized interview that included an assessment of 14 adverse childhood experiences. Medical records relating to childhood were also retrieved and examined. The sample was divided into those meeting criteria for chronic widespread pain (CWP; another term for fibromyalgia), those with other pain, and those with no pain. The frequency of self-reported adverse events (illness among family members, parental loss, and abuse) was associated with increased odds of having CWP, but none of the odds ratios were significant. The odds were statistically significant for the association between CWP and self-reported hospitalization and surgery in childhood, but these associations were not upheld when medical records were used as the measure of childhood exposure to hospitalizations and surgery. Clearly this study suggests that recall bias cannot be excluded in this field.

Raphael and her colleagues (2001) provided further evidence of the influence of this bias using a prospective cohort design that eliminated the possibility of recall bias in assessing early adverse experience. The authors constructed a group with known, documented exposure to childhood neglect and sexual or physical abuse occurring prior to age 11 through examination of court records. This sample and a control group—matched according to age, sex, race, family, and social class—were followed into early adulthood (up to an age of about 30 years), giving a total sample of about 1,100 persons. When court records were used to assess the relationship between abuse and medically explained and unexplained pain symptoms, there was no relationship between abuse or neglect and pain symptoms. However, the odds of one or more unexplained pain symptoms being associated with abuse was significant when concurrent self-report of abuse was considered.

In summary, observations from clinical samples suggest a relationship between early adverse experience and pain, especially unexplained pain. This notion is partly confirmed by larger studies of nonclinic populations when self-report assessment of the early event is the measure, but the association is nullified when the measurement of the adverse event is based on documented evidence. Given the prospective design and the large sample used by Raphael et al. (2001), this study should be accorded particular prominence. If abuse is found to be associated with chronic pain it is unlikely that the association will be specific because substantial evidence has shown that abuse is also associated with other disorders (Kessler et al. 1997; Polivy and Herman 2002). Unraveling the relationship between events in childhood and adult chronic pain will require elaboration of possible intervening events and processes. In taking account myriad intervening events, we either must assume that they represent noise and can be ignored or we must investigate their influence, preferably by building models that specify how such events moderate or mediate the expression of the early experience. This process is necessarily complex, and other studies of child development have shown that even severe and moderately enduring neglect may not have a deleterious permanent effect on a child's intellectual and emotional development (Rutter 1998). The situation is further complicated by the need to examine the relationship between certain events and the environment in which they happen. For example, girls exposed to sexual abuse are also likely to live in more adverse environments that facilitate earlier sexualization of behavior. As a consequence, young women have higher rates of early consensual intercourse, multiple partners, and unprotected sexual activity, with the associated risks of pregnancy and sexually transmitted disease (Fergusson et al. 1997). Rutter et al. (2001) indicate that the problems in separating the influences of specific environmental risk mechanisms for psychopathology require study designs that "pull apart" variables that ordinarily go together, in order to test specific hypotheses of possible causal processes. Although the hypothesis that early adverse experience can lead to chronic pain is attractive, the case that it is related to increased prevalence of pain is not proven.

MODELING AND THE SOCIAL ENVIRONMENT

Children are required to learn a tremendous range of socialized behavior, and it seems unlikely that the amount and variety of learning required could be obtained via direct experience alone. Considerable evidence shows that many aspects of social behavior, including behavior that is regarded as psychopathological, such as fears and phobias, are acquired vicariously by observing others. The possibility that exposure to others who are experiencing pain will influence a child's experience and behavioral expression of pain has received some attention, but perhaps not as much as might be expected. Not only may such models influence the child's acquisition of pain experience and behavior, but they are also a path whereby a child may learn to experience and express his or her pain within culturally acceptable norms as well as the mechanism by which he or she may acquire resilience. This latter aspect appears to have been neglected in the research literature, where most work concerns the "pathological" influences of models.

Children have many opportunities both to experience pain and to observe others in pain. Most children will frequently witness parents, siblings, and their peer group experience minor accidents at play or in the household (Fearon et al. 1996). A significant proportion of children will experience parents who have recurrent episodic pain, such as headache, or chronic pain and somatic complaints. However, in many of these instances, unlike acute pain attributable to accidents, the provoking stimulus is not obvious to the observer, so other aspects of the context may come to serve as the discriminative stimulus for pain. By this process it is possible that distress and various aspects of the social environment acquire functional pain-eliciting power. Two main questions arise: First, what is the evidence that children's behavior is influenced by observing others? And second, is there evidence that this behavior either persists into adulthood or makes the person more vulnerable to the experience of pain or other adverse events in adulthood? There are several approaches to gathering answers to these questions.

STUDIES OF ADULTS WITH CHRONIC PAIN RECALLING THEIR CHILDHOOD

Several studies conclude that patients with pain are more likely than controls without pain to report that they have family members with chronic pain (for reviews see Payne and Norfleet 1986; Gamsa 1994; for particular studies see Turkat and Noskin 1983; Turkat et al. 1984; Ehde et al. 1991). As commentators have noted, these studies are fraught with methodological problems familiar from the previous discussion of cohort studies of abuse, including memory bias and sampling issues. These studies also raise another problem in that they frequently do not test alternative hypotheses related to the influence of genetics and the persistence of adverse environments. Separation of these factors is made more complex because individuals with shared genes tend to share environments. Whereas other fields, particularly developmental psychopathology, have made advances in study-ing the impact of early experience and the relative influence of "nature" and "nurture" (Rutter 1994; Rutter et al. 2001), the study of pain has barely begun to consider these issues in depth.

STUDIES OF CHILDREN OF ADULTS
WITH CHRONIC PAIN

The case for the influence of modeling would be strengthened if it could be demonstrated that the presence of chronic pain in the family is associated with variation in children's current behavior. The modeling hypothesis makes the assumption that models have an immediate impact on the child, but there may be a "sleeper effect" with no change in the child at the time, but a sensitizing of his or her response to later exposure to adversity. However, the sleeper effect has not been considered in current research. If the model-ing is a significant influence then we might expect that in families where at least one of the adults has chronic pain, the children would show an in-creased rate of pain behavior when compared to children from other families in which the appropriate control for chronic illness in the absence of pain is made. To avoid biases such studies should ideally include direct observa-tions of the target child or inclusion of data collected by a third party, such as a teacher. Finally, the context of the observations needs to be carefully considered and assessed because learning theory suggests that learned be-havior is strongly influenced by environmental context. Studies vary in the extent to which they meet these requirements (Dura and Beck 1988; Rickard 1988; Mikail and von Baeyer 1990; Chun et al. 1993), but they consistently demonstrate an effect of living in a family in which one parent has pain. Children of such families have been variously shown to be less socially competent, to have more child-parent behavior problems, to have a higher frequency of health behavior problems, and to be more somatically focused. It is not yet clear whether these effects are attributable to pain per se or to the level of disability shown by parents. The evidence for an increased rate of specific pain behaviors in children is not strong. It seems that what may be transmitted socially is a model of illness behavior rather than a specific model of pain. Walker and colleagues' (2002) observations of pediatric patients with recurrent abdominal pain (RAP) highlight the occurrence of potential subtle interactions. They demonstrated the importance of the children's evaluation of their self-worth and academic competence. When these were low the impact of social factors on symptom maintenance was stronger. The authors concluded that children's success in their normal so-cial roles might affect the extent to which they identify with the sick role and find it a rewarding alternative. Thus success in roles other than the sick role may be an important pathway in establishing resilience.

As with studies of abuse, large-scale population-based studies are relatively scarce, and most findings are based on fairly small clinical samples. A recent exception is a study by Kovacs and colleagues (2003), who examined the risk factors for low back pain in 16,000 adolescents (13–15 years old) and their parents. Low back pain was associated with several behaviors, but there was no association in the incidence of this chronic pain problem between the generations.

STUDIES OF CHILDREN IN CHRONIC PAIN AND THE FAMILY ENVIRONMENT

A third source of evidence comes from several pertinent studies of children who have persistent pain. Terre and Ghiselli (1997) reported a study of a large sample of children and adolescents in which they related aspects of family functioning to bodily complaints. The data revealed consistent associations between family environment and somatic complaints, depending on the age of the child. For example, children in school grades 6–8 (11–14 years old) who perceived their families as more disorganized and less cohesive were more likely to have somatic complaints.

The causal direction of these associations is not clear: Is the child's pain learned from the parents, or is the parents' behavior a consequence of observing their offspring in distress? Dunn-Geier et al. (1986) approached this problem by investigating individual differences in mother-child interaction among adolescents who were or were not coping successfully with chronic benign intractable pain. Behavioral observations indicated that unsuccessful copers engaged in significantly more negative behavior than did successful copers. Unsuccessful copers also expressed more pain and stayed on task less often than did successful copers. Importantly, mothers of unsuccessful copers more frequently discouraged coping behavior. These observations could not be explained by differences on family or personality measures.

Another approach to clarifying causal relationships is to separate studies in which the child's pain is attributable to a known biomedical cause such as juvenile rheumatoid arthritis (JRA) from those in which the biomedical disease process is uncertain—the so-called "functional" pains such as RAP as well as chronic fatigue syndrome (CFS). It may be argued that the latter examples provide a stronger test of possible modeling influences. For example, Brace et al. (2000) hypothesized that parental encouragement of illness behavior correlates with psychosocial dysfunction in adolescents with chronic illness. Brace compared small samples of adolescents with CFS, adolescents with JRA, and healthy adolescents on a range of self-report measures. As predicted, the adolescents with CFS scored statistically higher on measures of depression, total competence, and the number of school days missed in the previous 6 months. Children with JRA scored significantly lower than the CFS group on the measure of parental reinforcement of illness behavior. The healthy group produced intermediate scores. Osborne et al. (1989) examined specific relationships between the presence of pain models and unexplained pain by interviewing children with sickle cell anemia and a comparison group of children with unexplained pain. Parents were also interviewed. The data indicated that children with unexplained pain and their parents were more likely to identify models of pain or illness from their environment than were the children with sickle cell pain.

Perhaps the most widely examined model of childhood chronic pain is recurrent abdominal pain. The original study of this syndrome (Apley and Naish 1957) in 1,000 schoolchildren reported that 46% of the RAP sample had physically ill family members compared with 8% of the non-RAP group. In reviewing this and succeeding studies, Hotopf (2002) notes the remarkable consistency of the findings over the subsequent 30–40 years. Parents of children with RAP report more "physical symptoms, *especially pain* [italics added], worse general physical health, higher rates of peptic ulceration, and more life events relating to physical health" (Hotopf 2002). The studies reviewed by Hotopf include several with large community samples.

Recently Bode and colleagues (2003) reported another large community-based study ($n = 1,221$) that also sought to test a plausible rival hypothesis to the modeling hypothesis. Bode and his colleagues obtained information on the children's medical history and recurrent abdominal pain symptoms and on family demographics using a standardized questionnaire. They also obtained information on whether or not the child was infected by *Helicobacter pylori*, which has been proposed as a possible cause of RAP. Their analysis showed that infection with *H. pylori* was not associated with RAP, but the authors found clear relationships between the incidence of RAP and living in a single-parent household, a parental history of peptic ulcer, and a parental history of nonulcer gastrointestinal disorders.

EXPERIMENTAL STUDIES

While the above studies support the social learning hypothesis, the case for this mechanism would be further strengthened if it could be established experimentally that the observation of an adult in pain differentially changes a child's response to a pain-eliciting event. In adults there is good experimental evidence that several aspects of a model's behavior can be transmitted to an observer. For example, Prkachin and Craig (1986) demonstrated that observing another person experiencing electric shock systematically modified the experienced threshold of the observer. In other studies the model's behavior has been controlled by experimental instruction (Craig and Prkachin 1978; Turkat et al. 1983; Turkat and Guise 1983) and was shown to influence the observer's facial expression and their behavioral persistence at a problem-solving task. However, there appears to be a dearth of experimental studies in children.

Thastum et al. (1997) examined responses to experimental cold pressor pain in JRA patients and healthy children, each of whom was accompanied by one of their parents. The data showed a correlation between the pain scores of children and their parents for both pain intensity and tolerance. More direct evidence comes from a study (Goodman and McGrath 2003) in which mothers were exposed to the cold pressor test while the children observed them. Children then completed the test while their facial display was recorded on video. The essential component of this study was that the mother's own behavior was experimentally manipulated. Mothers were randomly assigned to conditions where they were asked to minimize or exaggerate pain, and to a control condition with no instructions. The data provide initial evidence that the child's response is a function of observing the mother's display. Children assigned to the "exaggerate" condition had lower thresholds than did children in the control group. Children in the "exaggerate" and control groups showed more pain-related facial action in the first minute of their exposure to the cold pressor. These results suggest that modeling has an impact on a child's pain behavior.

DOES CHILDHOOD PAIN PERSIST?

Determining whether childhood pain persists requires cohort studies in which individuals can be followed for many years into adulthood. Such studies are not usually designed directly to answer questions about chronic pain or to investigate hypotheses about specific childhood experiences and later development (Turk and Rudy 1988). Thus, investigators must develop proxy measures of likely diagnoses in both childhood and adulthood. Nevertheless, the data from these studies offer important pointers to determining whether childhood pain persists after exposure to early illness. Hotopf and his colleagues have reported two analyses of different cohorts addressing questions of continuity between child and adult health. In the first study, Hotopf et al. (1998) examined data from the U.K. Medical Research Council national survey of health and development that followed a cohort born in

1946. The investigators constructed a proxy measure of recurrent abdominal pain, accessed information on several aspects of personal and family functioning in childhood, and obtained data from a standardized psychiatric interview when the participants were 36 years old. The analysis of childhood health replicated early observations that children with RAP were more likely to come from families with higher rates of reported physical illness and psychological symptoms, but these children were not greatly at risk of developing physical symptoms, including pain, in adulthood. They were, however, at considerably greater risk for developing psychiatric disorders in adulthood.

The second study (Fearon and Hotopf 2001) used data collected in 1991 from a cohort of 17,000 adults from the U.K. national child development study of children born in 1958. The focus of study was the association between frequent headaches in childhood and adult adjustment. Children with frequent headaches were more likely to have a mother with physical illness, or to have a family member with mental illness. At the age of 33 years, study participants who had experienced frequent headaches in childhood were more likely to report excessive headache and other physical and psychiatric symptoms. Fearon and Hotopf (2001) showed that childhood headache was still associated with adult headache even when childhood symptoms and adult psychiatric morbidity were controlled statistically.

Despite the differences in their findings, the studies suggest that recurrent pain in childhood does have an impact on adult functioning; however, there may be different trajectories for abdominal pain and headache. While there were some methodological differences between the studies, Fearon and Hotopf suggest that two plausible broad hypotheses. First, although headache is associated with adversity in childhood, it may also be characterized by a more stable phenotype. Second, differences may also partly reflect variation in the way in which parents, teachers, and health professionals responded to distress in childhood. Such responses would constitute a social learning mechanism.

CONCLUSIONS

Despite the inherent attractiveness of the idea that childhood experiences influence and shape the course of chronic pain, it is difficult to demonstrate the impact of those influences empirically. There are many complex methodological reasons for this difficulty, of which a major feature is the predominantly retrospective measurement of the key construct of "childhood experience." Many of the studies are dependent on studying associations between dichotomous measures of early experience and pain. Of necessity this process means reducing complex and multidimensional experiences of both the predictor and the outcome to binary scores. While this simplification is a necessary first step, it is possible that it may obfuscate possible crucial mechanisms. For example, evidence indicates that chronic pain patients should not be regarded as a homogeneous group. One might consider variation with respect to one of a number of indices of psychological adjustment such as those based on psychological constructs like depression (Banks and Kerns 1996; Pincus and Morley 2002) that are independent of chronic pain. Alternatively, investigators might consider classifications based on specific features of responding to the experience of pain (Turk and Rudy 1988), or might be interested in a theoretical analysis of fear in chronic pain (Vlaeyen and Linton 2000). These models of chronic pain suggest different associations of types of early experience with later adjustment to chronic pain. Theorists developing unambiguous specifications of key variables including potential moderators and mediators, and identifying additional probable confounding variables, could make a significant contribution to the field. Indeed, it would be surprising if childhood experiences did not have an impact on chronic pain. Nevertheless, is it the case that such events have a specific impact on chronic pain rather than creating a general vulnerability to a number of predominantly psychological disorders such as eating disorders, depression, and psychosis? If an event is not specific to pain, theoretical formulations will need to incorporate explanatory constructs that explain why chronic pain rather than another disorder is the outcome.

The cynical observer of the current state of play might reasonably ask why one would want to spend resources in answering the question posed in the title of this chapter. After all, it seems unlikely that, given the present state of knowledge, specific preventive measures akin to childhood vaccination could be easily targeted and applied to the population. There are several responses to the cynic. First, there is the issue of intellectual curiosity and the desire to develop etiological explanations for the development of chronic pain and the heterogeneity of the chronic pain experience. Second, it is possible that childhood experience continues to have an impact on chronic pain experience, either as part of a maintenance mechanism or as factors that may interfere with the effective delivery of treatment. For example, victims of childhood sexual abuse may find it more difficult to engage in physical therapy (avoiding physical touch because of a residual sense of dread) or to establish and maintain close interpersonal relationships that may be advantageous in effective psychological treatment. The relatively high base rate of abuse in the population implies that a significant proportion of people with chronic pain will have experienced abuse at some point in their lives. The absence of strong evidence that causally links this experience to the incidence of pain is not absence of evidence that prior experiences have some impact on the current predicament of pain sufferers or on their responses to treatment environments. Sensitive clinicians will develop practice-based evidence to guide their interactions. Third, chronic pain patients seek a reasoned account of why they suffer, and it is our moral imperative as researchers and clinicians to provided an accurate explanation wherever possible.

ACKNOWLEDGMENTS

I would like to thank Chris Eccleston and Amanda Williams, who let me ramble a while; David Owens, for some enlightening conversations on simple tables and their interpretation; the editors, for their remarkable patience; and finally, Alison, for sharing busy weekends.

REFERENCES

Apley J, Naish N. Recurrent abdominal pains: a field study of 1,000 school children. *Arch Dis Child* 1957; 32:165–170.

Banks SM, Kerns RD. Explaining high rates of depression in chronic pain: a diathesis-stress framework. *Psychol Bull* 1996; 119:95–110.

Bode G, Brenner H, Adler G, Rothenbacher D. Recurrent abdominal pain in children: evidence from a population-based study that social and familial factors play a major role but not *Helicobacter pylori* infection. *J Psychosom Res* 2003; 54:417–421.

Boisset-Pioro MH, Esdaile JM, Fitzcharles MA. Sexual and physical abuse in women with fibromyalgia syndrome. *Arthritis Rheum* 1995; 38:235–241.

Brace MJ, Scott Smith M, McCauley E, Sherry DD. Family reinforcement of illness behavior: a comparison of adolescents with chronic fatigue syndrome, juvenile arthritis, and healthy controls. *J Dev Behav Pediatr* 2000; 21:332–339.

Brewin CR, Andrews B, Gotlib IH. Psychopathology and early experience: a reappraisal of retrospective reports. *Psychol Bull* 1993; 113:82–98.

Chun DY, Turner JA, Romano JM. Children of chronic pain patients: risk factors for maladjustment. *Pain* 1993; 52:311–317.

Colegrave S, Holcombe C, Salmon P. Psychological characteristics of women presenting with breast pain. *J Psychosom Res* 2001; 50:303–307.

Collett BJ, Cordle CJ, Stewart CR, Jagger C. A comparative study of women with chronic pelvic pain, chronic nonpelvic pain and those with no history of pain attending general practitioners. *Br J Obstet Gynaecol* 1998; 105:87–92.

Craig KD, Prkachin KM. Social modeling influences on sensory decision theory and psychophysiological indexes of pain. *J Pers Soc Psychol* 1978; 36:805–815.

Drossman DA, Leserman J, Nachman G, et al. Sexual and physical abuse in women with functional or organic gastrointestinal disorders. *Ann Int Med* 1990; 113:828–833.

Dunn-Geier BJ, McGarth PJ, Rourke BP, et al. Adolescent chronic pain: the ability to cope. *Pain* 1986; 26:23–32.

Dura JR, Beck SJ. A comparison of family functioning when mothers have chronic pain. *Pain* 1988; 35:79–89.

Dworkin RH, Banks SM. A vulnerability-diathesis-stress model of chronic pain: herpes zoster and the development of postherpetic neuralgia. In: Gatchel RJ, Turk DC (Eds). *Psychosocial Factors in Pain: Critical Perspectives*. New York: Guilford Press, 1999, pp 247–269.

Ehde DM, Holm JE, Metzger DL. The role of family structure, functioning, and pain modeling in headache. *Headache* 1991; 31:35–40.

Fearon P, Hotopf M. Relation between headache in childhood and physical and psychiatric symptoms in adulthood: national birth cohort study. *BMJ* 2001; 322:1145.

Fearon I, McGrath PJ, Achat H. 'Booboos': the study of everyday pain among young children. *Pain* 1996; 68:55–62.

Fergusson DM, Horwood LJ, Lynskey MT. Childhood sexual abuse, adolescent sexual behaviors and sexual revictimization. *Child Abuse Negl* 1997; 21:789–803.

Fitzgerald M, Walker S. The role of activity in developing pain pathways. In: Dostrovsky JO, Carr DB, Koltzenburg M (Eds). *Proceedings of the 10th World Congress on Pain*, Progress in Pain Research and Management, Vol. 24. Seattle: IASP Press, 2003, pp 185–196.

Gamsa A. The role of psychological factors in chronic pain. I. A half century of study. *Pain* 1994; 57:5–15.

Goldberg RT, Goldstein R. A comparison of chronic pain patients and controls on traumatic events in childhood. *Disabil Rehabil* 2000; 22:756–763.

Goldberg RT, Pachas WN, Keith D. Relationship between traumatic events in childhood and chronic pain. *Disabil Rehabil* 1999; 21:23–30.

Goodman JE, McGrath PJ. Mothers' modeling influences children's pain during a cold pressor task. *Pain* 2003; in press.

Hotopf M. Childhood experience of illness as a risk factor for medically unexplained symptoms. *Scand J Psychol* 2002; 43:139–146.

Hotopf M, Carr S, Mayou R, et al. Why do children have chronic abdominal pain, and what happens to them when they grow up? Population based cohort study. *BMJ* 1998; 316:1196–1200.

Imbierowicz K, Egle UT. Childhood adversities in patients with fibromyalgia and somatoform pain disorder. *Eur J Pain* 2003; 7:113–119.

Ingram RE, Miranda J, Segal ZV. *Cognitive Vulnerability to Depression*. New York: Guilford Press, 1998.

Kessler RC, Davis CG, Kendler KS. Childhood adversity and adult psychiatric disorder in the US National Comorbidity Survey. *Psychol Med* 1997; 27:1101–1119.

Kovacs FM, Gestoso M, Gil del Real MT, et al. Risk factors for non-specific low back pain in schoolchildren and their parents: a population-based study. *Pain* 2003; 103:259–268.

Lampe A, Sollner W, Solder E, Hausler A. Severe sexual abuse and its relationship to the etiology of chronic pelvic pain in women. *Psychosomatics* 1997; 38:84.

Lampe A, Solder E, Ennemoser A, et al. Chronic pelvic pain and previous sexual abuse. *Obstet Gynecol* 2000; 96:929–933.

Linton SJ. A population-based study of the relationship between sexual abuse and back pain: establishing a link. *Pain* 1997; 73:47–53.

Linton SJ. A prospective study of the effects of sexual or physical abuse on back pain. *Pain* 2002; 96:347–351.

McBeth J, Macfarlane GJ, Benjamin S, et al. The association between tender points, psychological distress, and adverse childhood experiences: a community-based study. *Arthritis Rheum* 1999; 42:1397–1404.

McBeth J, Morris S, Benjamin S, et al. Associations between adverse events in childhood and chronic widespread pain in adulthood: are they explained by differential recall? *J Rheumatol* 2001; 28:2305–2309.

Melzack R, Scott TH. The effects of early experience on the response to pain. *J Comp Physiol Psychol* 1957; 50:155–161.

Mikail SF, von Baeyer CL. Pain, somatic focus, and emotional adjustment in children of chronic headache sufferers and controls. *Soc Sci Med* 1990; 31:51–59.

Nickel R, Egle UT, Hardt J. Are childhood adversities relevant in patients with chronic low back pain? *Eur J Pain* 2002; 6:221–228.

Osborne RB, Hatcher JW, Richtsmeier AJ. The role of social modeling in unexplained pediatric pain. *J Pediatr Psychol* 1989; 14:43–61.

Payne B, Norfleet MA. Chronic pain and the family: a review. *Pain* 1986; 26:1–22.

Pincus T, Morley S. Cognitive appraisal. In: Linton SJ (Ed). *New Avenues for the Prevention of Chronic Musculoskeletal Pain and Disability,* Pain Research and Clinical Management, Vol. 12. Amsterdam: Elsevier Science, 2002, pp 123–141.

Polivy J, Herman CP. Causes of eating disorders. *Annu Rev Psychol* 2002; 53:187–213.

Prkachin KM, Craig KD. Social transmission of natural variations in pain behaviour. *Behav Res Ther* 1986; 24:581–585.

Raphael KG, Widom CS, Lange G. Childhood victimization and pain in adulthood: a prospective investigation. *Pain* 2001; 92:283–293.

Rickard K. The occurrence of maladaptive health-related behaviors and teacher-rated conduct problems in children of chronic low back pain patients. *J Behav Med* 1988; 11:107–116.

Rutter M. Beyond longitudinal data: causes, consequences, changes, and continuity. *J Consult Clin Psychol* 1994; 62:928–940.

Rutter M. Developmental catch-up, and deficit, following adoption after severe global early privation. English and Romanian Adoptees (ERA) Study Team. *J Child Psychol Psychiatry* 1998; 39:465–476.

Rutter M, Pickles A, Murray R, Eaves L. Testing hypotheses on specific environmental causal effects on behavior. *Psychol Bull* 2001; 127:291–324.

Schofferman J, Anderson D, Hines R, et al. Childhood psychological trauma and chronic refractory low-back pain. *Clin J Pain* 1993; 9:260–265.

Taddio A, Katz J, Ilersich AL, Koren G. Effect of neonatal circumcision on pain response during subsequent routine vaccination. *Lancet* 1997; 349:599–603.

Taylor ML, Trotter DR, Csuka ME. The prevalence of sexual abuse in women with fibromyalgia. *Arthritis Rheum* 1995; 38:229–234.

Terre L, Ghiselli W. A developmental perspective on family risk factors in somatization. *J Psychosom Res* 1997; 42:197–208.

Thastum M, Zachariae R, Scholer M, et al. Cold pressor pain: comparing responses of juvenile arthritis patients and their parents. *Scand J Rheumatol* 1997; 26:272–279.

Turk DC, Rudy TE. Toward an empirically derived taxonomy of chronic pain patients: integration of psychological assessment data. *J Consult Clin Psychol* 1988; 56:233–238.

Turkat ID, Guise BJ. The effects of vicarious experience and stimulus intensity on pain termination and work avoidance. *Behav Res Ther* 1983; 21:241–245.

Turkat ID, Noskin DE. Vicarious and operant experiences in the etiology of illness behavior: a replication with healthy individuals. *Behav Res Ther* 1983; 21:169–172.

Turkat ID, Guise BJ, Carter KM. The effects of vicarious experience on pain termination and work avoidance: a replication. *Behav Res Ther* 1983; 21:491–493.

Turkat ID, Kuczmierczyk AR, Adams HE. An investigation of the aetiology of chronic headache: the role of headache models. *Br J Psychiatry* 1984; 145:665–666.

Vlaeyen JW, Linton SJ. Fear-avoidance and its consequences in chronic musculoskeletal pain: a state of the art. *Pain* 2000; 85:317–332.

Walker E, Katon W, Harrop-Griffiths J, et al. Relationship of chronic pelvic pain to psychiatric diagnoses and childhood sexual abuse. *Am J Psychiatry* 1988; 145:75–80.

Walker EA, Gelfand AN, Gelfand MD, Katon WJ. Psychiatric diagnoses, sexual and physical victimization, and disability in patients with irritable bowel syndrome or inflammatory bowel disease. *Psychol Med* 1995; 25:1259–1267.

Walker LS, Claar RL, Garber J. Social consequences of children's pain: when do they encourage symptom maintenance? *J Pediatr Psychol* 2002; 27:689–698.

Correspondence to: Stephen Morley, PhD, Academic Unit of Psychiatry and Behavioural Sciences, School of Medicine, University of Leeds, Leeds LS2 9JT, United Kingdom. Tel: 44-113-343-2733; Fax: 44-113-243-3719; email: s.j.morley@leeds.ac.uk.

Psychosocial Aspects of Pain: A Handbook for Health Care Providers, Progress in Pain Research and Management, Vol. 27, edited by Robert H. Dworkin and William S. Breitbart, IASP Press, Seattle, © 2003.

26

Risk Factors for Chronic Pain in Patients with Acute Pain and Their Implications for Prevention

Ellen L. Poleshuck[a] and Robert H. Dworkin[b]

Departments of [a]Psychiatry and [b]Anesthesiology, University of Rochester School of Medicine and Dentistry, Rochester, New York, USA

The experience of acute pain is common. An unfortunate minority of individuals, however, undergo the transition to chronic pain when their acute pain fails to resolve. Understanding the differences between those who do and do not develop chronic pain has important implications for theory and practice. Recognition of risk factors for chronic pain may facilitate the identification of prevention strategies for those individuals most likely to develop chronic pain. In addition, the identification of individuals with an increased risk of developing chronic pain would make it possible to deliver interventions to those most in need of preventive efforts. Finally, knowledge of risk factors for chronic pain may advance our understanding of the pathogenesis of chronic pain.

Studies in different pain conditions have examined a variety of putative risk factors for chronic pain. In this chapter, we will discuss three categories of risk factors for chronic pain—the severity of acute pain, psychological distress and mental disorders, and other psychosocial factors. These risk factors were selected based on the range and quality of the literature available. We will focus primarily on the results of prospective studies because they provide data that directly lend themselves to the study of risk factors in chronic pain by following individuals both prior to and following the development of chronic pain. Although demanding of time and resources, a prospective research design is necessary to identify risk factors for chronic pain because studies of patients who are already suffering from chronic pain and its deleterious effects cannot differentiate the antecedents of chronic pain from its consequences. The confounding of potential antecedents of chronic pain with its negative consequences is most evident when we consider psychological factors. For example, it has frequently been reported that a substantial number of chronic pain patients suffer from depression, but studies of depression in chronic pain patients cannot resolve whether depression is a risk factor for chronic pain or whether living with chronic pain causes patients to become depressed.

We will begin by reviewing risk factors for the development of chronic pain in patients with three types of acute pain. Each of these acute pain conditions—acute postoperative pain, herpes zoster, and acute low back pain—allow for the prospective study of the development of chronic pain. This chapter is not intended to be a comprehensive review of the literature on risk factors for chronic pain, and we will focus on these conditions, which represent chronic pain developing as a consequence of medical treatment, illness, and injury. We will then present a model of the development of chronic pain that attempts to integrate these different risk factors, and will briefly discuss implications for the development of strategies to prevent chronic pain.

SEVERITY OF ACUTE PAIN

The severity of acute pain has consistently emerged as one of the most reliable predictors of chronic pain, as evidenced by research on postoperative pain, herpes zoster, and low back pain (Dworkin 1997a,b). Among patients undergoing breast surgery, hernia repair, lateral thoracotomy, and amputation, the severity of acute postoperative pain predicts the likelihood of developing chronic pain (Katz 1997a; Perkins and Kehlet 2000; Jung et al. 2003). Most of these studies assessed acute pain severity using ratings by patients of the intensity of their acute pain following surgery. However, some studies used the consumption of analgesics during the immediate postoperative period to assess pain severity. For example, results showed that patients who required more analgesics during the immediate postoperative period following thymectomy, coronary bypass surgery, or breast cancer surgery were more likely to develop chronic pain (Perkins and Kehlet 2000; Kalso et al. 2001).

In patients with a herpes zoster (shingles) infection, the intensity of acute pain is now considered a well-established risk factor for the development of postherpetic neuralgia (PHN), the chronic pain syndrome that is diagnosed when the acute pain that accompanies herpes zoster fails to resolve. Various study designs, pain measures, and approaches to examining persisting pain have been used in research on risk factors for PHN, but the results of approximately 20 prospective studies are remarkably consistent in showing that patients with more severe acute pain during herpes zoster have a greater risk of developing PHN (Dworkin and Schmader 2001). Most of these studies examined the persistence of pain over a 6-month follow-up period, but one study found greater acute pain to be a risk factor for PHN nine years after herpes zoster (M.W. McKendrick et al., unpublished data).

Similar results have been found among patients with acute low back pain. In a study of patients with first episodes of acute back pain, greater acute pain intensity predicted chronic back pain at a 6-month follow-up (Philips et al. 1991). Another prospective study found that among patients with an acute episode of low back pain, greater acute pain and disability predicted which patients at 6-month and 1-year follow-up assessments were disabled and unable to return to work (Gatchel et al. 1995a,b). When acute pain and the disability associated with it are examined as a composite measure, it is unclear whether one or both variables increase the risk of developing chronic pain. A study of men with low back pain that examined both variables independently found that disability, but not pain intensity, contributed significantly to the transition from acute to chronic pain (Epping-Jordan et al. 1998). The authors of this study suggest that severe pain intensity alone may not be sufficient to place individuals at risk for chronic low back pain and disability.

Determining whether it is greater acute pain intensity or the accompanying disability that causes pain to become chronic has important implications. Resolution of this issue would not only increase understanding of the mechanisms involved in the development of chronic pain but also influence clinical practice. If pain intensity is the major risk factor, then pathophysiological mechanisms such as central sensitization and excitotoxic damage to central pain pathways may play an important role in the development of chronic pain. If the disability associated with acute pain accounts for the development of chronic pain, however, then processes such as physical deconditioning may augment acute pain and prevent recovery. Identifying the mechanisms underlying risk factors for chronic pain has clear implications for developing preventive interventions, as will be discussed below. For example, if central sensitization underlies chronic pain, then aggressive analgesic interventions in acute pain patients may prevent chronic pain; however, if the disability associated with severe acute pain underlies the development of chronic pain, then reducing acute disability might be an effective preventive intervention.

PSYCHOLOGICAL DISTRESS AND MENTAL DISORDERS

Psychological distress and mental disorders have been identified as risk factors for the development of chronic pain in studies of patients with acute pain. Symptoms of depression, anxiety, emotional distress, and loneliness have all been found to predict the transition from acute to chronic pain. Furthermore, a history of alcohol and other substance abuse, current or past mood or anxiety disorders, and psychological and psychiatric treatment are risk factors for one or more chronic pain syndromes (Deyo and Diehl 1988; Fordyce et al. 1992; Gatchel 1995a,b; Turk 1997; White et al. 1997).

The most extensive research regarding psychological variables and the transition from acute to chronic pain has been conducted in patients with low back pain. Psychological distress and psychopathology are significant problems in such patients, of whom 45% have concurrent depression and 65% report a lifetime history of depression (Gachtel and Dersh 2002); such data, however, do not address whether depression is a risk factor for or a consequence of chronic low back pain. A recent literature review found that in prospective studies, psychological variables were related to the onset of pain and to acute, subacute, and chronic pain in patients with back and neck pain (Linton 2000). Stress, distress, anxiety, depression, substance abuse, and personality disorder are all associated with the development of chronic back pain (Philips et al. 1991; Gatchel et al. 1995a,b; Feyer et al. 2000; Linton 2000). Recently, it was reported that anxiety, insomnia, and social dysfunction are also associated with the transition to chronic back pain (Fransen et al. 2002). However, psychological distress and mental disorders can also follow the onset of pain, and therefore may function both as risk factors for and consequences of chronic pain (Atkinson et al. 1991; Polatin et al. 1993).

Measures of psychological distress and various illness-related beliefs predicted the development of PHN in two prospective studies in patients with herpes zoster (Dworkin et al. 1992; J. Katz et al., unpublished manuscript). The results of studies examining the role of psychological distress and mental disorder as risk factors for chronic pain in patients undergoing surgery have been less consistent. Neither depression nor anxiety has emerged as a consistent risk factor for the development of chronic postoperative pain (Perkins and Kehlet 2000). The results of several studies, however, suggest that psychological distress may be a risk factor for greater pain in the postoperative period. For example, in a recent study of women undergoing modified radical mastectomy, preoperative anxiety and depression predicted total analgesic consumption postoperatively, as well as patients' satisfaction with their level of analgesic control (Ozalp et al. 2003). In addition, in women undergoing hysterectomy, preoperative anxiety predicted postoperative pain during recovery in the hospital, which in turn predicted pain at home (Kain et al. 2000). These studies did not examine the transition to chronic pain. However, the finding that preoperative anxiety is associated with increased postoperative pain, which as discussed above is a robust risk factor for chronic pain, suggests the need for further research examining which types of psychological distress may be risk factors for which types of chronic postoperative pain.

OTHER PSYCHOSOCIAL RISK FACTS FOR CHRONIC PAIN

A variety of other psychosocial factors, including demographic variables, social support, and stress and trauma, have been examined as potential risk factors for the development of chronic pain.

DEMOGRAPHIC VARIABLES

The association between age and the development of chronic pain has been examined in a number of pain conditions. In patients with herpes zoster, it has been known for many years that increased age is a risk factor for the development of PHN (Dworkin and Schmader 2001). For example, in one study the risk of pain at 2 months after onset of herpes zoster was 27 times higher in patients aged 50 years and older compared with younger patients (Choo et al. 1997). In general, studies of individuals with chronic back pain also suggest that older individuals are less likely to return to the same level of functioning they had prior to the onset of their pain (Turk 1997). In contrast, studies examining the relationship between age and the development of chronic postoperative pain have been less consistent; indeed, some data suggest that younger patients may be at greater risk than older patients for some chronic postoperative pain syndromes (Kalso et al. 2001; Jung et al. 2003).

Findings have been variable regarding the role of gender differences in accounting for which patients with acute pain are most likely to develop chronic pain. Some evidence indicates that men are more likely to develop chronic pain than women, whereas women are more likely to become disabled than men. Turk (1997) has suggested that the role of sex in the transition from acute to chronic pain is confounded by other variables such as the nature of the patient's work at the time he or she developed acute pain. Although demographic risk factors such as age and sex have no obvious implications for preventive interventions because they cannot be changed, they may provide clues for preventive efforts if the mechanisms by which they increase the risk of chronic pain can be determined.

SOCIAL SUPPORT

Although the roles of family, partner relationships, and social support have been widely studied in individuals with chronic pain, few prospective studies have examined these variables in patients with acute pain as potential risk factors for chronic pain. Although several studies have found that being single is associated with chronicity in low back pain (Westerin et al. 1972; Murphy and Cornish 1984; Lehmann et al. 1993; Baldwin et al. 1996), Baldwin et al. (1996) found that being single predicted disability for men but not women, and that being married predicted disability for women but not men. Moreover, several studies have failed to find an association between marital status and the chronicity of low back pain (Feuerstein and Thebarge 1991; Lancourat and Kettelhut 1992; Gatchel et al. 1995a,b).

Studies examining social support more generally have reported a relationship between social support and chronicity in back pain patients (Cunningham and Kelsey 1984; Lehmann et al. 1993; Hasenbring et al. 1994), although there is little consensus on how to conceptualize social support and its measurement. The limited evidence available suggests that being single, in a conflictual relationship, or isolated with limited support may increase the risk of developing chronic pain.

STRESS AND PSYCHOLOGICAL TRAUMA

Stress-related variables, particularly those related to work, may also predict which individuals with acute pain develop chronic pain. Several prospective studies have found job dissatisfaction and work stress to be risk factors for the development of low back pain (Papageorgiou et al. 1997; Krause et al. 1998; Linton 2001; Johnston et al. 2003). These findings suggest that improving psychosocial work environments, such as by reducing job scheduling demands and work intensity, may decrease the risk of both acute and chronic pain among employees (Johnston et al. 2003).

A study of patients undergoing lumbar spine surgery found that childhood psychological trauma of various sorts was a risk factor for unsuccessful outcomes (Schofferman et al. 1992). Patients who had three or more of five serious childhood traumas—physical abuse, sexual abuse, substance abuse in primary caregivers, abandonment, and emotional neglect or abuse—had an 85% likelihood of an unsuccessful surgical outcome as compared to 5% in patients with none of these experiences. An association between chronic pain and self-reported physical and sexual abuse has been well documented, and individuals with abuse histories report higher disability levels and greater utilization of health care resources than do patients without histories of abuse (Scarinci et al. 1994; Walling et al. 1994). Although the role of abuse is more difficult to examine prospectively, in one population-based study the risk of new episodes of back pain was increased by four to five times in women who reported physical or sexual abuse (Linton 2002).

BIOMEDICAL RISK FACTORS

It is beyond the scope of this chapter to review biomedical risk factors for the development of chronic pain in patients with acute pain. In patients with herpes zoster, various indications of a more aggressive viral infection—for example, the presence of a prodrome and a more severe rash—are risk factors for PHN (Dworkin and Schmader 2001). Prospective studies of patients with acute back pain, however, have generally failed to find evidence that measures of physical pathology make a major contribution to the development of a chronic pain syndrome (Dworkin 1997a). It is likely that the relative contributions of biomedical and psychosocial risk factors and the underlying processes they reflect vary in different chronic pain syndromes. For example, pathophysiological mechanisms may play a greater role in PHN than in the development of chronic back pain, for which psychosocial processes may be predominant.

MODELS OF RISK FACTORS FOR CHRONIC PAIN

Based on the risk factors for the development of chronic pain that have been identified in studies of patients with acute pain, various biopsychosocial models have been proposed to explain the processes by which chronic pain develops. It has been suggested that the overall severity of acute pain reflects its sensory and affective components, and that these are determined by pathophysiological mechanisms and psychosocial processes (Dworkin 1997a). In this model, severe acute pain is considered a "final common pathway" by means of which pathophysiological mechanisms and psychosocial distress jointly contribute to the development of chronic pain. Similarly, other investigators have suggested that the transition from acute to chronic pain involves emotional, cognitive, and behavioral components (Linton 2000) and reflects an interaction between physical and psychosocial variables (Waddell 1987; Turk 1997).

Gatchel has proposed a model of the transition from acute to chronic pain with an evolution of three stages of psychosocial processes (Gatchel 1996; Gatchel and Dersch 2002). During the acute stage of pain, the individual has emotional responses such as anxiety or fear as a consequence of his or her perception of pain. Then, if the pain persists for as long as 2–4 months, a wider range of behavioral and psychological responses can develop—for example, depression, anxiety, and substance abuse—with the specific form of these responses depending on premorbid psychosocial functioning and current social context. The third stage, when the pain has become chronic, reflects the patient's acceptance of the sick role and the development of a persisting pattern of illness behavior.

Dworkin and Banks (1999) have proposed a vulnerability-diathesis-stress model of the development of chronic pain that not only includes biological, psychological, and social factors but also makes it possible to examine hypothesized interactions among these risk factors (Fig. 1). In this model, the development of chronic pain originates in neurobiological and psychosocial vulnerability factors that precede the onset of pain and increase the risk of chronicity. The neurobiological factors that predispose to the development of chronic pain are likely to be very diverse, including genetic factors and physiological and structural abnormalities resulting from prior disease or injury or their treatment.

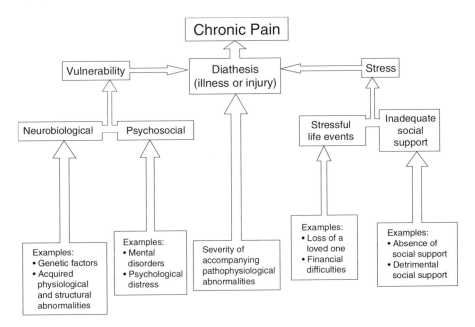

Fig. 1. Vulnerability-diathesis-stress model of the development of chronic pain.

The psychosocial factors that predispose to chronic pain are also likely to be diverse, and include psychological distress, mental disorders, inadequate social support, and stress and psychological trauma, as discussed above. In addition, the individual's prior experiences with pain may also be a psychosocial vulnerability factor, although it is also possible that such experiences result in physiological changes and are therefore neurobiological vulnerability factors. Other pain-relevant personality traits, attitudes, beliefs, and behaviors that develop during childhood and adolescence are also likely to be psychosocial vulnerability factors.

In this model of chronic pain, the neurobiological and psychosocial risk factors that precede the development of chronic pain constitute the vulnerability component of the model. This vulnerability is conceptualized as a continuum to which both the neurobiological and psychosocial factors contribute, and individuals therefore range from low to high in their vulnerability to the development of chronic pain. Neurobiological and psychosocial factors combine to constitute an enduring vulnerability to chronic pain that interacts with subsequent events—specifically, the onset of a diathesis and psychosocial stress at the time the diathesis occurs. The diathesis for chronic pain is an illness or injury (e.g., herpes zoster, an acute low back injury, surgery) that causes acute pain, which in turn places an individual at risk for the subsequent development of chronic pain. This acute pain reflects, at least in part, pathophysiological processes that, strictly speaking, are the diatheses for chronic pain; unfortunately, however, current knowledge of the pathophysiology of chronic pain is limited, and our ability to directly measure the severity of the damage or dysfunction underlying both acute and chronic pain is minimal. Although the illness or injury that is the diathesis for chronic pain is either present or absent in an individual, when present the diathesis should be considered a continuum of severity along which individuals vary from low to high with respect to their risk of developing chronic pain. For many diatheses, this continuum may be reflected in the severity of the acute pain that accompanies the illness or injury.

The diathesis for chronic pain interacts with the degree of psychosocial stress experienced during the months directly preceding an injury or illness. Dohrenwend and Dohrenwend (1981) propose that the "life-stress process" includes not only recent stressful life events but also the relative absence of ongoing social supports. Many life events involve important changes in an individual's relationships, and so stressful life events often involve decreases in social support. Indeed, Moos (1992) has argued that life events and social supports are so closely related that an integrated approach to their assessment is necessary. For this reason, the stress component of the vulnerability-diathesis-stress model of chronic pain comprises both stressful life events and the relative absence of social support (and any detrimental effects of its presence).

In the vulnerability-diathesis-stress model, an individual's risk for developing chronic pain is determined by the interaction between his or her level of neurobiological and psychosocial vulnerability, the severity of the diathesis, and the psychosocial stress at the time the illness or injury occurs (Dworkin and Banks 1999). For example, individuals with high levels of psychosocial and neurobiological vulnerability, a severe diathesis, and considerable psychosocial stress at the time of their illness or injury are very likely to develop chronic pain. Because vulnerability, diathesis, and stress interact, it is important to note that in this model low levels of vulnerability and stress and high levels of social support serve to protect the individual from developing chronic pain even when the diathesis is severe.

IMPLICATIONS FOR PREVENTION

The results of the studies of risk factors and the models reviewed above have important implications for the prevention of chronic pain in individuals with acute pain. As Roberts (1983) suggested in discussing the treatment of chronic pain: "Perhaps the greatest single need at this time is to shift our focus to prevention rather than treatment. Prevention programs should be developed for patients at risk to develop chronic pain." Although this statement is as true today as it was 20 years ago, increased knowledge of risk factors for chronic pain now provides a foundation for developing such preventive efforts.

INTERVENTIONS THAT TARGET ACUTE PAIN

The research reviewed in this chapter indicates that severe acute pain is a major risk factor for chronic pain. An important implication is that acute pain should be minimized, both by reducing its intensity and shortening its duration. For example, it has been predicted that the combination of antiviral therapy and aggressive analgesic treatment in patients with acute herpes zoster will reduce neural damage and acute pain and thereby lessen the risk of PHN (Dworkin et al. 2000; Dworkin and Schmader 2003).

In patients undergoing thoracotomy, preoperative initiation of thoracic epidural analgesia significantly reduced the risk of acute and chronic post-surgical pain (Senturk et al. 2002). In patients undergoing amputations, continuous epidural blockade for 72 hours before surgery reduced the incidence of phantom limb pain 6 months later (Bach et al. 1988). Moreover, continuous postoperative regional analgesia for 72 hours after amputation was followed by the complete absence of phantom pain in a sample of 11 patients up to 1 year later (Fisher and Meller 1991). However, a controlled trial comparing continuous epidural morphine and bupivacaine with a saline control administered before and during amputation found no differences in pain up to 12 months after surgery (Nikolajsen et al. 1997).

Jensen and Nikolajsen (2000) concluded that pre-emptive pain treatment of short duration might not be sufficient to prevent chronic phantom pain and proposed that persisting central sensitization may be caused by intense afferent input before, during, and after amputation. Efforts to prevent the development of functional and structural nervous system abnormalities during and after surgery would then be important in minimizing the risk of chronic pain following amputation. It has also been suggested that the combined use of preoperative spinal analgesia and general anesthesia for amputations would be expected to reduce the development of chronic phantom pain by blocking somatosensory and cognitive pain memory systems (Katz 1999).

Many of the issues involved in the prevention of chronic pain in individuals with acute pain have been considered in discussions of the benefits of pre-emptive analgesia. The literature reviewed in this chapter is certainly consistent with recent efforts to decrease postoperative pain by reducing perioperative pain. The inconsistent results of studies investigating the benefits of pre-emptive analgesia in hastening postoperative recovery and decreasing pain duration suggest that future studies of pre-emptive analgesia should evaluate the effects of providing preoperative, intraoperative, and postoperative analgesia (Katz 1997b; Kissin 2000).

INTERVENTIONS THAT TARGET PSYCHOSOCIAL FACTORS

The literature reviewed above suggests that various psychosocial factors are associated with an increased risk of transitioning from acute to chronic pain and that these risk factors may be associated with decreased resilience for coping with pain and with increased vulnerability to experiencing severe acute pain. The risk of developing chronic pain thus might be attenuated by reducing the psychological distress that accompanies acute pain.

Recent discussions of preventive interventions for low back pain have suggested that medical personnel should attend to the psychological characteristics of their acute back pain patients in order to prevent prolonged disability (Gatchel et al. 1995a) and that preventive interventions should be "early, active, and oriented toward health behaviors" (Linton and Bradley 1996). It is likely that these recommendations are applicable to *all* individuals with acute pain who have an increased risk of developing chronic pain, not just to those with acute back pain. Decreasing the psychological distress that often accompanies acute pain and addressing psychosocial factors such as social support to improve individuals' ability to cope with acute pain might decrease the risk of developing chronic pain. Various techniques could be used to reduce distress and improve coping with acute pain, including relaxation exercises, training in various coping strategies, patient education programs, hypnosis, and brief counseling or psychotherapy.

When practitioners consider interventions for acute pain, however, typically their emphasis is on its treatment rather than on the prevention of chronic pain. Most often, acute pain is treated "passively" with traction, heat, ice, manipulations, medications, instruction, education, and reassurance (Gatchel and Dersh 2002). For individuals who do not return to their baseline level of functioning after such care, treatment can shift to preventing chronic disability, physical deconditioning, and secondary psychological symptoms (Gatchel and Dersh 2002). Such interventions tend to involve strategies such as pacing, relaxation training, and reassurance. Only when individuals develop a chronic pain syndrome are they likely to receive an integrated interdisciplinary program of treatment, such as that provided in many pain clinics. Unfortunately, by the time such a treatment program is implemented, many individuals have already developed chronic pain that significantly interferes with physical and emotional functioning and overall quality of life. The longer the duration of pain and the greater the number of treatments, the worse the prognosis appears to be (Frymoyer 1992; Nachemson 1992). A shift of focus to prevention might therefore reduce the personal suffering and societal financial costs caused by chronic pain.

Several studies of patients with acute back pain have examined the efficacy of interventions designed to prevent the development of chronic back pain. In a classic study, Fordyce and his colleagues (1986) examined a sample of 107 patients with acute back pain treated either with analgesics and recommendations for rest and activity restrictions as needed, or with an intervention that emphasized behavioral time contingencies so that pain behaviors would not be reinforced and chronic pain would be prevented. The authors found that individuals in the prevention group returned to the levels of functioning they had prior to their episode of acute pain, whereas the usual treatment group displayed increased levels of impairment compared to their baseline functioning.

One recent study implemented a six-session group intervention using cognitive-behavioral therapy (see Waters et al., this volume) for patients with acute or subacute spinal pain (Linton and Andersson 2000). The intervention focused on patients' behaviors and beliefs regarding their pain. Outcomes included absenteeism, health care use, pain severity, function, and fear-avoidance beliefs. Although both the treatment and comparison groups reported benefits, the reduction in long-term absenteeism was nine times greater in the treatment group, which also reported significant decreases in the frequency of physician and physical therapy visits.

Another recent study of individuals with acute back pain compared cognitive-behavioral therapy and biofeedback to standard-of-care treatment (Hasenbring et al. 1999). Cognitive-behavioral therapy was superior to biofeedback, and both were superior to standard of care in reducing pain, disability, and depression and improving work performance. However, 32% of the patients referred to cognitive-behavioral therapy declined the intervention, which raises the important question of how receptive patients with acute pain may be to psychotherapeutic treatments. Such treatments may need to be structured differently for patients with acute pain than they have been for patients with chronic pain, not only to increase patients' willingness to participate but also to maximize their motivation and adherence to the intervention (Pulliam et al. 2003).

These studies have evaluated whether cognitive and behavioral therapies can reduce the likelihood that individuals with acute pain will develop a chronic pain syndrome. As discussed above, there is reason to believe that reduced social support, job stress and dissatisfaction, and psychological trauma may increase the risk of chronic pain. Interventions that focus on strengthening and expanding social support systems, on developing stress management skills, and on alleviating psychological distress may further decrease the patient's risk for developing chronic pain and should be considered for inclusion in future studies of chronic pain prevention.

In discussing the prevention of chronic pain, Linton and Bradley (1996) recommend that intervention protocols emphasize what patients should be doing rather than what they should be avoiding. In particular, such interventions should prevent the reinforcement of specific illness-promoting behaviors and thoughts. In addition, the authors suggest that preventive interventions should incorporate the patient as an active partner in the intervention, because motivation is essential to adherence to treatment protocols. Moreover, interventions that promote good communication skills are important because they will improve the patient's interactions with family members, coworkers, and health care providers. Finally, Linton and Bradley recommend that an important component of any prevention effort should be a follow-up plan that includes "booster" sessions for flare-ups and other methods of ensuring maintenance of strategies used to prevent chronic pain.

CONCLUSIONS

In discussing research on risk factors for chronic pain and the development of interventions for its prevention, we have not specified how chronic pain has been defined. It would not be at all surprising if different risk factors and preventive interventions were ultimately identified for different chronic pain outcomes—for example, presence of any pain, however mild; pain of moderate or greater intensity accompanied by minimal disability or distress; and pain accompanied by significant disability and/or psychosocial distress.

The selection of the specific chronic pain outcome to be examined in studies of risk factors and prevention will depend on the primary goal of the research. If the primary goal is understanding the pathogenesis of prolonged pain, then any pain—regardless of its intensity and whether or not it is accompanied by disability—may be the outcome of greatest interest. If the primary goal, however, is to design preventive interventions and identify those most in need of such efforts, then outcomes characterized by greater personal suffering and social costs must also be examined. Such a focus is necessary because screening and prevention programs will be costly, especially with prevalent conditions such as low back pain and herpes zoster. Of course, with a large sample and with enough measures administered at the baseline and follow-up assessments, it would be possible to compare risk factors for different chronic pain outcomes within a single study.

Our review of the literature suggests that severe acute pain, biomedical risk factors, psychological distress and mental disorders, and psychosocial stressors such as poor social support, stressful life events, and psychological trauma may all contribute to an increased risk of chronic pain in patients with acute pain. Although the extent to which each of these risk factors is causal rather than simply a marker of increased risk is unknown, some evidence suggests that preventive strategies targeting several of these risk factors may reduce the development of chronic pain.

Some individuals with acute pain will develop chronic pain regardless of intervention (Macrae 2001). Nevertheless, the number of individuals who develop chronic pain syndromes may be reduced by developing preventive interventions that simultaneously seek to attenuate multiple risk factors, perhaps combining aggressive analgesia to reduce acute pain, relaxation training to improve pain management skills, and a brief psychosocial intervention to decrease distress and increase social support. A conceptual shift by health care providers, patients, and the health care system alike is needed to embrace a preventive model of intervention for individuals at risk for chronic pain. Ultimately, we believe that such preventive efforts will minimize the long-term suffering, disability, and social costs currently associated with chronic pain.

REFERENCES

Atkinson JH, Slater MA, Patterson TL, et al. Prevalence, onset, and risk of psychiatric disorders in men with chronic low back pain: a controlled study. *Pain* 1991; 45:111–121.

Bach S, Noreng MF, Tjellden NU. Phantom limb pain in amputees during the first 12 months following limb amputation, after preoperative lumbar epidural blockade. *Pain* 1988; 33:297–301.

Baldwin ML, Johnson WG, Butler RJ. The error of using return-to-work to measure the outcome of healthcare. *Am J Ind Med* 1996; 29:632–641.

Choo P, Galil K, Donahue JG, et al. Risk factors for postherpetic neuralgia. *Arch Intern Med* 1997; 157:1217–1224.

Cunningham LS, Kelsey JL. Epidemiology of musculoskeletal impairments and associated disability. *Am J Public Health* 1984; 74:574–579.

Deyo RA, Diehl AL. Psychosocial predictors in patients with low back pain. *J Rheumatol* 1988; 15:1557–1564.

Dohrenwend BS, Dohrenwend BP. Life stress and illness: formulation of the issues. In: Dohrenwend BS, Dohrenwend BP (Eds). *Stressful Life Events and Their Context*. New York: Prodist, 1981, pp 1–27.

Dworkin RH. Which individuals with acute pain are most likely to develop a chronic pain syndrome? *Pain Forum* 1997a; 6:127–136.

Dworkin RH. Toward a clearer specification of acute pain risk factors and chronic pain outcomes. *Pain Forum* 1997b; 6:148–150.

Dworkin RH, Banks SM. A vulnerability-diathesis-stress model of chronic pain: herpes zoster and the development of postherpetic neuralgia. In: Gatchel RJ, Turk DC (Eds). *Psychosocial Factors in Pain: Critical Perspectives*. New York: Guilford Press, 1999, pp 247–269.

Dworkin RH, Schmader KE. The epidemiology and natural history of herpes zoster and postherpetic neuralgia. In: Watson CPN, Gershon AA (Eds). *Herpes Zoster and Postherpetic Neuralgia,* 2nd ed. New York: Elsevier Press, 2001, pp 39–64.

Dworkin RH, Schmader KE. Treatment and prevention of postherpetic neuralgia. *Clin Infect Dis* 2003; 36:877–882.

Dworkin RH, Harstein G, Rosner HL, et al. A high-risk method for studying psychosocial antecedents of chronic pain: the prospective investigation of herpes zoster. *J Abnorm Psychol* 1992; 101:200–205.

Dworkin RH, Perkins FM, Nagasako EM. Prospects for the prevention of postherpetic neuralgia in herpes zoster patients. *Clin J Pain* 2000; 16(Suppl):S90–S100.

Epping-Jordan JE, Wahlgren DR, Williams RA, et al. Transition to chronic pain in men with low back pain: predictive relationships among pain intensity, disability, and depressive symptoms. *Health Psychol* 1998; 17:421–427.

Feuerstein M, Thebarge RW. Perceptions of disability and occupational stress as discriminators of work disability in patients with chronic pain. *J Occup Rehab* 1991; 1:185–195.

Feyer AM, Herbison P, Williamson AM, et al. The role of physical and psychological factors in occupational low back pain: a prospective cohort study. *J Occup Environ Med* 2000; 57:116–120.

Fisher A, Meller Y. Continuous postoperative regional analgesia by nerve sheath block for amputation surgery: a pilot study. *Anesth Analg* 1991; 72:300–303.

Fordyce WE, Brockway JA, Bergman JA, Spengler D. Acute back pain: a control-group comparison of behavioral vs traditional management methods. *J Behav Med* 1986; 9:127–140.

Fordyce WE, Bigos SJ, Battie MC Fischer LD. MMPI Scale 3 as a predictor of back injury report: what does it tell us? *Clin J Pain* 1992; 8:222–226.

Fransen M, Woodward M, Norton R, et al. Risk factors associated with the transition from acute to chronic occupational back pain. *Spine* 2002; 27:92–98.

Frymoyer JW. Predicting disability from low back pain. *Clin Orthop* 1992; 79:101–109.

Gachtel RJ. Psychological disorders and chronic pain: cause-and-effect relationships. In: Gatchel RJ, Turk DC (Eds). *Psychological Approaches to Pain Management: A Practitioner's Handbook.* New York: Guilford Press, 1996, pp 33–52.

Gatchel RJ, Dersh J. Psychological disorders and chronic pain: are there cause-and-effect relationships? In: Gatchel RJ, Turk DC (Eds). *Psychological Approaches to Pain Management: A Practitioner's Handbook,* 2nd ed. New York: Guilford Press, 2002, pp 30–51.

Gatchel RJ, Polatin PB, Kinney RK. Predicting outcome of chronic back pain using clinical predictors of psychopathology: a prospective analysis. *Health Psychol* 1995a; 14:415–420.

Gatchel RJ, Polatin PB, Mayer TG. The dominant role of psychosocial risk factors in the development of chronic low back pain disability. *Spine* 1995b; 20:2702–2709.

Hasenbring M, Marienfeld G, Kuhlendahl D, Soyka D. Risk factors of chronicity in lumbar disc patients: a prospective investigation of biologic, psychologic, and social predictors of therapy outcome. *Spine* 1994; 24:2759–2765.

Hasenbring M, Ulrich HW, Hartmann M, Soyka D. The efficacy of a risk factor-based cognitive behavioral intervention and electromyographic biofeedback in patients with acute sciatic pain: an attempt to prevent chronicity. *Spine* 1999; 24:2525–2535.

Jensen TS, Nikolajsen L. Pre-emptive analgesia in postamputation pain: an update. *Prog Brain Res* 2000; 129:493–503.

Johnston JM, Landsittel DP, Nelson NA, et al. Stressful psychosocial work environment increases risk for back pain among retail material handlers. *Am J Ind Med* 2003; 43:179–187.

Jung BF, Ahrendt GM, Oaklander AL, Dworkin RH. Neuropathic pain following breast cancer surgery: proposed classification and research update. *Pain* 2003; 104:1–13.

Kain ZN, Sevarino F, Alexander GM, et al. Preoperative anxiety and postoperative pain in women undergoing hysterectomy: a repeated-measures design. *J Psychosom Res* 2000; 49:417–422.

Kalso E, Mennander S, Tasmuch T, Nilsson E. Chronic post-sternotomy pain. *Acta Anaesth Scand* 2001; 45:935–939.

Katz J. Perioperative predictors of long-term pain following surgery. In: Jensen TS, Turner JA, Wiesenfeld-Hallin, Z (Eds). *Proceedings of the 8th World Congress on Pain,* Progress in Pain Research and Management, Vol. 8. Seattle: IASP Press, 1997a, pp 231–240.

Katz J. Phantom limb pain. *Lancet* 1997b; 350:1338–1339.

Katz J. Phantom limb pain. In: Block AR, Kremer EF, Fernandez E (Eds). *Handbook of Pain Syndromes: Biopsychosocial Perspectives.* Hillsdale, NJ: Erlbaum, 1999, pp 403–434.

Kissin I. Preemptive analgesia. *Anesthesiology* 2000; 93:1138–1143.

Krause N, Ragland DR, Fisher JM, Syme SL. Psychosocial job factors, physical workload, and incidence of work-related spinal injury: a 5-year prospective study of urban transit operators. *Spine* 1998; 23:2507–2516.

Lancourat J, Kettelhut M. Predicting return to work for lower back pain patients receiving worker's compensation. *Spine* 1992; 17:629–640.

Lehmann TR, Spratt KF, Lehmann KK. Predicting long-term disability in low back injured workers presenting to a spine consultant. *Spine* 1993; 18:1103–1112.

Linton SJ. A review of psychological risk factors in back and neck pain. *Spine* 2000; 25:1148–1156.

Linton SJ. Occupational psychological factors increase the risk for back pain: a systematic review. *J Occup Rehabil* 2001; 11:53–66.

Linton SJ. A prospective study of the effects of sexual or physical abuse on back pain. *Pain* 2002; 96:347–351.

Linton SJ, Andersson T. Can chronic disability be prevented? A randomized trial of a cognitive-behavior intervention and two forms of information for patients with spinal pain. *Spine* 2000; 25:2825–2831.

Linton SJ, Bradley LA. Strategies for the prevention of chronic pain. In: Gatchel RJ, Turk DC (Eds). *Psychological Approaches to Pain Management: A Practitioner's Handbook.* New York: Guilford Press, 1996.

Macrae WA. Chronic pain after surgery. *Br J Anaesth* 2001; 87:88–98.

Moos RH. Understanding individuals' life contexts: implications for stress reduction and prevention. In: Kessler M, Goldston SE, Joffe JM (Eds). *The Present and Future of Prevention.* Newbury Park, CA: Sage, 1992, pp 196–213.

Murphy KA, Cornish RD. Prediction of chronicity in acute low back pain. *Arch Phys Med Rehabil* 1984; 65:334–337.

Nachemson AL. Newest knowledge of low back pain: a critical look. *Clin Orthop* 1992; 279:8–20.

Nikolajsen L, Ilkjaer S, Krøner K, et al. Randomized trial of epidural bupivacaine and morphine in prevention of stump and phantom pain in lower-limb amputation. *Lancet* 1997; 350:1353–1357.

Ozalp G, Sariogl R, Tuncel G, et al. Preoperative emotional states in patients with breast cancer and postoperative pain. *Acta Anaesth Scand* 2003; 47:26–29.

Papageorgiou AC, Macfarlane GJ, Thomas E, et al. Psychosocial factors in the workplace—do they predict new episodes of low back pain? Evidence from the South Manchester back pain study. *Spine* 1997; 22:1137–1142.

Perkins FM, Kehlet H. Chronic pain as an outcome of surgery: a review of predictive factors. *Anesthesiology* 2000; 93:1123–1133.

Philips HC, Grant L, Berkowitz J. The prevention of chronic pain and disability: a preliminary investigation. *Behav Res Theory* 1991; 29:443–450.

Polatin PB, Kinney RK, Gatchel RJ, et al. Psychiatric illness and chronic low-back pain: the mind and the spine—which goes first? *Spine* 1993; 18:66–71.

Pulliam C, Gatchel RJ, Robinson RC. Challenges to early prevention and intervention: personal experiences with adherence. *Clin J Pain* 2003; 19:114–120.

Roberts AH. Contingency management methods in the treatment of pain. In: Bonica JJ, Lindblom U, Iggo A (Eds). *Proceedings of the Third World Congress on Pain,* Advances in Pain Research and Therapy, Vol. 5. New York: Raven Press, 1983, pp 789–794.

Scarinci IC, Haile JM, Bradley LA, Richter JE. Altered pain perception and psychosocial features among women with gastrointestinal disorders and history of abuse: a preliminary model. *Am J Med* 1994; 97:107–118.

Schofferman J, Anderson D, Hines R, et al. Childhood psychological trauma correlates with unsuccessful lumbar spine surgery. *Spine* 1992; 17:S138–S144.

Senturk M, Ozcan PE, Talu GK, et al. The effects of three different analgesia techniques on long-term postthoracotomy pain. *Anesth Analg* 2002; 94:11–15.

Turk DC. The role of demographic and psychosocial factors in transition from acute to chronic pain. In: Jensen TS, Turner JA, Wiesenfeld-Hallin Z (Eds). *Proceedings of the 8th World Congress on Pain,* Progress in Pain Research and Management, Vol. 8. Seattle: IASP Press, 1997, pp 185–213.

Waddell G. A new clinical model for treatment of low back pain. *Spine* 1987; 12:632–644.

Walling MK, Reiter RC, O'Hara MW, et al. Abuse history and chronic pain in women: 1. Prevalences of sexual abuse and physical abuse. *Obstet Gynecol* 1994; 84:193–199.

Westerin DG, Hirsch C, Lindegard B. The personality of the back patient. *Clin Orthop* 1972;
    87:209–216.
White CL, LeFort SM, Amsel R, Jeans M. Predictors of the development of chronic pain. *Res
    Nurs Health* 1997; 20:309–318.

Correspondence to: Robert H. Dworkin, PhD, Department of Anesthesiology, University of Rochester School of Medicine and Dentistry, University of Rochester, 601 Elmwood Avenue, Box 604, Rochester, NY 14642, USA. Email: robert_dworkin@urmc.rochester.edu.

Psychosocial Aspects of Pain: A Handbook for Health Care Providers, Progress in Pain Research and Management, Vol. 27, edited by Robert H. Dworkin and William S. Breitbart, IASP Press, Seattle, © 2004.

27

Sex Differences in Pain Perceptions, Responses to Treatment, and Clinical Management

Christine Miaskowski[a] and Jon D. Levine[b]

Departments of [a]Physiological Nursing and [b]Oral and Maxillofacial Surgery, University of California, San Francisco, San Francisco, California, USA

In the past decade, attention has been drawn to the existence of sex differences in pain perceptions, in responses to analgesic medications, and in the clinical management of pain. While their biological and psychological bases are not completely understood, these sex differences have important implications for the assessment and management of acute and chronic pain. This chapter provides a summary of the research findings on sex differences in pain perceptions and responses to analgesic medications, as well as a synthesis of the studies that have reported on sex differences in the clinical management of acute and chronic pain. The chapter concludes with a discussion of the implications of these findings for clinical practice and research.

SEX DIFFERENCES IN PAIN PERCEPTION

Studies of sex differences in pain perception can be categorized into two groups. The first group consists of experimental pain studies that evaluated for sex differences in pain thresholds and tolerance and drew conclusions about sex differences in pain sensitivity (for reviews, see Fillingim and Maixner 1995; Riley et al. 1998, 1999). The second group of studies evaluated for sex differences in pain intensity scores for a variety of acute and chronic pain problems or investigated sex differences in the prevalence of a variety of chronic pain problems.

EXPERIMENTAL STUDIES OF SEX DIFFERENCES
IN PAIN SENSITIVITY

An initial review of sex differences in experimentally induced pain (Fillingim and Maixner 1995) concluded that the literature supported sex differences in responses to noxious stimuli, with women displaying greater sensitivity. However, Berkley (1997) suggested that the failure of a number of studies to reach statistical significance suggested that the effect might be small and of little clinical significance. In order to provide quantitative evidence to address the magnitude of the sex differences observed in response to experimentally induced pain, Riley and colleagues (1998) performed a meta-analysis of 22 pertinent studies. The effect size for these studies ranged from moderate to large, depending on whether pain threshold or pain tolerance was measured and on which method of stimulus administration was used. The effect sizes for pressure pain and electrical stimulation were the largest, for both the threshold and tolerance measures. With studies that used a threshold measure, the effect of thermal pain was smaller and more variable. Based on the results of this meta-analysis, Riley and colleagues concluded that women were more sensitive to experimentally induced pain than men. In addition, they found that given the estimated effect size of 0.55 for threshold and 0.57 for tolerance, a minimum of 21 participants per gender are necessary to provide adequate power (i.e., 0.70) to test for sex differences in experimental pain. They noted that the discrepancies in the studies published to date were due partially to the fact that many of the studies lacked adequate power to detect sex differences in pain sensitivity.

In a recent study of experimentally induced pressure pain, Chesterton and colleagues (2003) evaluated for sex differences in the magnitude of pressure pain and determined the effect of 14 repeated measures on any recorded sex differences. A sex difference of 28% was observed, with women exhibiting a lower pressure threshold. In addition, this sex difference in pain threshold was maintained across the 14 measurements, which were taken over a period of 1 hour.

One potential mechanism for these sex differences in sensitivity to experimentally induced pain is physiological differences between men and women. In an effort to determine the influence of sex steroid hormones on pain sensitivity, Riley and colleagues (1999) performed a meta-analysis on 16 published studies that had reported on differences in pain thresholds and tolerance in women across the phases of the menstrual cycle. The results of this meta-analysis suggest that relatively consistent patterns exist in a woman's sensitivity to painful stimuli across the phases of the menstrual cycle and that the patterns are similar across the various types of painful stimuli except for electrical stimulation. For pressure stimulation, cold pressor pain, thermal heat stimulation, and ischemic muscle pain, a clear pattern emerged, with the follicular phase of the menstrual cycle demonstrating higher thresholds than the luteal phase. This pattern was similar for measures of pain tolerance. In contrast, electrical stimulation showed the highest thresholds during the luteal phase. The authors concluded that the effect of the menstrual cycle on pain perception in women is too large to ignore and that authors of both experimental and clinical studies of acute and chronic pain need to consider these effects in the design and implementation of future studies.

CLINICAL STUDIES OF SEX DIFFERENCES IN ACUTE AND CHRONIC PAIN

While experimental pain studies are important to help us elucidate some of the basic physiological and psychological mechanisms that may underlie sex differences in responses to painful stimuli, studies of sex differences in clinical pain problems may provide additional information about how men and women perceive and respond to the human experience of pain. The existing clinical studies of sex differences in acute and chronic pain can be grouped into two broad categories. The first group consists of large epidemiological studies that have evaluated for sex differences in the prevalence of chronic pain in the general population as well as for the sex distribution of specific chronic pain problems. The second group of clinical studies have investigated differences in pain characteristics (e.g., pain intensity and number of pain locations) between men and women with a variety of acute and chronic pain problems.

Two excellent reviews (Unruh 1996; LeResche 2000) provide perspectives on the evidence for sex differences in the prevalence and distribution of a number of chronic pain problems. Both Unruh (1996) and LeResche (2000) summarized the findings from epidemiological studies that evaluated for the prevalence of common recurrent pain problems in men and women. The most common recurrent pain problems reported by both men and women were headache, migraine, oral or facial pain, musculoskeletal pain, back pain, and abdominal pain. However, as shown in Table I, which summarizes data from epidemiological studies of the general population, several chronic pain problems appear to have a specific sex distribution, and many of these pain syndromes are more prevalent in women than in men.

In Table I, the prevalence rates for the pain problem in women compared to men, in the same population, is shown as a ratio. A number greater than 1 indicates a higher rate in women than in men (e.g., a ratio of 1.2 indicates that the rate is 20% higher in women than in men). As shown in

Table I
Gender prevalence ratios for various pain conditions
from studies of the adult general population

Pain Site/Condition	No. Studies	F:M Prevalence Ratio	
		Range	Median
Headache (general)	15	1.1–3.1	1.3
Migraine	14	1.6–4.0	2.5
Temporomandibular pain	10	1.2–2.6	1.5
Burning mouth pain	2	1.3–2.5	1.9
Neck pain	5	1.0–3.3	1.4
Shoulder pain	5	1.0–2.2	1.3
Back pain	4	0.9–1.3	1.2
Knee pain	4	1.0–1.9	1.6
Abdominal pain	4	1.2–1.3	1.25
Fibromyalgia	4	2.0–6.8*	4.3

Source: Adapted from Le Resche (2000).
* All cases were female in one study.

Table I, the median prevalence ratios indicate that many of these chronic pain problems are more common in women. However, LeResche (2000) noted that some of the studies of neck, shoulder, back, and knee pain reported equal prevalence rates for men and women and in one case a higher prevalence rate in men (i.e., a ratio of 0.9 for one study of back pain). In addition, LeResche (2000) suggested that prevalence ratios greater than or equal to 2.0 may indicate substantial sex differences in risk that warrant further investigation.

Several themes emerge from examination of the findings from clinical studies of acute and chronic pain that report on sex differences in various pain characteristics. Findings from these studies of common clinical problems suggest that compared to men, women report greater pain with the same pathology (Moulin et al. 1988; Warnell 1991; Cleeland et al. 1994), greater pain with a similar degree of tissue injury (Savedra et al. 1993; Puntillo and Weiss 1994), and a greater number of painful sites (Andersson et al. 1993; Lester et al. 1994), and are more likely to develop a chronic pain syndrome after equivalent trauma (Von Korff et al. 1990; Ektor-Andersen et al. 1993).

The findings from one additional clinical study of acute postoperative pain (Faucett et al. 1994) are worth noting because this study represents a large-scale clinical investigation of sex differences in pain intensity scores following extractions of third molars (wisdom teeth). Data were obtained from 543 patients who underwent third molar extractions using a standard operative procedure by the same oral surgeon. Women reported significantly higher pain intensity scores (mean = 44.3 on a 0–100 visual analogue scale [VAS]) than men (mean = 34.6) regardless of ethnic group (i.e., Asian, Black American, European, Latino), age, education, or difficulty with surgical extraction.

POSSIBLE EXPLANATIONS FOR THE SEX DIFFERENCES IN PAIN PERCEPTIONS

The findings from the studies of experimental pain, from the large-scale epidemiological studies on sex differences, and from the clinical studies of acute and chronic pain suggest that women are more sensitive to pain stimuli than men, that they report pain problems more frequently than men, and that the characteristics of acute and chronic pain differ between men and women. Several authors (Unruh 1996; Berkley 1997; Fillingim and Ness 2000; LeResche 2000; Mogil et al. 2003) have attempted to explain these findings.

Numerous biological and psychological factors may influence the sex differences reported in several large-scale epidemiological studies. First, when women and men were surveyed and asked to recall how frequently they access a health care system for a variety of health problems, women reported more visits (Verbrugge 1985; Dawson and Adams 1986; Verbrugge and Wingard 1987; Henderson et al. 1993; Nolan 1994) and more return visits (Brit et al. 1993) than did men. However, when a prospective design was used to evaluate for gender differences in health care utilization, both Berkanovic and colleagues (1981) and Rakowski and colleagues (1988) found no sex differences in the number of health care visits. Therefore, one needs to consider that sex differences in participants' memory of health care visits and in their willingness to report them may have some bearing on the outcomes of retrospective epidemiological studies of clinical pain problems conducted to date.

Another factor that must be considered when interpreting the findings from large-scale epidemiological studies on pain is that several investigators have reported that women tend to perceive and report more physical symptoms than men (Grove and Hughes 1979; Gijsbers van Wijk et al. 1991). This tendency may bias the results of epidemiological studies on pain prevalence.

An additional factor that may influence the pain experience of women is the fact that women routinely experience nonpathological pain that occurs with menstruation, ovulation, pregnancy, and childbirth. Such pain may occur occasionally or on a recurrent basis. For example, approximately 50% of all girls in early adolescence experience some menstrual pain, and by late adolescence, 75% of all girls have menstrual pain (Windholm 1979; Shye and Jaffe 1991). In contrast, men do not experience nonpathological pain on a routine basis.

While a variety of psychosocial factors may be used to explain sex differences in pain perceptions, another explanation for these differences is the contribution of gonadal hormones. In an excellent review, Fillingim and Ness (2000) described the studies that evaluated the influence of sex steroid hormones on pain sensitivity in animals and humans. They noted that the human studies that examined changes in the perception of experimental pain across the menstrual cycle found enhanced pain sensitivity during the luteal phase for most forms of painful stimuli tested, with the exception of electrical pain (Riley et al. 1999). In addition, Fillingim and Ness (2000) noted that little is known about the influence of exogenous hormones on pain responses in humans. Findings from the limited number of experimental studies conducted to date suggest that the use of oral contraceptives may obviate the effects of the menstrual cycle on pain perception and may be associated with diminished pain sensitivity. Additional research is warranted to determine the effects of hormone replacement therapy on pain responses in postmenopausal women, as well as the effects of estrogen and androgen ablation on pain responses in men and women with hormonally responsive cancers.

Age may interact with sex to influence sex differences in acute and chronic pain. LeResche (2000) noted that age- and sex-specific prevalence rates for certain pain problems are evident in some of the published studies. For example, joint pain, chronic widespread pain, and fibromyalgia all appear to increase in prevalence with age in both sexes at least up to the age of 65 years, and all show higher prevalence rates in women compared to men. Additional studies are needed to evaluate the interaction between age and sex in relationship to the prevalence rates for and the characterization of various acute and chronic pain problems.

Another possible explanation for sex differences in pain sensitivity concerns genetic factors. Evidence suggests that several chronic pain disorders involve genetic influences, including migraine headache (Ogilvie et al. 1998, Ziegler et al. 1998; Ulrich et al. 1999), rheumatoid arthritis (Reveille 1998; Perdriger et al. 1999), and fibromyalgia (Yunus et al. 1999). As noted by Fillingim and colleagues (2000), these disorders are more prevalent in women, which raises the possibility that their genetic contributions may be sex-linked. In addition to these genetic associations with painful disorders, Mogil and colleagues have generated considerable animal research that indicates that genetic factors affect experimental pain sensitivity and that these influences appear to be sex-related (Mogil 1999). In a recent publication, Mogil and colleagues (2003) presented findings that suggest that the melanocortin-1 receptor gene mediates female-specific mechanisms of analgesia in mice and in humans. Additional research is warranted to determine the multiple mechanisms that underlie sex differences in pain perception.

SEX DIFFERENCES IN RESPONSES TO ANALGESIC MEDICATIONS

Sex differences in the pharmacokinetics and pharmacodynamics of various analgesic medications have not been investigated in great detail. In a recent review, Pleym and colleagues (2003) noted that only 11 reviews have been published on the impact of gender on various aspects of clinical pharmacology and therapeutics. Of note, three of these reviews (Miaskowski and Levine 1999; Kest et al. 2000; Meibohm et al. 2002) have reported on sex differences in the analgesic effects of opioids. This section summarizes the data on sex differences in analgesic responses to non-opioid and opioid analgesics and in the side effects of analgesic medications.

NONOPIOID ANALGESICS

Sex differences in the effects of acetaminophen were evaluated in two studies (Abernethy et al. 1982; Miners et al. 1983). Following the intake of a single dose of 650 mg of acetaminophen (Abernethy et al. 1982), women displayed an approximately 30% lower clearance and volume of distribution of the drug than did men. In another study (Miners et al. 1983), a single dose of 1 g of acetaminophen was given to young, healthy men and women, including women who were taking oral contraceptives. The findings related to the clearance and volume of distribution of acetaminophen in men and in women who were not taking oral contraceptives were identical to those from the study by Abernethy and colleagues (1982). Of note, women who were taking oral contraceptives had a 50% higher clearance of acetaminophen compared to the other two groups.

Several studies evaluated differences in the pharmacokinetics of acetyl-salicylic acid (ASA, aspirin) (Pleym et al. 2003). The major sex differences include a longer time to maximum serum concentrations of ASA in women compared to men (54 minutes versus 32 minutes; Miaskiewicz et al. 1982; Greenblatt et al. 1986), higher peak plasma concentrations of ASA in women compared to men (50% higher; Trnavska and Trnavsky 1983), and lower oral clearance of ASA (40–60% lower) in women compared to men (Trnavska and Trnavsky 1983).

While nonsteroidal anti-inflammatory drugs (NSAIDs) are frequently used to manage acute and persistent pain problems, only one study (Walker and Carmody 1998) has investigated sex differences in the pharmacokinetics and pharmacodynamics of an NSAID, namely ibuprofen. Using electrical stimulation of the earlobe, the investigators evaluated pain detection thresholds and maximal pain tolerance in young, healthy participants. Only the male participants demonstrated a statistically significant analgesic response to ibuprofen. The sex differences in analgesic response could not be attributed to differences in any pharmacokinetic parameter. Additional studies are warranted to investigate sex differences in analgesic responses to other NSAIDs, as well as to selective cyclooxygenase-2 (COX-2) antagonists.

OPIOID ANALGESICS

The opioid analgesics available for clinical use can be divided into two major classes, μ and κ, based on the predominant opioid receptor subtype at which they are thought to produce analgesic effects. Most of the experimental studies on sex differences in the effectiveness of opioid analgesics have evaluated κ-opioid agonists (e.g., pentazocine, nalbuphine, and butorphanol).

Two recent reviews (Miaskowski and Levine 1999; Miaskowski et al. 2000) summarized data from 14 papers that reported on the results of 18 studies that evaluated for sex differences in analgesic consumption during the postoperative period. The primary aim of most of these studies was to evaluate the pharmacokinetic and/or pharmacodynamic properties of one or more opioid analgesics. Only two of the studies that were reviewed (Gourlay et al. 1988; Burns et al. 1989) stated that one of their specific aims was to investigate sex differences in postoperative use of opioid analgesics. Based on the results of this analysis (Miaskowski and Levine 1999), as well as on data from our studies that used relatively selective κ-opioid agonists described below, we concluded that opioid analgesics are more effective in women.

A recent prospective study of postoperative pain (Chia et al. 2002), which was not part of our original review (Miaskowski and Levine 1999), evaluated sex differences in the use of morphine for the first three postoperative days in 1,444 women and 854 men. Morphine was administered through a patient-controlled analgesia device for 3 days following primarily abdominal and orthopedic surgery. Sex was the strongest overall predictor of postoperative morphine requirements; men needed 24%, 38%, and 30% higher doses of morphine than women for each of the three study days, respectively.

A review of the literature on sex differences in analgesic medications by Pleym and colleagues (2003) drew similar conclusions regarding sex differences in opioid analgesia. The authors stated that "although the clinical studies are less clear, they indicate that males require a higher dose of morphine to achieve adequate pain relief. On average, the difference in dose requirements seems to be at least 30% to 40%."

All of our studies (Gordon et al. 1995; Gear et al. 1996a,b, 1999) that evaluated for sex differences in κ-opioid analgesia were conducted using the same postoperative pain paradigm. All patients underwent standardized surgery by the same surgeon for the removal of third molar teeth. The surgical procedure always included the removal of at least one bony impacted mandibular third molar. This procedure is associated with moderate to severe postoperative pain.

Prior to surgery, patients received intravenous diazepam and a local anesthetic without a vasoconstrictor to obtain a nerve block of short duration. After surgery, each patient was randomly assigned, in an open double-blinded fashion, to receive a test drug through an intravenous line. The drug was administered at least 80 minutes after the onset of the local anesthetic and was only given if the patient had a pain intensity rating that was greater than 2.5 cm on a 10-cm VAS. Baseline pain intensity was defined as the VAS pain rating just prior to the administration of the test drug. The duration of most of the experiments was 5 hours. After administration of the study drug, pain ratings were taken every 20 minutes for a total of 2.5 hours. The magnitude of the analgesic response for each patient was defined as the difference between the pain rating at each time point following test drug administration and the baseline VAS pain rating (Miaskowski et al. 2000).

The first study (Gordon et al. 1995) evaluated the effects of preoperative administration of baclofen on the analgesia produced by postoperative administration of morphine (predominantly a μ-opioid agonist) or pentazocine (predominantly a κ-opioid agonist). The results showed that the analgesic efficacy of morphine was enhanced by the preoperative administration of baclofen. No sex differences were found in the analgesic responses to either morphine alone or morphine given in combination with baclofen. In contrast, in the pentazocine experiments, regardless of drug group (i.e., pentazocine alone or pentazocine with baclofen), women reported consistently better analgesic effects. These data suggest that the administration of an analgesic that relieves pain by an action at the κ-opioid receptor produced better analgesia in women compared to men. This experiment was confirmed with another study that evaluated for sex differences in the analgesic effects of pentazocine administered intravenously (Gear et al. 1996a). Again, the analgesic efficacy of pentazocine was greater in women than in men.

To determine whether sex differences were associated with κ-opioid agonists, the analgesic effects of two additional drugs in this class, namely nalbuphine and butorphanol, were compared in men and women who underwent surgery for removal of third molar teeth (Gear et al. 1996b). In accordance with the findings from our previous studies (Gordon et al. 1995, Gear et al. 1996a), 10 mg of nalbuphine administered intravenously prolonged the duration of analgesia in women significantly more than it did in men. Similar sex differences were observed with 2 mg of butorphanol (Gear et al. 1996b).

The next study was conducted to determine whether, within a range of doses usually administered in clinical practice, the observed sex differences in analgesia produced by nalbuphine were due to a rightward shift in the dose-response relationship for men compared to women (Gear et al. 1999). Specifically, we tested the hypothesis that men, given a sufficiently large dose of nalbuphine, would experience analgesia equivalent to that observed in women. Because there were no previous studies of analgesic efficacy with κ-opioids, we compared the analgesic effects produced by nalbuphine with those produced by placebo within each sex. In addition, we evaluated for sex differences in placebo responses. Different groups of male and female patients who were experiencing moderate to severe postoperative pain were given either placebo (0.9% saline) or one of three doses of nalbuphine (5, 10, or 20 mg).

No sex differences were found in responses to placebo. However, women experienced a significantly greater analgesic response than men for all of the doses of nalbuphine. Unexpectedly, men who received the 5-mg dose of nalbuphine experienced significantly *greater* pain than those who received placebo. Only the 20-mg dose of nalbuphine in men produced significant analgesia compared to placebo. While no antianalgesic effect was observed in women, only the 10-mg dose of nalbuphine produced significant analgesia compared to placebo (Gear et al. 1999). Taken together, the results of these studies (Gordon et al. 1995; Gear et al. 1996a,b, 1999) support the hypothesis that among patients experiencing postoperative pain, women obtain better analgesia than men from opioid analgesics of the κ-opioid class.

In a recent study, Sarton and colleagues (2000) evaluated for sex differences in responses to the analgesic effects of morphine in the setting of experimentally induced pain. Young, healthy men and women received an intravenous injection of morphine (0.1 mg/kg followed by an infusion of 0.03 mg/kg/hour for 1 hour). Pain threshold and pain tolerance were tested in response to a gradual increase in transcutaneous electrical nerve stimulation. The results indicated sex differences in the analgesic effects of morphine, with greater morphine potency but slower speed of onset and offset in women. Given the paucity of studies on sex differences in the effectiveness of analgesic medications, additional research is warranted to evaluate for sex differences in responses to other opioid analgesics.

SEX DIFFERENCES IN THE SIDE EFFECTS OF ANALGESIC MEDICATIONS

Two studies have evaluated for sex differences in the side effects of analgesic medications (Dahan et al. 1998; Zun et al. 2002). The first study evaluated for sex differences in the respiratory effects of morphine (Dahan et al. 1998). This study was a randomized, double-blind, placebo-controlled trial that evaluated steady-state ventilatory responses to intravenous morphine (a bolus dose of 100 µg/kg followed by a continuous infusion of 30 µg/kg/hour) in a sample of 12 men and 12 women. Sex differences were noted in the respiratory effects of morphine, with women having a decreased hypoxic sensitivity to morphine compared to men.

The second study (Zun et al. 2002) evaluated sex differences in the incidence of nausea and vomiting following the administration of an opioid agonist in the emergency department. Significantly more women required the administration of an antiemetic following the administration of an opioid analgesic for pain management. Given the fact that only two studies were found that evaluated for sex differences in side effects associated with opioid analgesics, additional research is warranted in this area.

SEX DIFFERENCES IN THE MANAGEMENT OF ACUTE AND CHRONIC PAIN

Studies on sex differences in the prescription of analgesic medications by physicians and on the administration of analgesic medications by nurses are limited in number. In a study performed over a decade ago, Calderone (1990) investigated whether the frequency of administration of pain and sedative medications to patients following coronary artery bypass surgery differed according to the sex of the patient. The medical records of 30 male and female patients were reviewed. Patients were matched on age, number of coronary artery bypass grafts, and the location of the graft donor sites. The frequency of administration of pain and sedative medications to these patients was evaluated for 12–72 hours after surgery. The results revealed that the male patients received pain medications significantly more frequently but received sedative medications significantly less frequently than the female patients. While these results are interesting and indicate the need for additional research in this area, no data were provided on the effectiveness of the analgesic and sedative medications in these patients.

Two studies of patients with persistent pain (Cleeland et al. 1994; Breitbart et al. 1996) evaluated gender differences in analgesic prescriptions. In a prospective study of cancer pain in 1,308 outpatients with metastatic cancer (Cleeland et al. 1994), female oncology patients were found to be at greater risk for inadequate prescription of analgesics and were significantly more likely to experience inadequate pain management than male patients. A similar study of patients with acquired immunodeficiency syndrome (AIDS) and AIDS-related pain (Breitbart et al. 1996) found that women were at increased risk for inadequate prescription of analgesics and were significantly more likely to experience inadequate pain management than men. Again, these findings suggest the need for systematic investigations regarding the potential sex bias in the prescription and administration of analgesic medications.

IMPLICATIONS FOR CLINICAL PRACTICE AND RESEARCH

Sechzer and colleagues (1994) conducted surveys of both the animal and human studies to systematically evaluate the sex bias in biomedical and behavioral research. In their excellent review, the authors point out the pervasiveness of sex bias throughout science. A large proportion of animal and human research has been done primarily with males. Current thinking suggests that this approach influences research findings and often leads to inappropriate generalizations, usually from males to females.

Similar conclusions can be drawn regarding research in pain management. However, recent findings from experimental and clinical studies of sex differences in pain perception, analgesic responses, and clinical management have opened the eyes of pain clinicians and researchers. An entirely new area of basic and clinical research has developed and is producing exciting results. Many of the investigations are moving beyond descriptive studies to begin to elucidate the biobehavioral mechanisms that may underpin these sex differences in pain.

REFERENCES

Abernethy D, Divoll M, Greenlatt D. Obesity, sex, and acetaminophen disposition. *Clin Pharmacol Ther* 1982; 31:783–790.

Andersson HI, Ejlertsson G, Leden I, et al. Chronic pain in a geographically defined general population: studies of differences in age, gender, social class, and pain localization. *Clin J Pain* 1993; 9:174–182.

Berkanovic E, Telesky C, Reider S. Structural and social psychological factors in the decision to seek medical care. *Med Care* 1981; 19:693–709.

Berkley KJ. Sex differences in pain. *Behav Brain Sci* 1997; 20:371–380.

Breitbart W, Rosenfeld BD, Passik SD, et al. The undertreatment of pain in ambulatory AIDS patients. *Pain* 1996; 65:243–249.

Brit H, Miles DA, Bridges-Webb C, et al. A comparison of country and metropolitan general practice. *Med J Aust* 1993; 159:514–557.

Burns JW, Hodsman NBA, McLintock TT, et al. The influence of patient characteristics on the requirements for postoperative analgesia: a reassessment using patient-controlled analgesia. *Anesthesia* 1989; 44:2–6.

Calderone KL. The influence of gender on frequency of pain and sedative medication administered to postoperative patients. *Sex Roles* 1990; 23:713–725.

Chesterton LS, Barlas P, Foster NE, Baxter GD, Wright CC. Gender differences in pressure pain threshold in healthy humans. *Pain* 2003; 101:259–266.

Chia YY, Chow LH, Hung CC, et al. Gender and pain upon movement are associated with the requirements for postoperative patient-controlled IV analgesia: a prospective study of 2,298 Chinese patients. *Can J Anaesth* 2002; 49:249–255.

Cleeland CS, Gonin R, Hatfield AK, et al. Pain and its treatment in outpatients with metastatic cancer. *N Engl J Med* 1994; 330:592–596.

Dahan A, Sarton E, Teppema L, et al. Sex-related differences in the influence of morphine on ventilatory control in humans. *Anesthesiology* 1998; 88:903–913.

Dawson DA, Adams PF. Current estimates from the National Health Interview Survey: United States, 1986. Hyattsville, MD: National Center for Health Statistics, 1986.

Ektor-Andersen J, Janzon L, Sjolund B. Chronic pain and the sociodemographic environment: results from the Pain Clinic at Malmö General Hospital in Sweden. *Clin J Pain* 1993; 9:183–188.

Faucett J, Gordon N, Levine JD. Differences in postoperative pain severity among four different ethnic groups. *J Pain Symptom Manage* 1994; 9(6):383–389.

Fillingim RB, Maixner W. Gender differences in the responses to noxious stimuli. *Pain Forum* 1995; 4(4):209–221.

Fillingim RB, Ness TJ. Sex-related hormonal influences on pain and analgesic responses. *Neurosci Biobehav Rev* 2000, 24:485–501.

Fillingim RB, Edwards RR, Powell T. Sex-dependent effects of reported familial pain history on recent pain complaints and experimental pain responses. *Pain* 2000; 86:87–94.

Gear RW, Gordon NC, Heller PH, et al. Gender difference in analgesic response to the kappa-opioid pentazocine. *Neurosci Lett* 1996a; 205:207–209.

Gear RW, Miaskowski C, Gordon NC, et al. Kappa-opioids produce significantly greater analgesia in women than in men. *Nat Med* 1996b; 2:1248–1250.

Gear RW, Miaskowski C, Gordon NC, et al. The kappa-opioid nalbuphine produces gender- and dose-dependent analgesia and antianalgesia in patients with postoperative pain. *Pain* 1999; 83:339–345.

Gijsbers van Wijk CM, van Vliet KP, Kolk AM, Everaerd WT. Symptom sensitivity and sex differences in physical morbidity. *Women Health* 1991; 17:91–124.

Gordon NC, Gear RW, Heller PH, et al. Enhancement of morphine analgesia by the GABA-B agonist baclofen. *Neuroscience* 1995; 69:345–349.

Gourlay GK, Kowalski SR, Plummer JL, Cousins MJ, Armstrong PJ. Fentanyl blood concentrations–analgesic response relationship in the treatment of postoperative pain. *Anesth Analg* 1988; 67:329–337.

Greenblatt DJ, Abernethy DR, Boxenbaum HG, et al. Influence of age, gender, and obesity on salicylate kinetics following single doses of aspirin. *Arthritis Rheum* 1986; 29:971–980.

Grove W, Hughes M. Possible causes of apparent sex differences in physical health. *Am Sociol Rev* 1979; 44:126–146.

Henderson G, Akin J, Zhiming L, et al. Equity and the utilization of health services: report of an eight-province survey in China. *Soc Sci Med* 1993; 39:687–699.

Kest B, Sarton E, Dahan A. Gender differences in opioid mediated analgesia: animal and human studies. *Anesthesiology* 2000; 93:539–547.

LeResche L. Epidemiologic perspectives on sex differences in pain. In: Fillingim RB (Ed). *Sex, Gender, and Pain,* Progress in Pain Research and Management, Vol. 17. Seattle: IASP Press, 2000, pp 233–249.

Lester N, Lefebvre JC, Keefe, FJ. Pain in young adults. I: Relationship to gender and family pain history. *Clin J Pain* 1994; 10:282–289.

Meibohm B, Beierle I, Derendorf H. How important are gender differences in pharmacokinetics? *Clin Pharmacokinet* 2002; 41(5):329–342.

Miaskiewicz SL, Shively CA, Vesell ES. Sex differences in absorption kinetics of sodium salicylate. *Clin Pharmacol Ther* 1982; 31:30–37.

Miaskowski C, Levine JD. Does opioid analgesia show a gender preference for females? *Pain Forum* 1999; 8:34–44.

Miaskowski C, Gear RW, Levine JD. Sex-related differences in analgesic responses. In: Fillingim RB (Ed). *Sex, Gender, and Pain,* Progress in Pain Research and Management, Vol. 17. Seattle: IASP Press, 2000, pp 209–230.

Miners J, Attwood J, Birkett D. Influence of sex and oral contraceptive steroids on paracetamol metabolism. *Br J Clin Pharmacol* 1983; 16:503–509.

Mogil J. The genetic mediation of individual differences in sensitivity to pain and its inhibition. *Proc Natl Acad Sci USA* 1999; 96:7744–7751.

Mogil JS, Wilson SG, Chesler EJ, et al. The melanocortin-1 receptor mediates female-specific mechanisms of analgesia in mice and humans. *Proc Natl Acad Sci USA* 2003; 100(8):4867–4872.

Moulin DE, Foley KM, Ebers GC. Pain syndromes in multiple sclerosis. *Neurology* 1988; 38:1830–1834.

Nolan B. General practitioner utilization in Ireland: the role of the socioeconomic factors. *Soc Sci Med* 1994; 38:711–716.

Ogilvie AD, Russell MB, Dhall P, et al. Altered allelic distributions of the serotonin transporter gene in migraine without aura and migraine with aura. *Cephalalgia* 1998; 18:23–26.

Perdriger A, Guggenbuhl P, Chales G, et al. Positive association of the HLA DMB1*0101-0101 genotype with rheumatoid arthritis. *Rheumatology (Oxford)* 1999; 38:448–452.

Pleym H, Spigset O, Kharasch ED, et al. Gender differences in drug effects: implications for anesthesiologists. *Acta Anaesthesiol Scand* 2003; 47:241–259.

Puntillo K, Weiss SJ. Pain: its mediators and associated morbidity in critically ill cardiovascular surgical patients. *Nurs Res* 1994; 43:31–36.

Rakowski W, Julius M, Hickey T, Verbrugge LM, Halter JB. Daily symptoms and behavioral responses: results of a health diary with older adults. *Med Care* 1988; 26:278–295.

Reveille JD. The genetic contribution to the pathogenesis of rheumatoid arthritis. *Curr Opin Rheumatol* 1998; 10:187–200.

Riley JL, Robinson ME, Wise EA, Myers CD, Fillingim RB. Sex differences in the perception of noxious experimental stimuli: a meta-analysis. *Pain* 1998; 74:181–187.

Riley JL, Robinson ME, Wise EA, Price DD. A meta-analytic review of pain perception across the menstrual cycle. *Pain* 1999; 81:225–235.

Sarton E, Olofsen E, Romberg R, et al. Sex differences in morphine analgesia—an experimental study in healthy volunteers. *Anesthesiology* 2000; 93:1245–1254.

Savedra MC, Holzemer WL, Tesler MD, Wilkie DJ. Assessment of postoperation pain in children and adolescents using the adolescent pediatric pain tool. *Nurs Res* 1993; 42:5–9.

Sechzer JA, Rabinowitz VC, Denmark FL, et al. Sex and gender bias in animal research and in clinical studies of cancer, cardiovascular disease, and depression. *Ann NY Acad Sci* 1994; 736:21–48.

Shye D, Jaffe B. Prevalence and correlates of premenstrual symptoms: a study of Israeli teenage girls. *J Adolesc Health* 1991; 12:217–224.

Trnavska Z, Trnavsky K. Sex differences in the pharmacokinetics of salicylates. *Eur J Clin Pharmacol* 1983; 25:679–682.

Ulrich V, Gervil M, Kyvik KO, Olesen J, Russell MB. Evidence of a genetic factor in migraine with aura: a population-based Danish twin study. *Ann Neurol* 1999; 45:242–246.

Unruh AM. Gender variations in clinical pain experience. *Pain* 1996; 65:123–167.

Verbrugge L. Gender and health: an update on hypotheses and evidence. *J Health Soc Behav* 1985; 26:156–182.

Verbrugge LM, Wingard DC. Sex differentials in health and mortality. *Women Health* 1987; 12:103–145.

Von Korff M, Dworkin SF, LeResche L. Graded chronic pain states: an epidemiological evaluation. *Pain* 1990; 40:279–291.

Walker JS, Carmody JJ. Experimental pain in healthy human subjects: gender differences in nociception and in response to ibuprofen. *Anesth Analg* 1998; 86:1257–1262.

Warnell P. The pain experience of a multiple sclerosis population: a descriptive study. *Axone* 1991; 13:26–28.

Windholm O. Dysmenorrhea during adolescence. *Acta Obstet Gynecol Scand* 1979; 87(6):61–66.

Yunus MB, Khan MA, Rawlings KK, et al. Genetic linkage analysis of multicase families with fibromyalgia syndrome. *J Rheumatol* 1999; 26:408–412.

Ziegler DK, Hur YM, Bouchard JR TJ, Hassanein RS, Barter R. Migraine in twins raised together and apart. *Headache* 1998; 38:417–422.

Zun LS, Downey LV, Gossman W, Rosenbaumdagger J, Sussman G. Gender differences in narcotic-induced emesis in the ED. *Am J Emerg Med* 2002; 20:151–154.

Correspondence to: Christine Miaskowski, RN, PhD, FAAN, Department of Physiological Nursing, University of California, 2 Koret Way, Box 0610-N631Y, San Francisco, CA 94143-0610, USA. Tel: 415-476-9407; Fax: 415-476-8899; email: chris.miaskowski@nursing.ucsf.edu.

Psychosocial Aspects of Pain: A Handbook for Health Care Providers, Progress in Pain Research and Management, Vol. 27, edited by Robert H. Dworkin and William S. Breitbart, IASP Press, Seattle, © 2004.

28

Placebo Analgesia

Howard L. Fields

Department of Neurology, University of California, San Francisco, San Francisco, California, USA

In a patient experiencing pain, the belief that an effective treatment has been administered is sufficient to produce significant pain relief. This is the placebo analgesic response. The treatment manipulation can take a variety of forms: a dummy tablet, surgical procedure, or topical cream. The critical parameter for the analgesic effectiveness of a placebo is the patient's expectation that it is an effective treatment. It is implied in the concept of placebo that there is a mismatch between the patient's belief in the treatment and its intrinsic efficacy, which in turn implies that the patient has been deceived. The deception can be intentional or unintentional. Furthermore, the deception can be a matter of degree. Thus, under some circumstances (such as a low dose of morphine), part of the effectiveness of an active treatment is due to expectation rather than to the direct action of the treatment itself on the body. Even though the active treatment cannot be called a placebo in the strict sense, the analgesic response it elicits in the patient may be said to have a placebo component.

The placebo analgesic response has attracted broad interest among pain researchers and clinicians. The subject has also drawn widespread interest from psychologists, social scientists, the media, and the general public. The attraction stems in part from the mysterious and counterintuitive "observation" that the mind can "heal" the body. While there is now no question that expectation can produce a powerful analgesic effect, in a typical clinical situation it is usually not obvious whether the improvement observed in a patient is due to a placebo response. This is true even when the patient is known to have received a placebo treatment. Failure to appreciate this point has bedeviled placebo research from its beginning and has generated widespread confusion about the phenomenon. Because of this, the first part of this chapter will deal at length with definitions and with the phenomena that are most commonly confused with placebo analgesic responses.

TERMINOLOGY

A first step toward clarity about the placebo is a definition of terms. The term means "I shall please" in Latin. But as Patrick Wall pointed out (1999), inherent in our use of the term is a pejorative connotation of self-serving deceit, in particular, telling people what they want to hear. Wall quotes the following phrase from Chaucer: "Flatterers are the devil's chaterlaines for ever singing placebo." It is widely appreciated that there are dishonest health professionals who knowingly deceive patients by giving them fake treatments. These intentionally fake treatments clearly reflect the original meaning of the term *placebo* as it applies to the health professions. Over the years, however, the concept has expanded.

For most of the history of the healing arts, treatments were based on theories of disease. Subsequent research has rendered all early theories of disease obsolete, so it is no surprise that when treatments based on those theories were put to the test in prospective, randomized, placebo-controlled trials, the vast majority were proven ineffective. Despite the fact that these treatments were ultimately shown to be inactive for the conditions treated, many of the patients recovered, and they erroneously attributed their recovery to these ineffective treatments. Thus, in spite of the bogus underpinnings of their trade, physicians have been able to maintain their position of authority and their incomes. Part of the reason their patients recovered was no doubt due to the effect of suggestion, as was widely accepted by the medical savants of the time. For example, John Burton (1628) writes in the *Anatomy of Melancholy*: "An empiric often times, or a silly chirurgeon, doth more strange cures than a rational physician because the patient puts more confidence in him."

In this chapter I will differentiate between the placebo, the placebo effect, and the placebo response. The *placebo* itself is a dummy treatment such as sham surgery, a sugar pill, or magnets. The *placebo effect* is the difference between two treatment groups—one that has received a placebo treatment and another that has received no treatment. The *placebo analgesic response* refers to the pain relief in an individual that is due to expectation produced by administration of the placebo. It is the placebo response of the individual that is the most interesting and informative object of study. Furthermore, understanding the psychological and neural mechanisms underlying the placebo analgesic response will be a major step toward improving the care of pain patients.

COMMON CONFUSION: THE IMPORTANCE
OF THE NATURAL HISTORY OF ILLNESS

The placebo is much maligned and widely misunderstood, largely due to those who have used it deliberately. To a large degree the fact that it is misunderstood is an accident of modern medicine. With the development of clinical trials as the gold standard for evaluating treatment efficacy, the use of comparison groups who receive a dummy treatment has become commonplace. These dummy treatments were called placebos because, in fact, they were meant to resemble, as closely as possible, the active treatment but without the active ingredient. The idea was to deceive both the subject and the person giving the treatment. Often, subjects in the placebo group improved. The confusion began with the assumption that the reason they improved was because they received a placebo. As will be seen below, this assumption is often unwarranted.

Despite the growth of interest in and study of the placebo effect, many early investigators failed to appreciate what is required to demonstrate the occurrence of a placebo response. The most common error is to attribute to placebo administration a change that reflects the natural history of the underlying pain problem. For example, you will frequently read statements to the effect that a certain percentage of subjects or patients in a treatment trial were placebo responders. In most cases, this statement ignores the very real possibility that many of the patients would have improved with no treatment (Fig. 1). Thus, if a placebo treatment is given, the improvement observed might have nothing to do with that treatment. If the improvement is not due to the expectation of relief but to the time course of the underlying pain mechanism, it is not a placebo response.

To illustrate this problem, consider the common condition of idiopathic headache. In most people, the headaches they experience will arise and subside completely without treatment. Thus, any treatment (or no treatment) given at the peak of headache severity will inevitably be followed by improvement. This is true whether the treatment is a dummy tablet or an active analgesic.

To appreciate just how elusive the occurrence of a placebo analgesic response can be, consider the following thought experiment. Assume that we can time travel and repeat the same day over again. The subject of the experiment is a headache patient who is first seen at the time of his peak headache severity. We observe that his pain gradually subsides over 3 hours in the absence of any treatment. Now imagine that we can play the same day over again. This time we administer a placebo to the patient and observe that the time course of the pain is identical to the first day. We have given a

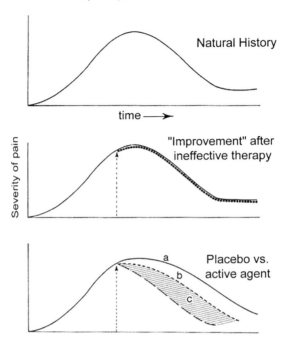

Fig. 1. Finding the placebo effect. The top panel illustrates a hypothetical painful episode such as an idiopathic headache, which starts at a low level and subsides in the absence of treatment. Giving a placebo (middle panel; vertical interrupted line with arrowhead indicates time) is followed by improvement, but this is exactly what would have happened in the absence of treatment. Lower panel: Under some circumstances, due to anticipation of pain relief, administration of a placebo results in a more rapid improvement than with no treatment. The difference in pain levels between no treatment (a) and placebo (b) is the placebo analgesic effect. An active analgesic agent produces an even more rapid or complete pain reduction (c) compared to placebo. (From Fields and Levine 1984, with permission.)

placebo and the pain has improved. Had we not known that the pain was going to gradually improve, we might have erroneously attributed the improvement to the placebo treatment. In fact, this is the most common misconception in the interpretation of placebo research. For example, in the typical randomized, placebo-controlled clinical trials of headache treatment (e.g., De Craen et al. 2000), large numbers of patients in the placebo control group report improvement. In these reports, the authors typically conclude that this result represents a high placebo response rate. However, because these trials do not include a no-treatment group, there is no way to know what proportion of these placebo "responders" would have improved without any treatment. The absence of a no-treatment group in clinical trials means that there is really no way to ascertain either the proportion of placebo responders or the magnitude of the placebo response in an individual. This problem is exemplified by Beecher's (1955) survey of clinical analgesic trials. The author's widely quoted conclusion that an average of 30% of patients respond to placebo treatments clearly had no scientific basis.

It is also important that in the case of a condition that spontaneously improves, a treatment that in fact produces a slight worsening of pain might be interpreted as providing relief (Fig. 2, top). A corollary of this idea is that the concept of "success rate" for a treatment is almost always misleading. A treatment that is totally without effect on the pathophysiology of the pain-generating mechanism, or even produces a slight worsening through its direct action on the body or nervous system, might be interpreted as beneficial by patient and physician if improvement is the natural history of the pain-producing process. By the same logic, a treatment given to a patient with a condition having a natural history characterized by worsening of pain would be interpreted as ineffective or harmful, even if it had a mild pain-relieving effect (Fig. 2, bottom).

Many chronically painful illnesses are relapsing and remitting over time. Given this variability, unless the onset of a treatment effect is immediate, it is often difficult to know whether a given treatment has had any effect. Individuals judge the effectiveness of a treatment against a running average of the time course of their own previous untreated episodes. Clearly, the "response" to treatment is an inference, not an observation. If the "effect" of a placebo treatment is itself highly variable, the difficulty of attributing relief to the placebo treatment is even greater.

REGRESSION TO THE MEAN

The statistical phenomenon of regression to the mean provides an important and clinically relevant illustration of the confounding of natural history with the placebo response. The phenomenon is a primary consideration in painful conditions with a relapsing and remitting course. Consideration of regression to the mean illustrates the importance of the timing of treatment initiation.

The phenomenon of regression to the mean is most prominent in painful conditions such as headache and low back pain that are episodic and vary widely in intensity from episode to episode. Assuming that episode severities for an individual are normally distributed, most episodes will have a severity near the average (Fig. 3). Furthermore, if episode severity is normally

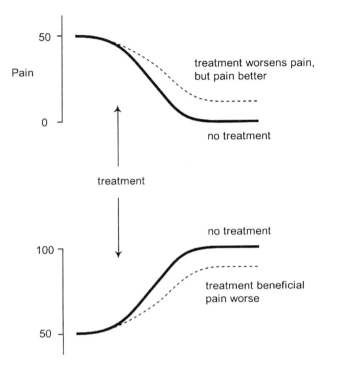

Fig. 2. A thought experiment to illustrate the relationship of natural history to the attribution of treatment effects. In the top panel a treatment is given that worsens the pain (interrupted line), but the natural history (solid line) is steady improvement such that the net effect (treatment + natural history) is improvement. The tendency in this situation is to attribute the improvement to the treatment, even though the effect of the treatment is to worsen the pain. In the converse situation, the natural history is a worsening of pain; the treatment effectively reduces pain but the net effect is increased pain. In this case the worsening will be erroneously attributed to the treatment. (From Fields and Price 1997, with permission.)

distributed, the relatively rare severe episode is most likely to be followed by the more common average intensity episode (central tendency). Severe episodes are uncommon but are most likely to cause the person to seek medical consultation and to be treated or entered into a clinical treatment trial. Thus, the pain episodes immediately *following* the one that precipitated the physician consultation are likely to be less severe. In the circumstance where treatment is initiated quickly, this phenomenon might lead to the erroneous conclusion that the improvement is treatment related, regardless of whether the treatment is an active analgesic, a surgical procedure, or a placebo. If there is a longer delay between the severe episode and the physician visit, the patient may cancel the appointment or come in and say, "Doc, it's funny but since I made my appointment, my pain got much better."

The relevance of regression to the mean to common chronic pain syndromes is beautifully illustrated by the work of Whitney and Von Korff (1992). They initiated a population- and clinic-based study of temporomandibular disorders (TMD) in members of the Group Health Cooperative of Puget Sound, a 320,000-member health maintenance organization (HMO) in the United States. In their investigation, they studied a consecutive series of 147 patients who had been referred for treatment of "facial ache or pain in the jaw muscles, the joint in front of the ear or inside the ear (excluding infection)." This group was compared with 95 "community cases" identified in a random sample survey of Group Health members who reported the same complaints but did not seek treatment. All subjects rated their pain severity at study entry and a year later. In all groups, the mean pain severity

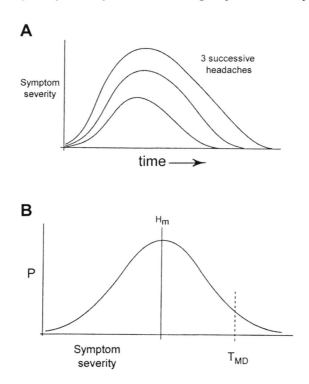

Fig. 3. The concept of regression to the mean. (A) In some relapsing/remitting conditions like headache, successive episodes vary widely in their peak intensity (three episodes are shown). (B) A hypothetical situation in which the distribution of peak intensities around a mean value (H_m) has a normal distribution. Because average values are more common than extreme values (close to no pain or extremely high levels), the most severe episodes are likely to be followed by less intense episodes (central tendency). Assuming that there is a high threshold for seeking medical care (T_{MD}), it is very likely that the episodes immediately following the physician visit will be of lower intensity. Thus an "ineffective" or "placebo" treatment initiated at that visit is likely to be followed by improvement.

at 1 year was much less than at entry. The greatest improvement occurred in the groups with the highest level of pain at study entry. When the subjects were matched for initial pain severity, there was no difference in pain levels at 1-year follow-up between treatment and no-treatment groups. It is of interest that the same authors report preliminary data indicating that at 4–6 weeks, a large number of the TMD patients reported that they had improved, and 85% attributed their improvement to the treatment received. In this case, there was no obvious treatment effect, even though most subjects improved and attributed the improvement to the treatment.

Beyond the relevance of natural history effects for interpretation of placebo studies, the consideration of regression to the mean is important in the evaluation of new and unproven treatments. Because they are often treatments of last resort in patients with very severe pain, any improvement observed should be interpreted with caution. Attribution of causality should be received with skepticism, and randomized, prospective, placebo-controlled trials should be demanded before widespread use of any treatment is recommended.

IS THERE A PLACEBO ANALGESIC RESPONSE AND, IF SO, HOW POWERFUL IS IT?

Because of the problem of natural history it is usually difficult in a clinical setting to determine if and when a placebo analgesic response has occurred. On the other hand, several studies have specifically investigated the placebo response by including a no-treatment control group. Based on these studies of clinical and experimental pain it is possible to state with confidence that placebo analgesic responses do occur. Furthermore, the evidence is compelling that placebo administration can produce considerable improvements in severely painful conditions.

Consistent analgesic responses to placebo administration have been demonstrated for dental postoperative pain, post-thoracotomy pain, and experimental limb pain caused by exercise under ischemic conditions. In dental postoperative pain and the limb ischemia model, the underlying pain-generating mechanisms produce a pain that gradually rises from low levels into the range of 5–8 out of 10 on a visual analogue scale (VAS). In all untreated subjects using these paradigms, the reported pain rises steadily. When a placebo is administered, the pain either stays the same or decreases. Thus, in this situation it is possible to identify the placebo analgesic response in an individual and to assess its probability and magnitude. In the dental postoperative pain model, we found that about 40% of subjects showed a placebo response (Levine et al. 1978, 1979), and about 27% of subjects responded to a placebo manipulation in the tourniquet pain model. The percentage of responders should be considered an arbitrary and highly variable figure, and several factors will influence this probability. For example, a subcutaneously injected placebo appears to be more effective than an orally administered placebo (De Craen et al. 2000). In the clinical situation the enthusiasm and belief of the physician and what is verbally communicated to the patient are critical, as are conditioning effects due to prior exposure to an active (or inactive) analgesic drug (see below). Other factors that probably influence the placebo effect include the physical properties of the placebo and how it is administered. In the research setting, consent forms, training, instruction, and experimental design will all affect placebo effect magnitude.

The magnitude of the placebo analgesic response can be quite large in an individual responder. The important point to keep in mind is that there are two aspects to magnitude. First, there is the placebo analgesic *effect* magnitude, which is the mean effect across all subjects receiving placebo compared to a no-treatment condition. This effect is an average that includes both responders and nonresponders. Another way to look at magnitude is to ask: "In individuals who show a placebo analgesic *response,* how big is the response in those individuals?" Benedetti (1996), using the ischemic tourniquet test, showed that by 30 minutes from the onset of the stimulus, mean pain levels had reached a mean of about 9.5 on a 10-point VAS in the no-treatment group compared to slightly over 5 in the placebo group—a dramatic reduction. Similarly, in our studies of dental postoperative pain, we found that the reduction of pain in placebo responders averaged about 5 points on a 10-point VAS. It is of interest that this magnitude in individual responders was identical to that of morphine (Levine et al. 1979). The difference was that at higher doses of morphine, almost all subjects responded, compared to the 40% who responded to placebo. Thus the mean magnitude of the analgesic effect across all subjects, including nonresponders, is greater in the morphine group than the placebo group because a higher percentage of individuals respond. As will be discussed below, the mean magnitude of the placebo analgesic effect can be markedly enhanced by conditioning. On the other hand, it is not clear whether this effect represents an increase in the magnitude of an *individual* placebo analgesic response or is explained by an increase in the proportion of responders.

CONDITIONING

Conditioning plays a powerful role in determining the magnitude of the placebo effect (Wickramasekera 1980). The clearest evidence for conditioning effects in the clinical situation is derived from placebo-controlled crossover trials of analgesic medications. In a study of acute pain in hospitalized patients, Kantor et al. (1966) and Laska and Sunshine (1973) compared placebo and several different doses of an active analgesic. What they found was a clear conditioning effect. When placebo was given as a second "drug" 24 hours after administration of an active analgesic, the magnitude of placebo analgesia was positively correlated with the dose of the previously administered active medication. These results suggest that there was a conditioning effect of the treatment context (the hospital, the physician, the nurse, the capsule) and the analgesic effect of the drug through its direct action on the central nervous system. This effect is formally identical to classical conditioning as described by Pavlov (1927). In one of his famous experiments, he would ring a bell just before feeding his dogs. In time, the bell (the conditioned stimulus) would elicit salivation (the unconditioned response) in the absence of the food (the unconditioned stimulus). In the placebo analgesia example, the contextual cues (white coat, pill, or needle) are the conditional stimuli, the direct drug effect on the brain is the unconditioned stimulus, and the analgesic effect is the unconditional response. Amanzio and Benedetti (1999) tested this idea in normal volunteers using duration of tolerance for ischemic arm pain as the outcome measure. In the absence of treatment the mean pain tolerance was about 13 minutes. In subjects who were given a saline infusion but were told it was a powerful painkiller, mean pain tolerance increased to about 17 minutes, compared to a 25-minute mean in subjects receiving 0.12 mg/kg morphine. After subjects were conditioned with two trials of the morphine infusions during pain tolerance testing, the analgesic effect of a subsequent placebo infusion was significantly enhanced (to about 20 minutes).

These studies indicate that analgesic effects can be conditioned by presenting contextual and specific treatment-related cues concurrently with analgesic drug administration. But experimental studies show that analgesic drug effects are not required to condition placebo analgesic responses. Voudouris and colleagues (1990) were able to produce conditioned analgesia by *simulating* an analgesic effect. They first applied a noxious stimulus to the skin to determine the subject's pain threshold. They then applied an inert cream to the skin and re-applied the stimulus but surreptitiously reduced its intensity in order to suggest to the subject that the cream had an analgesic effect. After this simulated analgesia, the placebo "analgesic" cream was applied and the original noxious stimulus was delivered to the same area of skin. Compared to a group given the cream with no conditioning, the conditioned group obtained significant pain reduction from the placebo cream. These results show that in addition to direct drug-conditioning effects, the experience of reduced pain per se can have a dramatic analgesic effect when the same manipulation is performed later.

RESPONSE EXPECTANCY

As we have seen, if a manipulation is associated with a pain experience that is less intense than expected, subjects will attribute pain-relieving efficacy to that manipulation. If this process of attribution is accompanied by subjective awareness on the part of the subject, the next time the manipulation is carried out in the presence of a noxious stimulus, the subject will have the conscious expectation of less intense pain. For some investigators, this conscious expectancy of less pain is the key mediator of placebo analgesia.

To address the extent to which placebo analgesia depends on this process, Montgomery and Kirsch (1997) directly manipulated conscious expectancy following conditioning. In a conditioning procedure similar to the Voudouris paradigm, the investigators used reduced stimulus intensity in the presence of an inert cream to generate a virtual analgesic effect. Some of the subjects were then informed verbally that the cream was inert and that the apparent effect was due to stimulus intensity reduction during the conditioning. As in the Voudouris study, if the subjects did not know about the stimulus manipulation, their pain ratings were markedly diminished by the conditioning procedure. However, when subjects were informed about the experimental design and learned that the cream was inert, the placebo effect disappeared. Despite conditioning, removing conscious expectation prevented placebo analgesia.

Using similar methodology, Price and colleagues (1999) took this idea one step further by explicitly asking subjects about their expectancy. They found that the conditioning procedure did indeed markedly reduce the subject's expectation of how much pain he or she would experience when the placebo cream was applied before the stimulus. Furthermore, they found that the extent to which the placebo cream diminished pain intensity was positively correlated with the subject's expectancy for reduced pain. The investigators also made the interesting discovery that the analgesic efficacy of placebo as remembered a few minutes after testing was much greater than the effect measured immediately after testing. This memory enhancement of placebo analgesia would be likely to have a major impact on the efficacy of subsequent, physically similar placebo manipulations.

Manipulations of expectancy by verbal instruction are also important in clinical pain models. Benedetti's group studied this issue in a group of patients being treated with buprenorphine for post-thoracotomy pain (Pollo et al. 2001). All patients initially received sufficient buprenorphine for pain control and then were started on a saline infusion. Patients were divided into three groups based on what they were told about the infusion. One group was told it was a hydrating solution, the second group that it could be either a painkiller or a placebo (double-blind administration), and the third group that the infusion was a powerful painkiller (deceptive administration). Pain ratings were made every hour for 40 hours, and patients were instructed to ask for buprenorphine if they needed it for pain control. All groups had the same mean pain levels, but patients in the double-blind group needed less buprenorphine than those who were told the infusion was saline. Not surprisingly, the deceptive administration group requested the least amount of buprenorphine. Clearly, substantial positive effects of verbal instruction on placebo analgesia are possible without specific conditioning.

In summary, both conditioning and verbal suggestion have demonstrably powerful actions on the magnitude of the placebo effect. In a comprehensive review of placebo analgesia studies, Vase et al. (2002) concluded that the effects of conditioning and suggestion are additive. The evidence suggests that both verbal suggestion and conditioning effects are mediated by expectancy; however, this point has not been definitively resolved.

THE NOCEBO

No discussion of placebo analgesia would be complete without mention of its evil twin, the nocebo. The nocebo is the opposite of the placebo; it is the reduced effect of a treatment based on the expectation that it is ineffective or will make the pain worse. An extensive literature demonstrates that expectation of pain, and attention to it, will increase its intensity (Sawamoto et al. 2000; see Villemure and Bushnell [2002] for a brief review). One clear example of the role of expectation is the study of Dworkin and colleagues (1983) on the effect of nitrous oxide on pain elicited by tooth pulp stimulation. Using verbal instruction, these investigators were able to turn the effect of nitrous oxide from analgesia to hyperalgesia. As with placebo analgesia, the evidence indicates that conditioning can reduce analgesic efficacy in clinical situations. One of the clearest examples of this phenomenon in a clinical pain model is a clinical trial of a long-acting morphine preparation in a group of chronic musculoskeletal pain patients (Moulin et al. 1996). This study had a placebo-controlled crossover design, so that half the subjects had a 6-week trial of placebo before being placed on the morphine compound. When given as the first drug in the trial, the morphine preparation was significantly more effective than placebo as an analgesic. However, when given as the second drug after a 6-week placebo trial, the morphine was no more effective than placebo. Obviously, preconditioning patients with an inactive substance had markedly reduced the effectiveness of the morphine.

The neural mechanisms underlying nocebo pain enhancement have not been studied extensively. The contribution of conditioning and expectancy to both placebo and nocebo effects suggests that there are overlapping pathways in the central nervous system that contribute to both effects.

THE NEUROBIOLOGY OF PLACEBO ANALGESIA

Knowing that conditioning and expectancy are critical parameters in the generation of placebo analgesic responses, we can now turn our attention to the issue of the underlying neurobiology. As discussed above, direct manipulations of expectancy have powerful effects on pain (see above and Fields 2000). Either through conditioning or verbal instruction, neutral contextual cues associated with a tissue-damaging stimulus or with a reduction in the intensity of a painful state can change activity in the pain transmission pathway. There are two steps: first, the conditioning process by which neutral cues acquire salience; and second, the expression process by which these cues enhance or reduce pain intensity.

Functional imaging studies show that when pain reports are enhanced or reduced by suggestion, noxious stimuli evoke increased or decreased activity in both the insular and anterior cingulate cortices (Petrovic et al. 2002; Villemure and Bushnell 2002). Obviously, language areas are required to interpret the message, but beyond the language decoding process we have no idea about how the phrase "this is a powerful analgesic" influences pain transmission. In straight conditioning studies, pain expectancy prior to delivery of the noxious stimulus is correlated with activation in the anterior cingulate cortex (ACC) rostral to the region that is activated by noxious stimuli (Ploghaus et al. 1999; Sawamoto et al. 2000). Presumably, direct connections between caudal cingulate neurons activated by noxious stimuli and rostral cingulate anticipatory neurons play a role in the conditioning that mediates the development of the expectancy response. The rostral ACC appears to be involved in a general way in anticipatory responses across a variety of behavioral situations.

The circuitry involved in the expectancy of *reduced pain* is obviously more relevant to the placebo situation. Unfortunately, we know even less about the regions of the brain involved in this computation. The simplest way to conceptualize the process is to understand that through conditioning or verbal instruction, contextual cues (e.g., placebo-associated stimuli) come to be predictive of reduced activity in pain transmission pathways. Placebo analgesia would result when such stimuli activate circuitry that suppresses the neural activity evoked by the tissue-damaging stimuli. It is unclear which neural structures mediate the associative process by which contextual stimuli become predictive of pain relief. It is very likely that limbic system brain structures are involved, including the amygdala, ventral striatum, ACC, and prefrontal cortex. In fact, Petrovic and colleagues (2002) have shown that activity in the rostral ACC is correlated with placebo analgesia. They did not, however, specifically address the issue of expectancy. In any case, once the associations are formed, the question becomes: "How do the relevant limbic circuits modulate pain?" The site of modulation could be the thalamo-cortical pathways that mediate pain sensation. However, there is reason to believe that the analgesic effect of expectation is mediated by a pain-modulating pathway that includes brainstem structures that project to and control pain transmission at the level of the trigeminal and spinal dorsal horn.

PAIN-MODULATING CIRCUITRY

The key structure of the most extensively studied pain-modulatory system is the midbrain periaqueductal gray (PAG, Fig. 4). The first evidence of a selective pain-modulatory system was the serendipitous discovery in rodents that electrical stimulation of the PAG produces analgesia (see Fields and Basbaum 1999 for review). This discovery in animals was extended to human subjects with clinically significant pain (for example, see Baskin et al. 1986). The PAG is best thought of as the primary outflow to the brainstem and spinal cord of the limbic forebrain and hypothalamus. The limbic fore-brain is connected to the PAG directly and via the central nucleus of the amygdala and hypothalamus. The PAG in turn is connected via the dorsolateral pons and ventromedial medulla (VMM) to the spinal and trigeminal dorsal horn (Fields and Basbaum 1999). The projection from the brainstem is targeted selectively to those neurons that receive input from primary afferent nociceptors and project to supraspinal sites. This pain-modulating network has high concentrations of endogenous opioid peptides and opioid receptors. Animal studies have demonstrated that this pathway is required for the optimal analgesic effect of opioid analgesics such as morphine. Sites in the prefrontal cortex, amygdala, PAG, and VMM are sensitive to locally applied opioids, and their inactivation shifts the systemic morphine dose-response curve to the right.

The amygdala → PAG → VMM → spinal cord pathway has also been implicated in the analgesia associated with stress and fear conditioning (Kim et al. 1993; Helmstetter and Tershner 1994). A human functional imaging study is consistent with a role for this pain-modulating pathway in mediating placebo analgesia. Exploiting the animal studies demonstrating that the pathway mediates opioid analgesia, Petrovic and colleagues (2002) used positron emission tomography to map brain regions activated by the powerful short-acting opioid analgesic remifentanil. These areas included the rostral

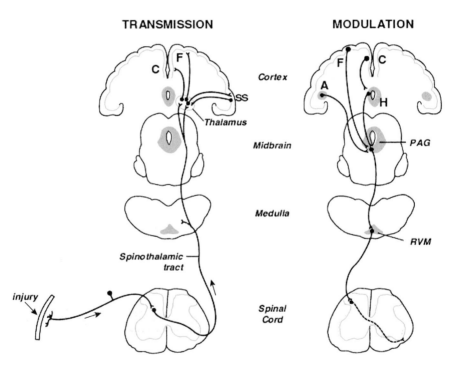

Fig. 4. Pain transmission and modulation: distinguishing transmitting (left) from modulating (right) circuitries. In the lower left, activation of a primary afferent nociceptor leads to activity in the spinothalamic tract which is distributed by the thalamic receiving nuclei to the anterior cingulate cortex or ACC (C), the frontal insular cortex (F), and the somatosensory cortex (SS). Modulatory inputs arise from the ACC, other frontal regions associated with the limbic system, and the amygdala (A) and hypothalamus (H), sending a limbic forebrain output to the midbrain periaqueductal gray (PAG), which then controls dorsal horn nociceptive neurons via the rostral ventromedial medulla (RVM). (From Fields 2000, with permission.)

ACC and other frontal cortical areas as well as midbrain and pontomedullary regions that overlap with known components of the pain-modulatory system. Importantly, the investigators demonstrated that both placebo and opioid administration produce highly significant covariation of activity in the rostral ACC with the activity in brainstem pain-modulatory relay nuclei in the midbrain, pons, and medulla. This finding specifically implicates connections between the cingulate and brainstem pain-modulatory regions in both placebo and opioid analgesia.

Animal studies have demonstrated that the PAG $\to$ VMM $\to$ dorsal horn links require endogenous opioids (Roychowdhury and Fields 1996; Bodnar 2000). If the same circuitry mediates opioid and placebo analgesia in humans, administration of the opioid antagonist naloxone should significantly reduce or block the placebo analgesic effect. In fact, Jon Levine, Newton Gordon, and I tested this hypothesis directly in 1978 using the dental postoperative pain model. We showed that 10 mg of naloxone completely blocked placebo analgesia. While other investigators have confirmed and extended this finding, there are circumstances where naloxone reversal is only partial (Grevert et al. 1983; Fields and Levine 1984; Amanzio and Benedetti 1999).

In conclusion, while our knowledge of the neural circuitry underlying placebo analgesia is far from complete, a sketchy outline is emerging (Fields and Basbaum 1999; Petrovic and Ingvar 2002). Contextual cues predictive of an analgesic response produce an expectancy state. This expectancy state probably involves neurons in the limbic forebrain including the rostral ACC. These structures activate pain-modulating circuitry in the PAG and VMM, which, via opioid links, inhibit pain transmission neurons in the dorsal horn.

THE PLACEBO RESPONSE IN CLINICAL PRACTICE

Very little information has been published on the extent to which placebo effects contribute to outcome in clinical practice. By definition, clinical practice occurs outside the research setting. In a very controversial meta-analysis of clinical trials, Hrobjartsson and Gotzsche (2001) concluded that placebo effects were small to nonexistent. However, in most clinical trials, patients are told (or led to believe) that placebos are ineffective. Furthermore, because patients believe they have only a 50% chance of receiving an effective treatment, it is likely that active drug analgesic efficacy is reduced under conditions of a placebo-controlled trial. To address this issue, Vase and colleagues (2002) performed a meta-analysis comparing clinical analgesic trials with studies explicitly designed to investigate placebo analgesia using a no-treatment control. They found that placebo effects were quite large when patients were explicitly led to believe that the placebo manipulation was an effective treatment (i.e., in the studies directed at placebo analgesia). Based on what we know about experimental studies of placebo analgesia, this result is no surprise. It is important, however, to point out that in clinical practice the deliberate use of placebo is usually accompanied by the care provider's suggestion and/or the patient's expectation that patients are receiving an active drug.

Thus, in contrast to the conclusion of Hrobjartsson and Gotzsche, it is likely that in clinical practice placebo analgesic effects are quite significant. It seems obvious that expectancy plays a significant role in clinical practice. Both patient and care provider enter the treatment situation with a set of expectations about the course of the illness and the efficacy of various treatment approaches. Because pain is subjective, and its perceived intensity is affected by a variety of pathophysiological mechanisms, including expectancy, one never knows how much of a patient's response (or lack thereof) depends upon natural history, placebo, or nocebo and how much is due to a direct effect of the treatment manipulation on the pain-generating process. However, there are several obvious factors that can have an important impact on treatment outcome.

First, the more ineffective treatments a patient receives, the more likely are future treatments to fail. Therefore, it is important to find the optimal therapy as rapidly as possible. It is important for patients to believe that they can improve, and often this is the biggest challenge, especially for patients with chronic pain. Second, it is important for those providing the treatment to have a firm grasp on why they think the treatment they are giving will work and to communicate this clearly to the patient. The practitioner may have reason to be doubtful about the efficacy of the treatment, and problems can arise if these doubts are communicated to the patient. In this case, total honesty may not be in the patient's best interest. Third, explaining the effect of expectancy to patients may be helpful, particularly if there is reason to believe that expectancy may be worsening the patient's pain or reducing the efficacy of a treatment. Fourth, the use of prognostic drug infusions may be helpful. For example, with the use of lidocaine or opioid infusions, high plasma levels of drug can be obtained rapidly, thus demonstrating to the patient that relief is possible. It is also possible that such infusions have a conditioning effect, which can add to the initial efficacy of the same class of drug when given orally. Of course, if the infusions are ineffective, the same medications given orally will be much less likely to be effective and the conditioning will work in the wrong direction.

SUMMARY AND CONCLUSIONS

The expectation of pain relief can exert a powerful analgesic effect. This effect can be produced even in clinical situations characterized by severe pain. Depending upon conditioning and verbal instruction, a placebo analgesic effect can be elicited acutely in a very large percentage of individuals in severe pain. We are beginning to understand the neurobiology of placebo analgesia. The evidence indicates that verbal communication or contextual cues predictive of analgesia activate a circuit that includes the anterior cingulate gyrus and an opioid-mediated brainstem pathway that controls dorsal horn pain transmission neurons. A fuller understanding of the placebo analgesic response could lead to new treatments that exploit behavioral methods for activating pain-modulating circuitry. Ironically, once such an approach is demonstrated to be effective, it would no longer constitute a placebo manipulation.

REFERENCES

Amanzio M, Benedetti F. Neuropharmacological dissection of placebo analgesia: expectation-activated opioid systems versus conditioning-activated specific subsystems. *J Neurosci* 1999; 19:484–494.

Baskin DS, Mehler WR, Hosobuchi Y, et al. Autopsy analysis of the safety, efficacy and cartography of electrical stimulation of the central gray in humans. *Brain Res* 1986; 371(2):231–236.

Beecher HK. The powerful placebo. *JAMA* 1955; 159:1602–1606.

Benedetti F. The opposite effects of the opiate antagonist naloxone and the cholecystokinin antagonist proglumide on placebo analgesia. *Pain* 1996; 64:535–543.

Bodnar RJ. Supraspinal circuitry mediating opioid antinociception: antagonist and synergy studies in multiple sites. *J Biomed Sci* 2000; 7:181–194.

De Craen AJM, Tijssen JGP, de Gans J, Kleijnen J. Placebo effect in the acute treatment of migraine: subcutaneous placebos are better than oral placebos. *J Neurol* 2000; 247:183–188.

Dworkin SF, Chen AC, LeResche L, Clark DW. Cognitive reversal of expected nitrous oxide analgesia for acute pain. *Anesth Analg* 1983; 62:1073–1077.

Fields HL. Pain modulation: expectation, opioid analgesia and virtual pain. In: Mayer EA, Saper CB (Eds). *The Biological Basis for Mind Body Interactions,* Progress in Brain Research, Vol. 122. Amsterdam: Elsevier, 2000, pp 245–254.

Fields HL, Basbaum AI. Central nervous system mechanisms of pain modulation. In: Wall P, Melzack R (Eds). *Textbook of Pain,* 4th ed. Edinburgh: Churchill-Livingstone, 1999, pp 309–329.

Fields HL, Levine JD. Placebo analgesia—a role for endorphins? *Trends Neurosci* 1984; 7:271–273.

Fields HL, Price DD. Toward a neurobiology of placebo analgesia. In: Harrington A (Ed). *The Placebo Effect: An Interdisciplinary Exploration.* Cambridge, MA: Harvard University Press, 1997, pp 93–116.

Grevert P, Albert LH, Goldstein A. Partial antagonism of placebo analgesia by naloxone. *Pain* 1983; 16:129–143.

Helmstetter FJ, Tershner SA. Lesions of the periaqueductal gray and rostral ventromedial medulla disrupt antinociceptive but not cardiovascular aversive conditional responses. *J Neurosci* 1994; 14:7099–7108.

Hrobjartsson A, Gotzsche PC. Is the placebo effect powerless? An analysis of clinical trials comparing placebo with no- treatment. *N Engl J Med* 2001; 344:1594–1602.

Kantor TG, Sunshine A, Laska E, Meisner M, Hopper M. Oral analgesic studies: pentazocine hydrochloride, codeine, aspirin, and placebo and their influence on response to placebo. *J Clin Pharm Ther* 1966; 7:447–454.

Kim JJ, Rison RA, Fanselow MS. Effects of amygdala, hippocampus, and periaqueductal gray lesions on short and long-term contextual fear. *Behav Neurosci* 1993; 107:1093–1098.

Laska E, Sunshine A. Anticipation of analgesia: a placebo effect. *Headache* 1973; 13:1–11.

Levine JD, Gordon NC, Fields HL. The mechanism of placebo analgesia. *Lancet* 1978; 2:654–657.

Levine JD, Gordon NC, Bornstein, JC, Fields HL. Role of pain in placebo analgesia. *Proc Natl Acad Sci USA* 1979; 76:3528–3531.

Montgomery GH, Kirsch I. Classical conditioning and the placebo effect. *Pain* 1997; 72:107–113.

Moulin DE, Iezzi A, Amireh R, et al. Randomised trial of oral morphine for chronic non-cancer pain. *Lancet* 1996; 347:143–147.

Pavlov IP. *Conditioned Reflexes.* London: Oxford University Press, 1927.

Petrovic P, Ingvar M. Imaging cognitive modulation of pain processing. *Pain* 2002; 95:1–5.

Petrovic P, Kalso E, Petersson KM, Ingvar M. Placebo and opioid analgesia-imaging a shared neuronal network. *Science* 2002; 295:1737–1740.

Ploghaus A, Tracey I, Gati JS, Clare S, et al. Dissociating pain from its anticipation in the human brain. *Science* 1999; 284:1979–1981.

Pollo A, Amanzio M, Arslanian A, et al. Response expectancies in placebo analgesia and their clinical relevance. *Pain* 2001; 93:77–84.

Price DD, Milling LS, Kirsch I, et al. An analysis of factors that contribute to the magnitude of placebo analgesia in an experimental paradigm. *Pain* 1999; 83:147–156.

Roychowdhury SM, Fields HL. Endogenous opioids acting at a medullary mu-opioid receptor contribute to the behavioral antinociception produced by GABA antagonism in the mid-brain periaqueductal gray. *Neuroscience* 1996; 74(3):863–872.

Sawamoto N, Honda M, Okada T, et al. Expectation of pain enhances responses to nonpainful somatosensory stimulation in the anterior cingulate cortex and parietal operculum/posterior insula: an event-related functional magnetic resonance imaging study. *J Neurosci* 2000; 20:7438–7445.

Vase L, Riley JL, Price DD. A comparison of placebo effects in clinical analgesic trials versus studies of placebo analgesia. *Pain* 2002; 99:443–452.

Villemure C, Bushnell MC. Cognitive modulation of pain: how do attention and emotion influence pain processing? *Pain* 2002; 95:195–199.

Voudouris NJ, Peck CL, Coleman G. The role of conditioning and verbal expectancy in the placebo response. *Pain* 1990; 43:121–128.

Wall PD. The placebo and the placebo response. In: Melzack R, Wall PD. *Textbook of Pain,* 4th ed. Edinburgh: Churchill Livingstone, 1999, pp 1419–1430.

Whitney CW, Von Korff M. Regression to the mean in treated versus untreated chronic pain. *Pain* 1992; 50:281–285.

Wickramasekera I. A conditioned response model of the placebo effect: predictions from the model. *Biofeedback Self-Regul* 1980; 5:5–18.

Correspondence to: Howard L. Fields, MD, PhD, Department of Neurology, Box 0453, University of California, San Francisco, San Francisco, CA 94143, USA. Email: hlf@itsa.ucsf.edu.

Index

Progress in Pain Research and Management Series